Handbook of Measurement and Evaluation in Rehabilitation

Handbook of Measurement and Evaluation in Rehabilitation

Fourth Edition

Edited by
Brian F. Bolton
and
Randall M. Parker

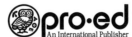

An International Publisher

8700 Shoal Creek Boulevard
Austin, Texas 78757-6897
800/897-3202   Fax 800/397-7633
www.proedinc.com

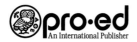

© 2001, 2008 by PRO-ED, Inc.
8700 Shoal Creek Boulevard
Austin, Texas 78757-6897
800/897-3202 Fax 800/397-7633
www.proedinc.com

Library of Congress Cataloging-in-Publication Data

Handbook of measurement and evaluation in rehabilitation / edited by
Brian F. Bolton and Randall M. Parker.—4th ed.
    p. cm.
  Includes bibliographical references and index.
  ISBN-13: 978-1-4164-0258-9
  1. Rehabilitation counseling.   2. Psychometrics.   I. Bolton, Brian,
1939–   II. Parker, Randall M., 1940–
  HD7255.5.H35 2007
  361'.06—dc22

                                        2007005568

Art Director: Jason Crosier
Designer: Sandy Salinas
This book is designed in Bembo and Futura.

Printed in the United States of America

1 2 3 4 5 6 7 8 9 10   17 16 15 14 13 12 11 10 09 08

Contents

PART 2 REVIEWS OF INSTRUMENTS

Chapter 4
Intelligence Testing 91
Elizabeth O. Lichtenberger, James C. Kaufman, and Alan S. Kaufman

Chapter 5
Aptitude Testing 121
Randall M. Parker

Chapter 6
Assessment of Personality 151
Samuel E. Krug

Chapter 7
Assessment of Psychopathology 175
Rodney L. Lowman and Linda M. Richardson

Contributors

Norman L. Berven, PhD
Professor
Department of Rehabilitation Psy-
  chology and Special Education
University of Wisconsin–Madison
Madison, Wisconsin

Nancy E. Betz, PhD
Professor
Department of Psychology
The Ohio State University
Columbus, Ohio

Terry L. Blackwell, PhD
Professor
Montana State University–Billings
Billings, Montana

Brian F. Bolton, PhD
University Professor Emeritus
Department of Rehabilitation Educa-
  tion and Research
University of Arkansas
Fayetteville, Arkansas

Walter C. Borman, PhD
Professor
Department of Psychology
University of South Florida
  and Personnel Decisions
  Research Institutes
Tampa, Florida

Jeffrey B. Brookings, PhD
Professor and Chair
Department of Psychology
Wittenberg University
Springfield, Ohio

Nancy M. Crewe, PhD
Professor Emeritus
Counseling, Educational Psychology,
  and Special Education
Michigan State University
East Lansing, Michigan

Richard H. Dana, PhD, ABPP
Research Professor (Honorary)
Regional Research Institute
Portland State University
Portland, Oregon

Nadya A. Fouad, PhD
Professor
Department of Educational Psychology
University of Wisconsin–Milwaukee
Milwaukee, Wisconsin

John T. Gallagher, EdD
Licensed Psychologist
John T. Gallagher & Associates
Portage, Michigan

**Darlene A. G. Groomes, PhD,
  CRC**
Research Associate
Project Excellence Adjunct Faculty
Michigan State University
Ease Lansing, Michigan

Amy Guillen, MS
Ames, Iowa

Sandra E. Hansmann, PhD, CRC
Assistant Professor
Department of Rehabilitation
The University of Texas Pan American
Edinburg, Texas

Mary Ann Hanson, PhD
President
Center for Career and Community
   Research
St. Paul, Minnesota

Neeta Kantamneni, MS
Milwaukee, Wisconsin

Alan S. Kaufman, PhD
Clinical Professor of Psychology
Yale University School of Medicine
New Haven, Connecticut

James C. Kaufman, PhD
Director, Learning Research Institute
Psychology and Human Development
California State University at San
   Bernardino
San Bernardino, California

Samuel E. Krug, PhD
President
MetriTech, Inc.
Champaign, Illinois

Stephen J. Leierer, PhD
Counseling, Educational Psychology
   and Research
The University of Memphis
Memphis, Tennessee

Elizabeth O. Lichtenberger, PhD
Alliant International University
San Diego, California

Rodney L. Lowman, PhD
Provost and Vice President for
   Academic Affairs
Alliant International University
San Diego, California

Kim L. MacDonald-Wilson, ScD
Assistant Professor
University of Maryland
College Park, Maryland

**Leonard N. Matheson, PhD, CVE,
CRC**
Associate Professor
Director, Work Performance Clinical
   Laboratory
Washington University School of
   Medicine
St. Louis, Missouri

Patricia B. Nemec, PsyD
Clinical Associate Professor
Department of Rehabilitation Counseling
Boston University
Boston, Massachusetts

Randall M. Parker, PhD
Professor
Department of Special Education
The University of Texas at Austin
Austin, Texas

Jeanne B. Patterson, EdD, CRC
Professor and Program Director
Health Science–Rehabilitation Counsel-
   ing Program
University of North Florida
Jacksonville, Florida

Linda M. Richardson, PhD
Mental Health Program Head
County of Los Angeles–Department
   of Mental Health
Juvenile Justice Mental Health Services
Downey, California

Ronald M. Ruff, PhD, ABPP
Director of Neurobehavioral
   Rehabilitation
St. Mary's Medical Center
Associate Clinical Professor of Physical
   Medicine and Rehabilitation
Stanford University
Associate Adjunct Professor of Neuro-
   surgery and Psychiatry
University of California
San Francisco, California

Shawn P. Saladin, PhD, CRC, CPM
Assistant Professor
Department of Rehabilitation
The University of Texas Pan American
Edinburg, Texas

James C. Schraa, PsyD
Clinical Neuropsychologist
Craig Hospital
Englewood, Colorado

Melissa K. Smothers, MA
Milwaukee, Wisconsin

Douglas C. Strohmer, PhD
Chair
Counseling, Educational Psychology
   and Research
The University of Memphis
Memphis, Tennessee

Robert M. Thorndike, PhD
Professor
Department of Psychology
Western Washington University
Bellingham, Washington

Tracy Thorndike-Christ, PhD
Assistant Professor
Woodring College of Education
Department of Special Education
Western Washington University
Bellingham, Washington

Richard T. Walls, PhD
Professor
Educational Psychology Program
   and the International Center
   for Disability Information
West Virginia University
Morgantown, West Virginia

David J. Weiss, PhD
Professor
Department of Psychology
University of Minnesota
Minneapolis, Minnesota

William R. Wiener, PhD
Vice Provost for Research and Dean
   of the Graduate School
Marquette University Graduate School
Milwaukee, Wisconsin

Irla Lee Zimmermann, PhD, ABPP
Clinical Psychologist (Retired)
Private Practice
Whittier, California

Preface

All professionals in rehabilitation recognize that comprehensive client assessment provides the strategic foundation for the provision of rehabilitation services to persons with disabilities. The fourth edition of the *Handbook of Measurement and Evaluation in Rehabilitation* was prepared for use by practitioners whose primary function is to translate the results of client assessment into an effective program of rehabilitation services. Thus, the major purpose of the *Handbook* is to serve as a textbook for undergraduate and graduate courses in rehabilitation assessment, psychological testing, and vocational evaluation. Secondary objectives are to serve as a resource for specialists who conduct psychological and vocational evaluations of persons with disabilities and for researchers who design projects to evaluate the efficacy of rehabilitation service programs.

The fourth edition of the *Handbook* discusses the current status of the rehabilitation discipline of client assessment, which is defined as the application of psychological measurement principles and practices to the appraisal of persons with disabilities. The four principal terms in the volume's title indicate what role the book will play in client evaluation. It is a "handbook" (not an encyclopedic reference book but a comprehensive manual for practitioners and students) of "measurement" (the standardized procedure for gathering psychologically and vocationally relevant information about people) and "evaluation" (synonymous with assessment or individual appraisal, the systematic use of measurement results in planning services for clients) in "rehabilitation" (the range of psychological and vocational services that are provided to persons with disabilities to restore them to optimal functioning).

The 20 chapters of the *Handbook* are organized into three parts. Part 1, Fundamentals of Measurement, reviews basic psychometric concepts, including scores and norms, reliability, and validity. The first chapter also includes a brief introduction to test interpretation and an overview of additional sources of information. Part 2, Reviews of Instruments, summarizes the state of the art in five areas: intelligence tests, multifactor aptitude tests, personality inventories, psychopathology instruments, and vocational inventories. Part 3, Applications in Rehabilitation, contains chapters that describe measurement systems and models, summarize special assessment areas, and detail procedures for the appraisal of special populations.

The focus of the 20 chapters of the fourth edition is identical to that in the third edition, with at least some of the coauthors of 19 chapters continuing to the fourth edition. Hence, there is excellent professional continuity in this latest edition. The fourth edition of the *Handbook* is quite literally the product of many years of clinical and research experience. The authors are recognized experts in psychology and rehabilitation, and their contributions are greatly appreciated.

Editors' Note

The royalties generated through the sales of this book are being contributed to the Donald D. Hammill Foundation, which funds a variety of innovative projects that serve people with disabilities.

PART 1

Fundamentals of Measurement

Chapter 1

Scores and Norms

Brian F. Bolton, Randall M. Parker, and Jeffrey B. Brookings

The first three chapters of the *Handbook* provide succinct overviews of basic psychometric theory and issues (such large topics cannot be covered thoroughly in such a small space). This chapter addresses four main questions: What is a psychological test or measure? What are the important characteristics of test scores? How are test scores interpreted or given meaning? What are the basic principles of test use in rehabilitation? Advanced subjects such as test construction, scaling, and equating are not covered in this chapter; however, readers interested in learning more will find references for these and other topics. The second and third chapters deal with two essential properties of tests: reliability and validity. Generally speaking, reliability refers to the precision of the measuring process, whereas validity is concerned with determining how accurately a test measures the trait or construct it claims to quantify.

Measurement and Testing

Definitions and Terminology

Psychological measurement may be defined as the assignment of numbers to attributes of persons according to rules. The rules, or procedures for assigning numbers, must be stated explicitly. It is important to emphasize that psychological measurement is concerned with abstract aspects of human behavior (e.g., intelligence, personality, motivation), qualities that are inferred from various types of observable performance. The trait or attribute that is measured is referred to as a psychological construct, a term discussed in some detail in Chapter 3.

Cronbach (1990) defined a test as "a systematic procedure for observing behavior and describing it with the aid of numerical scales or fixed categories" (p. 32). A systematic or *standardized* procedure requires detailed rules for administration, observation, and scoring of the examinee's performance. Standardization exists when different examiners can use the test to obtain similar results. Tests consist of tasks, items, or stimuli that provide a basis for the observation of behavior.

Cattell (1986) defined a test in a manner that stresses its use: a standard stimulus situation, containing a defined instruction and mode of response, in which a person is measured on the response in a predefined way, the measure being used to predict or make inferences about other behavior of the person. Consistent with this definition, Cattell argues that properly constructed tests indicate the examinee's positions on one or more unitary psychological dimensions, or source traits, which are the underlying causal influences that determine or explain observed behavior.

According to Newland (1980), "Testing is the controlled observation of the behavior of an individual to whom stimuli of known characteristics are applied in a known manner" (p. 76). He expanded the definition by specifying six assumptions underlying testing:

1. The examiner is adequately skilled to administer and score the test.
2. The sampling of behavior in the test situation is both adequate in amount and representative in scope.
3. Subjects being tested have been exposed to comparable, but not necessarily identical, acculturation.
4. Error is assumed to be present in the measurement of human behavior.
5. Only present behavior is observed.
6. Future behavior of the subject is inferred.

Because these assumptions or requirements are essential to the proper interpretation of testing instruments used in conducting the comprehensive diagnostic evaluation in rehabilitation, they are discussed in some detail in subsequent chapters of the *Handbook*.

Cronbach's well-known distinction between tests of *maximum* performance and tests of *typical* performance is especially useful in discussing testing issues. On tests of maximum performance, the examinee demonstrates possession of knowledge or ability to do something by answering questions or solving problems that have preestablished correct solutions; these are tests of intelligence, achievement, aptitude, or skill. In contrast, tests of typical behavior involve items or stimuli that require opinions about the test taker and others; these questionnaires measure personality, attitudes, interests, or values. Although most measures of typical performance are self-report instruments, some entail ratings by trained observers.

The measurement of differences among persons, referred to as *interindividual* differences, is the fundamental purpose of psychological measurement: This is all that is accomplished by unidimensional instruments (i.e., instruments that measure a single trait). However, most tests and questionnaires described in the *Handbook* generate multiscore profiles, which summarize an individual's strengths and deficits in aptitudes, personality, or independent living skills. Instruments that provide score profiles, called multifactor or multidimensional tests, provide scores that can be used to describe *intraindividual* differences, or relevant variability within the individual. As explained in Chapter 2, caution must be exercised in interpreting scale differences within a profile because of the diminished reliability of difference scores.

Although there are distinctions among the terms *measurement, assessment, evaluation,* and *appraisal,* these terms are used interchangeably in the *Handbook*. However, it should be noted that *measurement* refers to the scientific process of quantifying psychological characteristics, whereas the other three words include the process of developing an integrated picture of the individual based on a wide variety of test and nontest information. The words *test, measure,* and *instrument* are also used interchangeably; although these terms may denote any type of measuring procedure, *inventory* and *questionnaire* usually refer to tests of typical performance and rarely to measures of abilities, aptitudes, or skills.

Standardized tests and measures, therefore, can be said to have five advantages over unstandardized observations and clinical judgment (Nunnally & Bernstein, 1994):

1. *Objectivity:* Standardized measures are not dependent on the personal opinions of examiners.
2. *Quantification:* Numerical precision enables finer discriminations on the dimension of interest to the assessor.
3. *Communication:* Communication among professionals is enhanced when standardized measures are used.
4. *Economy:* Standard procedures can often be administered by aides or computers, giving professionals more time to interpret results and to plan rehabilitation strategies.
5. *Scientific generalization:* Standardized measures are essential in the formulation of scientific principles that explain human behavior.

Features of Standardized Tests

Parts 2 and 3 of this volume describe a wide variety of measuring instruments, such as intelligence and aptitude tests, personality questionnaires, interest inventories, assessment interviews, and rating scales of functional skills and competencies. Every instrument can be classified with respect to major features of administration, scoring, and interpretation. The categories described in the following may be used to classify and facilitate comparisons among available measuring techniques.

- *Individual versus group administration:* Individually administered tests allow opportunities for the examiner to use judgment in adapting to the unique disabling condition of the examinee and to gather clinically relevant information during the testing session. Group-administered tests are much more economical and generally provide data of good reliability and validity, although typically not as good as data from individually administered instruments. Many tests and inventories that were originally designed for group administration have been programmed for individualized administration by computer, thus constituting a third category.
- *Timed versus untimed administration:* Many tests of maximum performance are carefully timed because speed of performance is considered to be an essential component of the attribute being measured. Evidence suggests that some examinees' abilities are seriously underestimated by speeded tests; these persons typically do much better on untimed or

power tests. Measures of typical performance are usually not timed, and examinees work at their own pace.

- *Keyed versus impressionistic scoring:* Most group-administered ability tests and almost all questionnaires and inventories are scored by clerks using keys or by machine. In contrast, many individually administered instruments, such as the Stanford-Binet, Wechsler, Rorschach, Bender Gestalt, and sentence completion techniques, require the subjective judgment of highly trained examiners to translate responses into scores.
- *Normative versus ipsative scoring:* Tests of maximum performance consist of a series of questions or problems that are independently answered and scored (i.e., item independence generates normative scores). In contrast, some inventories and questionnaires require the examinee to choose among several stimuli; both selected and nonselected items are scored (on different scales). The result is that if respondents score high on some scales, they must score low on other scales (i.e., forced-choice items generate ipsative score profiles).
- *Examiner versus computer-generated interpretation:* Most psychological and vocational instruments are accompanied by manuals, handbooks, code books, or other similar compilations of research designed to assist the examiner with the interpretation of test scores. However, an increasing number of tests can be interpreted by computer programs—that is, a narrative report is produced by selecting interpretive statements from an assembled "library" using a series of "rules."
- *Absolute versus culture-relative interpretation:* The majority of rehabilitation clients come from the broadly defined American middle class and, therefore, test interpretation using general population norm groups is usually reasonable and appropriate. (Norm groups are representative samples of people that provide a comparative basis for giving meaning to test scores. Normative score interpretation is discussed later in this chapter.) However, it is well-established that disabilities occur disproportionately among minority and disadvantaged segments of society, necessitating for some examinees more flexible test interpretation that takes into account limited opportunities for development of aptitudes, occupational interests, and suitable work values.

Each of these issues has implications for the selection and use of tests in assessing people with disabilities. For example, an ipsatively scored interest inventory may be required with individuals who tend to like all activities (or, conversely, who dislike almost everything). Although there is nothing wrong with liking everything, a "flat" interest profile is of little diagnostic value in vocational counseling. In general, group-administered, objectively scored tests are favored for reasons of cost and efficiency, but with clients of high "case difficulty," individually administered tests that provide a standardized format for obtaining detailed, clinically relevant material may be a good investment. Various aspects of these distinctions among tests are discussed throughout the *Handbook*.

Levels of Measurement

The purpose of psychological measurement is to quantify or convert to numerical form attributes or characteristics of people. Test scores are almost always composed of the sum of responses to stimuli or tasks that are thought to adequately represent the attribute being measured. An issue of special importance to psychometricians, and one that has clear implications for the interpretation of test scores, concerns the quality or meaningfulness of the numerical scores that result from psychological and vocational instruments. The problem of quality of scores is addressed through scaling techniques and is a central and continuing topic in measurement theory. Four measurement scales typically are recognized, although the lowest level is not really a scale in the technical sense of the term.

1. A *nominal* scale simply uses numbers as labels to identify individuals, as when consecutive case file numbers are assigned to persons applying for rehabilitation services. The numbers obviously do not represent quantities or magnitudes of attributes, only sequential order. Numerical labels may also be used to designate classes or categories, as in psychiatric diagnosis using the *Diagnostic and Statistical Manual of Mental Disorders–Fourth Edition, Text Revision* (DSM–IV–TR; American Psychiatric Association, 2000)—for example, delusional disorder (297.1), obsessive–compulsive disorder (300.3), and schizoid personality disorder (301.2). When individuals are identified with numbers that are assigned arbitrarily, the numerical property of the scale has no relevance. Although no psychological test "measures" at the nominal level, the resulting interpretation may entail nominal assignments, such as diagnostic categories, occupational groups, and remedial training programs.

2. An *ordinal* scale allows persons in a testing group to be ordered only based on rank for the measured attribute. Ordinal scales do not convey information about the magnitude of the differences among individuals or the absolute magnitude of the characteristic. Because ordinal scale information would not be particularly useful to counseling practitioners, few measuring procedures use ordinal scales. Sociometric techniques (in which group members identify peers who possess specified characteristics) are a rare example of standardized measurements that generate strictly ordinal data, but many psychological tests produce scores that possess only ordinal meaning with respect to a normative population.

3. An *interval* scale has a standard unit of measurement that allows for estimating the magnitude of differences among individuals as well as showing simply that one person possesses more (or less) of the trait than another person. So an interval scale may be thought of as an ordinal scale with an established unit of measurement; however, the interval scale does not indicate the absolute magnitude of the attribute. For example, if a mechanical aptitude test approximates an interval scale, the difference between scores of 58 and 53 would be equivalent to the difference between scores of 45 and 40. However, a score of 0 would not signify an absolute absence of mechanical aptitude. A familiar example is the Fahrenheit thermometer that measures temperature with a standard unit; however, 0° has no particular significance.

4. A *ratio* scale includes the properties of an interval scale (i.e., it has a standard unit of measurement) and also has an absolute zero point. None of the instruments discussed in this volume measure attributes on a ratio scale, so this scale will not be discussed further. In fact, the only procedures in psychology that are considered to approach the ratio scale are certain psycho-physical methods that are used to determine thresholds and scale values for stimuli that can be ordered on a physical continuum (see Nunnally & Bernstein, 1994).

Most psychological and vocational tests and inventories measure on a scale somewhere between the ordinal and interval levels, depending on the particular instrument. It should be obvious from the previous descriptions that measurement on an interval scale is desirable, all other considerations being equal. Measurement at the interval level is valuable to counselors because scores can be regarded as measured distances (i.e., number of standard units) on the trait from a fixed reference point such as the mean, whereas ordinal scale scores only indicate relative position in a normative reference group. However, the construction of interval scales of measurement is a complex procedure (see DeVellis, 2003; Magnusson, 1967; Netemeyer, Bearden, & Sharma, 2003; Nunnally & Bernstein, 1994; Torgerson, 1958).

Most authorities in psychometrics would agree that tests of maximum performance, and especially individually administered intelligence tests, come closer to an interval scale of measurement than do tests of typical performance (e.g., personality questionnaires, interest inventories, projective techniques, vocational rating scales). There is no disagreement, however, that tests of maximum performance generally measure with greater precision and accuracy than do tests of typical performance. As Parts 2 and 3 of the *Handbook* explain, however, the various typical performance instruments are extremely useful tools in rehabilitation planning with persons with disabilities. The rehabilitation practitioner would be advised to exercise somewhat more caution in interpreting measures of typical performance.

Strategies and Issues in Score Interpretation

Interpretation of Scores

Raw scores, which are usually sums of keyed item responses, are meaningless without additional knowledge concerning the instrument. At the very least, information about the nature and number of items composing the test, the response format used, and the range of possible scores is essential. With most standardized measures, it is necessary to have carefully described reference groups as a basis for giving meaning to scores. The simplest form of instrument, the problem checklist, can be used to identify a client's significant areas of difficulty. The results of a checklist may be reported simply as a list of problems requiring attention. Another measurement situation in which raw scores might appropriately be interpreted directly is with interest inventories; Cronbach (1990, p. 474) advocates the use of raw scores for interpreting interest profiles because absolute preference for a particular type of work is more meaningful than relative standing on interest scales.

Three strategies for interpreting test scores are available: domain-referenced (or content-referenced) interpretation, norm-referenced interpretation, and criterion-referenced (or predictive) interpretation. A fourth interpretive strategy, which transcends these three specific approaches, is trait-referenced interpretation. As the name suggests, trait-referenced interpretation is concerned with the nature of the underlying trait that the test or scale purports to measure. The psychometric basis for trait-referenced interpretation is the empirically determined construct validity of the instrument. As explained in Chapter 3, construct validation procedures identify and explicate the psychological trait (or construct) that accounts for variability in scores on the test.

Because trait-referenced interpretation usually occurs in conjunction with one of the other three interpretive strategies, it is not discussed separately in this chapter. When trait-referenced interpretations are implied in the following illustrations, however, they are indicated as such.

1. *Domain-referenced score interpretation:* This interpretive approach reports the examinee's performance as a proportion of essential skills mastered. The strategy requires that the test content be a representative sample of the performance domain to be measured. The domain-referenced tests most familiar to readers are academic achievement tests and competency tests for measuring skill acquisition. In rehabilitation, domain-referenced tests have been used most extensively in the measurement of daily living skills but have become increasingly popular in the evaluation approach known as functional assessment (see Halpern & Fuhrer, 1984). The critical aspect of domain-referenced tests is the adequacy of the sampling plan; the validity of the instrument depends to a great extent on the representativeness of the content. Obviously, the tasks and items composing the instrument must be directly relevant to the provision of rehabilitation services. Scores on domain-referenced tests are often reported as percentages of items correctly answered or tasks mastered.

2. *Norm-referenced score interpretation:* This approach to test interpretation locates the examinee in comparison to a large, representative sample of persons. The sample of persons is representative of a carefully defined *normative population,* and the compilation of test scores for the comparison sample is called test "norms." Norm tables, then, are simple statistical devices for converting raw scores into scores with comparative meaning, called "derived scores." Derived scores are reported on standard scales with known properties; the topic of derived scores is considered in greater detail in the next section. The important point

to emphasize about norm-referenced scores is that they are predicated on the identification of a relevant normative population. For example, a language usage score at the 85th percentile in a norm group of high school seniors might be located at the 15th percentile of graduate students in English. Because there may be several relevant populations for interpretive purposes, many instruments have several normative samples tabled. Selection of appropriate norms depends on the types of decisions to be made in rehabilitation planning. Normative samples should always be fully described on demographic characteristics, such as sex, age, education, and disabilities represented. When performance differences exist among subgroups, separate norm tables or adjustment calculations should be provided. The subject of choosing the proper norm groups for interpreting test results for persons with disabilities is discussed in several chapters in the *Handbook*.

3. *Criterion-referenced score interpretation:* This interpretive strategy translates the examinee's score (or score profile) directly into an estimate of success on an external criterion, such as completion of a training program or satisfactory performance in an occupation. Criterion-referenced score reports typically convert test scores into *probabilities* or predicted levels of given behavioral outcomes, using experience tables, multiple regression equations, or multiple cutoff criteria based on established minimum competency scores. The translation of personality profiles from inventories such as the *Minnesota Multiphasic Personality Inventory* (MMPI) and *Clinical Analysis Questionnaire* into diagnostic categories using high-point codes or indexes of profile similarity is also regarded as criterion-referenced interpretation, when the characteristics of the diagnostic groups have been determined independently. To use the criterion-referenced interpretive approach, the test must be predictive of subsequent performance on relevant criteria and the empirical relationships must be appropriately quantified.

Derived Standard Scores

Derived standard scores are used to report the results of test performance because the distributions of these scores have known characteristics. Hence, the meaning of derived scores is readily understood and easily communicated, and score comparisons across different instruments (when warranted by identical or comparable norms) are facilitated. Three types of derived standard scores are described in this section: percentiles, linear standard scores, and normalized standard scores.

The simplest kind of derived score is the *percentile* or percentile rank. The percentile scale ranges from a low score of 1 to a high score of 99; each scale point or centile indicates the proportion of the normative population that is exceeded by the examinee. For example, a person who achieves a percentile score of 72 (or who is located at the 72nd percentile) exceeds 72% of the people in the normative population. Conversion of raw scores to percentile scores does not entail any assumptions about the distribution of the measured trait; regardless of the nature of the raw score distribution, the percentile distribution is always *rectangular* in form. Stated somewhat differently, the percentile distribution consists of 99 points that partition a score distribution into 100 categories of equal size (except for the end categories, which are half-size).

Conversion to percentile ranks may result in some loss of measurement precision. This generally means that the percentile scale exaggerates raw score differences near the center of the distribution and tends to diminish raw score differences at the extremes. This distortion of the raw score scale is illustrated in Figure 1.1, which depicts a mathematical curve called the normal (or Gaussian) distribution. Most values in a normal distribution cluster around the central

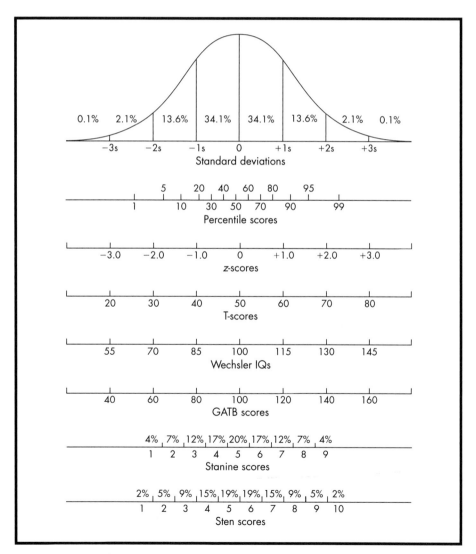

FIGURE 1.1. Standard scores in the normal distribution.

point, or average, with fewer values at greater distances from the average. The normal curve is a theoretical frequency distribution that is *approximated* by many biological and psychological variables, such as height and measured intelligence; it is not "a fact of nature." It can be observed in Figure 1.1 that the percentile scores are compressed at the middle of the distribution and stretched out at the ends. Despite the fact that percentile ranks constitute only an ordinal level of measurement, the percentile scale is a highly useful reporting device because it is so readily understood by practitioners and clients, yet it should be realized that ease of interpretation may be achieved at the expense of measurement precision (i.e., equal-interval data may be lost).

In contrast to percentile ranks, *linear* standard scores preserve the scale units and the form of the raw score distribution. Linear standard scores are calculated by subtracting the mean (*M*) from each score and dividing by the standard deviation (*SD*) of the distribution. The result is a transformed distribution of z scores that has a mean of 0 and standard deviation of 1.0. The standard z scores indicate how far above or below the mean a given score is located in standard deviation units (e.g., a z score of 1.5 *SD* is one and one-half standard deviations above the mean). Because z scores may contain negative values and decimals (e.g., $z = -1.2$), they are not convenient for reporting test scores. The most commonly used standard scores for normative test interpretation are *T*-scores, which have a mean of 50 and standard deviation of 10. Other well-known standard distributions are the Wechsler IQ scale, with a mean of 100 and standard deviation of 15, and the *General Aptitude Test Battery* (GATB) scale, with a mean of 100 and standard deviation of 20.

If the distribution of raw scores is approximately normal in shape (i.e., the histogram of scores when smoothed looks similar to the curve in Figure 1.1), then the linear standard scores described earlier may be converted to percentile ranks to facilitate interpretation. But if the distribution of raw scores departs substantially from the normal curve, conversion from linear standard scores to percentiles using the normal curve table will not be accurate. If it is reasonable to assume that a psychological trait is normally distributed (see Chapter 8 in Hays, 1963), the raw score distribution may be *normalized* in conjunction with the calculation of standard scores; the resulting distribution consists of normalized standard scores. This procedure assumes that score distributions depart from normal form because the measuring procedure distorts or inaccurately quantifies the psychological characteristic; hence, it is argued that normalizing the raw score distribution simply recaptures the "true" metric of the trait.

At this point, the reader may wonder why it is necessary to go to the trouble of calculating normalized standard scores just to have available the percentile interpretation, when percentiles can be calculated directly from the raw score distribution. The answer is that the *assumption* of a normally distributed psychological trait provides one basis for the derivation of an interval scale of measurement (see Magnusson, 1967) and, therefore, *differences* among individuals at different locations on normalized standard score scales can be compared because the unit of measurement is the same throughout the scale. In other words, with normally distributed test score distributions, both standard scores and percentiles convey important information and are useful interpretive vehicles.

Two often-used normalized score reporting formats with greatly simplified scales are stens (standard-*ten*) and stanines (standard-*nine*), which range from 1 to 10 and 1 to 9, respectively. As can be seen in Figure 1.1, the score categories of both the sten and stanine scales are one-half standard deviation wide (except for the end categories) and approximate the normal distribution. Each of these standard score scales has the advantage of expressing test performance as positive, whole numbers.

Two other "standard" scores that are sometimes used to report test performance are mental age equivalent scores and grade equivalent scores. The former typically are used to indicate level of intellectual development, whereas the latter are often used to report the results of academic achievement testing. Both of these scales are controversial because they are prone to misinterpretation and, consequently, should be avoided in reporting test results.

Examples of Score Interpretation

In this section, the three interpretive strategies outlined previously are illustrated, using instruments that either have been developed for use with persons with disabilities or have been successfully applied in rehabilitation settings.

Domain-Referenced Interpretation

The *Independent Living Behavior Checklist* (ILBC; Walls, Zane, & Thvedt, 1979) is a list of 343 independent living skills that are organized into six categories: Mobility Skills, Self-Care Skills, Home Maintenance and Safety Skills, Food Skills, Social and Communication Skills, and Functional Academic Skills. In a defined situation or condition, performance of the specified behavior is observed and judged as either satisfactory or unsatisfactory according to the specified criterion.

All 343 items are written in a standard format that facilitates reliable observation of the examinee's performance. An example from Mobility Skills is "bathtub":

> Condition: Given a bathtub
>
> Behavior: Client steps into the tub, sits down, stands up, and steps out of the tub.
>
> Standard: Behavior within 30 seconds. A handrail or other objects may be used to help with stepping into the tub, sitting down, standing up, or stepping out of the tub.

The Mobility Skills scale of the ILBC contains 42 items that measure independent living skills ranging from getting in and out of bed and traveling up and down steps to moving about the community. The examiner may delete skill items considered inappropriate for a given client or irrelevant for a particular rehabilitation program; needed skill items may be added to the ILBC.

The results of an ILBC assessment are summarized on a *Skill Summary Chart,* which lists applicable skills for the individual and indicates whether the task was completed successfully. A *Skill Objective Profile* reports the client's relative status in all six areas by calculating the percentage of skill objectives that have been mastered in each category and portraying the percentages in a graphical, thermometer-like figure. If an examinee mastered 14 of 33 mobility skills deemed relevant, then the percentage score would be 42%. Scores in other areas might be higher or lower, providing some indication of relative status or progress.

The primary applications of the ILBC in rehabilitation settings are to diagnose deficiencies and difficulties as a basis for program planning and to assess progress in skill mastery via repeated measurements. The logic of domain referencing should be emphasized in these applications: use of the ILBC and similar instruments is predicated on the adequacy and completeness of the definition of the skills that compose the behavioral domain (e.g., mobility skills, social and communication skills). It should also be noted that observer–rating instruments assume that judgments can be made reliably; with the ILBC, interobserver agreement for the typical skill item averages 99%.

Norm-Referenced Interpretation

The *Personal Opinions Questionnaire* (POQ) is a self-report measure of intrapersonal empowerment developed for use with rehabilitation clients (Bolton & Brookings, 1998). Intrapersonal empowerment refers to how people think about their capacity to influence social and political systems important to them. The POQ measures four components of intrapersonal empowerment: Personal Competence, Group Orientation, Self-Determination, and Positive Identity as a Person with a Disability.

The POQ consists of 64 statements to which the examinee responds "true" or "false." Half of the items are phrased positively and half negatively to control for acquiescence. The following items are examples from the Group Orientation subscale:

- I do not like to work in groups.
- I can achieve most of my goals by working with others.
- I prefer to do things by myself.
- I rarely participate in community activities.
- I like to work on projects that help the community.

Raw scores are calculated by counting one point for each response in the keyed direction. In other words, the scoring procedure gives one point for "true" responses to positively stated items and one point for "false" responses to negatively phrased items. Thus, raw scores on the Group Orientation scale may range from 0 to 15 because the scale consists of 15 items.

The POQ is the only instrument that measures the extent to which people with disabilities have acquired the values and attitudes associated with the philosophy of empowerment. Norms for the POQ are based on the responses of 473 candidates for rehabilitation services provided through the state and federal vocational rehabilitation program. Because men and women did not have significantly different scores on the POQ scales, a single normative table with sexes combined was assembled (Brookings & Bolton, 2000). Using the norm table, raw scores on the POQ are converted to normalized percentile scores, thus locating an examinee's position on the four POQ subscales and providing a total score relative to the normative sample.

For example, assume that a respondent achieved raw scores on the four subscales and total score of 19, 6, 10, 9, and 44, respectively. These raw scores translate to percentile equivalents of 55th percentile, 20th percentile, 65th percentile, 95th percentile, and 60th percentile, respectively. The normative interpretation of this individual's POQ protocol is that, although she is only slightly above average in overall empowerment (60th percentile), her profile is quite differentiated. She scored highest on Positive Identity (95th percentile), indicating that she accepts her disability realistically. She scored slightly above average on Self-Determination (65th percentile) and Personal Competence (55th percentile), suggesting that she is typical in standing up for her rights and assuming responsibility for herself. Finally, her low score on Group Orientation (20th percentile) indicates that she prefers to work alone. This information should be useful in rehabilitation program planning.

Criterion-Referenced Interpretation

The MMPI is the most widely used personality inventory in assessment practice. The MMPI-2 (Butcher et al., 1989) is the current version of the instrument that was developed in the late 1930s and early 1940s. The MMPI-2 consists of 567 true/false items that are scored on 3 validity scales and 10 clinical scales: Faking (L), Infrequency (F), Defensiveness (K), Hypochondriasis (Hs), Depression (D), Hysteria (Hy), Psychopathic Deviate (Pd), Masculinity–Femininity (MO), Paranoia (Pa), Psychasthenia (Pt), Schizophrenia (Sc), Hypomania (Ma), and Social Introversion (Si).

Raw scale scores are converted to standard *T*-scores with a mean of 50 and standard deviation of 10 (see Figure 1.1), based on a national normative sample of 2,600 men and women. Higher scale scores are indicative of the various types of emotional maladjustment suggested by the names of the scales. *T*-scores of 65 or greater are typically regarded as "clinically significant."

Interpretation of the MMPI-2 is a complex process involving three interrelated issues: validity of the protocol, elevation of the individual clinical scales, and analysis of the configuration of the clinical profile. Critical items, content scales, and other supplementary information may be used to interpret the protocol. Although each of the clinical scales has interpretive value, it is the combination or configuration of scores in the profile that assumes greater importance in the interpretation of the MMPI-2.

One of the most widely used strategies for interpreting the MMPI-2 profile is that of high-point codes. As the name suggests, high-point codes focus on the two (or three) highest scores in the individual's profile. The procedure entails identifying one or more *criterion* groups that have the same high-point scale combinations as the individual does. To illustrate the concept of criterion-referenced interpretation, three different two-high-point code descriptions were extracted from more extensive material compiled by Graham (1990).

- *Code* D-Pt: These individuals are anxious and tense, worry excessively, and exhibit symptoms of clinical depression. They are extremely pessimistic and brood about their problems. They harbor feelings of inadequacy and insecurity and tend to be docile and dependent in their relationships with other people.
- *Code* Pa-Sc: These individuals are suspicious and distrustful of other people. They are often deficient in social skills and are most comfortable when alone. Other people regard them as irritable, unfriendly, and negativistic. Their thinking typically is autistic, fragmented, and bizarre.
- *Code* Pd-Ma: These individuals are narcissistic, self-indulgent, and impulsive. They often exhibit poor judgment and fail to learn from experience. They harbor feelings of anger and hostility. They are unwilling to accept responsibility, and they blame their difficulties on other people.

A client with the two highest scale scores (in either order) corresponding to one of these code groups may possess some of the clinical symptomatology present in the description. In other words, the MMPI-2 two-high-point code *similarity* establishes a basis for inferring shared behavioral features. The extra-test behavioral correlates contained in the descriptions, which were accumulated from clinical studies and empirical research on the code groups, constitute the content of the criterion-referenced interpretation. It should be emphasized that the inferred behavioral similarities are treated as *hypotheses* to be evaluated by the MMPI-2 interpreter.

The MMPI-2 code type interpretation illustrates the strategy called the multiple cutoff method, meaning that the two highest scores in the profile must both be T scores of 65 or greater. The interpreter must exercise judgment in cases where critical scores lie near the cutoff levels, and this includes taking into account the unreliability of the scale scores (see Chapter 2). Other statistical devices for translating test scores into criterion performance estimates are experience tables, expectancy charts, and multiple regression equations. In contrast to the multiple cutoff strategy, these procedures treat criterion performance as a continuous variable, generating either a probability estimate or an estimated score on a standard scale.

Scores of Doubtful Validity

It is almost impossible, and certainly an extremely rare occurrence, for an examinee to achieve an erroneously high score on an ability test by guessing or "faking good." However, examinees' performance on ability tests may be influenced detrimentally by test anxiety or by lack of motivation to perform at their best (i.e., to make a maximal effort). Lack of motivation may be addressed through careful test instructions that stress the importance of doing one's best because of the positive implications of higher test scores, such as expanded educational and occupational opportunities. The presence of test anxiety in an examinee may be a more serious and generalized inhibiting factor, requiring therapeutic treatment for successful modification (see Sarason, 1980; Zeidner, 1998). In any case, it is important that ability test scores be accompanied by the examiner's observations concerning potentially invalidating circumstances. Here, invalidity refers to the negative effects of test-taking attitudes and response styles that render the accuracy of an individual's score doubtful. This usage is consistent with the definition of test validity given earlier in this chapter and elaborated on in Chapter 3. Any condition or factor that diminishes the accuracy with which an instrument measures the trait or construct it purports to measure is a source of invalidity.

Tests of typical performance, especially self-report inventories and questionnaires, are potentially susceptible to a variety of irrelevant response factors or "styles" (i.e., test behaviors that produce scores that may not accurately reflect respondents' true interests, personality, or values). The most straightforward invalidating test behavior is *faking.* Occasionally an examinee will make a conscious and concerted effort to present a favorable self-description or, conversely, attempt to appear disturbed by endorsing numerous items symptomatic of difficulties. However, some respondents may answer questionnaire items in the *socially desirable* or socially approved direction, not with the intent to deceive or portray themselves inaccurately, but simply because the response style is consistent with their personalities. In fact, it has been argued that social desirability responding is the major source of interindividual variation on personality inventories (see Edwards, 1970). Still another response style that may produce inaccurate scores is *acquiescence,* the general tendency of some examinees to say "true" or "yes" to personality questionnaire items or to check "like" for interest inventory items.

Several strategies have been devised by measurement specialists to identify and estimate the extent of faking and social desirability responding, and some instruments even incorporate procedures for adjusting or "correcting" the obtained scores to remove the unwanted influence. Two standard techniques for dealing with response sets are (a) disguise the purpose of the instrument with an innocuous, if not misleading, title and statement of purpose (although this may raise ethical questions); and (b) use a forced-choice format, where the alternatives have been previously equated for social desirability. A third strategy that is applicable only with empirically keyed instruments is reliance on "subtle" items—that is, items for which the socially approved response is not obvious.

Numerous verification scales have been developed for questionnaires and inventories (e.g., the so-called Lie or Faking [L] scale of the MMPI, the Motivational Distortion scale of the *Sixteen Personality Factor Questionnaire,* and the Good Impression scale of the *Adult Personality Inventory*). Most inventories that do not use a forced-choice format count the total number of endorsements and/or the uncertain responses. It is sufficient at this point to emphasize that valid scores depend greatly upon the establishment of a cooperative relationship ("rapport") between counselor and client, so that clients understand that it is in their best interest to respond honestly and carefully to inventory items as well as interview questions. Readers desiring an in-depth analysis of the subject of response sets and a review of the empirical research on supplementary validity keys are referred to Nunnally and Bernstein (1994).

General Guidelines for Test Usage

Using Tests in Rehabilitation

The topic of diagnostic assessment in rehabilitation is addressed in considerable detail in the chapters in Part 3 of the *Handbook.* This brief section presents a general overview of test interpretation in counseling in the form of a set of preliminary suggestions that establishes a foundation for subsequent discussions. These suggestions also extend the strategies outlined and illustrated in previous sections to the practical activity of counseling clients with disabilities.

The ultimate purpose of assessment interpretation is to translate scores and associated observations into a comprehensive rehabilitation plan that optimizes the probability of the client's successful vocational adjustment (in the competitive labor market, if feasible) and makes possible suitable living arrangements in the least restrictive environment. The counselor and client work together to develop a mutually acceptable plan, based substantially on knowledge derived through client evaluation procedures.

To establish a foundation for rehabilitation planning, it is essential that the assessment results be shared with the client in a feedback interview. The feedback interview has four goals: presenting information in a nonthreatening manner, interpreting results so that the client understands the implications, eliciting the client's response to test results, and developing alternative courses of action.

It follows that test interpretation in rehabilitation involves two interrelated processes: assembling the assessment data into a coherent written report and discussing the assessment results with the client. The objective of this activity is to organize and synthesize test and interview information into a comprehensive, integrated summary of the client's rehabilitation potential. An optimal strategy is for the counselor to outline a preliminary report and use this rough draft as the framework for conducting the feedback interview with the client. The final written report should incorporate the client's reactions and suggestions into the recommendations section of the report.

Vash (1981) and Vash and Crewe (2004) discuss three reasons for involving the client in the test interpretation process: (a) explaining the purpose of assessment to clients encourages them to become active participants; (b) sharing assessment results with clients gives them some responsibility for acting on the results; and (c) because clients are lifelong experts on themselves, they bring a wealth of self-knowledge to assessment interpretation. The authors conclude with the following advice for counselors: When in doubt, consult the expert, the client.

There are several basic principles and strategies of test interpretation that can facilitate the task of translating assessment results into implications for rehabilitation planning. The following suggestions were taken from three primary sources (Bolton, 1998; McGowan & Porter, 1967; Moriarty, Minton, & Spann, 1981).

Preparing the Written Report

1. The interpretation of assessment data requires clinical judgment and expertise with assessment instruments. Clinical expertise is based on experience conducting assessments and knowledge about the research foundations of the instruments used. In other words, counselors need supervised *practice* interpreting assessment data and *knowledge* about the technical features of the tests and inventories used.

2. Interpretation begins with immersion in the raw assessment data, which include the interview protocol, scores from tests and inventories, and other sources of information. The salient results should be reduced to a manageable set of hypotheses using a variety of interpretive resources, such as test manuals and handbooks. The assessment report should cover the client's background, disability factors, intelligence, interests, personality, vocational skills, and recommendations for rehabilitation planning.

3. Many assessment instruments generate a profile of scores that should be interpreted simultaneously. There are three distinct steps involved. First, the overall level of the profile should be examined—do the scores tend to be above average, average, or below average? Second, the overall variability of the scores should be noted—do the scores tend to be about the same, or is there substantial intraindividual variation? Third, the highest and lowest scores in the profile should be identified to describe the client. Multiscore profiles provide important information about the organization of the client's traits.

4. Look for convergence across scales, instruments, work history, and interview data in developing hypotheses about the client. Interpretation

of scale scores should be based on construct validity evidence and examination of instrument content—that is, the client's responses to the test items that produced the score. It should be emphasized that all score interpretation is trait referenced, meaning that the foundation of interpretation is the evidence that indicates that the test score measures what it purports to measure.

5. It is important to remember that test scores are estimates of the client's performance potential, so allowance should be made for unreliability of the measurement process. The proper strategy for doing this is to report test scores as bands or intervals, using the standard error of measurement to establish the width of the interval (see Chapter 2 for details), rather than as single values.

6. As the basis for formulating recommendations, begin by listing the client's strengths and deficits in selected relevant areas. Do the strengths offset the deficits? Can the deficits be remediated? Start with simpler, more straightforward explanations. Translate assessment results into implications for client service planning.

Providing Feedback to Clients

1. Use short, concise methods of explaining to clients the purposes of the tests taken and the meaning of scores. Describe test results in functional terms in relation to rehabilitation planning.

2. Encourage clients to participate in test interpretation. Test results should help clients achieve a better understanding and acceptance of their strengths and weaknesses.

3. Discussion of assessment results should subsume all other relevant information, including work history, education, motivation, and disability issues. Test scores can be really useful only when considered in the larger context of the client's life circumstances, aspirations, and goals.

4. Assessment data become meaningful to the client when the results are related directly to the client's past experiences, current behavior, and future plans. Emphasize concrete implications of test scores, rather than abstract assessment issues.

5. Explain low test performance or unpleasant information honestly, while maintaining a broader perspective. Do not dismiss low scores as unimportant, but place more emphasis on the client's strengths. At the same time, give clients the opportunity to talk about low scores and their relevance for rehabilitation planning.

6. Remember that the purpose of the feedback interview is to involve the client in the test interpretation process and to enhance the client's self-understanding as a basis for joint rehabilitation service planning. Respect the client's role in the problem-solving task by sharing responsibility for the activity. Conclude with a brief summary that stresses the positive features of the assessment results.

Testing Job Applicants With Disabilities

Employment testing of job applicants with disabilities is central to the goals of rehabilitation practitioners. In contrast to assessment in rehabilitation, which focuses on clients' assets and potentials, as well as deficits that can be remediated through training, employers are concerned almost exclusively with identifying and hiring applicants who will perform optimally. However, employers are required by law to make certain that the tests and test procedures they use do not discriminate unfairly against job applicants with disabilities. This section (a) outlines the relevant federal legislation and regulations; (b) describes possible modifications of tests and testing procedures to accommodate job applicants with disabilities; and (c) evaluates the potential impact of such modifications on the psychometric properties of employment tests, in light of the *Standards for Educational and Psychological Testing* (American Psychological Association, 2000).

Federal Laws and Regulations

Section 504 of the Rehabilitation Act of 1973 prohibited discrimination against job applicants with disabilities by those receiving federal grants. The act was amended in 1978 to include all federal agencies, and Title I of the Americans with Disabilities Act of 1990 (ADA) extended this provision to the private sector. Included in the legislation is the requirement to consider reasonable accommodations of employment tests for applicants with mental or physical limitations.

The ADA further prohibits employers from administering "medical tests" until an offer of employment has been made. In 1994 the Equal Employment Opportunity Commission (EEOC) issued guidelines for determining if a psychological test is medical (this issue is discussed in detail under "Unresolved Issues").

Test Modifications

A common modification entails changing the way the test is presented. For example, test takers who are visually impaired may use modified materials produced in larger type or braille, use materials recorded on audiocassette, or hear materials read aloud. If the applicant is hearing impaired, the test materials may be presented via a sign language interpreter.

A second type of modification pertains to response format. Applicants who are speech impaired could be accommodated by having them write out their responses to items that otherwise require a verbal response, whereas oral responses would be allowed for examinees with disabling conditions that prevent them from making motor responses to items. Finally, for individuals with both speech and motor impairments, it may be necessary to limit responses to a simple yes/no format.

It also may be necessary to change the environment in which tests are administered. For example, applicants with visual impairments may require modified lighting to read the test materials properly, and some applicants may have to be tested individually in their homes, rather than at the employment setting. Other modifications of tests or testing procedures may include shortening the test by eliminating items or subtests, rephrasing or replacing items, or even substituting one test for another.

Finally, because persons with disabling conditions may not be able to clearly formulate or articulate answers to some types of test items, examiners may need to incorporate the "acculturation" of applicants into their interpretation of test responses.

Unresolved Issues

When the ADA was passed (1990) there was little empirical evidence on the effects of test modifications on test validity, and measurement specialists warned that strict interpretations of ADA provisions would create problems for employers making good-faith efforts to comply with the provisions. Specifically, Division 5 (Evaluation, Measurement, and Statistics) of the American Psychological Association issued a statement called "Psychometric and Assessment Issues Raised by the Americans with Disabilities Act (ADA)" (1993). The statement identified four important psychometric questions raised by the ADA.

1. Do applicants' scores on a modified test accurately reflect the scores they would have obtained on the original (i.e., unmodified) test under standardized conditions, assuming the absence of a disabling condition?
2. Do modified tests measure the same constructs as standardized tests and predict job behavior with comparable accuracy?
3. Should those responsible for making employment decisions be informed that scores were obtained from a modified test?
4. Are personality or "temperament" measures properly considered part of a medical examination, which may be given, under the ADA, only *after* an offer of employment has been made to the applicant?

With respect to Questions 1 and 2, the Educational Testing Service conducted a series of studies comparing standard and modified versions of the Scholastic Aptitude Test and Graduate Record Examination for persons with disabling conditions (e.g., learning disabilities; physical, visual impairment). The standard and modified versions were generally comparable, except for modifications involving test timing (see Willingham et al., 1988, for a detailed presentation of the findings).

Cohen and Swerdlik (1999) addressed Question 3 in their proposal that an "Accommodation Addendum" be added to psychological test reports for which the test or test procedure was modified to accommodate an examinee. The proposed addendum would include (a) a clear description of how the test or test procedure was modified; (b) a psychometric justification—supported by references from scholarly literature—for the accommodation; and (c) other information that might be relevant to the interpretation of test scores. *Not* included is a description of the examinee's disability. It should be noted that the *Standards for Educational and Psychological Testing* (American Psychological Association, 2000) stipulates that scores on modified tests should not be flagged if there is evidence that the standard and modified test versions are comparable (see later in this chapter).

Finally, prohibiting medical examinations until after a "contingent" offer of employment (i.e., contingent on further screening, such as for requisite physical abilities) has been made helps ensure that employers will not use knowledge of disabilities as a basis for rejecting job applicants and is a provision with which test professionals generally agree. What *is* problematic, however, is the definition of "medical examination" (Question 4). The American Psychological Association's (1994a) position is that tests should be defined based on how they are used. That is, if a company uses a personality test to predict job performance, rather than to diagnose psychological disorders, it should be allowed to administer the test *before* making an offer of employment. The EEOC guidelines, however, imply that if a test was *designed originally* for clinical diagnosis (e.g., the MMPI) and/or is administered by a "health care professional" (which includes psychologists), it is properly considered part of a medical examination and could therefore be used only after a job offer has been tendered. Consequently, employers may not assess the mental stability of job applicants—even for jobs with public safety responsibilities—until a contingent job offer has been extended (American Psychological Association, 1994b).

Standards for Testing Individuals with Disabilities

Ideally, modifications of tests and testing procedures would be informed by systematic research documenting the impact of the modifications on the psychometric properties of the tests. This is recognized explicitly in the *Standards for Educational and Psychological Testing* (American Psychological Association, 2000), which makes the following stipulations:

- All of those involved in the testing enterprise (e.g., test developers, test users) are responsible for minimizing the effects of construct-irrelevant factors, such as the effects of disabling conditions on the test scores of persons with disabilities.
- Those who modify tests for persons with disabilities should have access to the relevant psychometric expertise *and* knowledge about the effects of disabling conditions on test performance.
- Test manuals should include a detailed description of the test modification rationale and procedures. If evidence on the validity of the modification is not available, cautions regarding inferences from scores on the modified test should be included as well.
- If possible, modified tests should be pilot tested to determine the appropriateness of the modifications and their effects on the validity of the test for the intended population(s).

- Changes in time limits for modified versions of speeded tests should be based on empirical evidence, and possible fatiguing effects of extended time limits on examinees should be investigated as well.
- Where possible, those investigating the effects of test modifications on examinee scores should also administer the standard unmodified test for comparison purposes.
- Professionals who administer tests to persons with disabilities should be knowledgeable about the availability of modified tests and pass the information on to applicants, and they should have the psychometric expertise to select appropriate norms for reporting test scores.
- Scores on modified tests need not be "flagged" if there is evidence that the standard and modified versions of the test are comparable. However, if this evidence is not available, test users should be informed— as permitted by law—about the nature of the modification.

Testing Job Candidates with Disabilities: Recommendations

The Society for Industrial and Organizational Psychology (2003) issued a set of recommendations for the responsible assessment of job candidates with disabilities by businesses and corporate entities. These recommendations include the following:

- Organizations should have access to expertise regarding the potential impact of candidates' disabilities on selection measure performance and whether psychometrically sound modifications of their measures are available. In situations where the effects of the disability on selection measure performance are nontrivial, the company may then choose to modify the current measure, develop a new one, or substitute other job-relevant information for the measure.
- In most organizations, the number of job applicants and employees is too small to permit proper validation research. However, to the extent possible, employers should pilot test modified or substitute procedures on samples of comparable candidates and generate realistic estimates of their reliability and the validity of employment decisions made from them.
- All modifications, including data bearing on their psychometric properties and the scores of candidates who take them and—where possible—the original measures, should be specifically and thoroughly documented in writing. The identities of job applicants who take a modified form of a selection measure should be recorded but kept separate from the assessment data used by the organization to make employment decisions. Revealing such information to decision makers may be prohibited by law.
- Test users should undertake analyses of the extent to which a modified or substitute measure allows assessment of a candidate's standing on the construct of interest, independent of his/her disability. Included in the

procedure outlined for this purpose is a conversation with the applicant about the kinds of accommodations that are desirable and feasible.

- Finally, because the purpose of preemployment testing is to predict job performance, not to assess disabling conditions, the selection procedures used for candidates with disabilities should be as similar as possible to the procedures used for all other candidates.

Ethical Principles of Assessment

It is imperative that rehabilitation professionals observe the ethical standards that govern the selection, administration, and interpretation of psychological and vocational tests and inventories. All major professional organizations promulgate ethical codes that guide the behavior of their members. The rules of professional conduct that apply to testing and assessment activities in rehabilitation listed in the following were taken from the *Code of Professional Ethics for Rehabilitation Counselors* published by the Commission on Rehabilitation Counselor Certification (CRCC; 2001). Rehabilitation professionals should also be familiar with the ethical codes of closely related professions, especially those for counselors (American Counseling Association, 2005) and psychologists (American Psychological Association, 2002).

The CRCC ethical standards pertaining to assessment state that rehabilitation professionals will promote the welfare of clients in the selection, use, and interpretation of assessment measures. The principles are elaborated in a series of "Enforceable Standards of Ethical Practice" that specify the essential behaviors that constitute responsible assessment practice. To be in compliance with the code, rehabilitation professionals will do the following:

- Inform clients of the purpose of testing and the explicit use of the results before test administration.
- Recognize the limits of their competence and perform only those functions for which they are trained.
- Cautiously consider the specific validity, reliability, technical limitations, and appropriateness of tests when selecting them for a specific individual in a particular situation.
- Administer tests under standard conditions, except when accommodating clients with disabilities.
- Use caution in evaluating the performance of individuals with disabilities, members of culturally diverse groups, or persons who are not represented in the norm groups.
- Interpret test results with full consideration of the effects of age, gender, marital status, disability, sexual orientation, ethnicity, race, religion, culture, and accommodations on test scores.
- Explain the results of assessment to clients in a language they can understand.

- Ensure that the administration, scoring, and interpretations produced by electronic methods produce accurate results for the individual.
- Maintain the integrity and security of tests and other assessment procedures in accordance with legal and contractual obligations.
- Recognize that assessment results may become outdated and prevent the misuse of obsolete instruments.

Sources of Additional Information

More than 50 psychological tests regarded as useful for assessing the intelligence, abilities, personality, interests, and functional skills of persons with disabilities are described in Parts 2 and 3 of this book. It is the expert judgment of the chapter authors that these are the best instruments currently available for the purposes specified. But this sample of tests and measures is only a small fraction of those that could be used in rehabilitation settings. Consequently, this section cites important sources of further information, including basic textbooks, volumes containing independent evaluative reviews, technical reference books, academic journals, and other references concerning assessment in rehabilitation.

It should be emphasized that the primary source of information about tests is the accompanying test manual. In some cases, the test manual is supplemented by one or more reference volumes, such as handbooks for the test. Good test manuals, which are periodically updated, include thorough research summaries of reliability and validity studies and information about administration, scoring, and interpretation. The inherent problem with test manuals is that they are written by the test author and distributed by the test publisher; hence, strengths and positive features are stressed, whereas difficulties and negative features tend to be minimized.

The only adequate remedy for the natural inclination of test authors and publishers to "put their best foot forward" is to provide independent, critical reviews of psychological tests—a solution that the late Oscar Buros recognized more than 60 years ago. The product of his insight was a series of *Mental Measurements Yearbooks* (MMYs), which are now published and distributed by the University of Nebraska Press. Of most value to contemporary professionals are the *Thirteenth MMY* (Impara & Plake, 1998), the *Fourteenth MMY* (Plake & Impara, 2000), and the *Fifteenth MMY* (Plake, Impara, & Spies, 2003). Another major compilation of expert test reviews is the *Test Critiques* (TCs) series (Keyser, 1984–2005), which provides more detailed test descriptions than the MMYs.

A useful collection of test reviews reprinted from the MMYs, the TCs series, and other sources is *A Counselor's Guide to Career Assessment Instruments* (Kapes & Whitfield, 2001). Finally, a comprehensive index of hundreds of tests and inventories not published commercially is available in the multivolume

Directory of Unpublished Experimental Mental Measures (Goldman & Mitchell, 1997).

More than a dozen professional journals publish technical articles about measurement and/or test reviews; especially valuable for rehabilitation practitioners are *Applied Psychological Measurement, Journal of Personality Assessment, Journal of Psycho-Educational Assessment, Measurement and Evaluation in Counseling and Development, Psychological Assessment, Journal of Career Assessment,* and *Vocational Evaluation and Work Adjustment Bulletin.* Four textbooks, written by Anastasi and Urbina (1997), Cronbach (1990), Walsh and Betz (2000), and Urbina (2004), provide basic introductions to testing issues and evaluative descriptions of numerous tests, whereas Linn (1989), Nunnally and Bernstein (1994), and Thorndike (1982) address technical topics in test theory. Two additional general sources concerning the professional use of tests are the *Standards for Educational and Psychological Testing* (American Psychological Association, 2000) and the *Policy Statement on Responsibilities of Users of Standardized Tests* (American Counseling Association, 1989).

Numerous books, chapters, and monographs focus on instruments and practice especially suitable for use in rehabilitation assessment. Many of these instruments are *not* reviewed in the reference volumes listed previously, which are typically limited to commercially published tests. Bolton's (2004) chapter describes 22 instruments useful in measuring rehabilitation counseling outcomes. The resource volume by Harrison, Garnett, and Watson (1981) describes in substantial detail 40 older instruments that measure employment potential, independent living skills, and other client characteristics. The volume edited by Glueckauf, Sechrest, Bond, and McDonel (1993) contains chapters on theory, validity, utility, training, and applications in rehabilitation assessment. The book of collected readings by Bolton and Cook (1980) reprints 25 classic articles in rehabilitation client assessment, whereas Parker and Bolton's (2005) chapter provides a current overview of the subject. The volume edited by Cushman and Scherer (1995) addresses psychological assessment in medical settings. Parker and Schaller's (2003) chapter discusses a variety of issues concerning vocational assessment and disability. Finally, the recent textbook by Power (2006) is a good introduction to the use of tests in the vocational appraisal of people with disabilities. More specialized reference sources are given in several chapters of the *Handbook.*

Conclusion

This chapter has defined important terms in measurement and assessment, discussed salient features of standardized tests, illustrated major strategies in test interpretation, described basic types of standard scores, discussed scores of doubtful validity, presented guidelines for using tests in rehabilitation, specified standards for modifying tests for people with disabilities, listed ethical principles of assessment for rehabilitation practitioners, and reviewed sources of additional information about testing in rehabilitation. Because these topics are fundamental to the development of professional competence in rehabilitation assessment, readers should be thoroughly conversant with the subjects before proceeding to Parts 2 and 3 of the *Handbook*.

References

American Counseling Association. (1989). *Policy statement on responsibilities of users of standardized tests.* Alexandria, VA: Author.

American Counseling Association. (2005). *ACA code of ethics.* Alexandria, VA: Author.

American Psychiatric Association. (2000). *Diagnostic and statistical manual of mental disorders* (4th ed., text rev.). Washington, DC: Author.

American Psychological Association. (1994a). *Psychological Science Agenda, 7*(5).

American Psychological Association. (1994b). *Psychological Science Agenda, 7*(6).

American Psychological Association. (2000). *Standards for educational and psychological testing* (4th ed.). Washington, DC: Author.

American Psychological Association. (2002). *Ethical principles of psychologists and code of conduct.* Washington, DC: Author.

American Psychological Association Division of Evaluation, Measurement, and Statistics. (1993). Psychometric and assessment issues raised by the Americans with Disabilities Act (ADA). *The Score, 15*(4), 1–16.

Americans with Disabilities Act of 1990, 42 U.S.C. § 12101 *et seq.* (1990).

Anastasi, A., & Urbina, S. (1997). *Psychological testing* (7th ed.). Upper Saddle River, NJ: Prentice Hall.

Bolton, B. (1998). Rehabilitation client assessment. In R. M. Parker & E. M. Szymanski (Eds.), *Rehabilitation counseling: Basics and beyond* (3rd ed., pp. 411–435). Austin, TX: PRO-ED.

Bolton, B. (2004). Counseling and rehabilitation outcomes. In F. Chan, N. L. Berven, & K. R. Thomas (Eds.), *Counseling theories and techniques for rehabilitation health professionals* (pp. 444–465). New York: Springer.

Bolton, B., & Brookings, J. B. (1998). Development of a measure of intrapersonal empowerment. *Rehabilitation Psychology, 43,* 131–142.

Bolton, B., & Cook, D. (Eds.). (1980). *Rehabilitation client assessment.* Baltimore: University Park Press.

Brookings, J. B., & Bolton, B. (2000, July). Confirmatory factor analysis of a measure of intrapersonal empowerment. *Rehabilitation Psychology, 45,* 292–298.

Butcher, J. N., Dahlstrom, W. G., Graham, J. R., Tellegen, A. N., & Kaemmer, B. (1989). *MMPI–2: Manual for administration and scoring.* Minneapolis: University of Minnesota Press.

Cattell, R. B. (1986). Structured tests and functional diagnoses. In R. B. Cattell & R. C. Johnson (Eds.), *Functional psychological testing: Principles and instruments* (pp. 3–14). New York: Bruner/Mazel.

Cohen, R. J., & Swerdlik, M. E. (1999). *Psychological testing and assessment: An introduction to tests and measurement* (4th ed.). Mountain View, CA: Mayfield.

Commission on Rehabilitation Counselor Certification. (2001). *Code of professional ethics for rehabilitation counselors.* Schaumburg, IL: Author.

Cronbach, L. J. (1990). *Essentials of psychological testing* (5th ed.). New York: HarperCollins.

Cushman, L. A., & Scherer, M. J. (Eds.). (1995). *Psychological assessment in medical rehabilitation.* Washington, DC: American Psychological Association.

DeVellis, R. (2003). *Scale development: Theory and applications* (2nd ed.). Thousand Oaks, CA: Sage.

Edwards, A. (1970). *The measurement of personality traits by scales and inventories.* New York: Holt, Rinehart & Winston.

Glueckauf, R. L., Sechrest, L. B., Bond, G. R., & McDonel, E. C. (Eds.). (1993). *Improving assessment in rehabilitation and health.* Newbury Park, CA: Sage.

Goldman, B. A., & Mitchell, D. F. (Eds.). (1997). *Directory of unpublished experimental mental measures* (Vols. 1–7). Washington, DC: American Psychological Association.

Graham, J. R. (1990). *MMPI–2: Assessing personality and psychopathology.* New York: Oxford University Press.

Halpern, A. S., & Fuhrer, M. J. (Eds.). (1984). *Functional assessment in rehabilitation.* Baltimore: Brookes.

Harrison, D. K., Garnett, J. M., & Watson, A. L. (1981). *Client assessment measures in rehabilitation.* Ann Arbor: University of Michigan, Rehabilitation Research Institute.

Hays, W. L. (1963). *Statistics for psychologists.* New York: Holt, Rinehart & Winston.

Impara, J. C., & Plake, B. S. (Eds.). (1998). *The thirteenth mental measurements yearbook.* Lincoln: University of Nebraska Press.

Kapes, J., & Whitfield, E. (Eds.). (2001). *A counselor's guide to career assessment instruments* (4th ed.). Columbus, OH: National Career Development Association.

Keyser, D. J. (Ed.). (1984–2005). *Test critiques* (Vols. 1–11). Austin, TX: PRO-ED.

Linn, R. L. (Ed.). (1989). *Educational measurement* (3rd ed.). New York: Macmillan.

Magnusson, D. (1967). *Test theory.* Reading, MA: Addison-Wesley.

McGowan, J. F., & Porter, T. L. (1967). *An introduction to the vocational rehabilitation process* (Rev. ed.). Washington, DC: Department of Health, Education, and Welfare.

Moriarty, J. B., Minton, E. B., & Spann, V. (1981). *Preliminary Diagnostic Questionnaire, module 4: Feedback and interpretation.* Morgantown: West Virginia Rehabilitation Research and Training Center.

Netemeyer, R., Bearden, W., & Sharma, S. (2003). *Scaling procedures: Issues and applications.* Thousand Oaks, CA: Sage.

Newland, T. E. (1980). Psychological assessment of exceptional children and youth. In W. M. Cruickshank (Ed.), *Psychology of exceptional children and youth* (4th ed., pp. 74–135). Englewood Cliffs, NJ: Prentice Hall.

Nunnally, J. C., & Bernstein, I. H. (1994). *Psychometric theory* (3rd ed.). New York: McGraw-Hill.

Parker, R., & Bolton, B. (2005). Assessment in rehabilitation counseling. In R. Parker, E. Szymanski, & J. Patterson (Eds.), *Rehabilitation counseling: Basics and beyond* (4th ed., pp. 307–334). Austin, TX: PRO-ED.

Parker, R., & Schaller, J. (2003). Issues in vocational assessment and disability. In E. Szymanski & R. Parker (Eds.), *Work and disability: Issues and strategies in career counseling and job placement* (2nd ed., pp. 155–200). Austin, TX: PRO-ED.

Plake, B. S., & Impara, J. C. (Eds.). (2000). *The fourteenth mental measurements yearbook.* Lincoln, NE: University of Nebraska Press.

Plake, B., Impara, J., & Spies, R. (Eds.). (2003). *The fifteenth mental measurements yearbook.* Lincoln: University of Nebraska–Lincoln.

Power, P. (2006). *A guide to vocational assessment* (4th ed.). Austin, TX: PRO-ED.

Rehabilitation Act of 1973, 29 U.S.C. § 701 *et seq.*

Sarason, I. G. (Ed.). (1980). *Test anxiety: Theory, research, and applications.* Hillsdale, NJ: Erlbaum.

Society for Industrial and Organizational Psychology. (2003). *Principles for the validation and use of personnel selection procedures* (4th ed.). Bowling Green, OH: Author.

Thorndike, R. L. (1982). *Applied psychometrics.* Boston: Houghton Mifflin.

Torgerson, W. (1958). *Theory and methods of scaling.* New York: Wiley.

Urbina, S. (2004). *Essentials of psychological testing.* Hoboken, NJ: Wiley.

Vash, C. L. (1981). *The psychology of disability.* New York: Springer.

Vash, C., & Crewe, N. (2004). *Psychology of disability* (2nd ed.). New York: Springer.

Walls, R. T., Zane, T., & Thvedt, J. E. (1979). *The Independent Living Behavior Checklist.* Morgantown: West Virginia Rehabilitation Research and Training Center.

Walsh, W. B., & Betz, N. E. (2000). *Tests and assessment* (4th ed.). Englewood Cliffs, NJ: Prentice Hall.

Willingham, W. W., Ragosta, M., Bennett, R. E., Braun, H., Rock, D. A., & Powers, D. E. (1988). *Testing handicapped people.* Needham Heights, MA: Allyn & Bacon.

Zeidner, M. (1998). *Test anxiety: The state of the art.* New York: Plenum Press.

Chapter 2

Reliability

Robert M. Thorndike and Tracy Thorndike-Christ

Generalizing From Test Scores

Whenever measurements are made, there is some purpose for which they will be used. In the area of rehabilitation, the purposes for measurement range from research to diagnosis to prognosis. Whatever the purpose, almost all psychological measurements are indirect indicators of the characteristics that are really of interest. The scores that result from using the *Wechsler Adult Intelligence Scale–Third Edition* (WAIS-III; Wechsler, 1997) to measure a client's intellectual functioning are not, in themselves, intelligence. They are not the behaviors about which the therapist or counselor wishes to draw conclusions. Rather, they are indirect and imperfect indicators of intelligence. The test scores are a small sample of behavior in an artificial context. The practical user of these measurements wants to draw conclusions about the person's functioning at other times and in other situations.

Every psychological measurement involves a sample behavior. The items on a test are a restricted sample of possible behaviors, and the fact that the measurement is taken at one point in time is a further limitation on the sample. An important question that the user of tests must ask is "What generalizations are reasonable and appropriate from this information?"

Generalizations are of two basic kinds. The first is "over time." The test behavior occurs on a single occasion. Is the performance at Time 1 a good indicator of performance at Times 2, 3, and 4? This aspect of generalization concerns the stability of the test performance and, by inference, the underlying trait over time.

The second form of generalization that concerns the user of test information is generalization from the specific test items to other items or other indicators of behavior. For example, WAIS-III scores are of little inherent interest. The counselor uses them as indicators of other nontest behaviors or behavior potentials. There is a continuum of generalization across content from other items very like those on the test, through test-based measures of other behaviors, to nontest behaviors in school, work, and family situations.

This chapter concerns a limited set of generalizations that have traditionally gone under the heading of reliability. The generalizations that fall in this domain are those relating to time and to behavior on similar test items. Generalizations to other types of tests and to nontest behaviors fall in the category called validity and are covered in Chapter 3.

In a sense, the reliability of an instrument is its ability to predict itself, whereas its validity is the test's ability to predict something else. Both of these topics involve the quality of measurement obtained from an instrument; however, reliability refers to quality in an isolated sense, whereas validity involves the usefulness of the instrument for other purposes. There are several ways to evaluate reliability, each appropriate to some practical situations. An instrument must show some form of internal quality (reliability) before it can be expected to have external utility (validity).

Classical Test Theory

Early in the history of psychological measurement, investigators of human differences became aware that they were dealing with rather difficult subject populations. It seems to be part of human nature to be inconsistent in performance. Human behavior is so variable that the infant science of psychology quickly found itself dealing with measurement problems that older, more mature sciences had not yet needed to confront. Astronomers, chemists, and physicists had not had to be deeply concerned about consistency of measurement because the phenomena they studied occurred in such a regular fashion that subtle inconsistencies were not detected by their measuring devices. The reliability of observation was almost taken for granted, and the results could be replicated quite easily because it was assumed that the act of measurement did not alter the object being measured. Also, successive observations of new samples showed high degrees of consistency.

Prototypic psychological measures, such as those of Binet, were coarse and inaccurate, in an absolute sense, compared with those of the other sciences. However, the variability of human performance, both between groups at one time and within an individual person over time, is so great that even the unrefined instruments of 100 years ago detected this variability. A few years later their hard-science counterparts followed suit when the latter had developed instruments that detected the subtle variations in their observations. Today, all of the sciences are concerned with the reliability of their measures, but the problems are still most acute for psychology because the magnitude of variation, relative to the units of measure, is still greatest in the study of human behavior.

Repeated Measures and True Scores

Two concepts form the cornerstones of the classical model of test-score reliability. The first is that each person has some amount of the attribute to be measured. The representation of a person's amount of the attribute, as reflected by a given instrument, is the person's *true score* on that instrument. People differ in their true scores on a measure, but the true score for a person is assumed to be constant across successive administrations of the same or equivalent instruments. For example, if a test of general intelligence were given to the same person on several occasions, it is assumed that some underlying and constant level of intelligence would enter the score every time the test is taken. (It should be emphasized that this is an assumption. There are times when this assumption is not met, and there are times when it is inappropriate.)

Error of Measurement

The second cornerstone of the classical model of reliability is that each observation includes some component of error, called an *error of measurement*. There is an error of measurement associated with each observation of each person. It is assumed in classical test theory that each occurrence of an error of measurement is independent of all other errors of measurement. Furthermore, it is assumed that the errors for people are random deviations from their true scores (which means that the errors have a mean of zero and their distribution is normal in shape). Thus, the observed score for each person is composed of the individual's true score plus an error of measurement.

An intimate perspective on the way the classical model of reliability functions may be obtained by constructing a simplified example. Suppose the golfing ability of John Duffer is being measured, and the particular aspect of John's game under study is how far he can hit the ball with a driver. The first time John hits the ball he drives it 225 yards. This is John's "score" on this administration of the golfing test, but every experienced golfer knows that any particular shot is a combination of true ability and error. A second shot, even under the same conditions, will never precisely replicate the first. To get a better estimate of John's true ability, we have him hit another shot, then another and another until he has a fairway (and perhaps the rough) littered with golf balls. Each time John hits the ball, the distance of his drive is measured and recorded. Each observation is an independent estimate of John's ability. (Some assumptions have been made here—for example, that John has been making the same effort on each shot, that no learning has been taking place, and that fatigue has not set in.)

How should John's performance be summarized? From a practical point of view, the summary statement of John's ability should predict his future performance as accurately as possible—that is, the next time he steps to the tee, a reasonably accurate prediction could be made about how far he will hit the ball. A large number of observations showing substantial intrapersonal variation have been recorded. Assuming that the data cover the range of possible outcomes and that John's behavior conforms to the model, the best guess about his next drive will be the mean of the distribution of scores. True score is operationally defined as the mean of a distribution of scores obtained on successive testings using the same or equivalent measures. This has the advantage of permitting prediction of future performance with the least average error.

Standard Error of Measurement

The distribution of John's scores on the golfing test has another important property, the variation in scores, in addition to its mean as the definition of true score. True score is defined as the mean of a series of independent repeated measures, but each observed score is defined as a combination of true score and some random error of measurement:

$$X_{oi} = T_i + e_{oi}$$ (Eq. 1)

where the observed score of individual i on occasion o (X_{oi}) is the sum of the constant true score (T_i) and the random error of measurement associated with this observation (e_{oi}) Because T_i is the mean of the distribution, the standard deviation of observed scores is also the standard deviation of the errors of measurement. A special term, *standard error of measurement (SEM)*, has been given to this concept, and it is defined as the standard deviation of the distribution of errors of measurement.

An important change in the definition has just been made possible. The situation described for John Duffer resulted in the *SEM* being the standard deviation of observed scores on repeated independent measures of the same person. This is a valid and important definition, but it is not very practical. There are very few situations where a large number of independent repeated measures can be taken. Not only are humans variable as scientific subjects, but they also have a habit of remembering what they did in the test situation the last time. This problem affects the golfing example to some degree, but it presents particular difficulties when it comes to performance on psychological tests. In fact, the only place where the classical model can be expected to be reasonably appropriate for individual human performance is in those situations where fine discriminations are required and there is no feedback to the examinee about success or failure, such as some problems in classical psychophysics.

Take another look at the revised definition: The standard error of measurement is the standard deviation of the distribution of errors of measurement. Stated in this way, the definition permits the use of a number of individuals, each measured once. Each person has an observed score (X_1), which is composed of the true score and a random error component as shown in Equation 1. It may be reasonably assumed that the subjects in this sample will show some variation in their observed scores on the measure, that there is variability among them in their true scores, and that each one has been measured with some (random) error. Because the errors are independent of the true scores (by assumption), the variance of observed scores can be represented as the sum of the variance of true scores and the variance of errors, or:

$$S_X^2 = S_T^2 + S_e^2$$

from which it can be seen that:

$$S_e^2 = S_X^2 - S_T^2 \qquad \text{(Eq. 2)}$$

The distribution of the errors of measurement for the group will be normal in shape with a mean of zero and a variance of S_e. Because the ideal in measuring someone is to obtain as accurate an estimate as possible of that person's true score, it will be profitable to reduce S_e relative to S_X in any way possible.

Definition of Reliability

The problem with the foregoing definition of the *SEM* is that it is a verbal definition only. In any given observation, that portion of performance that is the result of true score cannot be separated from that which is the result of error. There is no way of estimating ei, and hence there is no way of computing S_e. This problem is overcome in the following way.

Assume that there are two equivalent measures of a characteristic. Tests are defined as equivalent if they are designed to measure the same characteristic, have equal means and standard deviations, and have equal *SEMs* (Feldt & Brennan, 1989). It can be shown (Thorndike & Thorndike, 1994) that:

$$r_{x_1 x_2} = \frac{S_T^2}{S_X^2}$$

(Eq. 3)

That is, the correlation between two equivalent forms of a test is equal to the ratio: the variance of true scores divided by the variance of observed scores.

The result obtained in Equation 3 is important for several reasons. First, it provides the basic definition of reliability as an index of the accuracy or consistency of measurement. Because true scores are constant from one administration of the test to another and across equivalent forms of the test, reliability has the following two properties:

1. Reliability is that portion of observed score variance among subjects that is the result of true score differences.
2. Reliability is that portion of a subject's performance that will remain constant over time.

The second property of reliability is discussed later. Now, some of the implications of Equation 3, as they are reflected in the first property, are considered.

SEM Revisited

Simple manipulation of Equations 2 and 3 permits an expression for the *SEM* in terms of obtainable quantities:

$$S_e = S_x \sqrt{1 - r_{x_1 x_2}}$$

(Eq. 4)

This provides a practical means of estimating the *SEM* that allows us to reexamine and extend its interpretations and uses. The value obtained from Equation 4 is an estimate of the standard deviation of errors of measurement for a group of individuals, but it is also an estimate of what the standard deviation of the distribution of observed scores for repeated measurements of an individual would be if such measures could be obtained. In this sense, the *SEM* provides an index of the absolute stability of measurement. Variation in the person's performance is estimated. The reliability coefficient, however, is an index of relative stability. It is a correlation coefficient and, as such, it indicates the degree to which each individual maintains the same relative position in the group on the two test administrations. Although the reliability coefficient is the index most frequently used to compare tests, the *SEM* is the most important for interpreting individual scores. It is useful to know that an instrument will order the members of a group consistently, but it is vital in areas such as rehabilitation counseling and educational placement to know how much error is likely to be made in using a test score for diagnostic or placement purposes. When the concern is with individual assessment, an index of the absolute consistency of measurement is of prime importance.

The distribution of errors of measurement is normal in shape with a mean of zero and a standard deviation of *Se*. Therefore, the most probable value for the error on any single observation is zero, and a person's observed score can be taken as a best estimate of his or her true score[*] but with full knowledge that there is a risk of being wrong by some amount. The *SEM* provides a means of estimating how large the error is likely to be. It permits a confidence band to be placed around an observed score such that one may be reasonably certain, with a specified probability of error, that the range covered by the confidence band includes the person's true score.

An example will help to clarify both this point and the computations associated with true and error score variances. Suppose that there is a test with the following characteristics: Mean = 110, S_X = 14.5, reliability = .80. From this information, the *SEM* is:

$$S_e = 14.5 \sqrt{1 - .80} = 14.5(0.4472) = 6.4846$$

$$S_e^2 = (6.48)^2 = 42.05$$

and from Equation 3 the variance of true scores is:

$$S_T^2 = .80(14.5)^2 = 168.2$$

The observed score variance may be broken down as:

$$S_X^2 = S_T^2 + S_e^2$$

$$210.25 = 168.2 + 42.05$$

which shows that 80% of the observed score variance is the result of variation in true scores.

Now, imagine that a client, Betty, has obtained a score of 97 on this test. By using the *SEM,* several things can be determined about Betty. Her most

---

[*]Technically, the best estimate of an individual's true score is obtained by regressing his or her observed score toward the mean. See Lord and Novick (1968, Chapter 7) or Feldt and Brennan (1989) for a complete discussion.

probable true score is 97, but the normal distribution property of errors can be used to conclude that the chances are two in three that her true score lies between 90.52 and 103.48 (97 ± 6.48). This band can be extended to any desired level of confidence by using the formula:

$$(X_i - z_p S_e) \leq T_i \leq (X_i - z_p S_e) \qquad \text{(Eq. 5)}$$

where X_i is the person's observed score, Ti is the person's true score, and Z_p is the normal deviate associated with the two-tailed probability p. Thus, for the 95% confidence band on Betty's score, one finds:

$$97 - 1.96(6.48) \leq T_i \leq 97 + 1.96(6.48)$$

$$84.30 \leq T_i \leq 109.70$$

There is a 95% probability that the interval 84.30 to 109.70 includes Betty's true score.

It might also be useful to determine the probability that Betty's true score is at least as great as some particular value, such as the group's mean. This can be done by the same general procedure as that for finding z scores:

$$z = \frac{97 - 110}{6.48} = \frac{-13}{6.48} = -2.01$$

$$P_z = 0.022$$

The probability that Betty's true score is at least as large as the group's mean is slightly greater than 1 in 50.

The foregoing discussion illustrates a feature of psychological measurement that is all too often overlooked by test users. Even when a test has a reliability as high as .80 (or even .95), the variability of human behavior is such that caution must be exercised in interpreting a client's scores. In the last example, the range of reasonably possible scores for Betty was 25.40 units wide. With a test as highly respected as the WAIS-III, the *SEM* is about 4 units, which yields a 95% confidence interval that is about 15 units wide. When treatment decisions are based on test scores, this is an uncomfortably large possible error. Under such conditions, it is often wise to evaluate the probability that the decision indicated by the test is wrong and to weigh this probability against the consequences for the client of using one procedure or another. See Charter (2003) for a discussion of the implications of different levels of reliability for clinical decision making.

Variation in Test Scores

The classical test theory model recognizes two types of variation that influence scores on a test. There is variation among people in their true levels of the trait being measured, and there is variation within each person's performance be-cause of error of measurement. Beginning in the 1940s, several developments led to a modification and refinement of the classical model and recognized additional factors that can affect test performance. These advances have been summarized by Cronbach, Gleser, Nanda, and Rajaratnam (1971) and Feldt and Brennan (1989). Consideration of these sources of variation allows one to evaluate the information contained in the several varieties of reliability coefficients discussed in the next section.

Sources of Variation

Six broad sources of test score differences were enumerated by R. L. Thorndike (1951). It is assumed that each will have some effect on the scores on a particular administration of a particular test. Some of them are appropriately considered contributions to true score differences between examinees, whereas others represent errors of measurement.

1. *Lasting general characteristics:* The first source of variation includes those features of the person that pervade performance on a variety of tests over relatively long periods. Aspects such as general intelligence and ability in broad areas such as verbal fluency, number ability, and spatial relations are included here. A second source of this long-term kind is general test-taking skills and personality characteristics related to behavior in testing situations. Ability to understand and follow test directions also has a widespread influence on test performance. In a sense, each of these three features is likely to have an essentially constant value for a given individual across several tests and over a substantial period. Any relatively stable and general characteristics of the person that affect performance on the test, such as attitudes and anxieties about tests or willingness to guess, will be inextricably bound to the true level on the trait.

2. *Lasting specific characteristics:* Some characteristics of a person will remain constant over a period of time but will be specific to a particular test. The characteristics that form this category may be divided into two subcategories: (a) those that affect the test as a whole and (b) those that function only for particular items.

   Under the first subcategory come characteristics such as ability or knowledge on a trait that is unique to the test, such as aspects of performance found in single cells of Guilford's structure of intellect model (Guilford, 1985). Also included here are abilities related to particular types of items. If a test is composed of only one type of item, such as multiple choice or short answer, differences in ability with that item type will appear as consistent differences among individuals. When a variety of item types are present in the test, abilities of this kind will have a smaller effect in creating stable differences among individuals.

There are times when a person will possess a particular piece of information that makes it possible to answer an unusually difficult item correctly and without guessing. This is most likely to happen with a test of knowledge of specific facts, such as a spelling test, but it may also occur in tests of general intelligence or scholastic aptitude. Sometimes isolated aspects of people's experiences have caused them to learn the meaning or spelling of obscure terms so that they get very difficult items correct while missing easier ones. These pieces of knowledge will increase their true scores on the test somewhat erroneously and are the kinds of things included in the second subcategory.

3. *Temporary general characteristics:* It is common to hear students complain that they would have received a better score on a test if they had felt better that day. Most comments of this kind are excuses for lack of adequate preparation; however, a certain amount of variation in test performance may be attributed to relatively short-term fluctuations in health and welfare. The variables included here, such as fatigue, motivation, and emotional strain, as well as health, are considered to be relatively short-term deviations from the person's normal level of functioning, lasting up to a few days. Factors in this category affect performance on all tests taken at a particular time but generally will change in a random manner if the person is retested days or weeks later.

   We may also include in this category the demand characteristics of the testing situation when these are subject to change. Some people approach a testing situation in a different manner when they are told that the test results will be used for personal guidance or for admission to a program, and this may be reflected in their performance. The way one views an evaluation, as either threatening or supportive, can be especially important for those who have had repeated unpleasant experiences with testing or who have feelings of inferiority. The effect of this variable on test performance can be minimized by attempting to give a consistently positive, nonthreatening set to all those being tested.

4. *Temporary specific characteristics:* In addition to those temporary features that affect a whole range of test performances, there are characteristics of the person that are temporary and reflected in performance only on one test or a part of a test. These features include variations in the comprehension of test instructions or item contents caused by fluctuations in attention, tricks, insights about the test discovered in the course of testing, and random events that occur in the testing situation and affect performance on a few items.

5. *Administration and appraisal of test performance:* Qualities of the measurement operation itself compose the fifth category of sources of variation

in test scores. Different test administrators vary in the way in which they read and explain test directions, in the amount of help they give, and in the care with which they maintain a standardized environment. If one tester pays close attention to time limits and ensures that everyone has the necessary materials and another does not, the result may be differences in test score that are not the result of differences in ability. To the extent that there are changes in the testing environment from one testing to another, there may appear to be greater instability in performance than really exists.

Also included here are variations resulting from lack of standardization in the evaluation of performance by graders or raters. Halo or other biases in the ratings of behavior provide examples of variation of this sort. If, as is usually the case, it is desired to eliminate these sources of variation, steps must be taken to improve the standardization of evaluation procedures. Making multiple evaluations and using the average of several of them is beneficial.

6. *Chance variance:* Whatever variation is left in test scores is attributed to chance and random effects. The most obvious contributor here is the increase in score obtained from being lucky in guessing the correct answer when knowledge is not present. Another source of variation of this type is the chance mismarking of an answer sheet either by the examinee or the examiner, as when the examinee gives the correct answer on an individual intelligence test but the examiner fails to give credit or records the answer in the wrong place. Variation of this type is specific to a particular occasion and, as such, represents a close approximation to pure error. The only way to reduce its effect is to take a larger sample of behavior.

Strategies of Data Collection

The variety of ways in which test scores can be affected by different aspects of tests and testing situations provides ample evidence that there is no single, true, and correct reliability for any test. Before the value of a statement that the reliability of test X is .85 can be judged, the user must have some idea of the test author's definition of true and error scores. Different ways of collecting data for a reliability study allocate the sources of variation outlined earlier to true and error scores differently. A test that is reported to have a high reliability may be unsuitable for certain purposes if the method used to estimate reliability is inappropriate for the use to which the test will be put.

Five experimental designs frequently used for collecting information about the reliability of a test can be described in terms of two dimensions. First, one may inquire whether the study involved a single form of the test or whether multiple equivalent forms (two or more) were administered; second, one may inquire whether there was a time interval between the first and second testing, and if so, how long it was. There are four obvious possibilities that result from this scheme: delayed test–retest (one form administered twice with an interval), immediate test–retest (one form administered twice without a time interval), delayed equivalent forms (two equivalent tests with an interval between administrations), and immediate equivalent forms (two equivalent forms with no time interval between administrations). Each of these procedures provides a means of obtaining two scores for each person so that a correlation may be computed.

A fifth alternative design is known as the split-half procedure. It has some features in common with both the single and equivalent forms designs, although it would properly be labeled an immediate equivalent forms method. When only one form of the test exists and it is unfeasible or unwise to administer it twice, two sets of scores may be obtained by dividing the test in half and scoring each half separately. The division may be done before testing to ensure that the two halves are equivalent, or it may be done after testing by scoring odd-numbered items as one test and even-numbered items as another. In either case, two different sets of items are used to obtain the two sets of scores, but there is generally no time interval between the tests.

Restrictions on Use of Half-Test Designs

If it is necessary to estimate reliability with a split-half procedure, several important restrictions must be kept in mind. Where items differ markedly in content or difficulty, care must be taken to ensure that these features are equated in the resulting scores. This may require that the items be assigned to halves of the test by blocks rather than by random division.

When speed of response is a major component of test score, as is the case with many clerical tests, a split-half procedure does not yield an appropriate index of reliability. In a pure speed test where all items are very easy and scores generally equal the number of items attempted, an odd-even split of the items will result in each examinee obtaining almost identical scores on both halves of the test, thereby yielding an inflated estimate of the test's reliability. The only way to overcome this restriction for speed tests is to time the two halves of the test separately. Otherwise, a test–retest procedure must be used.

A third aspect of the split-half design that restricts its value is the fact that scores are based on relatively few items. The reliability of a test score is dependent to some extent on the number of observations on which it is based. Correlations between half-test scores, therefore, will tend to be lower than would be correlations between scores based on twice as many items. It is possible to overcome this problem by correcting for the reduction in length using the Spearman-Brown formula, which estimates what the correlation would be between two full-length equivalent forms of the test. The Spearman-Brown estimate is given by the formula:

$$r_c = \frac{2r_{12}}{1 + r_{12}}$$

where r_c is the estimate of the reliability of the full-length test and r_{12} is the correlation between the two halves of the test. A thorough discussion of the use of the Spearman-Brown formula and of the benefits and dangers of split-half reliability estimates is given by Feldt and Brennan (1989).

Internal Consistency Coefficients

Another problem with the use of split-half methods for estimating reliability is not necessarily of direct concern to test administrators but has drawn the attention of measurement theorists. Any particular way of dividing the test in half is only one of a multitude of possible ways. Because there is no necessarily correct way of obtaining two equivalent halves and because different ways of splitting the test will ordinarily yield different estimates of the test's reliability, it is not possible to obtain a unique reliability estimate using split-half procedures. It is often desirable to be able to obtain a single index that reflects consistency of measurement for the test as a whole, regardless of variabilities that might be the result of using one split or another.

This problem was first attacked by Kuder and Richardson (1937), and their results were extended by Cronbach (1951). Kuder and Richardson's approach assumed that items were dichotomously scored (p = the proportion of correct responses; $q = 1 - p$, or the proportion of incorrect responses). By adding a number of additional assumptions, namely that all items in the test (a) have the same true score variance and observed score variance, (b) have equal correlations with all other items, and (c) measure the same trait, they derived a formula that provides a unique estimate of the reliability of a test from a single administration, known as KR_{20} reliability. With a test composed of n items, the KR_{20} reliability estimate is obtained from:

$$KR_{20} = \frac{n}{n-1}\left(1 - \frac{\sum pq}{S_X^2}\right) \qquad \text{(Eq. 6)}$$

where S_X^1 is the variance in observed scores and $\sum pq$ is the sum across items of the pq products. However, because pq is really just the variance of a dichotomously scored item, $\sum pq$ is the sum of the item variances. An additional simplifying assumption, that all items are of the same difficulty, leads to Kuder and Richardson's "formula 21":

$$KR_{21} = \frac{n}{n-1}\left(1 - \frac{\bar{X}\left[1 - \left(\bar{X}/n\right)\right]}{S_X^2}\right) \qquad \text{(Eq. 7)}$$

Here, the reliability estimate is calculated from only the mean ($\bar{X}$), the variance of test scores, and the number of items. Where its assumption of equal item difficulties is met, KR_{21} will yield the same results as KR_{20}. When this assumption is not met, the KR_{21} estimate is conservative.

Coefficient α (Cronbach, 1951) is the most general form for internal consistency coefficients and can be used for many types of items, not just those that are scored right or wrong. It is based on the idea that each item is a parallel form "mini-test," and the overall reliability is the average of all interitem correlations, corrected to the length of the total test. The formula, which bears noticeable and expected resemblance to Equations 6 and 7, is:

$$\alpha = \frac{n}{n-1}\left(1 - \frac{\sum S_i^2}{S_X^2}\right) \qquad \text{(Eq. 8)}$$

where $\sum S_i^2$ is the sum of the individual item variances. KR_{20}, KR_{21}, and coefficient α are estimates of the extent to which the items in the test are consistent in their "ordering" of the examinees, and, for this reason, all three are referred to as internal consistency coefficients. They provide statistical evidence of the homogeneity of the test.

Like the split-half procedures, the internal consistency estimates of reliability cannot be used with speeded tests. They require that all examinees respond to all items. In addition, it is assumed that the test is homogeneous in content. Failure of this second assumption generally will mean that the reliability estimate obtained by one of these internal consistency procedures will be too low. Note that the split-half, test-retest, and equivalent forms designs do not require homogeneous tests, merely equivalence of content. For a thorough discussion of these procedures, their assumptions, and restrictions, see Feldt and Brennan (1989).

Reliable Sources of Variance

Each of the five research designs yields an estimate of the reliability of measurement provided by the test, but the different designs result in different estimates. The sources of variation outlined earlier may be used to see why this variation in reliability estimates occurs. The main feature of this approach is that some sources of variation appear to be functioning as systematic or consistent sources of variance (contributing to true score variance or true differences among people) in some designs and as inconsistency or error variance in others.

The equivalent forms approach to reliability estimation requires two equivalent forms of the test. If the forms are truly equivalent, they will measure the same general abilities and require the same test-taking skills. However, care must be taken in their construction so they are sufficiently similar to measure the same specific abilities or factors but not so similar in their items that they call on the same pieces of information—that is, properly prepared equivalent tests should have sources 1 and 2a remaining constant for each person on both tests, but source 2b should not be constant for an examinee because the specific information required is different. When there is an interval separating the administration of the forms, the temporary factors affecting performance on the whole test (3) should change randomly for each individual from one testing to the next, whereas these same factors will result in consistent differences among subjects when there is no delay between testings. In either case, sources resulting from particular items or groups of items (4) and from chance factors (6) will function as error or random variation. The effect of administrative factors (5) depends on the skill of the administrator in providing a consistent testing environment and in carefully adhering to the time limits and administrative conditions. Differences in administration from one occasion to another may introduce a substantial error component. Careful attention to the details of test administration can eliminate this source of variance by making it essentially constant for all people on all occasions.

When two equivalent forms of the test are identical to the extent that they have the same items, we have a test-retest design. Obviously, sources 1 and 2a will appear as consistent differences among people and contribute to true score variance, but repetition of items means that factors specific to particular test items will also appear as consistent variation. Thus, source 2b will be added to the consistent component and be reflected as true score variation. It is the addition of this knowledge-for-particular-items factor (which is confounded with memory for the response chosen the last time the test was taken) that causes test-retest estimates of reliability to be generally higher than those obtained with a comparable equivalent forms administration. Of course, when no time interval occurs between administrations, the temporary factors influence consistency of performance in much the same way that they influence it in equivalent forms designs. However, the potential effect of memory for items on an immediate retest is also much greater than when the retest is delayed, so the use of test-retest design with no interval generally should be restricted to tests in which memory cannot play a significant role—for example, in tests of motor performance after a warm-up period.

The split-half and internal consistency designs are similar in the way that they allocate the sources of variation to true score and error components. They both include sources 1 and 2a as consistent components and, because both use a single administration of the test (no time interval), the temporary sources (3 and 4) also function as true score. The influence of temporary factors affecting less than the whole test is somewhat unclear because the effects on single items result in error variance, but effects on groups of items may contribute to systematic variation in performance. The split-half procedure will generally treat variation in category 2b as error, whereas the homogeneity restriction on internal consistency designs may result in some systematic variance arising from this source. The single administration used by both of these designs generally will mean that administration factors (5) are constant for a given group of examinees. They will appear as true group differences when data are pooled from different administrations. Chance factors (6) are considered error.

The magnitude of the reliability coefficient obtained for a particular test will be related to the number of sources of variation that can be considered to yield consistent or systematic differences among people. The equivalent forms design has the fewest sources that are classified as systematic, which means that with other things (such as care in administration) being equal, this design will yield the lowest or most conservative estimate of the test's reliability. A somewhat higher estimate will be obtained with no interval or with a delayed test-retest, the relative magnitude of these two depending on the length of the delay and the potency of the temporary and memory factors. The other designs generally will yield higher estimates of reliability, with the exception that the internal consistency methods are sensitive to violations of the homogeneity assumption. When this assumption is not at least approximately satisfied, an internal consistency coefficient may seriously underestimate the reliability of the test. Caution must be exercised in selecting the design for a reliability study and in interpreting the results of such studies.

Factors Affecting Reliability Interpretation

The proper interpretation of reliability coefficients requires more information than just the magnitude of the coefficient and the design used to obtain it. Various aspects of the distributions of test scores and the relationship of the test to other variables must be considered when evaluating reliability. In addition, the use to which the test will be put will affect the relative importance of one or another type of information about the quality of measurement.

Logical Factors

Each of the several designs for obtaining data on the reliability of a test provides information that is valuable for some testing situations but not for others. Three basic conditions are involved: the breadth of coverage of the test, the assumed nature of the trait that the test is intended to measure, and the way the test is to be used (concurrently or predictively). A test may appear to have promising reliability for some situations, but the information necessary to justify its use in others may be absent.

Breadth of Coverage
Breadth of coverage refers primarily to the homogeneity that the test is designed to have. When the score resulting from the measurement is claimed to reflect a narrow range of behavior, such as a single factor of ability, one may reasonably require that the internal consistency of the test be high. A low value could indicate that the test is measuring a complex composite of several dimensions. This inference would be supported if the test were found to have substantial temporal stability as measured by a delayed retest. However, high internal consistency would be inappropriate in a test that has been designed to measure a complex trait. One might rightfully be suspicious of a test claiming to measure "general psychomotor performance" in a single score and showing high

internal consistency because previous research has shown abilities of this type to be only moderately correlated. A test is not necessarily condemned by the fact that it may show low to moderate internal consistency. The design may be inappropriate for the particular situation.

Nature of the Measured Trait

Most tests are designed to measure traits that are relatively stable features of behavior. When the characteristics that the test is assumed to measure can be considered to change relatively little over time, it is appropriate and desirable to evaluate the temporal stability of the test scores by using a delay between one administration and another. However, it is possible to conceive of traits that fluctuate over time but are highly consistent at one point in time. For example, a measure of hypomania might yield very low temporal stability for a group of patients with cyclic manic depression but be highly internally consistent and a valid indicator of current status at any given point in time. Regardless of the way reliability is defined, the evaluation of a particular measuring device requires information about consistency of test scores that is appropriate for the assumed nature of the trait.

Use of the Test

Another aspect of the stability issue involves the way in which the test will be used. A test that is used to forecast behavior must be able to forecast itself. A test that is to act as a predictor must have temporal stability as shown by a delayed retest or delayed equivalent forms design. Otherwise, there is no assurance that anything other than temporary states of individuals are being measured. However, when a test is developed to act as an indicator of current status on the trait, as when a test is used as a substitute for a more costly and time-consuming evaluation procedure, assurances of temporal stability may not be necessary. It may generally be assumed that a test that is stable over the long term will also yield stable evaluations for immediate use, but evidence of short-term consistency is not a substitute for studies of long-term stability when long-range predictions are to be made.

Consideration of the factors discussed here leads to the conclusion that to evaluate adequately the reliability of a test for a particular purpose there must be data from a study (or, better yet, a series of studies) that utilize a design appropriate for the purpose. An internal consistency coefficient yields no information about the stability of measurement over time, and a stability coefficient may be inappropriate for evaluating the quality of measurement of traits that are subject to marked temporal fluctuations.

Statistical Factors

All other things being equal, reliability coefficients are higher in heterogeneous samples. In other words, as observed score variance increases, and assuming that error variance remains relatively constant, the reliability coefficient will increase. Formulas are available for estimating the reliability coefficient for a sample that differs in variability from the one in which the reliability study was performed (Feldt & Brennan, 1989).

Group Variability

Statistical considerations connected with group variability also affect the interpretation of reliability coefficients when there has been selection of the sample on a related variable. The effects of selection may lead to increased or decreased variability in the group, but the possible presence of this effect should not be overlooked when interpreting reports of reliability studies. If, for example, a reliability study for an intelligence test were performed on a group of 10-year-old children and the test is to be used with 6- to 14-year-olds (assuming the test is appropriate for a group this diverse and that age is related to intelligence), one might expect the test to have a higher reliability coefficient in the latter group. One may also estimate the reliability in the population when the sample has been selected on the basis of some other test. The necessary formula is given by R. L. Thorndike (1951).

The problem of assessing the effects of selection on the reliability of the test is more critical when the selection has greatly increased the variability of scores, so that the reliability coefficient is a rather gross overestimate of what the reliability would probably be in a population of interest. There are, for example, intelligence tests on the market for which claims of near-perfect reliability are made. At first glance it would appear that our problems have been solved, until one reads a little more closely and discovers that the test authors used small samples with age ranges of 40 or 50 years. The reliability coefficient of .98 that the authors might have found would be perfectly true and accurate for their sample, but it would greatly overestimate the reliability one might realistically expect to obtain in the more homogeneous populations with which test users generally work. Reliability studies of this type are Barnum-like demonstrations of how high a coefficient can be obtained with a particular test, rather than useful contributions to knowledge about the test. To be of maximum value for a particular application of a test, the reliability study should be performed with a group that is as similar as possible to the application or target group. This, of course, also means that care must be exercised in the interpretation of reliability coefficients when the target group is exceptionally high or low in its average level of the trait and the reliability study has been performed on a representative sample of the general population. The reliability of the test for special groups, such as children with brain damage or who are educationally handicapped, generally will be lower than the results from a study of non-disabled individuals would indicate.

Test Length

The length of the test is another factor that affects reliability. There may be times when it is not possible to give an entire test or when it is desirable to use more than one form of the test to increase the precision of measurement. In such cases, the general form of the Spearman-Brown formula makes it possible to estimate what the reliability of the reduced or expanded test is likely to be. The formula to use to estimate the reliability of a lengthened or shortened test is:

$$r_c = \frac{k r_{x_1 x_2}}{1 + (k - 1) r_{x_1 x_2}}$$ (Eq. 9)

where r_c is the new estimate, $r_{x_1 x_2}$ is the original estimate, and k is the ratio of the length of the new test to the length of the original test. For example, if the original test has 20 items and the new test has 50 items, then the value of k is 2.5. However, if the original test has 50 items and the reliability of a 20-item test is being estimated, then the value of .40 would be used for k. An original 50-item test with a reliability of .80 would thus be estimated to yield a 20-item test with a reliability of .62 $\left(\frac{.40(.80)}{1 + (.40 - 1)(.80)}\right)$. This formula permits one to determine whether a shorter test will have satisfactory reliability or whether the gain in reliability that will be achieved by lengthening the test is likely to be worth the time and expense involved.

Reliability of Difference Scores

Counselors and therapists often attempt to interpret the difference between two test scores. These differences may be interpreted as measures of either growth or change, as when the same or an equivalent test is given after some treatment or intervention, or they may be used in what has been called a configural approach to identify particular ability or personality patterns. Either kind of interpretation is hazardous and should be undertaken with caution.

The reason that caution is needed is that the reliability of differences between two measures is generally quite a bit lower than the reliability of either of the original measures. To see why this happens, consider two tests, X and Y, that are correlated. The fact of their correlation implies that they share some common variance (S_C^2). Each of them also has some reliable variance that is unique to that test ($S_{U_X}^2$ and $S_{U_Y}^2$, respectively) and some error variance ($S_{E_X}^2$ and $S_{E_Y}^2$)—that is, the observed variance in Test X is composed of common, unique, and error elements. True score variance is composed of the common and unique elements. Therefore, the reliability of test X is $\frac{S_C^2 + S_{U_X}^2}{S_{U_X}^2}$. The same relationship holds for test Y. However, the difference score ($X - Y$) does not contain the common variance, S_C^2, as part of true score; it contains only the unique and error components. Thus, the two error components will make up a larger portion of the variance in difference scores and the reliability of the differences will be lower than that of the original tests by an amount estimated as follows:

$$r_{X-Y} = \frac{\frac{1}{2}(r_{XX} + r_{YY}) - r_{XY}}{1 - r_{XY}} \qquad \text{(Eq. 10)}$$

From this formula it is clear that it is the correlation between the two tests that reduces the reliability of the difference scores. If two tests each have a reliability of .80 and their correlation is .40, then the reliability of the differences scores is .67. The situation becomes considerably worse as the correlation between the two tests increases or the average of their reliabilities drops. Clearly, if one is going to interpret and base decisions on difference scores, the original measures should have high reliabilities and there should be a low correlation between them. Because repeated measures (gain scores) are likely to show high correlations between the two tests, particular caution is needed to reach confident conclusions about growth or change. The fact that a client's score on a test has risen or dropped several points may be a large overestimate or underestimate of the true amount of change, making correct interpretation of the scores uncertain.

Reliability of Computer Adaptive Tests

In the past 25 years a number of tests have been developed that use a technology called computer adaptive testing (CAT) in their administration, scoring, and interpretation. These tests approach the concept of reliability in a different way. They use a procedure called item response theory (IRT) to develop item difficulty and discrimination statistics and select the most appropriate items to administer at any point in testing, based on the past performance of the particular examinee. The fundamental idea behind IRT and CAT is that an underlying trait is measured on which both test items and examinees can be located. The items are located by their ability requirements, and the examinees are located by their ability levels. Measurement provides the greatest amount of information about an examinee when the test items and the examinee are at the same place on the trait. This is the point where the examinee has a 50% probability of getting each item right. IRT provides the link between the ability level of the examinee and the ability demands of the item, and CAT is the process by which items are selected to yield the optimum match between item difficulty and examinee ability. In a computer adaptive test, each examinee receives a unique set of test items from a large pool of items. Because no two examinees take the same test, traditional measures of test reliability are not appropriate.

The problem is solved by using item information functions. An item's information function is an index, derived from the item–total score correlation, of how accurately the item is measuring examinees at particular ability levels. The total information provided about a given examinee by the adaptive test is the sum of the item information functions for the items that were administered to this examinee. The *SEM* for the test is then computed from the test information function. This *SEM* can be used to place a confidence interval on the ability estimate. No traditional index of reliability is reported.

A major advantage of the IRT–CAT approach to measurement is that testing is more efficient than with paper-and-pencil tests. In the usual test, examinees are exposed to items that are too easy for them and items that are too hard. These items yield little information. Often, a computer adaptive test can achieve the same level of measurement accuracy, the same *SEM,* with half as many items, which means that CAT can be administered in about half the time of conventional testing, or it can achieve substantially more accurate measurement in the same amount of time. For a detailed treatment of IRT, see Embretson and Reise (2000). See Kline (2005) for a comparison of classical and modern (IRT) approaches to reliability.

Conclusion

A reasonable level of reliability is a necessary quality for a psychological assessment instrument to possess. An instrument's reliability tells how much confidence can be placed in the score obtained by the examinee. Reliability, through its relationship with the standard error of estimate, allows the test interpreter to calculate a confidence band on a person's obtained score that has a specified probability of including the person's true score. The width of the confidence band should cause the counselor to interpret test scores with considerable caution.

There are several sources of variance that may affect test scores. The method by which reliability data are collected will determine which of these sources function as true differences between examinees and which function as errors of measurement. In evaluating reliability evidence, the test user must carefully consider whether the data collection design is appropriate for the uses to which the test will be put. This is particularly true when the testing procedure involves an element of speed of performance.

Classical reliability evidence, such as that described in the main part of this chapter, is appropriate for traditional testing formats such as paper-and-pencil tests and individually administered ability scales. However, testing with computers is becoming more common, which makes possible some innovative assessment strategies such as computer adaptive tests. Newer and more informative ways to assess reliability of measurement, such as item response theory, have been developed and will allow the test user to assess cognitive functioning in new and more informative ways in the near future.

References

Charter, R. A. (2003). A breakdown of reliability coefficients by test type and reliability method, and the clinical implications of low reliability. *The Journal of General Psychology, 130,* 290–299.

Cronbach, L. J. (1951). Coefficient alpha and the internal structure of tests. *Psychometrika, 16,* 297–334.

Cronbach, L. J., Gleser, G. C., Nanda, H., & Rajaratnam, N. (1971). *The dependability of behavioral measurements.* New York: Wiley.

Embretson, S. E., & Reise, S. (2000). *Item response theory for psychologists.* Mahwah, NJ: Erlbaum.

Feldt, L. S., & Brennan, R. L. (1989). Reliability. In R. L. Linn (Ed.), *Educational measurement* (3rd ed., pp. 105–146). New York: American Council on Education.

Guilford, J. P. (1985). The structure of intellect model. In B. B. Wolman (Ed.), *Handbook of intelligence* (pp. 225–266). New York: Wiley.

Kline, T. J. B. (2005). *Psychological testing: A practical approach to design and evaluation.* Thousand Oaks, CA: Sage.

Kuder, G. F., & Richardson, M. (1937). The theory of estimation of test reliability. *Psychometrika, 2,* 151–160.

Lord, F. M., & Novick, M. R. (1968). *Statistical theories of mental test scores.* Reading, MA: Addison-Wesley.

Thorndike, R. L. (1951). Reliability. In E. F. Lindquist (Ed.), *Educational measurement* (pp. 560–620). Washington, DC: American Council on Education.

Thorndike, R. L., & Thorndike, R. M. (1994). Reliability in educational and psychological measurement. In T. Husen & N. Postlethwaite (Eds.), *International Encyclopedia of Education* (2nd ed., pp. 4981–4995). New York: Pergamon Press.

Wechsler, D. (1997). *Manual for the Wechsler Adult Intelligence Scale–Third Edition* (WAIS-III). San Antonio, TX: Psychological Corp.

Chapter 3

Validity

Nancy E. Betz and David J. Weiss

There are many uses for psychological test data. For example, an ability test might be used to predict performance in an academic curriculum or success in performing a particular job. An achievement test might be used to determine the extent to which an individual has mastered a defined area of content. Personality and interest tests might be used by counselors to help them know more about an individual or to help individuals to know more about themselves. Each of these uses of tests implies a particular interpretation of a given test score. A high score on Test *X* frequently suggests good possibilities for job success. A high score on Test *Y* might indicate that an individual has little interest in social service occupations. Narrowly considered, validity information concerns the accuracy or soundness of each of these *specific* interpretations of a test score.

Regardless of the *particular* uses to which a test is to be put, however, psychological measurement—the process of converting psychological observations into numerical representations—occurs within the framework of the science of psychology. Tests are the instruments used by psychologists to quantify and study the behavior of people, just as balances and thermometers are instruments used by physicists to quantify and study the behavior of matter. In the broader context of science, validity concerns how much we know about all of the uses of a given instrument and the interpretations of its numerical values. Thus, the discussion of the validity of psychological tests should begin in this broader context, showing the importance and function of measurement, scientific theories, and validation in the pursuit of the goals of any science.

Measurement in the Context of Science

The goals of science are to describe; predict; and, most important, *explain* natural phenomena. To reach these goals, it is necessary first to make careful and precise observations of the phenomena; this is the process of *measurement*. Second, it is necessary to have some framework within which to interpret, or attribute meaning to, these measurements; the explanatory framework of science is *theory*. Finally, it is necessary to examine the truthfulness or soundness of the explanation or interpretation of the measurement; this is the process of *validation*.

Measurement

Measurement can be defined as a set of rules for assigning numbers to objects to represent quantities of attributes of those objects. In psychology, the objects are most frequently people (or animals); the attributes are variables of psychological interest, such as anxiety, intelligence, or motivation. That the process of measurement consists of the application of "rules" indicates that the procedures for assigning the numbers are explicitly formulated. Such explicit formulation of rules for measurement is essential to the *standardization* of a measuring instrument. An instrument is well-standardized if different people who use it obtain similar results. For example, an intelligence test is well-standardized if different examiners arrive at the same scores for a particular child.

Standardized measurements offer several advantages over unaided observations of phenomena. First, they permit *communicability* of findings. A key principle of science is that the findings of one scientist should be independently verifiable and usable by other scientists. This is not possible unless scientists can agree on the observation of empirical events. The use of standardized measuring instruments—those based on an explicitly formulated set of rules—permits independent scientists to observe the same events in the same way.

Second, the assignment of *numbers* to attributes makes it possible to report results in much finer detail than is possible otherwise. For example, a teacher might be able to classify children into categories of "bright," "average," and "below average." But intelligence test scores permit much more precise descriptions of any particular child and much more accurate and informative differentiations within a group of children. Using numbers to represent quantities of attributes permits the use of powerful methods of mathematical and statistical analysis in both the formulation of theories and in the evaluation of research results.

Thus, standardized measurement, although really only a refinement and systematization of the ordinary process of observation, is essential in science. Standardization is an *internal* requirement for the usefulness of a measure and is closely related to its reliability (or precision) because standardization is a prerequisite to obtaining reliable, repeatable, or precise measurements.

Measures must not only meet criteria of standardization and reliability/precision but also provide information that contributes to the understanding of real-world phenomena. Highly reliable measures *can* provide information that is essentially meaningless and of little practical utility. For example, the cephalic index, or ratio of head width to head length, was a well-standardized and highly reliable measure that early in the 20th century was thought to be related to intelligence (Anastasi, 1958), but no relationship was ever found between the cephalic index and intelligence or any other psychological variable. Scores on the cephalic index related to nothing other than themselves and thus had no *meaning*. It is the *meaning* of test scores—that is, their relationships to other variables of interest—that establishes their *validity,* and *theory* plays a vital role in the exploration of meaning.

Theory

Finding relationships among variables enhances scientific understanding when there is some basis for explaining *why* these relationships occur. For example, a correlation between job performance and job satisfaction could be explained by postulating that (a) higher levels of performance cause people to be more satisfied, (b) higher levels of satisfaction cause people to work harder and thus perform better, or (c) a third variable (e.g., the abilities required to perform the job) leads to both better performance and higher levels of satisfaction. Thus, a given relationship among variables can be explained in a variety of ways; *a theory* is the proposed interpretation or explanation of the observed relationships among variables.

The basic elements of a theory are (a) constructs, (b) hypotheses, and (c) operational definitions or measures, all of which can be represented in a "nomological network" (Cronbach & Meehl, 1955) or path diagram. Figure 3.1 shows an illustrative nomological network of a simple "theory" of intelligence.

The upper half of the figure shows the *constructs* and hypotheses of the theory. Constructs are words or phrases that describe postulated attributes or characteristics. Their most important property is that they are abstractions from observations and are themselves unobservable—they can also be called "latent," meaning invisible or intangible. For example, constructs such as anxiety and motivation might be postulated in a given theory. We cannot actually "see" anxiety or motivation because they are abstractions from observed behavior. In the theory shown in Figure 3.1, the constructs are school performance, intelligence, and learning ability.

Constructs are related to other constructs by hypotheses that specify the ways in which variation in one construct is assumed to be related to variation

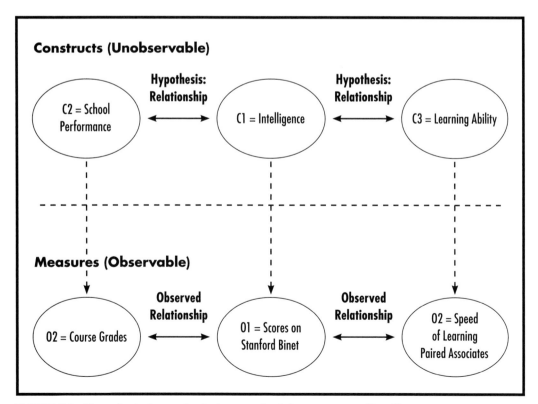

FIGURE 3.1. Hypothetical nomological network of the construct of intelligence.

in another construct. Hypotheses, which also are abstracted from observations, are the proposed interpretations of events and are the second basic element of a theory. When we have formulated one or more hypotheses relating to the "behavior" of a construct, we have begun to construct a theory of that construct. For the theory shown in Figure 3.1, the construct of intelligence is postulated to be related to both school performance and learning ability.

Following specification of our constructs and hypotheses, we need to translate our "theory" into phenomena that we can observe and study directly. Constructs are made observable in numerical form through "operational definitions" or measures. In the example in Figure 3.1, intelligence is "operationalized" as (or measured by) scores on the Stanford-Binet test; the operational definition of school performance is course grades, and that for learning ability is speed of learning paired associates. As should be evident, the hypotheses regarding relationships among constructs (upper half of the figure) imply a parallel system of observable relationships among the operational definitions or measures of the constructs (as shown in the bottom half of Figure 3.1).

Once the theory is completely specified, it can be *tested* by collecting data. To investigate the usefulness of the theory in Figure 3.1, the data would include school grades, Stanford–Binet test scores, and scores from a test of speed of learning paired associates in a large group of schoolchildren. The degree that *observed* relationships among the measures correspond to the *hypothesized* relationships among the underlying constructs provides evidence concerning the utility of the theory as a way of understanding the phenomena embedded in that theory.

Construct Validity

Although findings that the observed relationships among the measured variables correspond to hypothesized relationships among the constructs are essential evidence for the utility of the theory, they are also important to the ability to infer that the operational definitions of the constructs were appropriate. In other words, such findings are essential to our inferences that our measures actually reflect or represent the constructs they were designed to measure. If one or more of our measures is a poor operational definition of the construct it was designed to measure, then the theory might not receive empirical support no matter how great its potential utility. Thus, failure of the data to correspond to the theoretical expectation might result from errors in the theory or from the use of measures that did not measure the intended construct.

The degree to which the measure or test reflects the construct it was intended to reflect is known as *construct validity*. Although specific strategies for the study of the construct validity of a test will be discussed in the next section, it is important to note that the process of test validation is embedded within a theoretical framework defining tests as operational definitions of theoretical constructs. Construct validation and theory development are interrelated, interdependent processes; both are essential to describing; predicting; and, most important, understanding human behavior.

Types of Evidence for Validity

There are a variety of uses for psychological tests, and specific types of validity are important depending on the intended uses of a test. A committee of representatives from the American Educational Research Association, the American Psychological Association, and the National Council on Measurement in Education has developed a set of standards for test use, the *Standards for Educational and Psychological Testing* (2000). These standards provide guidelines for the sound and ethical use of tests, including recommended ways for evaluating the quality of tests and testing practices.

One major requirement for high quality in a test is demonstration of validity. There are three major types of validity: content validity, criterion-related validity, and construct validity. Content validity is the most frequent standard of evaluation applied to achievement tests but is also important in the evaluation of other types of tests and measuring instruments. Criterion-related validity is important when the test is to be used as a predictive device to aid in making practical decisions about people or predictions about their likely or probable behavior. Construct validity, of course, is essential when the psychologist wants to interpret test scores as indicants of some psychological variable or trait. Although the three major types of validity will be discussed separately in the sections to follow, it should be noted that content and criterion-related validity are really only specific but widely used approaches to the more general issue of construct validity. All of these approaches to validation address the question of whether the test measures the construct that it is intended to measure.

A fourth and conceptually unrelated type of validity, face validity, will also be discussed. Face validity is of concern when it is necessary to justify or convey the appropriateness of the test to potential users or examinees who are not familiar with the principles and procedures of psychological measurement.

Content Validity

Content validity refers to how well the particular sampling of behaviors (test questions/items) used to measure a trait or characteristic reflects performance or standing on the whole domain of behaviors that constitute that trait—that is, it concerns the behavior of a person as expressed in a variety of situations or toward a universe of possible content. However, when measuring anxiety, for example, it would be impossibly time-consuming to ask the examinee about every possible situation that might produce anxiety. Or if trying to quantify an individual's level of achievement in an American history course, it would be impossible to ask him or her questions about every event in the history of America. Instead, a sampling of the content of the trait or variable domain is taken, and the individual's behavior on that sample is used to generalize or make inferences about the examinee's level of anxiety or knowledge of American history. In establishing content validity, items should be chosen from a well-defined behavioral domain. Furthermore, the sampling of items from that domain should be broad and representative to allow direct inferences from the sample of items to the domain as a whole.

The achievement test situation, where there is a defined body of knowledge to be learned, provides the most obvious application of the principles of content validity. To attempt to meet the criteria for content validity, the test items should be taken from *that* body of knowledge and not some other, and the items should be taken systematically from each segment of the subject area so that specific gaps or emphases in the knowledge of any one individual will not have a disproportionate effect on the assessment of his or her knowledge of the domain. The more precisely the instructor has clarified and organized the relevant subject matter, the easier it will be to construct a test that adequately samples from that subject matter.

The principles of content validity are important, however, in the construction of any psychological measuring instrument because content validity is directly related to our conceptualization and definition of a construct. For example, in defining the construct of anxiety, it is necessary to specify what behaviors are indicative of anxiety (e.g., increased heart rate, sweaty palms, anxiety) and to specify a universe of situations in which anxiety might be felt. Some people might feel anxious in social situations, some in academic or job situations, some while driving a car or grocery shopping, and some in all of these situations. To obtain an estimate of a person's overall tendency toward becoming anxious (the trait or construct), it is important to sample from the entire range of situations in which the behavior could be exhibited. Thus, as in the achievement test situation, the more precisely the construct-related behaviors have been organized and clarified, the better able we will be to make generalizations to it from a measuring instrument that is a sampling of those behaviors.

Evidence in Support of Content Validity

Content validity is best achieved through careful definition of the construct prior to actual test construction. The more closely item development *follows,* and is *based on,* a careful definition and delineation of the construct, including distinguishing it from related constructs, the more likely the resulting measuring instrument will possess content validity. It is through this careful process of construct definition that scientific progress can also be made.

The kind of evidence most often presented in initial support of content validity is the subjective judgment of those who construct the test or of other "experts" familiar with the subject area or trait definition. This kind of evidence is usually qualitative and should be accompanied by a detailed definition of the behavioral domain of interest and by a clear specification of the item sampling methods used. In later stages of instrument development, these judgments can be quantified by having judges rate the appropriateness of each behavior sample or test item as a member of the domain and then calculating indices of interjudge agreement (Tinsley & Weiss, 2000) on the ratings of each item.

Content validity can be indirectly evaluated as the degree to which the test shows high internal consistency reliability or homogeneity. A high internal consistency reliability coefficient such as coefficient alpha or Kuder-Richardson Formula 20 indicates that each of the items reflects the same behavioral domain as does each other item and the total test score. What is still lacking, however, is the demonstration that the total score reflects the domain as a whole. For example, it would be possible to construct a highly internally consistent test of mathematics achievement that was composed only of addition items. All of the items could be highly related to each other and to the total score, but this total score would certainly not have great generalizability to the domain of mathematics achievement and would not have content validity relative to that domain.

Thus, high internal consistency shows that all of the items are related to each other and presumably measure the same variable. It provides some evidence that we are sampling from a domain of content. However, it remains for other methods, notably construct validation procedures, to establish that this domain of behavior represents the intended construct faithfully and completely.

Factor analysis (e.g., Gorsuch, 1983; Guttman, 1990; Velicer, Eaton, & Fava, 2000; Weiss, 1970, 1971) is a method that can also provide some evidence supporting the content validity of a measuring instrument. The results of a factor analysis of the intercorrelations of test items yield information about how many dimensions or traits are needed to describe or explain test performance. If a test is constructed to measure a single trait, and items are sampled only from behaviors reflecting that trait, a factor analysis yielding a single large "general" factor is evidence that test performance can be explained in terms of that single trait. However, if the factor analysis yields several factors, the conclusion must be that the test measures more than one trait. Conversely, factor analysis of the items of a test designed to measure several variables (e.g., anxiety, dependence, sociability) should result in factors identifiable as these variables, if the test is to have demonstrated content validity. Again, however, it remains for other validation methods to establish that the factors obtained are accurate and complete representations of the relevant constructs. Cluster analysis and multidimensional scaling can also be used to evaluate content validity and to link content and construct validity evidence (e.g., Deville, 1996; Sireci & Geisinger, 1992).

Thus, content validation is an essential *first* step in the establishment of construct validity because it presumes that we have given time and careful thought to a detailed yet comprehensive definition of the construct of interest. Although our notions of the construct might change as we collect empirical data describing the measure and its correlates (see Nunnally & Bernstein, 1994), we cannot begin the process of developing high-quality measures and testing theories without such careful initial definition. Further, our ability to interpret and to attribute psychological meaning to test scores depends on our knowledge of what behavioral domain the test items reflect. It is perhaps more straightforward to evaluate content validity in achievement tests than in other kinds of psychological tests because the domain consists of stated instructional goals within a defined body of content or knowledge. However, cognizance of the content validity of nonachievement constructs is valuable because it forces careful definition of the observable indicators of that construct. Furthermore, the content validity focus requires a specification of the means by which a sampling of those behaviors will permit generalizations to some broader explanatory construct or characteristic of behavior. Thus, emphasizing content validity in test construction greatly increases the chances that we will be measuring what we intended to measure and that test scores will be meaningful and useful.

Criterion-Related Validity

Criterion-related validity refers to the extent to which a measure of a trait is related to some external behavior or measure of interest. This external measure, called the criterion, represents the behavior in which we are actually interested—we want to use test scores or other measurements to *predict* status or performance on the criterion. For example, scholastic ability tests are used to predict success in completing a college curriculum. Success in college is the behavior of interest, but it is unobservable because it has not yet occurred. The magnitude of the correlation between test scores and success (once it can be observed) is an important index of the applied usefulness of the scholastic ability test in that application.

Some authors differentiate two types of criterion-related validity, and the difference between the types depends on the *temporal* relationship between collection of the predictor data and collection of the criterion data. *Predictive validity* is studied when the criterion is measured some time after scores are obtained on the predictor. It assesses how *present* status on the test predicts *future* status on the criterion variable. Thus, the correlation between the ability test scores of high school seniors and their grades as college juniors would be a predictive validity coefficient.

Concurrent validity is studied when both the predictor and criterion scores are obtained at the same time; it assesses the relationship between *present* status on the test and present status on the criterion. The observed relationship between scores on scales of the *Minnesota Multiphasic Personality Inventory* and present psychiatric diagnosis (as reflected in the *Diagnostic and Statistical Manual of Mental Disorders–Fourth Edition* classification) would be concurrent validity data. Similarly, correlations between ability test scores and present performance in school or on the job are examples of concurrent validity coefficients.

In a more general sense, however, criterion-related validity refers to the direction and extent of the observed relationships between a measure of a trait and other measures or variables that, according to the theory of the trait, should be correlated with that trait. It is in this sense that criterion-related validity can be seen as an integral step in the establishment of the construct validity of a trait measure. As indicated earlier, part of the process of establishing the construct validity of a measuring instrument involves showing that scores on the instrument are related to the behaviors the scale is intended to measure. School performance was originally considered an observable index of the intelligence of children, and it was necessary to show that a test of intelligence correlated with or predicted school performance. Similarly, it should be shown that self-report measures of the traits of anxiety or extroversion are related to other indices of these traits, such as ratings by psychologists or peers.

In addition, in the process of elaborating the theory of a construct or trait, we make hypotheses about the variables or traits that should show *no* relationship to scores on a given measuring instrument. For example, in elaborating the theory of the construct of anxiety, we might hypothesize that it should be independent of measured intelligence because there is no reason to expect that more anxious people should be more intelligent or less intelligent. Although intelligence is certainly not a "criterion" of anxiety, demonstrating that measured anxiety does *not* predict intelligence is consistent with a criterion-related validity approach.

Thus, two kinds of evidence are necessary for the demonstration of criterion-related validity. First, there should be a strong relationship shown between a measured variable and other measured variables that the first measured variable ought to predict (i.e., a "criterion"). Second, to be sure that the measuring instrument does not measure other variables that it ought not correlate with, scores on the test should not be related to variables that are not appropriate criteria. Because these potential relationships are best determined by appropriate theory, criterion-related validity becomes a special way of investigating the construct validity of a test.

Evidence Supporting Criterion-Related Validity

The basic evidence in support of criterion-related validity is that of a relationship between two variables. The two variables are the predictor (the operational definition of a central construct) and the criterion (the operational definition of another construct of theoretical or practical interest). The nature and magnitude of the relationship between the two variables is specified in the theory of the central construct.

The idea of a relationship between two variables implies a variety of statistical procedures designed to *describe* relationship or association. It is generally suggested (e.g., Cronbach & Meehl, 1955; Dunnette, 1966), however, that two different types of statistical data—data on mean differences between groups and correlational data—are relevant to establishing criterion-related validity. Although these two general classes of statistical methods do yield data relevant to criterion-related validity, the distinction between them is artificial. Both mean differences data and correlational data can be construed as measures of relationship or association. Both methods of analysis, then, are consistent with the contention that criterion-related validity is a special case of evidence for demonstrating construct validity. Criterion-related validity investigates a restricted range of hypotheses of association as specified by the theory of the construct being measured.

Score Differences Among Groups

One way of establishing criterion-related validity involves the extent to which the test or measuring instrument can differentiate among groups of people. In applied situations, we might want to use test scores to predict success or failure in a job or training program, to separate people with psychoses from those with neuroses, or to predict membership in a particular occupation. Or, our hypotheses about the nature of a construct might suggest that different groups of people should perform differently on a measure of that construct. For example, we might expect that an instrument constructed to measure extroversion should yield higher extroversion scores for a group of successful sales personnel than for a group of successful research scientists. In thinking of score differences among groups as an indicator of association, it is important to note that each of the previously mentioned situations involves two variables—test scores and group membership.

It is useful to express the relationship of the predictor measure to group membership by calculating the mean predictor score obtained by people in each group or category. The direction and significance of the difference between these mean scores can provide evidence of criterion-related validity. Thus, if people successful in a job have higher average scores on a test meant to predict job success than do people judged to be unsuccessful on that job, there is some evidence for the criterion-related validity of the test.

Figures 3.2 through 3.4 present hypothetical data on the mean test score differences between groups of successful and unsuccessful employees; three possible results from the analysis of group differences in test scores are shown. In these figures, scores on the vertical axis are test scores and the plotted points (△) are group mean or average scores. Figure 3.2 illustrates a case in which the successful group has a higher mean test score (50) than the unsuccessful group (35). If the test score measures a variable hypothesized to be related to success in this fashion, these data might be taken as positive evidence for criterion-related validity.

In Figure 3.3 both the successful and the unsuccessful groups obtain the same average score of 43. There is, in these data, no association or relationship between group classification and test score. The lack of association is reflected by the horizontal line connecting the means of the two groups. Figure 3.4 shows data where the unsuccessful group obtains a higher mean score on the test (50) than the successful group (35). Because the line joining the two means is not horizontal, there is an association between the two variables (group membership and test score), but whether these data represent validity data depends on the nature of the trait and its nomological net. If the test score represents num-

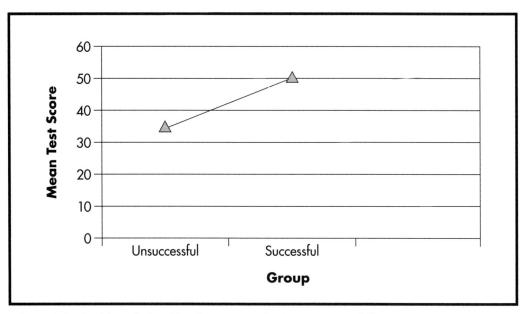

FIGURE 3.2. Positive relationship of scores to criterion success or failure.

ber of errors made in a clerical test, for example, and the groups are successful and unsuccessful clerks, the data in Figure 3.4 would be taken as evidence for criterion-related validity. However, if the test scores are number of words typed accurately in a typing test, the data in Figure 3.4 would be evidence that was contrary to criterion-related validity interpretation. Thus, criterion-related validity does not rest solely on the demonstration of group differences or association. Rather, the data must be in support of a hypothesis derived from the nomological net of the trait being measured.

In addition to meeting the criterion of theoretical relevance, criterion-related validity data must also satisfy the criteria of statistical significance and practical utility. The demonstration of statistical significance for the data in Figure 3.2 involves showing that the observed mean difference between two groups is not likely the result of chance. Thus, in Figure 3.2, under certain circumstances it is possible that the difference in group means (50–35) could have easily arisen by chance. It could then be concluded that the difference is not important—that is, that the difference is not *statistically significant.* However, a 15-point difference might be very unlikely to occur solely by chance. If this is true, the difference is probably the result of nonchance factors and is statistically significant. The search for statistically significant results for data of this type is, therefore, one of determining whether the observed mean difference is likely the result of chance factors or whether it represents a real difference between the groups. The methodology of inferential statistics, or how to determine whether the mean differences are statistically significant, is described in psychological statistics books (e.g., Glass & Hopkins, 1984; Hays, 1994).

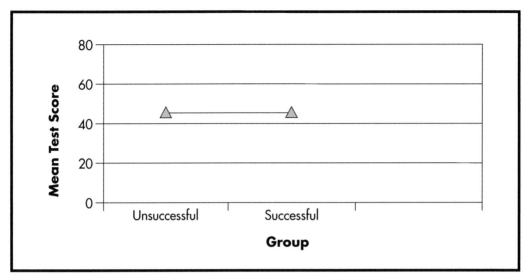

FIGURE 3.3. No relationship of scores to criterion success or failure.

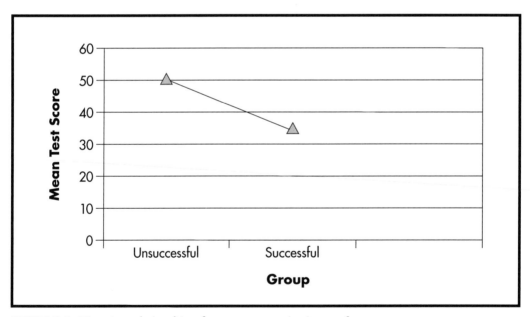

FIGURE 3.4. Negative relationship of test scores to criterion performance.

However, even a statistically significant difference between the mean scores of different groups on a test is not always a good indication of how useful the test is in a practical situation; with sufficiently large numbers of people in the groups, a *practically* unimportant difference between the groups can reach statistical significance. To get an idea of the *practical* usefulness of the test for making predictions about success based on test scores, it is useful to calculate effect sizes—for example, Cohen's (1988) *d*. Effect sizes of .20 to .50 generally indicate small to moderate effects, whereas those of .50 to .80 indicate moderate to large effects. Effect sizes of less than .20 likely indicate practically unimportant effects even if they are statistically significant.

Correlational Data

Correlational data are the other general type of statistical data used to investigate criterion-related validity. Correlations are designed to be indices of relationship or association. The logic of correlation, however, can derive from that of mean differences, as illustrated in Figure 3.2. As shown there, an *association* between two variables (group membership and test scores) exists when the means of two groups can be connected by a line that is not horizontal. When the two group means are the same, a line connecting them is horizontal and indicates that there is no association or relationship between group membership and test scores (see Figure 3.3).

When there are only two categories or groups, such as successful and unsuccessful, the classification variable is said to be dichotomous. The extent of relationship between test scores and a dichotomous criterion can be summarized by the point-biserial correlation coefficient. The point-biserial can be computed from the data on the mean differences between the two groups or from a product-moment correlation formula with the dichotomous variable coded 0-1 (McNemar, 1969). A positive point-biserial correlation would reflect the mean difference shown in Figure 3.2. The data in Figure 3.4 would result in a negative correlation. Because the means of the two groups in Figure 3.3 are the same, the point-biserial correlation would be zero, indicating that there is no relationship between group membership and test scores. A point-biserial correlation can vary from −1.0 to +1.0.

Related to the point-biserial is the biserial correlation, used when one variable is continuously distributed (e.g., test score) and the other is *dichotomized,* or artificially dichotomous. For example, if a distribution of continuous criterion scores (such as scores on a test of job knowledge) was arbitrarily divided at some point, and the top half was designated "successful" and the bottom half "unsuccessful," the biserial correlation would be an appropriate statistic to express the relationship between a set of continuous predictor scores and the dichotomized criterion variable of successful group versus unsuccessful group membership.

The Pearson product-moment correlation coefficient (*r*) is the most frequently used index of association. The use of *r* presumes the existence of two continuous (measured) variables. Thus, in contrast to the earlier examples where one variable was group membership, *r* assumes that both variables are scores from some measuring instrument or continuous variable. For example, *r* might be computed to predict from a test score to a *measured* criterion of success on a job. This criterion could be degree of job success as indicated by a test of job knowledge (but without dividing the score distribution into successful and unsuccessful groups). Or job success might be measured by a rating scale on which a supervisor of a group of employees rates each employee according to his or her degree of success. In these cases, the relationship between the two variables is expressed by computing the Pearson product-moment correlation coefficient, or *r*. The value of *r* for two continuous variables can be shown using a scatterplot, illustrated in Figure 3.5.

A positive correlation, shown in Figure 3.5 by the line moving upward to the right, shows that higher scores on the test of visual acuity are associated with better performance as an air traffic controller, at least as indicated by supervisors' ratings. This would be evidence of criterion-related validity for the test of visual acuity, assuming that it was contained in a nomological network postulating constructs related to successful performance in this occupation. A negative correlation would indicate that lower scores on one variable are associated with higher scores on the other. An *r* of zero indicates that there is no association between the two variables. When the correlation is near zero, just as in the biserial correlation, the scatterplot shows a line that is near to being horizontal, again as shown in Figure 3.5. However, when the means themselves do not approximate a straight line, the Pearson product-moment correlation coefficient will not accurately reflect the relationship that does exist. In this case it is necessary to use the general case of that coefficient, called the eta coefficient or the correlation ratio (Hays, 1994; McNemar, 1969), which indicates the amount of relationship between two variables regardless of whether the means fall on a straight line. Eta squared is also used as an indicator of effect size in advanced applications of the analysis of mean differences (Kirk, 1982; Tabachnick & Fidell, 1989)

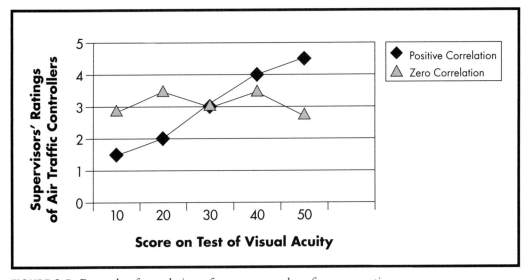

FIGURE 3.5. Example of correlation of test scores and performance ratings.

It is important to note that *correlation* (or the related case of mean differences) *does not imply causation*. Correlation indicates association between two variables; it means that the variables vary together. To demonstrate that one variable *causes* another requires an experimental design in which one variable is systematically manipulated while the other is free to vary. If the second variable can be shown to be experimentally dependent on the first variable, and if it can be shown that there are no other variables that account for this observed dependency, causation might be inferred. Correlational data, however, do not demonstrate experimental dependence and cannot, therefore, be interpreted in a causal framework.

Because correlational data and mean differences data are closely related, correlations between variables must also meet the tests of statistical significance and practical utility. Correlations based on very small samples tend to be considerably higher than they would be if sample sizes were larger. Thus, small sample results can lead to a false conclusion that there is a high relationship between two variables, when in fact that apparent relationship is spurious. It is, therefore, necessary for computed correlations (including eta correlations) to be tested for statistical significance (e.g., Glass & Hopkins, 1984; Hays, 1994) to determine if they are substantially different from zero. However, very large sample sizes will result in very small correlations that might be statistically different from zero. It is, therefore, necessary to examine correlational results for practical utility.

The usefulness of correlations can be based on the accuracy of predictions made from one variable to another based on an observed correlation. Such prediction involves estimation of an individual's probable score on one variable given his or her observed score on the other. For example, if the correlations were known between clerical test scores and job performance, the probable job performance level of a new employee could be estimated from knowledge of his or her clerical ability test score. Predictions of this type involve the use of a two-variable regression equation to obtain a predicted score on the criterion variable from an examinee's predictor score. Once the predicted score is obtained, an estimate of the amount of error in that prediction can be obtained for a given practical application by examining the distribution of actual criterion scores around the predicted criterion score. That distribution can be summarized by a quantity called the "standard error of estimate." This quantity gives an estimate of the reduction in errors of prediction from knowledge of the correlation between the two variables in comparison to predictions that would be made if the correlation were not known (Hays, 1994). This information can be used to determine the ability of an observed correlation for making predictions about individuals.

The demonstration of criterion-related validity is not based solely on significant mean differences or significant correlations. Virtually any statistical method of investigating a hypothesis of relationship can be used in the investigation of construct validity. These include, but are not limited to, chi-square analysis (Glass & Hopkins, 1984; Siegel, 1956), other methods of computing correlations (McNemar, 1969), the powerful techniques of experimental design

(Winer, 1971), and a variety of methods for the analysis of multivariate data (Bentler & Dudgeon, 1996; Loehlin, 1987; Long, 1983a, 1983b; Maruyama, 1998; Weiss, 1974).

Convergent and Discriminant Validity and the Multitrait–Multimethod Matrix

In addition to demonstrating that test scores are related to one or more criteria, as hypothesized in a theory, verifying a test's criterion-related validity also requires demonstrating that test scores are uncorrelated with theoretically unrelated variables. D. T. Campbell and Fiske (1959) introduced the terms "convergent" and "discriminant" to differentiate between these two aspects of criterion-related validity. Convergent validity is based on evidence that scores on the test correlate with independent measures of the same trait. Discriminant validity is based on evidence of a *lack of relationship* with irrelevant or unrelated variables.

One of the most pervasive influences on the results of psychological measurement is the *method* of measurement. High correlations between scores on two or more tests might result from the fact that the tests used the same method of measurement, *not* because they measure the same construct. For example, many tests of abilities use paper-and-pencil administration with computer-scored answer sheets and are administered under defined time limits. Individuals who are experienced in the use of these answer sheets and able to work quickly might have an advantage over those who do not have experience using the answer sheets or who work at a slower pace. Thus, characteristics of the method of measurement might lead to artificially high correlations among test scores. Score variability that is a result of the method of measurement rather than of the construct of interest is called "method variance." Method variance is *not* valid trait variance.

D. T. Campbell and Fiske (1959) have shown that to examine the effects of method variance and both convergent and discriminant validity for a measure, it is necessary to use a design in which two or more traits are each measured by two or more of the same methods. The correlations among all of the test scores are then the entries in what D. T. Campbell and Fiske called a multitrait–multimethod matrix. An example of such a design might include traits of anxiety, dominance, and extraversion each measured by self-report, peer ratings, and a situational test (i.e., six measurements observed on each of a number of persons). The extent to which different measures of the *same* trait are correlated indicates convergent validity, whereas a *lack* of correlation between different traits measured by the same methods indicates discriminant validity. If, however, there are significant correlations between different traits measured by the same methods, there is evidence of method variance.

A number of analytic methods have been proposed to simplify the interpretation of multitrait–multimethod matrices, especially confirmatory factor analyses (Schmitt & Stultz, 1986). Others have offered methods of determining whether two tests measure the same construct (Turban, Sanders, Francis, & Osburn, 1989). For further information on the use of multitrait–multimethod matrices, see Ivancevich (1977), Schmitt (1978), and Widaman (1985).

Special Problems in Criterion-Related Validity

Quality of the Criterion Measures. One problem that has always affected criterion-related validity studies is poor quality of measures of the criterion. If a criterion measure—for example, job performance—is of questionable reliability and/or validity, a well-conceived and well-developed predictor might not correlate with it. In such cases it might be concluded that the predictor is not valid when in fact the invalid measure is the criterion. To see the importance of examining criterion-related validity within the broader context of construct validity, consider the nomological network relevant to a relatively straightforward examination of criterion-related validity (Figure 3.6). Let's say we want to validate a measure of conscientiousness as a predictor of job performance (and there is strong evidence of this relationship in the literature; see Barrick & Mount, 1991). Conscientiousness and job performance are both at the construct (unobservable) level in our nomological network; assume that we have operationalized conscientiousness using the *NEO Personality Inventory–Revised* (NEO–PI–R; Costa & McCrae, 1992).

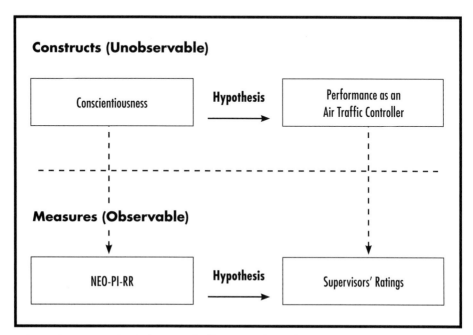

FIGURE 3.6. Nomological network illustrating hypothetical criterion-related validity study where validity of the criterion might be questioned.

Assume that the job in question is air traffic controller. We need to operationalize (measure) job performance, our criterion. We could define job performance by supervisors' ratings of performance, although we know that these are susceptible to rater biases (see Murphy & Davidshofer, 1991, for a review of rater biases and errors). To measure job performance, we could also count the number of airplanes guided to safe landings or the number of accidents occurring on the employee's shift, we could develop and administer a test assessing the assimilation of data from a radar screen, or we could develop a "performance test" simulating an accident (e.g., a midair collision) and see how well the employee responds to the crisis. There are obviously measurement issues with any of these criterion definitions—even the simple "counts" (e.g., of airplanes landed) would need to be validated as a measure of the overall construct of job performance.

One obvious answer to these problems of the reliability and validity of criterion measures is to either use or develop measures that are of high quality. In addition, multiple measures reflecting various aspects of criterion performance can be used. Ideally, this use should be guided by systematic investigation of the nature and dimensionality of criterion performance (e.g., J. P. Campbell, McCloy, Oppler, & Sager, 1993). Thus, when designing studies of criterion-related validity it is essential to select criterion measures that have been shown to have adequate psychometric quality (i.e., reliability and validity). If such measures are not readily available, then research should also be focused on the development and evaluation of one or more criterion measures.

Multiple Variables. Criterion variables to be predicted in applied validity studies are frequently complex variables. For example, job performance is frequently predicted from ability tests, but, because of the variety of factors that go into successful performance on a job, adequate validation of predictor tests requires the use of multiple predictor variables to predict a single criterion.

There are a variety of ways of combining data from several test scores to make a single prediction (Weiss, 1974). The most common of these, used when the predictors and the criterion are all measured variables, is multiple correlation, or multiple regression. Predictor scores are first weighted according to how well they each predict the criterion and then are summed to obtain a predicted criterion score. This predicted criterion score is a weighted sum of the predictor scores and can be expressed by the formula:

$$\hat{y} = b_1 x_1 + b_2 x_2 + \ldots + b_k x_k \qquad \text{(Eq. 1)}$$

In this formula, the bs (called "beta weights") are the weights attached to each of the k predictors, x, and $\hat{y}$ is the predicted criterion score or "variate." A variate can be defined as an artificial score constructed from some combination (in the multiple regression case, a weighted sum) of two or more other scores. The multiple correlation coefficient, R, is the Pearson product-moment correlation between the variate, $\hat{y}$, and the actually obtained criterion scores. The weights *(bs)* for each predictor variable are determined mathematically in such a way as to maximize *R*.

The multiple correlation coefficient, derived from the multiple regression equation, describes the relationship between the single criterion variable (e.g., job performance) and a combination of scores on the set of predictor variables (e.g., an ability test battery). The magnitude of this correlation, and the magnitude of the beta weights for specific predictor variables, can contribute to an interpretation of the criterion-related validity of specific predictors.

Cross-Validation. Regression equations are *developed* within a group where both predictor scores and criterion scores are known, but they are *used* in groups where only the predictor scores are known—that is, if we already know the criterion score for a given individual, we have no need to predict it.

Regression equations—and all other prediction equations—are influenced by sample-specific characteristics of the development group—that is, the correlation between the observed and predicted scores is higher than it should be because of factors unique to a given sample of examinees. Consequently, it is always important to make sure that the regression or prediction equation will yield a similar correlation between predicted and actual criterion scores in other groups of people from the same population. This is done by using a procedure called cross-validation, which involves applying the regression or prediction equation derived from one group of examinees to the predictor scores of another group of people. If the predicted criterion scores obtained in this way show a similar degree of relationship to the actual criterion scores of people in the new group, then we have some assurance that the equation will have more general predictive usefulness. The correlation between the predicted criterion (or variate) scores obtained in this way and the new group's actual criterion scores is called the cross-validated prediction coefficient. This cross-validated correlation gives a more realistic estimate of the degree of relationship between the predictors and the criterion because the inflation from sample-specific error has been eliminated.

Moderator Variables. Another important problem in the demonstration of criterion-related validity results from the fact that some groups or types of people are more or less "predictable" than other groups of people—that is, the predictive validity of a test or battery of tests might differ depending on the composition of the group in which the validity coefficient is obtained. For example, Seashore (1961) summarized data showing that the school grades of women in both high school and college were more predictable than those of men; there was a higher correlation between scholastic ability and scholastic achievement in groups of women. Grooms and Endler (1960) found that the grades of anxious college students were more predictable *(r = .63)* from ability and achievement test data than were those of nonanxious students *(r = .19)*.

Also, Stern, McCants, and Pettine (1982) found that the relationship between life change events and the severity of illness was stronger for uncontrollable events, such as death of a spouse, than for controllable events, such as divorce.

A moderator variable is a categorical (gender, race, marital status) or measured (anxiety level) variable that affects the direction and/or strength of the relationship between a predictor and a criterion. The discovery of moderator variables is important for several reasons. First, knowing how well we can predict for an individual might influence the types of decisions that are made about him or her. Second, if we know that the prediction for some person is less likely to be accurate, we might want to gather other types of information about him or her. Further, it might be found that one test is optimally predictive for one group of people but that a different test is optimally predictive of the same criterion for other people. The efficiency and accuracy of using test scores in prediction can thus be maximized by making use of this information. Finally, the types of moderator variables that are found have implications for our theoretical network of the constructs involved—the higher predictability of anxious students suggests something about the construct of ability and its relationship to performance on relevant criteria.

There are a number of ways that have been proposed for discovering which variables are moderators of a given predictor–criterion relationship. One way to discover moderator variables is to examine the composition of the sample or population of interest and hypothesize about whether there are individual difference variables that might be related to differential predictability among individuals. Gender is an obvious candidate for a moderator variable, but the theory of the construct might suggest others, such as anxiety level, abilities, age, or education.

Once a moderator variable is postulated there are several ways to analyze whether the variable is actually moderating predictor–criterion relationships. One way, that of statistically comparing the validity coefficients from two or more groups, has been criticized (e.g., Baron & Kenney, 1986; Nunnally & Bernstein, 1994) (a) on the basis of susceptibility to differences in variability within the groups, and (b) because this method does not allow for continuous moderators. A more generally useful method of analysis is moderated multiple regression (see Frazier, Tix, & Baron, 2004; Nunnally & Bernstein, 1994, for a detailed description of methods of analyzing moderator effects).

Moderator variables can also be found empirically by examining those variables that distinguish individuals whose actual criterion scores were close to their predicted criterion scores from individuals whose actual scores were further from those predicted for them. However, moderator variables found in this way capitalize on sample-specific characteristics and thus need to be cross-validated before they can be assumed to have more general predictive usefulness. In this case, cross-validation involves determining whether the moderator variable results in differential predictability in another sample. For more information concerning various approaches to discovering and using moderator variables, see a review by Baron and Kenney (1986) and Frazier et al. (2004).

Construct Validity

Finally, as was discussed earlier, construct validation addresses the question of the degree to which the test measures the construct it was intended to measure. Construct validation occurs within an overall framework of the development and evaluation of a theory of (or including) the construct of interest.

Evidence for Construct Validity

Broadly speaking, evidence for construct validity is provided by any type of empirical research leading to results that support the hypotheses of the theory. For example, if the theory of the construct includes the hypothesis that there should be no gender differences in a trait, then a *t* test of the significance of the difference between the means of men and women on our test that operationalizes the construct should yield no significant differences. Similarly, if it is hypothesized that the construct "intelligence" should be related to "ability to learn," then we should find a moderate to high positive correlation between scores on a test of intelligence and scores on a test of speed of learning paired associates.

If, as we hope, our empirical data support the theoretical predictions, there is evidence for *both* the construct validity of the measure and for the theory itself. For example, finding a high positive correlation between an intelligence test and a test of learning ability supports the construct validity of *both tests* as well as the validity of our theory of intelligence. If the data do *not* support the theory, however, there are several alternative explanations that lead to different courses of action. First, the intelligence test could lack construct validity—that is, the test was not measuring what it was designed to measure. Second, it is possible that the intelligence test measures the appropriate construct but that the theory was wrong—that is, hypotheses that seemed logical were based on insufficient understanding of the nature of the constructs. Third, the operational definitions of one or more of the other constructs may have been invalid—for example, the "learning" test may have actually measured attention. Fourth, the assignment of numbers to the behaviors sampled in the measuring instrument may have been based on faulty assumptions. For example, measurement may have been assumed to be on an equal-interval scale when it really was reflecting only ordinal (rank-order) differences. A fifth possibility is that the study had technical flaws that resulted in the inconsistent findings.

The researcher would follow different research strategies depending on which of these explanations seemed most appropriate. It might be best to give logical understanding the benefit of the doubt and carefully examine the methodology of the study, including methods of statistical analysis, before questioning either the test or the theory. The data might be analyzed differently or the study could be replicated or done again with variations meant to improve its quality or precision. If these approaches do not result in the findings predicted by the theory, a different way of operationalizing one or more of the noncentral constructs (e.g., the criterion) could be tried. If this proves unsuccessful, the next step would be to try another way of operationalizing the central construct. In this latter case we would have concluded that our original test lacked construct validity and that another approach to measurement should be tried. Only if several attempts to operationally define the central construct fail should we modify or reject a carefully developed, logically coherent theory of the construct.

Although empirical research provides evidence for the evaluation of construct validity, it is not possible to say that a test is "construct valid" or has a certain *amount* of construct validity. Rather, construct validation is a continual process of studying the empirical network of interrelationships of the test and of verifying, modifying, or proposing a theoretical system of constructs and hypotheses that provides logical meaning and interpretability to obtained empirical results. Construct validation is a slow, time-consuming process. As stated by Cronbach (1989), "For even one construct, developing a sturdy interpretation takes a long time. Nearly a century has elapsed between Binet's first efforts to characterize intelligence and our present modest understanding. As, slowly, a construction becomes more precise, elaborate and refined, probes into validity tend to repay the extra investment they require" (p. 163). A test has some degree of construct validity when we can say what the scores *mean* in practical terms and in terms that will enhance scientific understanding and explanation. The extent of construct validity, although it must be evaluated on a subjective rather than on a quantitative basis, depends on the solidity and variety of the relationships indicated in the supporting nomological network. It is primarily through the philosophy and methods of construct validation that psychological measurement contributes to the scientific enterprise. For a more recent reiteration of the ideas expressed by Cronbach and Meehl (1955), see Cronbach (1989).

Face Validity

Face validity concerns the extent to which the instrument appears to measure or "looks like" it measures what it is intended to measure. Probably the major reason for having a test with face validity is to ensure that it is acceptable to potential users and test takers. For example, if a test used to predict job performance has no obvious relationship to the job itself, personnel departments might be less likely to use it and job applicants might see the test as irrelevant, unfair, or both.

Face validity is *not* the same thing as content validity, although there is some similarity in their definitions. Face validity concerns judgment about a test *after* it has been constructed. Content validity, however, is the concern, *while* the test is being constructed, that the test's items are an adequate sample of a defined domain of content that defines the trait being measured. Some tests might have content validity but not face validity if the relationship of item content to the underlying trait is subtle or indirect.

Face validity is also irrelevant to criterion-related validity, in which empirical relationships are the important factor. Thus there are instances in which a test looks like it should correlate with a criterion but does not. There are also instances of instruments that bear no obvious relationship to a criterion but actually correlate well with it. Face validity might be helpful in formulating hypotheses about instruments that might predict a certain criterion—for example, a test of job performance that actually included elements of the job—but these hypotheses will be useful only if the test-criterion relationships are actually observed.

Because the construct validity of a measuring instrument is based on the evaluation of all the empirical data available on the instrument, face validity also has no relationship to construct validity. Consequently, face validity is not an appropriate kind of evidence for the evaluation of the validity of a measuring instrument. An instrument is *not* valid simply because it *appears* to be valid. Face validity is relevant to a test only as it establishes "rapport" between test taker and test administrator or ensures that the test will be appropriately used and it has no other influence in determining the validity of a measuring instrument.

Validity of Measurement and Practical Validity

Establishing the validity of psychological tests is essential. Only valid tests are useful in applied situations and contribute to our theoretical understanding of the important variables or constructs underlying the behavior of individuals. The issues and methods relevant to these two overall aims are somewhat different and sometimes conflicting.

Validity Evidence in Applied Situations

The major requirement for the usefulness of psychological tests in applied situations is demonstration that they predict some criterion measure or can distinguish among groups of people. In some of these situations there is no requirement that the test bear a common-sense relationship to that which it predicts or that there is a solid basis for interpreting the meaning of the test scores. In practical applications, test scores might only need to predict a criterion; in this case, a demonstration that they measure a construct is not necessary. However, concern about the adverse impact of using tests in selection on some gender or racial and ethnic groups, and developments in research on what is called "validity generalization," have led to an increased emphasis on the substantive relationships of predictors to more carefully conceptualized and measured criteria.

Test Bias

In the last decade, concerns have been voiced about the use of ability tests in selection, especially with racial and ethnic minorities. The major reason for this concern derives from the concept of "adverse impact," the situation where use of a test (usually a cognitive ability test) in selection results in the selection or hiring of proportionately fewer members of racial and ethnic minority groups or gender groups. Some writers have suggested that this adverse impact occurs because the tests are "biased against" some groups of individuals. Although adverse impact might exist for some measuring instruments, there is little or no evidence that it is the result of some form of bias, either content or selection (prediction), in the tests themselves.

Content bias would be present if test content were more familiar to white, middle-class examinees than to individuals from other racial and ethnic groups. One example would be test items relating to rural, farm-based life that might be unfamiliar to inner-city children. Although content bias might have been a problem in the past, now the content of most ability and achievement tests usually is reviewed for bias by panels of individuals representing the full range of racial, ethnic, and socioeconomic status groups, as well as both men and women and people with disabilities. Any content deemed potentially unfair or biased is removed.

In addition, most tests are empirically analyzed for differential item functioning (DIF). DIF is said to exist for a given test item if there is a difference in test performance in two groups (e.g., majority, minority) when the groups are equated for ability level (Holland & Wainer, 1993). Items that display statistically significant DIF are removed from a test, thereby eliminating or reducing potential test bias.

One hypothesized reason for adverse impact was *differential* predictive validity, also referred to as selection bias (Cole, 1981). Selection bias would result if a test has different degrees of predictive validity across racial and ethnic or gender groups—for example, some test critics have suggested that tests do not predict as well for minority group members as for majority group members and, in fact, *underpredict* the criterion performance of minority group members. In actuality, studies of differential prediction show that use of a common regression line (i.e., the same prediction equation) actually favors underrepresented groups because these equations overpredict rather than underpredict their performance (Niesser et al., 1996; Wagner, 1997). Thus, selection bias does not appear to be the cause of adverse impact.

Rather, the basis for adverse impact is the continuing tendency for members of some minority groups, at this time primarily African Americans and, secondarily, Hispanics, to obtain somewhat lower scores on cognitive ability tests (Niesser et al., 1996). There are many possible reasons for these lower scores (e.g., poorer school systems in poorer and/or urban neighborhoods; Card & Krueger, 1992; Rivkin, 1994; Yinger, 1995). Because of the lower scores, few current selection policies rely solely on ability tests to make selection decisions; in most, if not all, selection applications today, past indicators of achievement (e.g., high school rank) are used in addition to ability test scores. When such variables and the *goals* of diversity are included among the criteria used in selection, adverse impact should be minimized or eliminated. For example, Herrnstein and Murray's (1994) analyses suggest that in most graduate and professional school admissions decisions, racial diversity has higher priority than test scores. There are some excellent discussions of the use of ability tests with minority group members (e.g., Messick, 2000; Murphy & Davidshofer, 1991; Niesser, 1998; Niesser et al., 1996). The 2000 version of the *Standards for Educational and Psychological Testing* contains extensive discussions and recommended guidelines for such uses of tests.

Tests should not be discarded as tools for selection as placement. Rather, tests should be used in ways that, as far as possible, take advantage of the *utility* of test and other assessment data while also respecting a wide range of individual and cultural differences.

Meta-Analysis and Validity Generalization

One methodological advance in the study of validity is meta-analysis (Hedges & Olkin, 1985; Hunter & Schmidt, 1990; Schmidt & Hunter, 2003), a method of aggregating or summarizing findings across a series of studies. Schmidt and Hunter (1977) developed methods of combining validity coefficients from multiple studies to estimate the overall validity of tests and other selection methods. These methods, one of which is meta-analysis, are widely used in summarizing the data from multiple studies of the validity of selection methods. For example, Schmidt noted in 1992 that meta-analyses had been applied to more than 500 bodies of research in employment selection, most frequently in studies of the relationships of scores on cognitive ability tests to measures of overall job performance. Most recently, Schmidt and Hunter (1998) summarized the cumulative results of 85 years of research in personnel selection, covering meta-analyses of the relationships of 19 selection procedures, most notably general mental ability tests, to job and training performance.

Although meta-analysis is an increasingly popular method of summarizing findings across studies, it should be used in addition to, rather than instead of, careful logical analysis of differences in results across studies (Nunnally & Bernstein, 1994). Meta-analyses should also not be used in an attempt to compensate for poor-quality studies (e.g., studies using small sample sizes and/or unreliable measures) because it will simply provide a summary description of a series of unreliable findings. However, if it serves to stimulate *replications* of studies for the purposes of more precisely describing the effects, then it serves a useful purpose. For an understandable guide to conducting meta-analysis, see Cooper and Dorr (1996).

One outcome of this type of research has been the wide acceptance of the concept of validity generalization (Schmidt & Hunter, 1977; Schmidt, 1992) to describe the robustness of cognitive ability tests in predicting job performance across jobs and organizational settings. Meta-analyses of cognitive ability tests as predictors of job performance have demonstrated that some validity correlations can be generalized across a wide range of jobs, organizations, and settings

(Schmidt, 1992). Thus, there might be a limited need to determine whether a well-developed ability test will show validity for a new job–related application. The accumulated body of validation research might provide a clear basis for assuming that cognitive ability tests will show at least minimal validity as predictors of performance in virtually any job (Murphy, 1994, p. 64), although the data suggest that ability tests show higher validities in more cognitively demanding jobs (Gutenberg, Arvey, Osburn, & Jenneret, 1983; Hunter & Hunter, 1984). On the basis of their reviews, Schmidt and Hunter (1998, 2004) concluded that the variable most predictive of job performance was general mental ability (GMA). The validity coefficient of GMA alone was .51 for job performance and .56 for overall performance in job training programs (Schmidt & Hunter, 1998). However, the three combinations of variables with the highest validity across studies were GMA plus a work sample test (mean $R = .63$), GMA plus an integrity test (mean $R = .65$), and GMA plus a structured interview (mean $R = .63$).

The Utility of Psychological Tests

In 1965 Cronbach and Gleser stressed that the applied usefulness of a psychological test depends *not* on the absolute size of the criterion-related validity coefficient, but rather on the test's ability to aid in making correct decisions concerning the selection or placement of individuals. The *utility* of a test refers to its overall usefulness in decision making. This approach requires cognizance of the accuracy and importance of the decisions made. It also requires consideration of the costs involved both in constructing and using the test and in the effects of erroneous decisions.

Also influencing the utility of a psychological test is its "incremental validity," a term introduced by Sechrest (1963). Incremental validity concerns the extent to which the test improves on the accuracy of decision making that is possible using already available and perhaps less expensive methods. For example, a new test with a predictive validity of $r = .90$ will not have much utility if some older measure does nearly as good a job in prediction. However, even a test with a low predictive validity might have utility if there are no other bases on which to make the necessary decision.

The importance of decision making also leads to the use of data concerning mean score differences between groups and the overlap of their distributions rather than computation of simple correlation coefficients. This is because much decision making involves an accept–reject decision, and the extent to which a test can distinguish "successes" from "failures" is directly expressed by the overlap of the test score distributions of these two groups.

Other factors that must be taken into account in evaluating the utility of a test in a particular situation are the "base rates" and the "selection ratio." Base rates (Meehl & Rosen, 1955) are the expected a priori proportions of people who will fall into a given classification (e.g., success or failure on a job). The selection ratio, however, is the proportion of available applicants that must be selected to fulfill the needs of a given organization. Further considerations in the evaluation of the utility of psychological tests can be found in Cronbach and Gleser (1965). Their discussion emphasizes the need to consider a broad base of information in evaluating the applied usefulness of psychological tests.

Since Cronbach and Gleser's original conceptualization, a science of "utility" as applied to decision making has evolved. Called "utility analysis," this new specialty has been described as a family of theories and measures designed to describe, predict, or explain what determines the usefulness or desirability of decision options and to examine how information affects decisions (Boudreau, 1991, p. 621). For more information, see Boudreau (1991) or an excellent review by Murphy and Davidshofer (1991).

Finally, some writers suggest that the concept of validity be merged with notions of utility. In particular, Messick (1995, 2000) argued that validity should be conceived as a unified concept rather than as composed of subcategories such as content, criterion-related, and construct validity. Messick argued that test scores can be interpreted only in the context in which they are used. Meaning is contextual; validity is consequential. However, validity must remain at least in part a scientific issue, even as concerns about the use, and possible misuse, of psychological tests receive high priority from researchers and practitioners.

Validity of Trait Measurement

The scientific aims of psychology, as opposed to its practical applications, indicate the necessity for adequate psychological theories and theory-based research. The existence of appropriate theory leads to the measurement of constructs and the understanding of behavior in terms of these broad explanatory constructs. The procedures of construct validation lead to better understanding and interpretation of test scores and the instrument from which they are derived and also help to elucidate the nature and action of the important constructs of behavior. Following the rationale of construct validation, tests that have been shown to reflect meaningful psychological variables will be more generalizable to a variety of applied predictive needs. For example, a theoretical network describing the factors relevant to success or status on any particular criterion variable should make it possible to select those tests or predictors that, through construct validation procedures, have been shown to reflect precisely those factors. A construct-oriented approach to the selection of valid predictor instruments should be more efficient than an approach that is based on a trial-and-error search to identify those predictors that predict a criterion in a given applied situation.

Conclusion

This chapter stresses the overriding importance of theory-based measurement and construct validation procedures. If a measuring instrument is constructed to *measure* some important psychological variable, rather than just to *predict a* specific criterion, both its scientific and practical usefulness should be greatly enhanced. It is hoped that the present chapter will stimulate more attention to theory-based measurement and construct validation research.

References

American Educational Research Association, American Psychological Association, & National Council on Measurement in Education. (2000). *Standards for educational and psychological testing.* Washington, DC: American Educational Research Association.

Anastasi, A. (1958). *Differential psychology* (3rd ed.). New York: MacMillan.

Baron, R., & Kenney, D. (1986). The moderator–mediator variable distinction in social–psychological research. *Journal of Personality and Social Psychology, 51,* 1173–1182.

Barrick, M. R., & Mount, M. K. (1991). The big five personality dimensions and job performance: A meta-analysis. *Personnel Psychology, 44,* 1–26.

Bentler, P. J., & Dudgeon, P. (1996). Covariance structure analysis: Statistical practice, theory, and directions. *Annual Review of Psychology, 47,* 563–592.

Boudreau, J. W. (1991). Utility analysis for decisions in human resource management. In M. D. Dunnette & L. M. Hough (Eds.), *Handbook of industrial and organizational psychology* (2nd ed., Vol. 2, pp. 621–745). Palo Alto, CA: CPP.

Campbell, D. T., & Fiske, D. W. (1959). Convergent and discriminant validation by the multi-trait–multimethod matrix. *Psychological Bulletin, 56,* 81–105.

Campbell, J. P., McCloy, R. A., Oppler, S. H., & Sager, C. E. (1993). A theory of performance. In N. Schmidt & W. C. Borman & Associates (Eds.), *Personnel selection in organizations* (pp. 35–70). San Francisco: Jossey-Bass.

Card, D., & Krueger, A. B. (1992). Does school quality matter? The characteristics of public schools in the United States. *Journal of Political Economy, 100,* 1–40.

Cohen, J. (1988). *Statistical power analyses for the behavioral sciences* (2nd ed.). Hillsdale, NJ: Erlbaum.

Cole, N. S. (1981). Bias in testing. *American Psychologist, 36,* 1067–1077.

Cooper, H., & Dorr, N. (1996). Conducting a meta-analysis. In F. T. L. Leong & J. T. Austin (Eds.), *The psychology research handbook* (pp. 229–238). Thousand Oaks, CA: Sage.

Costa, P. T., & McCrae, R. R. (1992). *NEO–PI–R manual.* Odessa, FL: Psychological Assessment Resources.

Cronbach, L. J. (1989). Construct validity after thirty years. In *Intelligence: Measurement, theory, and public policy: Proceedings of a symposium in honor of Lloyd G. Humphreys* (pp. 147–171). Champaign: University of Illinois Press.

Cronbach, L. J., & Gleser, G. (1965). *Psychological tests and personnel decisions.* Urbana: University of Illinois Press.

Cronbach, L. J., & Meehl, P. E. (1955). Construct validity in psychological tests. *Psychological Bulletin, 52,* 281–302.

Deville, C. W. (1996). An empirical link of content and construct validity evidence. *Applied Psychological Measurement, 20,* 127–139.

Dunnette, M. D. (1966). *Personnel selection and placement.* Belmont, CA: Brooks/Cole.

Frazier, P. A., Tix, A. P., & Barron, K. (2004). Testing moderator and mediator effects in counseling psychology research. *Journal of Counseling Psychology, 51,* 115–134.

Glass, G. V., & Hopkins, K. D. (1984). *Statistical methods in education and psychology* (2nd ed.). Englewood Cliffs, NJ: Prentice Hall.

Gorsuch, R. L. (1983). *Factor analysis.* Hillsdale, NJ: Erlbaum.

Grooms, R. R., & Endler, N. S. (1960). The effect of anxiety on academic achievement. *Journal of Educational Psychology, 51,* 299–304.

Gutenberg, R. L., Arvey, R. D., Osburn, H. G., & Jenneret, P. R. (1983). Moderating effects of decision-making/information processing job dimensions on test validities. *Journal of Applied Psychology, 68,* 602–608.

Hays, W. (1994). *Statistics for psychologists* (5th ed.). New York: Holt, Rinehart & Winston.

Hedges, L. V., & Olkin, R. F. (1985). *Statistical methods for meta-analysis.* New York: Academic Press.

Herrnstein, P. J., & Murray, D. (1994). *The bell curve: Intelligence and class structure in American life.* New York: The Free Press.

Holland, P. W., & Wainer, H. (Eds.). (1993). *Differential item functioning: Theory and practice.* Hillsdale, NJ: Erlbaum.

Hunter, J. E., & Hunter, R. F. (1984). Validity and utility of alternative predictors of job performance. *Psychological Bulletin, 96,* 72–98.

Hunter, J. E., & Schmidt, F. L. (1990). *Methods of meta-analysis.* Newbury Park, CA: Sage.

Ivancevich, J. M. (1977). A multitrait-multimethod analysis of a behaviorally-anchored rating scale for sales personnel. *Applied Psychological Measurement, 1,* 523–532.

Kirk, R. E. (1982). *Experimental design: Procedures for the behavioral sciences* (2nd ed.). Belmont, CA: Brooks/Cole.

Loehlin, J. (1987). *Latent variable models: An introduction to factor, path, and structural analysis.* Hillsdale, NJ: Erlbaum.

Long, J. S. (1983a). *Confirmatory factor analysis.* Beverly Hills, CA: Sage.

Long, J. S. (1983b). *Covariance structure models.* Beverly Hills, CA: Sage.

Maruyama, G. M. (1998). *Basics of structural equation modeling.* Thousand Oaks, CA: Sage.

McNemar, Q. (1969). *Psychological statistics* (4th ed.). New York: Wiley.

Meehl, P. E., & Rosen, A. (1955). Antecedent probability and the efficiency of psychometric signs, patterns, or cutting scores. *Psychological Bulletin, 52,* 194–216.

Messick, S. (1995). Validity of psychological assessment. *American Psychologist, 50,* 741–749.

Messick, S. (2000). Consequences of test interpretation and use: The fusion of validity and values in psychological assessment. In R. D. Goffin & E. Helmes (Eds.), *Problems and solutions in human assessment* (pp. 3–20). Norwell, MA: Kluwer Academic.

Murphy, K. R. (1994). Meta-analysis and validity generalization. In N. Anderson & P. Herriott (Eds.), *Assessment and selection in organizations* (pp. 57–76). New York: Wiley.

Murphy, K. R., & Davidshofer, F. U. (1991). *Psychological testing: Principles and applications.* Englewood Cliffs, NJ: Prentice Hall.

Neisser, U. (Ed.). (1998). *The rising curve: Long-term gains in IQ and related measures.* Washington, DC: American Psychological Association.

Neisser, U., Boodoo, G., Bouchard, T. J., Boykin, A. W., Brody, N., Ceci, S. J., et al. (1996). Intelligence: Knowns and unknowns. *American Psychologist, 51,* 77–101.

Nunnally, J. C., & Bernstein, I. H. (1994). *Psychometric theory* (3rd ed.). New York: McGraw-Hill.

Rivkin, S. G. (1994). Residential segregation and school integration. *Sociology of Education, 67,* 279–292.

Schmidt, F. L. (1992). What do data really mean? Research findings, meta-analysis, and cumulative knowledge in psychology. *American Psychologist, 47,* 1173–1181.

Schmidt, F. L., & Hunter, J. E. (1977). Development of a general solution to the problem of validity generalization. *Journal of Applied Psychology, 62,* 643–661.

Schmidt, F. L., & Hunter, J. E. (1998). The validity and utility of selection models in personnel psychology. *Psychological Bulletin, 124,* 262–274.

Schmidt, F. L., & Hunter, J. E. (2003). Meta-analysis. In J. A. Schinka & W. Velicer (Eds.), *Handbook of psychology: Research methods in psychology* (pp. 533–554). Hoboken, NJ: Wiley.

Schmidt, F. L., & Hunter, J. E. (2004). General mental ability in the world of work: Occupational attainment and job performance. *Journal of Personality and Social Psychology, 86,* 162–173.

Schmitt, N. (1978). Path analysis of multitrait-multimethod matrices. *Applied Psychological Measurement, 2,* 157–174.

Schmitt, N., & Stultz, D. M. (1986). Methodology review: Analysis of multitrait–multimethod matrices. *Applied Psychological Measurement, 10,* 1–22.

Seashore, H. G. (1961, August). *Women are more predictable than men.* Presidential address, Division 17, American Psychological Association Annual Convention, New York.

Sechrest, L. (1963). Incremental validity. *Educational and Psychological Measurement, 23,* 153–391.

Siegel, S. (1956). *Nonparametric statistics for the behavioral sciences.* New York: McGraw-Hill.

Sireci, S. G., & Geisinger, K. F. (1992). Analyzing test content using cluster analyses and multidimensional scaling. *Applied Psychological Measurement, 16,* 17–31.

Stern, G. S., McCants, T. R., & Pettine, P. W. (1982). The relative contribution of controllable and uncontrollable life events to stress and illness. *Personality and Social Psychology Bulletin, 8,* 140–145.

Tabachnick, B. G., & Fidell, L. S. (1989). *Using multivariate statistics* (2nd ed.). New York: Harper & Row.

Tinsley, H. E. A., & Weiss, D. J. (2000). Interrater reliability and agreement. In H. E. A. Tinsley & S. Brown (Eds.), *Handbook of applied multivariate methods and mathematical modeling.* San Diego, CA: Academic Press.

Turban, D. B., Sanders, P. A., Francis, D. J., & Osburn, H. G. (1989). Construct equivalence as an approach to replacing validated cognitive ability selection tests. *Journal of Applied Psychology, 74,* 62–71.

Velicer, W., Eaton, C., & Fava, J.L. (2000). Construct explication through factor or component analysis. In R. D. Goffin & E. Helmes (Eds.), *Problems and solutions in human assessment.* (pp. 41–72). Norwell, MA: Kluwer Academic.

Wagner, R. K. (1997). Intelligence, training, and employment. *American Psychologist, 52,* 1059–1069.

Weiss, D. J. (1970). Factor analysis and counseling research. *Journal of Counseling Psychology, 17,* 477–485.

Weiss, D. J. (1971). Further considerations in applications of factor analysis. *Journal of Counseling Psychology, 18,* 85–92.

Weiss, D. J. (1974). Multivariate procedures. In M. D. Dunnette (Ed.), *Handbook of industrial and organizational psychology* (pp. 327–362). New York: Rand McNally.

Widaman, K. F. (1985). Hierarchically nested covariance structure models for multitrait–multimethod data. *Applied Psychological Measurement, 9,* 1–26.

Winer, B. J. (1971). *Statistical principles in experimental design* (2nd ed.). New York: McGraw-Hill.

Yinger, J. (1995). *Closed doors, opportunities lost: The continuing costs of housing discrimination.* New York: Russell Sage.

PART 2

Reviews of Instruments

Chapter 4

Intelligence Testing

Elizabeth O. Lichtenberger, James C. Kaufman,
and Alan S. Kaufman

Perhaps no area of psychology is so widely applied, practiced, and misunderstood as intelligence testing. Like a superhuman power, it has both the potential for great good as well as the potential for, if not evil, then great wrongdoing when in the wrong hands. Intelligence testing can categorize people into oblivion and be misread to support racist or sexist beliefs. However, with careful and intelligent use of intelligence testing, individuals can be specifically diagnosed and treated in the appropriate rehabilitation setting. Using cognitive assessment to assist in identifying clients' needs and directing rehabilitation is clearly beneficial (Johnstone, Schopp, Harper, & Koscuilek, 1999). However, it is important to consider specific cognitive abilities and the degree of decline in functioning in a cognitive assessment to obtain maximum benefit. Indeed, when the effects of many demographic variables are considered in a cognitive assessment, then specific intelligence and memory variables can provide valuable information to patients, families, and service providers with regard to returning to work after traumatic brain injury (O'Connell, 2000).

In this chapter, the history of intelligence testing will be surveyed. Current tests and perspectives will be addressed, with special attention paid to advances over the last 10 years. Finally, we will look toward the future, specifically to how intelligence testing can be beneficial in a rehabilitation setting.

Historical Perspectives

Earliest records regarding conceptions of human intellect date back to the 5th century B.C. (Watson, 1968), with Alcaeon of Croton's assertion that the brain was the center of intellectual behavior. Through the end of the 19th century, however, most writers did not distinguish intelligence from other human functions and phenomena, including the soul and human nature (Matarazzo, 1972). This failure to develop a clear and distinct concept of intelligence, separate from other psychological and metapsychological concepts, has continued to the present and accounts in part for the controversy and disagreement characterizing theory, research, and assessment of intelligence (Sternberg & Kaufman, 1998). Further confusing the picture regarding intelligence in adults is the observation that the precursors of the popular assessment instruments of today (Stanford-Binet IV, *Wechsler Adult Intelligence Scale–III* [WAIS-III]) were developed originally as children's scales or as tools to assess intelligence in the Army more than a half-century ago, with few alterations to accommodate the obvious differences between adult intelligence and child intelligence and between clinical assessment and military assessment, or to incorporate the large body of theory and research on intelligence that has accumulated since World War I.

Interest in the measurement of intelligence grew out of a recognition of individual differences in people and the need to determine the fitness of an individual for a particular occupation (Yoakum & Yerkes, 1920) and, in the case of children, to identify those who would profit from regular classroom instruction (Terman, 1916). Juan Huarte (1530–1589) generally is credited with first suggesting a formal approach to mental testing, with some emphasis given to the interpretation of test findings; however, this breakthrough came during a period in which a major philosophical debate arose concerning whether physical conditions or experiences could be measured in exact or mathematical terms.

Sir Francis Galton, however, is the founder of the intelligence test. It was the methods and conclusions of Charles Darwin, Galton's cousin, that introduced a new thrust in the study of the mind (Cronbach, 1984). Darwin stressed the concepts of variation, continuity, and function in his theory of evolution, and as evolution became the template for nearly all scientific endeavors, it was perhaps inevitable that Galton would seize upon Darwin's work as the rationale for his study of individual differences. Galton (1869) began by studying the distribution of ability among human beings and demonstrated that major differences could be observed among people as a function of their respective intellectual abilities. Along with the notion of individual differences and variation, Galton pressed into service the idea that intellectual capacity was an inheritable trait. Eventually, Galton (1883) devised a battery of tests including a series of sensory, motor, and reaction-time tasks, all of which produced reliable, consistent results, but none of which proved to be valid as measures of the construct of intelligence (Kaufman, 2000). Galton developed a statistic that was the forerunner of the coefficient of correlation and that proved to be his own undoing; shortly after his friend and biographer, Karl Pearson, perfected the statistic, a few studies revealed that the Galton intelligence test was misnamed because it did not correlate meaningfully with pertinent cognitive variables (such as grade point average).

During the same turn-of-the-century period in France, officials of the educational systems were recognizing the potential of the mental testing movement for assisting in placement decisions—to help identify those students who could not profit from "regular" academic instruction. It was in this context that Alfred Binet first received the opportunity to contribute significantly to the mental testing movement. For many years, Binet had argued that measuring elemental sensory and motor skills was inefficient and impractical as a means of assessing mental capacity. He contended that there were too many elements and their interrelationships were too poorly understood to offer any immediate hope of being successfully adapted to a routine use in assessing intelligence. In contrast, Binet proposed to measure higher order skills that could logically be linked to some objective index of mental capacity, such as academic achievement.

In 1895, Binet and his student Henri outlined the components and purposes of mental tests, which they suggested should assess variations among individuals in mental faculties as well as determine the covariation among the various mental faculties. As for what mental tests should measure, they recommended the following: memory, the nature of mental images, imagination, attention, the faculty of comprehension, suggestibility, aesthetic feeling, moral feelings, muscular strength and willpower, and motor skill and perceptual skill in spatial relations. In that same article, Binet and Henri (1895) made reference to certain requirements of testing: that it be simple, that it not require too much time, and that its results be independent of the examiner, so that results obtained by two different examiners for the same subject would be comparable. By 1905, Binet and Simon had developed for the French educational system a battery of measures that was used to identify schoolchildren who were unable to profit from regular classroom instruction. Binet's scales indexed mental capacity to age and reported findings in terms of "mental age." To his credit, Binet emphasized the distinction between what his scales measured and the more encompassing concept of intelligence and recommended that interpretations of scores be made in light of other, more qualitative information obtained during the examination.

While Binet's position regarding the measurement of mental functioning was logical and practical, Galton's approach was initially more widely embraced in Europe and the United States. During this pivotal era in testing, the measurement of mental functioning was primarily the province of psychologists, who still lacked total credibility within the academic and public communities as scientists. The rigor and purity of the sensorimotor tasks advocated by Galton strongly appealed to most psychologists. However, two studies conducted in the United States at the turn of the century had enormous impact upon the testing movement and later upon the preeminence of the Galton measures. Stella Sharp (1899) conducted an investigation into the methods of Galton and Binet and concluded that neither approach had as of that time succeeded in its promise of measuring intelligence. However, Sharp did indicate that the Binet method was superior to the Galton method, a conclusion not terribly surprising given that Sharp was a student of Tichenor, whose German gestalt training precluded any reductionist approach to studying human psychology. The second study, conducted by Clark Wissler (1901), was one of the first systematic uses of correlation with mental measures. Wissler focused primarily upon the Galton tasks of sensory and motor skills and reported two important findings. First, the extent to which the tasks of simple sensory and mental performance were found to be interrelated was uniformly small, with coefficients ranging from .1 to .2 being most common. This finding strongly suggested that the various tasks were measuring very different things. The second finding was that none of the sensory and mental measures correlated highly with academic marks obtained by the subjects of the study. Again, coefficients reported were typically below .2. By contrast, the intercorrelations found among academic marks for various courses of study were much higher, predominantly in the range of .5 to .6. Wissler concluded that measures of simple sensory skills and mental functions were poor candidates for predicting academic achievement.

At the time of their publication, these two studies called into question the value and validity of all attempts to measure mental functioning. Their findings strongly suggested that little relationship existed between these recently developed measures and the more global phenomena characterizing intelligence. One investigator who did not accept at face value the findings of these two studies was Charles Spearman (1863–1945), who found in his own research large, significant correlations among measures of simple sensory and computational tasks. Spearman (1904) criticized the Wissler study on the grounds that the subjects used (Columbia and Barnard College students) were too homogeneous to exhibit differences in the various sensory and mental tasks. When correction for attenuation was applied, the correlations Spearman found were much higher. Spearman went on to propose a two-factor theory of intelligence; his advocacy of the Galton-type measures, however, went generally unheeded. In retrospect, both Sharp's study and Wissler's study were flawed. Wissler used too homogeneous a sample, while Sharp's sample was far too small (seven students) and she chose to dramatically alter the tasks and the procedures for administering the tasks to accommodate the collection of repeated measures on her subjects. The short-term impact of these studies was to temporarily challenge the value of mental testing. The lasting impact was to turn most practitioners away from the Galton tradition and toward the Binet tasks for measuring mental functioning.

Binet followed the introduction of the 1905 version of his scale with a revised version in 1908. This version more closely linked the tasks to specific age ranges and allowed for the expression of intelligence of the child in terms of "mental age." In 1911, Binet again revised the scale to extend it through adulthood. In the United States, interest in the Binet-Simon scale quickly led to numerous translations into English versions. While many American psychologists developed their own form of the Binet-Simon scale (Goddard, 1911; Kuhlmann, 1912), it was Lewis Terman who eventually succeeded in creating the most popular form, largely as a result of his extensive efforts to standardize and develop adequate U.S. norms for the instrument. Terman's version of the Stanford revision of the *Binet-Simon Scale of Intelligence* was specifically designed to meet the needs of practitioners in the field (Terman, 1916). Terman incorporated the IQ concept for the first time, borrowing Sterns' definition of IQ as mental age, divided by chronological age, multiplied by 100.

A world event that significantly influenced the course of intelligence testing was World War I. For the first time in history, it was necessary to quickly and efficiently classify recruits and enlistees for various assignments, and the newly emergent mental tests were viewed as viable candidates for this selection process. However, one disadvantage of the popular Binet-type measures was the time and training required for their administration. To remedy this deficiency, paper-and-pencil versions were sought, and Arthur Otis, a student of Terman's, was able to provide the needed scales (Kaufman, 2000). Otis had worked on adapting the Binet scales to a group administration format, and the results of his efforts appeared directly in what came to be known as Army Alpha. Once the problem of mass testing was successfully addressed, another problem emerged. Many of the men tested had invalid scores due to language deficiencies attributable to their recent immigrant status or illiteracy. In response to this need, the group-administered Army Beta was developed.

Army Beta was composed of nonverbal and performance scales that minimized the role of language in testing. When it was discovered that some individuals could not be tested in group format even with the Army Beta, the

Army Individual Performance Scale was developed; this scale included tests called Digit Symbol, Picture Completion, Picture Arrangement, and so forth. These Army tests were the first IQ tests to be administered to huge samples (nearly 2 million), and the results demonstrated some basic validity: The tests were able to distinguish between officers and recruits (Kaufman, 1990; Yoakum & Yerkes, 1920).

During wartime, the need for group-administered tests of intelligence was critical, and the efforts to develop such tests were entirely legitimate. What followed the war's end was less defensible, as the development and use of group-administered tests of intelligence burgeoned. However, the Stanford-Binet remained the standard against which all other measures were compared, despite deficiencies (i.e., inadequate measurement of adult intelligence, nonrepresentative norming, unclear directions for administration and scoring, and a predominance of verbal tasks). The 1937 revision (Terman & Merrill, 1937) corrected many of these problems; for example, more nonverbal tests were added at the preschool levels, standardization was improved, and additional levels were added at the upper and lower ends of the scale.

While the Stanford-Binet enjoyed widespread popularity for many years, a challenge arose to its preeminence from the work of David Wechsler. Wechsler, a clinician who had participated in the army testing program during World War I, believed that while intelligence was appropriately conceptualized by Binet, its assessment was enhanced by the separate examination of Verbal and Performance scales. He reasoned that intelligence could be manifested in various fashions and that a measure of intelligence that relied entirely upon a single dimension of intelligence (such as verbal intelligence) would overlook important information regarding the global functioning of the individual. Wechsler made his first attempt at developing an intelligence test while he was chief psychologist of Bellevue Psychiatric Hospital, resulting in the *Wechsler-Bellevue Test* (Wechsler, 1939), which was designed to measure adult intelligence. Composed primarily of subtests found on the Army Alpha, the Army Beta, the Army Individual Performance Scale, the Binet scales, and several adapted measures (e.g., Kohs Blocks), the Wechsler-Bellevue was the first systematic attempt to measure verbal and nonverbal intelligence in the same individual and with a single instrument. Perhaps as important as the verbal-performance dichotomy in Wechsler's approach was his procedure for selecting the 11 subtests for his original 1939 Wechsler-Bellevue scale. Wechsler followed four steps in selecting his subtests: (a) All existing standardized tests were carefully analyzed for functions measured and reliability, (b) each reviewed test's validity claims were empirically assessed, (c) the clinical value of each test was subjectively determined, and (d) tryout data on the selected tests were collected over a 2-year period on individuals with known levels of intelligence (Wechsler, 1958, p. 63).

Wechsler experienced early difficulty in finding a publisher for his instrument because the Stanford-Binet appeared unassailable on the market. This led Wechsler to develop norms for his Wechsler-Bellevue on his own and required some ingenuity on his part in obtaining representative samples. All of the Wechsler scales used by clinicians during the past half-century, including the contemporary test batteries (1989 *Wechsler Preschool and Primary Scale of Intelligence–Revised,* 1991 *Wechsler Intelligence Scale for Children–III,* and 1997 WAIS-III), are derived either from the original Wechsler-Bellevue or from Form II of the Wechsler-Bellevue (Wechsler, 1946). The series of adult scales trace their lineage to Form I, and the children's scales trace to Form II. Wechsler also contributed a valuable new method of expressing the results of a test of intelligence when he introduced the deviation IQ to replace the mental age quotient. It was observed by Wechsler that adult intelligence was not a linear function of age, as appeared to be true of children, but rather tended to plateau and remain relatively stable over the adult years, declining in old age. Because the mental age quotient would systematically underestimate the intelligence of adults, he determined to express intelligence at each age level as a deviation from the mean or average values obtained at each age level. Later versions of the Stanford-Binet (1960) adopted Wechsler's innovative approach, although Binet authors resisted using Wechsler's choice of standard deviation (*SD*) of 15, opting for a value of 16 instead.

Current Perspectives

The clinical tests most commonly used to assess intellectual functioning in adolescents and adults have not changed much over the past 60 years. When the Binet was developed, there was little related theory or clinical evidence. Even when Wechsler assembled his first version of the Wechsler-Bellevue, no well-developed theories of intelligence existed and little pertinent clinical or neurological research had been conducted that could serve as a basis for his measure. It could be argued that the evolution of thought regarding the nature of intelligence has been more affected by the available measures of intelligence than those measures have been influenced by theory or research.

Had there been little significant progress in theory and research into the nature of intelligence over the intervening years, then the noted absence of progress in improving the available measures of intelligence might be justified. But the past 60 years have seen enormous developments in such areas as cognition, learning, child development, and neuropsychology. It has been only in the last 20 years that the works of R. Cattell, Horn, Luria, Sperry, Hebb, and other researchers have been utilized in the development of theory-based IQ tests. The older, more well-known tests, however, have resisted significant change, and the newer tests, while reaching a wide audience, have been unable to replace Wechsler's (Sternberg & Kaufman, 1996). Several other new theories of intelligence have emerged in the last 25 years, such as Robert Sternberg's triarchic approach (Sternberg, 1984) and Howard Gardner's theory of multiple intelligences (Gardner, 1983), but none of these have been successfully adapted into a workable, commercially published IQ test, nor is any adaptation likely to surface in the near future.

However, one of the most widely researched theories of cognitive abilities, the *Cattell-Horn-Carroll* (CHC) model (Flanagan & Ortiz, 2001; McGrew & Flanagan, 1998), has been successfully applied to the development of modern IQ tests. CHC theory was derived from the original Horn–Cattell theory, which posited broad fluid and broad crystallized dimensions (Horn & Cattell, 1966, 1967), and most cognitive tasks were readily categorized by these theorists into the fluid arena (if the task demanded new problem solving with minimal dependency on school learning or acculturation) or the crystallized domain (if the task was education dependent).

As Horn (1985, 1989, 1991) expanded *Gf-Gc* theory, he shifted his focus to an array of eight or nine abilities that were more "pure" in terms of what they measured. From current Horn theory, tasks are categorized as Fluid (Gf) only if they emphasize reasoning ability and as Crystallized (Gc) only if they stress knowledge base and comprehension. Previously, "contamination" with other abilities was acceptable; for example, many Gf tasks also depended on memory (short- and long-term), visualization, and speed, whereas numerous Gc tasks required short-term memory, auditory processing, quantitative thinking, and fluid reasoning. John Carroll (1943, 1993) examined and critiqued the voluminous results in the factor-analytic research on cognitive abilities, and ended up with a model of cognitive abilities that was consistent with those of Horn and Cattell. Thus, the separate but overlapping models of cognitive abilities were ultimately merged into a unified theory, dubbed CHC theory. Dawn Flanagan, Kevin McGrew, and Samuel Ortiz (2000; Flanagan & Ortiz, 2001) have well-articulated the details of CHC theory, which has driven the development of tests of intelligence in the recent years.

Below, the major test batteries, both classic and recent, are reviewed in greater detail. The WAIS-III (Wechsler, 1997), for ages 16 to 89 years, will be used to illustrate Wechsler's series of tests, the most commonly used measures worldwide. For thorough treatment of other popular Wechsler tests (Wechsler, 1991, 2002, 2003) consult Lichtenberger and Kaufman (2004) for administration, scoring, and interpretation of the WPPSI-III; Flanagan and Kaufman (2004) for administration, scoring, and interpretation of the WISC-IV; and Georgas, Weiss, van de Vijver, and Saklofske (2003) for the cross-cultural use of the WISC-III throughout the world. Following the discussion of the WAIS-III, three theory-based intelligence tests will be discussed: the *Kaufman Assessment Battery for Children–Second Edition* (KABC-II; Kaufman & Kaufman, 2004), for ages 3 to 18 years, based on CHC theory and Luria's neuropsychological theory; the *Cognitive Assessment System* (CAS; Naglieri & Das, 1997b), for ages 5 to 17 years, based on Luria's three functional blocks; and the *Stanford-Binet–Fifth Edition* (SB5; Roid, 2003), for ages 2 to 89 years, based on CHC theory.

WAIS-III

With the decline in popularity of the Stanford-Binet as a measure of adult intelligence (Brown & McGuire, 1976) came the concomitant increase in the use and popularity of the Wechsler scales: first the *Wechsler Adult Intelligence Scale* (WAIS; Wechsler, 1955), then the *Wechsler Adult Intelligence Scale–Revised* (WAIS-R; Wechsler, 1981), and the WAIS-III (Wechsler, 1997). Now on the horizon is the fourth edition of the WAIS, which is scheduled to be published in the next couple of years.

The WAIS-III is similar in format to the *Wechsler Intelligence Scale for Children–Fourth Edition* (WISC-IV; Wechsler, 2003), but it also has some important differences compared to this most recent version of the test for children ages 7 to 16. That is, the WAIS-III and WISC-IV both include four factor indexes, each with mean of 100 and *SD* of 15, and scaled scores on subtests (*M* = 10, *SD* = 3). Table 4.1 shows the WAIS-III subtests. Three of the four indexes are given the same name on both the WAIS-III and WISC-IV. On the WAIS-III, the indexes are Verbal Comprehension, Perceptual Organization, Processing Speed, and Working Memory (on the WISC-IV, the Perceptual Organization index is named *Perceptual Reasoning*). One of the key differences between the WAIS-III and the WISC-IV is that the WAIS-III offers three deviation IQs (Verbal, Performance, and Full Scale), but the WISC-IV offers only a single Full Scale IQ. As noted by Kaufman (1983, 2000; see also Kaufman & Lichtenberger, 1999), the reporting of a global IQ is consistent with Wechsler's notion about the nature of intelligence, despite the separate subtests and scales.

The organization of the two scales into four factors on WAIS-III represents a departure from Wechsler's clinical, armchair division of subtests into the

TABLE 4.1.
WAIS-III Subtests

Verbal Subtests	Performance Subtests
Verbal Comprehension	*Perceptual Organization*
Vocabulary	Picture Completion
Similarities	Block Design
Information	Matrix Reasoning
Working Memory	*Processing Speed*
Arithmetic	Digit–Symbol Coding
Digit Span	Symbol Search
Letter-Number Sequencing	*Excluded from indexes*
Excluded from indexes	Picture Arrangement
Comprehension	Object Assembly

Note. Object Assembly is supplementary and can replace a spoiled Performance subtest for ages 16–74.

Verbal and Performance scales. The WISC-IV has taken this one step further by completely removing the Verbal and Performance IQs, and it is likely that the forthcoming fourth edition of the WAIS will follow in the path of the WISC-IV by focusing on the indexes. Wechsler's decision to divide the subtests into two groupings was based on the fact that all Verbal subtests require both verbal comprehension and verbal expression, whereas all Performance subtests (although they demand following verbal directions) require nonverbal responding (or permit it on Picture Completion). The use of the four Factor Indexes, however, was an empirical decision based on the results of factor analysis, not a clinical decision. And just as the use of the four factors represents a psychometric departure from a clinical perspective, so, too, does the shift from the label Freedom from Distractibility (a term that denotes a behavior) to Working Memory reflect a shift toward research and theory. The introduction of four factors, divided equally between the Verbal and Performance scales, also has a facilitating effect on interpreting the profile of test scores by providing a built-in organization that proceeds from global to specific (IQs to Factor Indexes to scaled scores). Systematic, stepwise approaches to test interpretation have been developed to aid examiners in taking advantage of the new scale structure of the WISC-IV (Flanagan & Kaufman, 2004) and WAIS-III (Kaufman & Lichtenberger, 1999, 2006).

The WAIS-III was standardized on 2,450 adults, selected according to 1995 U.S. Census data and stratified for age, gender, race and ethnicity, geographic region, and education level. Thirteen age groups were created, ranging in age from 16 to 17 to 85 to 89. Each age group included between 100 and 200 people (Psychological Corporation, 1997). The WAIS-III standardization sample selection was carefully and precisely executed, leading to an overall well-stratified sample. The WAIS-III has proved itself a leader in the field of adult assessment, and it is likely that the forthcoming fourth edition will continue to follow in that tradition. The WAIS-III has strong reliability and validity for Verbal, Performance, and Full-Scale IQs.

Many visual and practical improvements were made in the development of the WAIS-III. With the clear and easy-to-read WAIS-III manual, administration is not difficult, and the record form has ample space and visual icons (Kaufman & Lichtenberger, 1999). The administration and scoring rules of the WAIS-III were made more uniform throughout the entire test, which reduces chances of examiner error, always a problem to be dealt with by examiners of any Wechsler test (Kaufman, 1990, Chapter 4).

Creators of the WAIS-III attempted to improve upon the floor and ceiling of the WAIS-R. Several step-down items have been added on each subtest for people with lower functioning. However, as in the WAIS-R, individuals who are extremely gifted or severely retarded cannot be adequately assessed with the WAIS-III because the range of possible Full-Scale IQs is only 45 to 155 (by contrast, the range for the *Wechsler Preschool and Primary Scale of Intelligence: Revised* [WPPSI-R] is 41 to 160, and the range for the WISC-III is 40 to 160). As on the WAIS-R, even if adults earn a raw score of zero on a subtest, they will receive one to five scaled-score points on that subtest.

The WAIS-III predecessors used a reference group (ages 20–34) to determine everyone's scaled scores, a practice that, happily, was dropped for the new test; the WAIS-III computes scaled scores for each individual based solely on his or her chronological age, the same procedure used for Wechsler's children's scales. The reference group technique was indefensible because use of this single reference group impaired profile interpretation below age 20 and above age 34, with the applicability of norms for ages 20–34 becoming extremely questionable for elderly individuals. Also, the WAIS-III manual and record form themselves provide the beginning of interpretation, with clearly laid out tables to calculate score discrepancies and so forth.

The failure to obtain construct validity evidence for all four factors for individuals aged 75 to 89 years is a problem for evaluating elderly populations. The Performance IQ appears to measure visual-motor speed more than problem solving for this group, bringing into question the construct validity of the entire Performance Scale and of the Perceptual Organization Factor as measures of cognitive ability for those aged 75 and older. In addition, an analysis of age differences in performance on the WAIS-III subtests and factors raises some issues about the interpretation of the Working Memory factor for individuals in their 50s through 80s. Each component subtest has a distinctly different relationship to age: Arithmetic is an ability that is maintained across most of the life span, whereas Digit Span shows the age-related vulnerability that is characteristic of short-term memory tasks and Letter–Number Sequencing demonstrates the dramatic decreases in old age that typify measures of fluid reasoning (Kaufman, Kaufman, & Lichtenberger, 1999, 2006).

If one were to evaluate the Wechsler scales from the vantage point of several popular theories of intelligence, they would fall short. Sternberg (1993) pointed out (the comments were made about the WISC-III, but they are applicable to the WAIS-III as well) that the Wechsler scales measure analytical intelligence but fail to capture creative or practical intelligence, the other two components of his triarchic theory of intelligence (Sternberg, 1985). In addition, Sternberg (1993) further indicates that the Wechsler scales cover only three of Gardner's (1983) multiple intelligences: linguistic, logical-mathematical, and spatial. These criticisms, however, could be applied to many intelligence tests that are actually used; these conceptions of intelligence have remained theoretical in nature and have only recently begun to be successfully applied to academic or business settings. For the WAIS-III, the most relevant theories are the ones that have generated the most pertinent research using Wechsler's subtests or related tasks: cerebral specialization theory and CHC theory (Flanagan, McGrew, & Ortiz, 2000; Kaufman & Lichtenberger, 2006).

Initial notions of the specialization of the two hemispheres of the brain focused on the verbal nature of the left hemisphere and the nonverbal–spatial nature of the right hemisphere (Reitan, 1955; Sperry, 1968). From that type of "content" interpretation, the Wechsler scales were a natural to reflect a strong theoretical basis (i.e., the verbal content matches up well with the left hemisphere, and the nonverbal matches up well with the right hemisphere). The prediction was that damage confined to a particular half of the brain should affect either Verbal IQ or Performance IQ but not both. The early researchers (e.g., Dennerll, 1964; Klove, 1959; Reitan, 1955) "validated" this hypothesis, but subsequent investigators noted methodological flaws in the preliminary research studies and offered results that were less supportive of the link between cerebral specialization theory and the Wechsler scales (e.g., Smith, 1966). An accumulation of studies with the WAIS and WAIS-R, with more than 1,400 patients having lesions to either the left or right hemisphere, indicated that Performance IQ does seem to be affected negatively by damage to the right hemisphere (10-point decrement) but that Verbal IQ is only trivially affected by damage to the left hemisphere (2.5-point decrement; Kaufman & Lichtenberger, 2006, Table 8.6).

The fact that the validation of the theory was only partial, however, may be due more to the failure of the initial theory to reflect the true specialization capacities of the two hemispheres. As more research was conducted by Sperry and his colleagues, the verbal versus nonverbal "content" distinction gave way to an analytic–sequential versus gestalt–holistic "process" distinction between the left and right hemispheres, respectively (Levy & Trevarthen, 1976). Wechsler organized his subtests into two scales based on the content demands—not the process demands—of each task, so the link between the IQ test and psychobiological theory was not as intuitive as Reitan and others had believed.

Matarazzo (1972) was probably the first to identify that Wechsler's Verbal IQ was a good measure of Gc ability; that the Performance IQ was a good measure of Gf ability; and that correspondence was accepted almost axiomatically by many researchers, especially those who were investigating IQ changes across the adult life span (Kaufman, 1990, Chapter 7). Since that time, researchers have applied the wider spectrum of CHC abilities to the interpretation of the WAIS-III and WISC-IV indexes (Flanagan & Kaufman, 2004; Flanagan, McGrew, & Ortiz, 2000; Kaufman & Lichtenberger, 2006). Using CHC theory, the Verbal Comprehension Index is interpreted as a measure of Crystallized Intelligence (Gc), the Working Memory Index is interpreted as a measure of Short-Term Memory (Gsm), the Perceptual Organization Index is interpreted as a measure of Fluid Reasoning (Gf) and Visual Processing (Gv), and the Processing Speed Index is interpreted as a measure of Processing Speed (Gs).

For a fuller analysis of the pros and cons of the WAIS-III, as well as its interpretation and clinical applications, see Kaufman and Lichtenberger (1999, 2006).

KABC-II

The KABC-II is based on two of the theories discussed in previous sections: the CHC model and Luria's model. The dual theoretical perspective that the KABC-II offers allows clinicians to select the model for each individual that is best suited to that person's background and reasons for referral. The constructs underlying the test provide useful insights into each individual's learning abilities and problem-solving strategies, and the dual theoretical model allows for process-oriented interpretations from either model depending on the needs of the clinician and the person being assessed.

The KABC-II has five scales. From Luria's perspective, the KABC-II scales assess Learning Ability, Sequential Processing, Simultaneous Processing, and Planning Ability. From a CHC perspective, the KABC-II measures Long-term Storage and Retrieval (Glr), Short-term Memory (Gsm), Visual Processing (Gv), Fluid Reasoning (Gf), and Crystallized Ability (Gc). The names of the KABC-II's scales reflect both the Luria process each is believed to measure and its CHC Broad Ability: Learning/Glr, Sequential/Gsm, Simultaneous/Gv, and Planning/Gf. However, the Knowledge/Gc scale only reflects Crystallized Ability from the CHC model because it is specifically excluded from the Luria process-oriented system.

The KABC-II yields two global scores: the Mental Processing Index (MPI) and the Fluid-Crystallized Index (FCI). The MPI is the global score based on the Luria model, while FCI is the global score based on the CHC model. The subtests that contribute to the Luria and CHC scales are identical, with the exception of the Knowledge/Gc subtests, which are only included in the CHC model. In addition to the FCI and MPI, the KABC-II has a Nonverbal Scale, with subtests that can be administered in pantomime and responded to motorically. This scale yields a global Nonverbal Index (NVI), which is especially useful in the assessment of individuals who are hearing impaired, have limited English proficiency, have moderate to severe speech or language impairments, or have other disabilities that make the Core Battery unsuitable.

The number of scales that the KABC-II yields varies slightly with age. For example, at age 3, only global scales are provided (i.e., FCI, MPI, or NVI). For ages 4–6, the global scales plus three or four scales are provided: Learning/Glr, Sequential/Gsm, Simultaneous/Gv, and Knowledge/Gc. For ages 7–18, the Planning/Gf scale joins the aforementioned scales, yielding either four (Luria) or five (CHC) scales.

The KABC-II includes a Core and an Expanded Battery. The expanded battery includes supplementary subtests to increase the breadth of the constructs that are measured by the Core battery. Scores earned on the supplementary subtests do not contribute to the client's standard scores on the KABC-II scales (except for the Nonverbal Scale). The *KABC-II Manual* and *Record Form* detail which subtests comprise the Core and Expanded Batteries at each age, and Table 4.2 provides a brief description of the KABC-II subtests.

The KABC-II is a psychometrically strong instrument. Detailed information on its reliability and validity are presented in the *KABC-II Manual* (Kaufman & Kaufman, 2004) and elsewhere (Kaufman, Lichtenberger, Fletcher-Janzen, & Kaufman, 2005), but we provide a summary here. The average internal consistency coefficients are .95 for the MPI at both ages 3–6 and ages 7–18; for the FCI the means are .96 for ages 3–6 and .97 for ages 7–18. Internal consistency values for individual subtests ranged from .69 for Hand Movements to .92 on Rebus (for ages 3–6); for the 7–18 age group, internal consistency values ranged from .74 on Gestalt Closure to .93 on Rebus. The median internal consistency value for the individual subtests was .84 for ages 3–6 and .86 for ages 7–18.

TABLE 4.2.
Description of KABC–II Subtests

Scale/Subtest		Age		
Sequential/ Gsm Subtests	**Core**	**Supplementary**	**Nonverbal**	**Description**
Word Order	3-18			The child touches a series of silhouettes of common objects in the same order as the examiner said the names of the objects; more difficult items include an interference task (color naming) between the stimulus and response.
Number Recall	4-18	3		The child repeats a series of numbers in the same sequence as the examiner said them, with series ranging in length from 2 to 9 numbers; the numbers are single digits, except that 10 is used instead of 7 to ensure that all numbers are one syllable.
Hand Movements		4-18	3-18	The child copies the examiner's precise sequence of taps on the table with the fist, palm, or side of the hand.
Simultaneous/ Gv Subtests				
Rover	6-18			The child moves a toy dog to a bone on a checkerboard-like grid that contains obstacles (rocks and weeds), and tries to find the "quickest" path—the one that takes the fewest moves.
Triangles	3-12	13-18	3-18	For most items, the child assembles several identical rubber triangles (blue on one side, yellow on the other) to match a picture of an abstract design; for easier items, the child assembles a different set of colorful rubber shapes to match a model constructed by the examiner.

(continues)

TABLE 4.2. Continued.

Scale/Subtest	Age			
Simultaneous/ Gv Subtests	**Core**	**Supplementary**	**Nonverbal**	**Description**
Conceptual Thinking	3-6		3-6	The child views a set of 4 or 5 pictures and identifies the one picture that does not belong with the others; some items present meaningful stimuli and others use abstract stimuli.
Face Recognition	3-4	5	3-5	The child attends closely to photographs of one or two faces that are exposed briefly, and then selects the correct face or faces, shown in a different pose, from a group photograph.
Gestalt Closure		3-18		The child mentally "fills in the gaps" in a partially completed "inkblot" drawing and names (or describes) the object or action depicted in the drawing.
Block Counting	13-18	5-12	7-18	The child counts the exact number of blocks in various pictures of stacks of blocks; the stacks are configured such that one or more blocks is hidden or partially hidden from view.
Planning/Gf				
Pattern Reasoning[a]	7-18		5-18	The child is shown a series of stimuli that form a logical, linear pattern, but one stimulus is missing; the child completes the pattern by selecting the correct stimulus from an array of 4 to 6 options at the bottom of the page (most stimuli are abstract, geometric shapes, but some easy items use meaningful shapes).
Story Completion[a]	7-18		6-18	The child is shown a row of pictures that tell a story, but some of the pictures are missing. The child is given a set of pictures, selects only the ones that are needed to complete the story, and places the missing pictures in their correct locations.

(continues)

TABLE 4.2. *Continued.*

Scale/Subtest	Age			
Learning/ Glr Subtests	Core	Supplementary	Nonverbal	Description
Atlantis	3-18			The examiner teaches the child the nonsense names for fanciful pictures of fish, plants, and shells; the child demonstrates learning by pointing to each picture (out of an array of pictures) when it is named.
Atlantis–Delayed		5-18		The child demonstrates delayed recall of paired associations learned about 15–25 minutes earlier during Atlantis by pointing to the picture of the fish, plant, or shell that is named by the examiner.
Rebus	4-18			The examiner teaches the child the word or concept associated with each particular rebus (drawing) and the child then "reads" aloud phrases and sentences composed of these rebuses.
Rebus–Delayed		5-18		The child demonstrates delayed recall of paired associations learned about 15–25 minutes earlier during Rebus by "reading" phrases and sentences composed of those same rebuses.
Knowledge/ Gc Subtests				
Riddles	3-18			The examiner provides several characteristics of a concrete or abstract verbal concept and the child has to point to it (early items) or name it (later items).
Expressive Vocabulary	3-6	7-18		The child provides the name of a pictured object.
Verbal Knowledge	7-18	3-6		The child selects from an array of 6 pictures the one that corresponds to a vocabulary word or answers a general information question.

Note. Descriptions are adapted from *KABC-II Manual* (Kaufman & Kaufman, 2004).

[a]At ages 5–6, Pattern Reasoning and Story Completion are categorized as Simultaneous/Gv subtests.

The KABC-II is a fairly stable instrument with average test-retest coefficients for the MPI of .86 (ages 3–5), .89 (ages 7–12), and .91 (ages 13–18). Average test–retest coefficients for the FCI were .90, .91, and .94 at ages 3–5, 7–12, and 13–18, respectively. Across the three broad age groups, the ranges of the stability values of Learning/Glr (.76–.81), Sequential/Gsm (.79–.80), Simultaneous/Gv (.74–.78), Planning/Gf (.80–.82), and Knowledge/Gc (.88–.95) denote adequate stability. The Simultaneous/Gv emerged as the least stable of all the composite scores.

The validity of the KABC-II was supported by factor analytic studies, correlational data, and special clinical group studies reported in the *KABC-II Manual*. Results of confirmatory factor analyses across age levels supported different batteries at different age levels. The confirmatory factor analyses also strongly supported the theory-based scale structure of the KABC-II. Correlations between the KABC-II and other major intelligence tests further indicated the test's validity. Correlations ranged from .71 to .91 between the global scales of the KABC-II and other intelligence tests (e.g., WISC-III, WISC-IV, WPPSI-III, KAIT, and WJ III).

The KABC-II does a good job of practically applying theory to practice and identifying cognitive strengths and weaknesses. It gives clinicians two well-defined models by which they can interpret the test results (CHC theory or Luria's Neuropsychological theory), and this flexibility is a great asset to clinicians. The interpretive process itself is clearly laid out in the manual and is expanded in other sources (Kaufman, Lichtenberger, Fletcher-Janzen, & Kaufman, 2005).

Cognitive Assessment System

The *Cognitive Assessment System* (CAS; Naglieri & Das, 1997b), for ages 5–17 years, is based on, and developed according to, the Luria-based *Planning, Attention, Simultaneous, and Successive* (PASS) theory of intelligence. The PASS theory is a multidimensional view of ability that is the result of the merging of contemporary theoretical and applied psychology (see summaries by Das, Naglieri, & Kirby, 1994, and Naglieri & Das, 1997a, 1997b). Naglieri and Das (1997b) linked the work of Luria (1966, 1973, 1980) with the field of intelligence when they suggested that PASS processes are the essential elements of human cognitive functioning. This theory proposes that human cognitive functioning is based on the four essential activities that employ and alter an individual's base of knowledge (Naglieri & Das, 1997b). According to this theory, human cognitive functioning includes four components: planning processes, which provide cognitive control, utilization of processes and knowledge, intentionality, and self-regulation to achieve a desired goal; attentional processes, which provide focused, selective cognitive activity over time; and simultaneous and successive information processes, which are the two forms of operating on information.

Planning processing provides the means to solve problems for which no solution is apparent. It applies to tasks that may involve attention, simultaneous and successive processes, and acquired knowledge. Success on planning tests should require the child to develop a plan of action or strategy, evaluate the value of the method, monitor its effectiveness, revise or reject an old plan as the task demands change, and control the impulse to act without careful consideration. Attention is "a mental process by which the individual selectively focuses on particular stimuli while inhibiting responses to competing stimuli presented over time" (Naglieri & Das, 1997b, p. 3). Successful performance on an attention task requires effort to be focused, selective, and sustained. Focused attention involves directed concentration on a particular activity. Selective attention requires concentrating on some stimuli and inhibiting responses to others that may be hard to ignore. Sustained attention refers to the performance over time, which can be influenced by varying amounts of effort.

Simultaneous and successive processing both involve mental integration. Simultaneous processing is when separate stimuli are integrated into a sole group, while successive processing takes stimuli and fits them into a specific order, forming a chainlike progression (Naglieri & Das, 1997b). Simultaneous processing allows for the integration of elements into a conceptual whole. Simultaneous processing has strong spatial components in nonverbal tasks and in language tasks involving logical–grammatical relationships. The spatial aspect involves both the perception of stimuli as a group and the internalized formation of complex visual images. The logical–grammatical dimension allows for the integration of words into ideas through the comprehension of word relationships to obtain meaning. Thus, simultaneous processes can be important to both nonverbal spatial as well as verbal tasks. Successive processing is involved when parts must follow each other in a specific order such that each element is related only to those that precede and follow it. Successive processing is most important in tasks with serial and syntactic components. The serial aspect involves both the perception of stimuli in sequence and the formation of sounds and movements in order (e.g., the serial organization of spoken speech and the synthesis of "separate sounds and motor impulses into consecutive series") (Luria & Tsvetkova, 1990, p. xvi). The syntactic aspect of successive processing allows for the comprehension of the meaning of narrative speech, especially when the "individual elements of the whole narrative always behave as if organized in certain successive series" (Luria, 1966, p. 78). Successive processing activities require perception and reproduction of the serial nature of stimuli, understanding of sentences based on syntactic relationships, and articulation of separate sounds in a consecutive series.

The CAS was designed to mirror the PASS theory, with subtests organized into four scales designed to provide an effective measure of each of the PASS cognitive processes. Planning subtests require the child to devise, select, and use efficient plans of action to solve the test problems, regulate the effectiveness of the plans, and self-correct when necessary. Attention subtests require the child to selectively attend to a particular stimulus and inhibit attending to distracting stimuli. Simultaneous processing subtests require the child to integrate stimuli into groups to form an interrelated whole. Successive processing subtests require the child to integrate stimuli in their specific serial order or appreciate the linearity of stimuli with little opportunity for interrelating the parts.

The CAS yields Planning, Attention, Simultaneous, Successive, and Full-Scale scales, which are normalized standard scores with a normative mean of 100 and *SD* of 15. All subtests are set at a normative mean of 10 and *SD* of 3. Interpretation of CAS also follows closely from the PASS theory, with emphasis on the scale-level rather than subtest-level analyses.

The CAS was standardized on 2,200 children ranging in age from 5 through 17 years and stratified by age, gender, race, ethnicity, geographic region, educational placement, and parent education according to recent U.S. Census reports, closely matching the U.S. population characteristics on the variables used. In addition to administration of the CAS, a representative sample of 1,600 included in the standardization sample was also administered achievement tests from the *WJ-R Tests of Achievement* (Woodcock & Johnson, 1989). This provided a rich source of validity evidence (e.g., the analysis of the relationships between PASS and achievement) and for the development of predictive difference values needed for interpretation of ability achievement discrepancies. Finally, 872 children from special populations (e.g., children with attention–deficit disorder, mental retardation, and learning disabilities) were tested for validity and reliability studies.

The internal consistency reliability estimates for the CAS Full-Scale are comparable with those of other tests of its kind. The CAS Standard Battery (12 subtests) average scale reliability coefficients for the entire standardization sample of children aged 5–17 years are as follows: Full-Scale .96, Planning .88, Simultaneous .93, Attention .88, and Successive .93. The average reliability coefficients for all ages in the standardization sample for the 12 subtests range from .75 to .89 (median = .82). The test-retest reliability for the CAS Full-Scale was .91, Planning .85, Simultaneous .81, Attention .82, and Successive .86 for 215 children aged 5–17 years (median interval = 21 days). Confirmatory factor analysis supports the construct validity of the four PASS components. Criterion-related validity was shown by the strong relationships between CAS scores and WJ-R achievement tests; correlations with achievement for special populations; and PASS profiles for children with attention–deficit and hyperactivity disorders, traumatic brain injury, and reading disability. Additionally, the utility of the PASS scores for treatment and educational planning is demonstrated (Naglieri & Das, 1997a).

Carroll (1995) provided two main criticisms of the PASS theory. First, he suggested that Planning is better described as a Perceptual Speed factor. Second, he argued that there was insufficient factorial support for the PASS as a measure of the constructs. Since the publication of Carroll's review, both of these criticisms have been addressed by data presented in the *Cognitive Assessment System Interpretive Handbook* (Naglieri & Das, 1997a), some of which will be summarized here. Naglieri and Das (1997a) provide strong evidence from confirmatory factor analytic investigations using the CAS standardization data that a four-factor PASS configuration of the 12 subtests provided the best fit to the data. Thus, it appears that Carroll's reanalyses of old experimental test data (some of the tests are not in the final version of the CAS) and smaller sample sizes led to the inconsistencies between his results and those provided in the manual.

Carroll's other criticism—that the Planning subtests really measure speed—merits further empirical investigation but is inconsistent with two sources of data. Naglieri and Das (1997a) show that approximately 90% of children in the entire standardization sample used strategies to solve the planning tests. These strategies show developmental changes and are differentially related to success on the subtests. Clearly, tests that have been shown to demand the generation, use, and monitoring of plans of action cannot be described as simple perceptual speed measures. More evidence that planning is not better described as perceptual speed is apparent when the relationship between planning and achievement is considered. Naglieri and Das (1997a) provide considerable information about the relationships between PASS and achievement for a large representative sample of 1,600 children who were administered the *WJ-R Tests of Achievement*. For example, they show that the correlations between planning and WJ-R Broad Mathematics and Mathematics Reasoning were substantial (median = .55), considerably higher than the median of .24 for the WJ-R Gs cluster for the large WJ-R standardization sample. The evidence for the use of strategies on planning tests and the strong and consistent correlations between CAS and math achievement do not support Carroll's reinterpretation of planning as speed.

Nonetheless, future research should explore the relationships between CAS Planning subtests with (a) pure perceptual speed tasks that involve minimal decision making and (b) tests of planning ability such as the Piagetian formal operations measures found on the KAIT. The results of such research studies should help clarify the degree to which the highly speeded visual–perceptual and visual–motor CAS Planning subtests are truly measures of Luria's Block 3 planning ability as opposed to perceptual speed as claimed by Carroll.

Esters, Ittenbach, and Han (1997) state that "attempts to establish the treatment validity of . . . the CAS have met with little success" (p. 217). This statement is inconsistent with evidence summarized by Naglieri and Das (1997a; see also Naglieri, 1999) and especially the papers published by Naglieri and Gottling (1995, 1997), who showed the relevance of PASS to math instruction. Naglieri and Gottling demonstrated that children who are poor in Planning improved considerably (80% over baseline) in math calculation taken directly from the classroom curriculum when provided an instruction that encouraged their use of strategies or plans. In contrast, children who were good in Planning showed modest improvement (about 40% over baseline) when provided exactly the same instruction. No similar relationships were found between Attention, Simultaneous, Successive, or Wechsler IQ scores.

The CAS provides an excellent translation of theory to test development. Although research is needed to clarify the precise construct measured by the Planning scale, Naglieri and Das have done an exemplary job of assessing the

Luria-based constructs and in demonstrating the possible link between theory-based assessment and educational intervention. For a fuller review of the research and theory behind the CAS, see Naglieri (1999).

Stanford Binet 5

The *Stanford-Binet Intelligence Scale—Fifth Edition* (SB5; Roid, 2003) is an individually administered measure of cognitive abilities for ages 2 to 89 years. The SB5 replaces the fourth edition of the Stanford-Binet (SB IV) that was published in 1986 (Thorndike, Hagen, & Sattler, 1986). Changes were made in the revision of the SB IV with the addition of a fifth factor (Visual–Spatial Processing), and with modification of the memory factor's content to more heavily emphasize working memory rather than short-term memory. The SB5 also increased the breadth of concepts measured by the Nonverbal IQ, which now covers five areas. The SB5 is based on the CHC theory of cognitive functioning and measures five of the 10 broad CHC abilities: Fluid Intelligence (Gf), Crystallized Knowledge (Gc), Quantitative Knowledge (Gq), Visual Processing (Gv), and Short-Term Memory (Gsm).

The SB5 is comprised of 10 subtests that yield a Full Scale IQ, two domain scores (Verbal IQ and Nonverbal IQ), and five factor indexes (Fluid Reasoning, Knowledge, Quantitative Reasoning, Visual–Spatial Reasoning, and Working Memory). Administration begins with two routing subtests (Vocabulary and Object Series/Matrices). These routing subtests determine the developmental starting point for the remaining subtests.

The five scales and the three IQs yield standard scores with a mean of 100 and standard deviation of 15. In contrast, scaled scores are calculated for the subtests ($M = 10$; $SD = 3$). Percentile ranks, confidence intervals, and age equivalents are also available scoring metrics. Change-Sensitive scores can be computed and provide a means to identify a person's change in scores over a period of time.

The SB5 was normed on a sample of 4,800 participants. The sample was stratified to match the 2001 Census data on the variables of sex, age, race/ethnicity, socioeconomic level, and geographic region. Strong reliability was indicated with average split-half reliability coefficients for the Nonverbal subtests ranging from .85 to .89 and coefficients for the Verbal subtests ranging from .84 to .89. Average reliability coefficients for the IQs were .98, .95, and .96 for the Full Scale, Nonverbal, and Verbal IQs, respectively. The factor index scores had reliabilities ranging from .90 for Fluid Reasoning to .92 for Knowledge, Quantitative Reasoning, and Visual-Spatial Processing. The test-retest reliability was examined in a series of studies and was found to be adequate across the age range of the test.

The construct validity of the SB5 was demonstrated in a principal components analysis. All SB5 subtests, across all ages, demonstrated average principal component loadings of greater than .70 on the *g*, or general factor, indicating that each subtest was a good measure of *g*. The proportion of SB5 variance accounted for by the *g* factor ranged from 56% to 61%, depending on the factoring method.

Each of the SB5 standard scores can be described qualitatively. The manual provides descriptive categories for each 10-point score range. The labels include the familiar Average, High Average, Low Average, Superior, and Borderline ranges, but they also included more detailed descriptions for individuals scoring ±2 *SD* above the mean. The SB5 results can be examined by using its CHC theoretical foundations. Each of the factor indexes measures a CHC Broad Ability and can be interpreted accordingly (or can be used in a more comprehensive cross-battery approach). The norm referenced standard scores provide a mechanism to determine how an examinee is performing relative to his or her peers. An examinee's profile of scores can also be examined to determine if it fits one of the 10 core profiles identified in the SB5 standardization. The SB5 presents these subtest profiles as an empirically supported method for interpretive analysis (Roid & Barram, 2004).

Although some key information is presented in the manual on interpretation, interpretive data in the SB5 technical manual and examiner's manual are limited (Johnson & D'Amato, 2005). In addition, to aid in interpretation, the 10 core profiles identified in the SB5 standardization sample need to be examined in future research to determine their stability and utility in regular and exceptional populations (Kush, 2005). Although the SB5 appears to be well-grounded in CHC theory, some question why the verbal/nonverbal dichotomy (not CHC-related) remains. Kush (2005) aptly points out: "It is not clear why an instrument so heavily influenced by CHC theory would include verbal and nonverbal abilities as neither is contained as a CHC Stratum I (Narrow) or Stratum II (Broad) ability. Certainly a test that includes a verbal/nonverbal dichotomy offers clinical advantages for certain types of referral questions (e.g., motor-impairment, limited English proficiency); however, the decision to retain this terminology is theoretically inconsistent. As a result, it is not clear when users of the SB5 should attempt to make test interpretations based on the two verbal/nonverbal domains or instead on the five factor scores" (p. 8).

Despite some of the SB5's weaknesses, the test has broadened the measurement of nonverbal abilities and added items to measure very low- and very high-functioning individuals. The working memory construct has been refined, and the five-factor structure is adequately supported with factor analytic data. The number of subtests was reduced from 15 on the SB IV to 10 on the SB5, a more manageable number when assessing individuals in a rehabilitation setting. The technical qualities of the SB5 are sound overall, appearing to have adequate reliability and validity.

Conclusion

Measures of intelligence are routinely included in the cognitive assessment of patients with traumatic brain injury and other related difficulties that lead to treatment in a rehabilitation setting (Martin, Donders, & Thompson, 2000). Measures of cognitive ability can contribute to the prediction of functional recovery, but many variables together must be considered to assist in creating a plan that successfully directs rehabilitation. Vocational rehabilitation programs can use neuropsychological evaluations most effectively for vocational planning by determining which specific abilities (e.g., intelligence, memory attention, cognitive processing speed, etc.) are most clearly related to vocational successes or difficulties so that the most appropriate rehabilitation plan can be developed (Johnstone, Schopp, Harper, & Koscuilek, 1999). Using an intelligent approach to testing, psychologists should consider the many variables that contributed to premorbid cognitive functioning when evaluating testing data to be used in developing a rehabilitation plan. Another component to using an intelligent approach in an assessment for rehabilitation is considering modern theories such as the CHC model of cognitive abilities that provide a solid theoretical foundation by which to interpret specific cognitive strengths and weaknesses evident on an intelligence test.

Despite the addition of newer, more modern theories of cognitive abilities and an ever-changing approach to interpreting test data, IQ tests have remained resilient. The IQ tests and the practices surrounding their use have been resistant to change but, nonetheless, have changed over time. If we think of Galton's test as being the first IQ test, in 1884, when he set up his laboratory at the International Health Exhibition (Sattler, 2001), then Galton's approach to intelligence reigned supreme for about 20 years. The torch was then passed to Binet and Terman, with the Binet-Henri system defining IQ measurement for about half a century; Wechsler's scales have carried the torch for the past 40 years, with the light still burning brightly as the new millennium begins. Test interpretation has undergone a comparable shift from the impersonal scientific statistical objectivity of Galton; to the developmental–psychometric approaches of Binet and Terman; to the clinical, flexible method embraced by Wechsler.

Wechsler's clinical tradition has always been at odds with the rigid ways in which local, state, and federal government agencies have forced school psychologists to make diagnostic and placement decisions. This basic conflict between the intelligent use of IQ tests (which fosters an understanding of a person's strengths and weaknesses and use of the evaluation results to *help* children) and how educational decisions are made has led to many controversies. This conflict still exists, so controversy and anti-testing sentiment are not likely to go away any time soon.

Will the Wechsler monopoly be broken? That is hard to answer. Its predecessors have each fallen out of favor eventually, yet school psychologists, clinical psychologists, and neuropsychologists have steadfastly resisted a wholesale switch from a Wechsler scale to a new or revised theory-based test. These other tests have been widely used throughout the United States and internationally, but often they are used alongside the WISC-IV or WAIS-III and not *instead* of Wechsler's tests. As excellent as some of the theory-based tests (e.g., the CAS, the KABC-II, the CHC-based *WJ-III Tests of Cognitive Ability*

[McGrew & Woodcock, 2001]) are, we do not expect that any of these tests will displace Wechsler's.

Yet computer technology is pervading nearly every aspect of life. Can computerized IQ tests geared to individual, clinical, psychoeducational, and neuropsychological assessment be too far off? Certainly not. At some point in the not-too-distant future, whether in 10 years or 20 years, a computerized IQ test will be nearly perfected. It will utilize the many possibilities of the multimedia capacities of CD-ROMs (or DVD-ROMs). It will make use of the Internet. It will have the potential to measure a person's response to stimuli with a level of perfection of which Galton could only have dreamed. It will use the point-and-click interactive capacity of the computer to take "verbal" measures in directions Binet could never have imagined.

And when that computerized IQ test finally hits the market, that test (or set of tests) may truly challenge the Wechsler domination of IQ measurement. It will be different from existing individual measures, and we believe that only something that represents radically different and new methodology has a chance of getting psychologists to abandon the tests they have grown up with, the tests that have benefited from more than 60 years of research (something that newer tests cannot boast, no matter how psychometrically sophisticated or theory driven they are).

But we believe the clinical approach of the Wechsler tests should not be abandoned completely. The examiner should remain an integral part of the test administration process; the child or adult being tested should not be left alone at a computer (or with a nonpsychologist). Test interpretation will, hopefully, still remain a function of integrating test behaviors with profiles of scores. Even if technology advances beyond our imagination, something will be lost the day that computerized assessment of IQ is reduced to evoked potentials, electroencephalograms, and eye blinks.

Whatever future tests are introduced and new controversies arise, we expect that IQ tests will continue on, even thrive, especially in the rehabilitation setting.

Authors' Note

The authors would like to dedicate this chapter to the memory of John Horn. The authors would like to acknowledge Julia H. Clark and Jim Flaitz, who contributed to an earlier edition of this chapter. The authors are also grateful to the following people for their contributions to this chapter: Drs. Nadeen L. Kaufman, Elaine Fletcher-Janzen, and Jack A. Naglieri. Nadeen and Elaine contributed primarily to the section on the KABC-II, and Jack contributed to the section on the Das-Naglieri CAS.

References

Binet, A., & Henri, V. (1895). La psychologie individuelle (Psychology of the individual). *L'Annee Psychologique, 2,* 411–465.

Brown, W. E., & McGuire, J. M. (1976). Current psychological assessment practices. *Professional Psychology, 7,* 475–485.

Carroll, J. B. (1943). The factorial representation of mental ability and academic achievement. *Educational and Psychological Measurement, 3,* 307–332.

Carroll, J. B. (1993). *Human cognitive abilities: A survey of factor-analytic studies.* Cambridge, UK: Cambridge University Press.

Carroll, J. B. (1995). Review of the book *Assessment of cognitive processes: The PASS theory of intelligence. Journal of Psychoeducational Assessment, 13,* 397–409.

Cronbach, L. J. (1984). *Essentials of psychological testing* (4th ed.). New York: Harper & Row.

Dennerll, R. D. (1964). Prediction of unilateral brain dysfunction using Wechsler test scores. *Journal of Consulting Psychology, 28,* 278–284.

Esters, I. G., Ittenbach, R. F., & Han, K. (1997). Today's IQ tests: Are they really better than their historical predecessors? *School Psychology Review, 26,* 211–223.

Flanagan, D. P. (1995). Review of the *Kaufman Adolescent and Adult Intelligence Test.* In J. C. Conoley & J. C. Impara (Eds.), *The twelfth mental measurements yearbook* (pp. 527–530). Lincoln, NE: Buros Institute of Mental Measurements of the University of Nebraska–Lincoln.

Flanagan, D. P., Alfonso, V. C., & Flanagan, R. (1994). A review of the *Kaufman Adolescent and Adult Intelligence Test*: An advancement in cognitive assessment? *School Psychology Review, 23,* 512–525.

Flanagan, D. P., & Kaufman, A. S. (2004). *Essentials of WISC-IV assessment.* New York: Wiley.

Flanagan, D. P., & McGrew, K. S. (1997). A cross-battery approach to assessing and interpreting cognitive abilities: Narrowing the gap between practice and cognitive science. In D. P. Flanagan, J. L. Genshaft, & P. L Harrison (Eds.), *Beyond traditional intellectual assessment: Contemporary and emerging theories, tests, and issues* (pp. 314–325). New York: Guilford Press.

Flanagan, D. P., McGrew, K. S., & Ortiz, S. (2000). *The Wechsler Intelligence Scales and Gf-Gc theory: A contemporary approach to interpretation.* Boston: Allyn & Bacon.

Flanagan, D. P., & Ortiz, S. (2001). *Essentials of cross-battery assessment.* New York: Wiley.

Galton, F. (1869). *Hereditary genius: An inquiry into its laws and consequences.* London: Macmillan.

Galton, F. (1883). *Inquiries into human faculty and its development.* London: Macmillan.

Gardner, H. (1983). *Frames of mind: The theory of multiple intelligences.* New York: Basic Books.

Georgas, J., Weiss, L. G., van de Vijver, F. J. R., & Saklofske, D. H. (Eds.). (2003). *Culture and children's intelligence: Cross-cultural analysis of the WISC-III.* San Diego, CA: Academic Press.

Goddard, H. H. (1911). A revision of the Binet Scale. *Training School, 8,* 56–62.

Golden, C. J. (1981). The Luria-Nebraska Children's Battery: Theory and formulation. In G. W. Hynd & J. E. Obrzut (Eds.), *Neuropsychological assessment of the school-age child* (pp. 277–302). New York: Grune & Stratton.

Horn, J. L. (1985). Old models of intelligence. In B. B. Wolman (Ed.), *Handbook of intelligence: Theories, measurements, and applications* (pp. 267–300). New York: Wiley.

Horn, J. L. (1989). Cognitive diversity: A framework of learning. In P. L. Ackerman, R. J. Sternberg, & R. Glaser (Eds.), *Learning and individual differences* (pp. 61–116). New York: Freeman.

Horn, J. L. (1991). Measurement of intellectual capabilities: A review of theory. In K. S. McGrew, J. K. Werder, & R. W. Woodcock (Eds.), *Woodcock-Johnson technical manual: A reference on theory and current research* (pp. 197–246). Allen, TX: DLM/Teaching Resources.

Horn, J. L., & Cattell, R. B. (1966). Refinement and test of the theory of fluid and crystallized intelligence. *Journal of Educational Psychology, 57,* 253–270.

Horn, J. L., & Cattell, R. B. (1967). Age difference in fluid and crystallized intelligence. *Acta Psychologica, 26,* 107–129.

Inhelder, B., & Piaget, J. (1958). *The growth of logical thinking from childhood to adolescence.* New York: Basic Books.

Johnson, J. A., & D'Amato, R. C. (2005). Test review of the Stanford-Binet Intelligence Scales (5th ed.). In R. A. Spies & B. S. Plake (Eds.), *The sixteenth mental measurements yearbook* [Electronic version]. Retrieved January 30, 2005, from http://www.unl.edu/buros

Johnstone, B., Schopp, L. H., Harper, J., & Koscuilek, J. (1999). Neurological impairments, vocational outcomes, and financial costs for individuals with traumatic brain injury receiving state vocational rehabilitation services. *Journal of Head Trauma Rehabilitation, 14*(3), 220–232.

Kaufman, A. S. (1983). Intelligence: Old concept—new perspectives. In G. W. Hynd (Ed.), *The school psychologist: An introduction* (pp. 95–117). Syracuse, NY: Syracuse University Press.

Kaufman, A. S. (1990). *Assessing adult and adolescent intelligence.* Boston: Allyn & Bacon.

Kaufman, A. S. (2000). Tests of intelligence. In R. J. Sternberg (Ed.), *Handbook of intelligence* (pp. 445–476). New York: Cambridge University Press.

Kaufman, A. S., & Horn, J. L. (1996). Age changes on tests of fluid and crystallized intelligence for females and males on the *Kaufman Adolescent and Adult Intelligence Test* (KAIT) at ages 17 to 94 years. *Archives of Clinical Neuropsychology, 11,* 97–121.

Kaufman, A. S., Ishikuma, T., & Kaufman, N. L. (1994). A Horn analysis of the factors measured by the WAIS-R, *Kaufman Adolescent and Adult Intelligence Test* (KAIT), and two new brief cognitive measures for normal adolescents and adults. *Assessment, 1,* 353–366.

Kaufman, A. S., Kaufman, J. C., Chen, T., & Kaufman, N. L. (1996). Differences on six Horn abilities for fourteen age groups between 15–16 and 75–94 years. *Psychological Assessment, 8,* 161–171.

Kaufman, A. S., & Kaufman, N. L. (1993). *Manual for Kaufman Adolescent &Adult Intelligence Test (KAIT).* Circle Pines, MN: American Guidance Service.

Kaufman, A. S., & Kaufman, N. L. (1997). The Kaufman Adolescent and Adult Intelligence Test (KAIT). In D.P. Flanagan, J. L. Genshaft, & P. L Harrison (Eds.), *Beyond traditional intellectual assessment: Contemporary and emerging theories, tests, and issues* (pp. 209–229). New York: Guilford Press.

Kaufman, A. S., & Kaufman, N. L. (2004). *Kaufman Assessment Battery for Children–Second Edition manual.* Circle Pines, MN: American Guidance Service.

Kaufman, A. S., & Lichtenberger, E. O. (1999). *Essentials of WAIS-III assessment.* New York: Wiley.

Kaufman, A. S., & Lichtenberger, E. O. (2006). *Assessing adult and adolescent intelligence* (3rd ed.). New York: Wiley.

Kaufman, A. S., Lichtenberger, E. O., Fletcher-Jansen, E., & Kaufman, N. L. (2005). *Essentials of KABC-II assessment.* New York: Wiley.

Keith, T. Z. (1995). Review of the *Kaufman Adolescent and Adult Intelligence Test.* In J. C. Conoley & J. C. Impara (Eds.), *The twelfth mental measurements yearbook* (pp. 530–532). Lincoln, NE: Buros Institute of Mental Measurements of the University of Nebraska–Lincoln.

Klove, H. (1959). Relationship of differential electroencephalographic patterns to distribution of Wechsler-Bellevue scores. *Neurology, 9,* 871–876.

Kuhlmann, F. (1912). A revision of the Binet-Simon system for measuring the intelligence of children. *Journal of Psych-Asthenics Monograph Supplement, 1,* 1–41.

Kush, J. C. (2005). Test review of the *Stanford-Binet Intelligence Scales–Fifth Edition*. In R. A. Spies & B. S. Plake (Eds.), *The sixteenth mental measurements yearbook* [Electronic version]. Retrieved January 30, 2005, from http://www.unl.edu/buros

Levy, J., & Trevarthen, C. (1976). Metacontrol of hemispheric function in human split-brain patients. *Journal of Experimental Psychology: Human Perception and Performance, 2*, 299–312.

Lichtenberger, E. O., & Kaufman, A. S. (2004). *Essentials of WPPSI-III assessment*. New York: Wiley.

Logie, R. H. (1995). *Visuo-spatial working memory*. Hove, East Sussex, UK: Erlbaum.

Luria, A. R. (1966). *Higher cortical functions in man*. New York: Basic Books.

Luria, A. R. (1973). *The working brain: An introduction to neuropsychology*. London: Penguin Books.

Luria, A. R. (1980). *Higher cortical functions in man* (2nd ed.). New York: Basic Books.

Luria, A. R., & Tsvetkova, L. S. (1990). *The neuropsychological analysis of problem solving* (A. Mikheyev & S. Mikheyev, Trans.). Orlando, FL: Paul M. Deutsch Press.

Martin, T. A., Donders, J., & Thompson, E. (2000). Potential of and problems with new measures of psychometric intelligence after traumatic brain injury. *Rehabilitation Psychology, 45*(4), 402–408.

Matarazzo, J. D. (1972). *Wechsler's measurement and appraisal of human intelligence* (5th ed.). Baltimore: Williams & Wilkins.

McGrew, K. S., & Flanagan, D. P. (1998). *The intelligence test desk reference (ITDR): Gf-Gc Cross-Battery assessment*. Boston: Allyn & Bacon.

Naglieri, J. A. (1999). *Essentials of CAS assessment*. New York: Wiley.

Naglieri, J. A., & Das, J. P. (1997a). *Cognitive Assessment System interpretive handbook*. Chicago: Riverside.

Naglieri, J. A., & Das, J. P. (1997b). *Das Naglieri Cognitive Assessment System*. Chicago: Riverside.

Naglieri, J. A., & Gottling, S. H. (1995). A cognitive education approach to math instruction for the learning disabled: An individual study. *Psychological Reports, 76*, 1343–1354.

Naglieri, J. A., & Gottling, S. H. (1997). Mathematics instruction and PASS cognitive processes: An intervention study. *Journal of Learning Disabilities, 30*, 513–520.

O'Connell, M. J. (2000). Prediction of return to work following traumatic brain injury: Intellectual, memory, and demographic variables. *Rehabilitation Psychology, 45*(2), 212–217.

Piaget, J. (1972). Intellectual evolution from adolescence to adulthood. *Human Development, 15*, 1–12.

Psychological Corporation. (1997). *WAIS-III and WMS-III technical manual*. New York: Psychological Corp.

Reitan, R. M. (1955). Certain differential effects of left and right cerebral lesions in human adults. *Journal of Comparative and Physiological Psychology, 48*, 474–477.

Reynolds, C. R. (1987). Playing IQ roulette with the Stanford–Binet–Fourth Edition. *Measurement and Evaluation in Counseling and Development, 20*, 139–141.

Richardson, J. T. E. (1996). Evolving concepts of working memory. In J. T. E. Richardson, R. W. Engle, L. Hasher, R. H. Logie, E. R. Stoltzfus, & R. T. Zacks (Eds.), *Working memory and human cognition* (pp. 3–30). New York: Oxford University Press.

Roid, G. H. (2003). *Stanford-Binet Intelligence Scales–Fifth Edition*. Itasca, IL: Riverside.

Roid, G. H. & Barram, R. A. (2004). *Essentials of Stanford-Binet Intelligence Scales (SB5) assessment*. New York: Wiley.

Sattler, J. M (2001). *Assessment of children: Cognitive applications* (4th ed.). San Diego, CA: Jerome M. Sattler.

Sharp, S. E. (1899). Individual psychology: A study in psychological method. *American Journal of Psychology, 10*, 329-391.

Smith, A. (1966). Verbal and nonverbal test performances of patients with "acute" lateralized brain lesions (tumors). *The Journal of Nervous and Mental Disease, 141,* 517–523.

Spearman, C. (1904). The proof and measurement of association between two things. *American Journal of Psychology, 15,* 72–101.

Sperry, R. W. (1968). Hemisphere deconnection and unity in conscious awareness. *American Psychologist, 23,* 723–733.

Sternberg, R. J. (1984). Toward a triarchic theory of human intelligence. *Behavioral and Brain Sciences, 7,* 269–287.

Sternberg, R. J. (1985). *Beyond IQ: A triarchic theory of human intelligence.* New York: Cambridge University Press.

Sternberg, R. J. (1993). Rocky's back again: A review of the WISC–III. In B. A. Bracken & R. S. McCallum (Eds.), *Journal of Psychoeducational Assessment monograph series, advances in psychoeducational assessment: Wechsler Intelligence Scale for Children–Third Edition* (pp. 161–164). Germantown, TN: Psychoeducational Corp.

Sternberg, R. J., & Kaufman, J. C. (1996). Innovation and intelligence tests: The curious case of the dog that didn't bark. *European Journal of Psychological Assessment, 12,* 167–174.

Sternberg, R. J., & Kaufman, J. C. (1998). Human abilities. *Annual Review of Psychology, 49,* 479–502.

Terman, L. M. (1916). *The measurement of intelligence.* Boston: Houghton Mifflin.

Terman, L. M., & Merrill, M. A. (1937). *Measuring intelligence.* Boston: Houghton Mifflin.

Thorndike, R. L., Hagen, E. P., & Sattler, J. M. (1986). *Technical manual for the Stanford Binet Intelligence Scale–Fourth Edition.* Chicago: Riverside.

Thurstone, L. L. (1938). Primary mental abilities. *Psychometric Monographs, 1.*

Watson, R. I. (1968). *The great psychologists from Aristotle to Freud* (2nd ed.). Philadelphia: Lippincott.

Wechsler, D. (1939). *Measurement of adult intelligence.* Baltimore: Williams & Wilkins.

Wechsler, D. (1946). *Manual for the Wechsler-Bellevue Intelligence Scale, Form II.* San Antonio, TX: Psychological Corp.

Wechsler, D. (1955). *Manual for the Wechsler Adult Intelligence Scale (WAIS).* San Antonio, TX: Psychological Corp.

Wechsler, D. (1958). *Measurement and appraisal of adult intelligence* (4th ed.). Baltimore: Williams & Wilkins.

Wechsler, D. (1981). *Manual for the Wechsler Adult Intelligence Scale Revised (WAIS-R).* San Antonio, TX: Psychological Corp.

Wechsler, D. (1991). *Manual for the Wechsler Intelligence Scale for Children–Third Edition* (WISC-III). San Antonio, TX: Psychological Corp.

Wechsler, D. (1997). *Manual for the Wechsler Adult Intelligence Scale–Third Edition* (WAIS-III). San Antonio, TX: Psychological Corp.

Wechsler, D. (2002). *Manual for the Wechsler Preschool and Primary Scale of Intelligence–Third Edition* (WPPSI-III). San Antonio, TX: Psychological Corp.

Wechsler, D. (2004). *Manual for the Wechsler Intelligence Scale for Children–Fourth Edition* (WISC-IV). San Antonio, TX: Psychological Corp.

Wissler, C. (1901). The correlation of mental and physical test (Monograph Supplement). *Psychological Review, 3*(6).

Woodcock, R. W. (1990). Theoretical foundations of the WJ-R measures of cognitive ability. *Journal of Psychoeducational Assessment, 8,* 231–258.

Woodcock, R. W., & Johnson, M. B. (1989). *Woodcock-Johnson—Revised, Tests of Cognitive Ability: Standard and supplemental batteries.* Chicago: Riverside.

Yoakum, C. S., & Yerkes, R. M. (1920). *Army mental tests.* New York: Henry Holt & Co.

Chapter 5

Aptitude Testing

Randall M. Parker

Aptitude tests are psychometric instruments designed to assess individuals' skills and abilities. Instruments falling within this category have been used by federal and state governments, private employers, and counseling and guidance professionals to improve the accuracy and efficiency of training and occupational plan development and in placement and selection decisions. Use of aptitude batteries may result in substantial savings in both human and financial costs. Schmidt and Hunter (1981), for example, estimated that if aptitude tests were uniformly used in selection, it would save $80 billion per year in 1980 dollars in national work force productivity. Furthermore, these tests have considerable potential in facilitating the planning and attainment of academic and vocational goals by persons with disabilities.

Using aptitude tests can be expensive and time-consuming. This fact leads to the question of whether they are worth the cost. Many rehabilitation professionals avoid formal aptitude testing by estimating the consumers' vocational abilities based on work history and the consumers' perceived strengths and weaknesses. These estimates then can be entered into computer programs that will list transferable skills and job possibilities.

Professionals may also use instruments that provide quick and easy assessment of an individual's interests and aptitudes. Many such instruments—for instance, the *Self-Directed Search* (SDS; Holland, Fritzsche, & Powell, 1994)—contain items asking individuals to rate their abilities. The SDS and similar tests are time efficient, easy to score, and highly regarded as reliable and valid instruments. There are, however, concerns about tests that involve consumer self-ratings of vocational aptitudes; such measures appear to contain more error and measure somewhat different constructs than traditional aptitude tests. Dunning (2005) reviewed the research on self-assessment and found that a large number of studies from many corners of psychology research suggest that, as a general rule, people's impressions of their abilities—whether arrogant or humble—are not anchored very closely to their actual level of skill. Across a large number of domains—from scholastic performance to leadership ability to clerical skills to professional knowledge—what people think about themselves can be quite distinct from the truth of their competence and expertise (p. 4).

A modest body of research on individuals' aptitude self-estimates suggests that such measures lack validity. Following a meta-analysis of 55 studies, Mabe and West (1982) reported that correlations between self-estimates of ability and test scores of college students and various workers averaged .29. Parker and Schaller (1994) studied the relationships between self-ratings and vocational aptitude and interest test scores. In their study, 564 students in the 8th grade from four middle schools rated 6 aptitudes and 12 interests and later completed the *Occupational Aptitude Survey and Interest Schedule* (OASIS; Parker, 1983). Correlations between the same-named constructs for self-ratings and test scores ranged from .10 to .56. More recently, in a study of the correspondence of interests, aptitudes, and occupational choice, Tracey and Hopkins (2001) found that rated abilities correlated about .44 with occupational choice.

This research suggests that aptitude self-ratings have relatively modest correlations with tested aptitudes and eventual occupational choice. The correlations suggest that there is substantial error in self-estimates and that self-ratings and aptitude scores measure somewhat different constructs. One cannot be substituted for the other without a substantial loss of information. Further research, however, is required to determine when self-ratings are adequate and when more formal psychometric measures are necessary in identifying vocational aptitudes. Until such research supports the use of self-ratings, rehabilitation professionals are taking a risk when they make decisions solely based on their clients' ratings of their aptitudes.

Although the issue of self-ratings versus tested aptitudes is an important topic, the emphasis of this chapter will be on definitions of aptitude, a brief history of aptitude testing, a description and evaluation of 10 aptitude batteries, and critical issues in aptitude assessment. The focus throughout is on multiple aptitude batteries that frequently prove useful in the vocational assessment of consumers in rehabilitation settings.

Definitions of Aptitude

There is considerable disagreement in the literature over the definition of the term *aptitude* and how it differs from *achievement*. Interestingly, aptitudes are regarded by many as relatively stable abilities that are innate or developed over a long period. For instance, Carroll (1985) stated that one should think of aptitude largely in terms of constitutional attributes of the individual (characteristics "built in" to the individual's brain and nervous system) that make for higher or lower degrees of success in learning. According to this view, an aptitude might be at least in part innate, or it could have developed over a long period as a result of the individual's experiences and activities. In any case, aptitudes are regarded as being relatively enduring (pp. 84–85).

Anastasi (1988) disagreed with this viewpoint. In comparing aptitude and achievement tests, she asserted that we should especially guard against the naive assumption that achievement tests measure the effects of learning, while aptitude tests measure "innate capacity" independent of learning. A useful concept that is coming to replace the traditional categories of aptitude and achievement in psychometrics is that of *developed abilities* (pp. 412–413).

Later, Carroll (1993) clarified his view of the differences between aptitude and achievement. An aptitude, he asserted, "helps in predicting degree of learning beyond a prediction from degree of prior learning" (p. 17). Achievement, however, refers to the "degree of learning in some procedure intended to produce learning such as a formal or informal course of instruction" (p. 17).

The notion that aptitude and achievement instruments are different is disputed by Aiken (2003). He asserted that it is now generally recognized that aptitude tests are measures of achievement, a complex product of the interaction between heredity and environmental influences. Conversely, if aptitude tests are psychometric instruments that can predict future accomplishments, then achievement tests that predict school marks and other performance criteria also qualify as measures of aptitude (p. 212).

Anastasi and Urbina (1997) present the predominant view today. They suggested that all tests of abilities, whether multiple aptitude batteries, general intelligence tests, or achievement tests, may be ordered along a continuum, ranging from specific to general, according to how much experiential background they presume. On this continuum, achievement tests are at one extreme, presuming highly specific experiences (e.g., completion of a course of study). Verbal intelligence and aptitude tests are closer to the general end of the spectrum, measuring basic cognitive skills that underlie individuals' performance in many activities. Finally, performance and cross-cultural ability tests lie at the end of extreme generality. These tests make the fewest presumptions regarding the individual's experiential background.

Brief History of Aptitude Testing

The notion that individuals possess varying levels of cognitive abilities may be traced back to the ancient Greeks and Chinese (DuBois, 1970). However, the first published empirical research on individual differences in mental abilities was done by Francis Galton (1869). His early findings suggested that intelligence tends to run in families. Galton's work inspired many early psychologists, including Charles Spearman.

Spearman proposed a theory asserting that all intellectual activities, including aptitudes, share a general factor he called *g* and that there were in addition numerous specific, or *s,* factors. Spearman's theory suggested that the goal of all intellectual tests should be to measure the general factor because this single general ability was common to all mental activities. Thus, a test measuring *g* would provide a single measure predictive of an individual's ability in a wide variety of endeavors (Anastasi, 1988).

Later theorists hypothesized the existence of multiple factors measuring different aspects of a person's aptitudes. Kelley (1928) indicated that there were several factors in the aptitude domain, including spatial, numerical, verbal, memory, and speed factors. Similarly, Thurstone (1938) proposed a set of primary mental abilities. Verbal comprehension, word fluency, number, space, associative memory, perceptual speed, and general reasoning were contained in his list of mental aptitudes. Subsequently, Guilford (1967) and Humphreys (1962) described more highly differentiated structures for aptitude and intellectual abilities. Not surprisingly, these theories and subsequent factor analytic studies led to the development of several multiple aptitude test batteries.

Description and Evaluation of Selected Aptitude Tests

To familiarize the reader with the major aptitude tests that may prove useful in rehabilitation settings, several aptitude batteries were identified for review. In selecting tests to present here, I relied heavily on Kapes and Whitfield's (2001b) *A Counselor's Guide to Career Assessment Instruments* and Aiken's (1998) *Tests and Examinations: Measuring Abilities and Performance.* Additional tests were identified from perusing volumes 12 through 16 of the *Mental Measurements Yearbook* (Conoley & Impara, 1995; Impara & Plake, 1998; Plake & Impara, 2001; Plake, Impara, & Spies, 2003; Spies & Plake, 2005).

Several criteria were used to develop a list of tests for review in this chapter. First, tests had to measure *vocationally relevant aptitudes,* as opposed to measures of intellectual or achievement-related constructs. Next, tests had to meet a criterion of *recency.* Tests with manuals that were published prior to 1990 were omitted (the *General Aptitude Test Battery* was an exception). Also, tests reviewed here were limited to those with *national norms for individuals of working age* and those judged to have *minimal technical information and research* supporting their reliability and validity. Finally, tests had to be *available for purchase* by qualified individuals (the *Armed Services Vocational Aptitude Battery* was an exception).

Of the multiple aptitude batteries, the *General Aptitude Test Battery* (GATB; U.S. Department of Labor, 1970), the *Armed Services Vocational Aptitude Battery* (ASVAB; U.S. Department of Defense, 1995, 1999), and the *Differential Aptitude Tests* (DAT; Psychological Corp., 1992) are the most widely used (Kapes & Whitfield, 2001a). Other multiple aptitude batteries reviewed include the *Ability Explorer* (AE; Harrington & Harrington, 1996), APTICOM (Harris & Danski, 1991), *Ball Aptitude Battery* (BAB; Ball Foundation, 1998a, 1998b, 1998c, 1998d), *CareerScope* (CS; Vocational Research Institute, 1998), *Career Planning Survey* (CPS; American College Testing Program, 1997, 1998, 1999), *Occupational Aptitude Survey and Interest Schedule–Third Edition* (OASIS-3; Parker, 2001), and PESCO 2001 (Loch, 1993a, 1993b, 1999). These 10 tests will be described and evaluated, and issues in aptitude assessment will be discussed in the remainder of this chapter.

GATB

The *General Aptitude Test Battery* (U.S. Department of Labor, 1970), whose validity has been seriously challenged in the last decade (Hartigan & Wigdor, 1989), is discussed here because it is primarily of historical interest. In my opinion it comprises the most sophisticated design and most rigorous scoring system related to job performance of any aptitude battery, although its norms are seriously out of date.

The GATB has nine aptitude factors, which were empirically derived through factor analytic studies and are measured by 12 subtests or parts. Eight of the subtests are paper-and-pencil tests, and four require manipulating objects (e.g., pegs in a pegboard). It takes approximately 2.5 hours to administer the complete GATB (U.S. Department of Labor, 1970). Table 5.1 shows the factors and subtests of the GATB.

The GATB incorporated two approaches to scoring and interpretation. The first involves multiple cutoff scores on the most relevant aptitudes for

TABLE 5.1.
GATB Factors and Their Subtests

GATB Factor	GATB Subtest
G—General Learning Ability	Part 3. Three-Dimensional Space
	Part 4. Vocabulary
	Part 6. Arithmetic Reason
V—Verbal Aptitude	Part 4. Vocabulary
N—Numeric Aptitude	Part 2. Computation
	Part 6. Arithmetic Reason
S—Spatial Aptitude	Part 3. Three-Dimensional Space
P—Form Perception	Part 5. Tool Matching
	Part 7. Form Matching
Q—Clerical Perception	Part 1. Name Comparison
K—Motor Coordination	Part 8. Mark Making
F—Finger Dexterity	Part 11. Assemble
	Part 12. Disassemble
M—Manual Dexterity	Part 9. Place
	Part 10. Turn

66 groups of jobs that are similar in requisite abilities. For each group, an Occupational Aptitude Pattern (OAP) has been developed containing cutoff scores on two to four aptitude factors indicating high, medium, and low levels of aptitudes necessary for the job. An individual's pertinent scores on the GATB may be compared to the cutoffs of the OAPs to determine which jobs the person will likely be able to perform successfully.

The second approach, referred to as the VG-GATB, was developed through a process called validity generalization (VG). The VG process determined that the nine GATB factors could be combined to form three composites without losing predictive power. The three composites and their factor components are Cognitive (G, V, N), Perceptual (S, P, Q), and Psychomotor (K, F, M). The three composite scores are then compared to the necessary level of composite aptitudes for five job families across 66 worker trait groups.

Data regarding the technical qualities of the GATB are so extensive that it is difficult to summarize. Suffice it to say that the test-retest and alternate form reliabilities for the 12 GATB subtests, as well as for the Cognitive, Perceptual, and Psychomotor composites, generally are high relative to those for other multiple aptitude tests. Validity evidence is similarly positive. Excellent critiques of the GATB and its psychometric properties can be found in Kirnan (2005), Hartigan and Wigdor (1989), and Bolton (1994).

Despite extensive research concerning the GATB and VG–GATB, serious limitations restricted their widespread use. One limitation is that the GATB is restricted for use by the United States Employment Service (USES) and is available only to nonprofit organizations that have personnel trained in GATB administration and scoring. Another limitation is that the subtests are highly speeded, putting certain groups at a disadvantage (i.e., people with certain disabilities and people unfamiliar with test taking). Additionally, the most recent forms, Forms C and D, were published in 1983. Moreover, the initial norms were developed in the 1950s to be representative of the populace as reflected in the 1940 census. More recent norms are based on convenience samples that are not representative of the groups they are intended to describe. A final issue concerns the GATB and VG–GATB's use of subgroup norms. Subgroup norming, which involved setting lower raw cutting scores for minority groups, caused a congressional political debate focusing on reverse discrimination. This debate, in turn, led to the passage of the Civil Rights Act of 1991 (P.L. 102-166), which prohibits subgroup norming (Urbina, 2004). The GATB is currently out of print and no longer used for job placement in government employment agencies (Anastasi & Urbina, 1997; Kirnan, 2005; Schmidt & Hunter, 2003).

Because of the difficulties concerning the GATB, the Department of Labor has replaced it with the O★NET Ability Profiler (AP), which was developed to improve the technical and operational characteristics of the GATB. The AP incorporates 11 of the GATB's 12 subtests; Form Matching was deleted. The AP contains (a) a reduced number of items and subtests, including items free from bias; (b) new instructions that include appropriate test-taking strategies for each of the subtests; (c) reduced speededness of certain subtests; (d) enhanced legibility and comprehension level of all written materials; (e) modernized typography and layout for test booklets, test items, answer sheets, and the Administration Manual; and (f) a self-interpretable O★NET Ability Profiler Score Report. The Score Report connects the users' results to O★NET occupations and information and compares examinees' profiles with typical ability profiles for workers in O★NET occupations (U.S. Department of Labor Employment and Training Administration, 2002).

Downloads of test materials, manuals, and scoring software are available at no cost at their Web site (http://www.onetcenter.org/AP.html). On the one hand, O★NET is to be commended for having the AP materials in the public domain. On the other hand, this circumstance creates concerns over test security and maintaining standards over who administers the battery. Although the *AP User's Manual* (U.S. Department of Labor Employment and Training Administration, 2002) contains considerable information about the development of the AP, it has not been separately reviewed in this chapter because the *AP Technical Manual,* containing information on reliability and validity, is still in development.

ASVAB

The *Armed Services Vocational Aptitude Battery* (ASVAB; U.S. Department of Defense, 1995, 1999), the most widely administered multiple aptitude battery, was developed for classification and selection of potential recruits between the ages of 16 and 23 for the U.S. military (U.S. Department of Defense, 1995, 1999). It contains 10 subtests (see Table 5.2) that require approximately 3 hours to administer. Rogers (2001) indicates that a computer adaptive testing (CAT) version of the test is in use.

Various composites have been developed for different purposes. For example, four subtests (AR, WK, PC, and MK) compose the *Armed Forces Qualification Test* (AFQT), which is used to screen potential recruits into the armed services. Profiles of the 10 scores may also be used by school counselors in educational and vocational guidance. Additional components include a Career Exploration Program and a computer adaptive testing version of the ASVAB.

Considerable information concerning the reliability and validity of the ASVAB with young adults is available. Alternate form reliabilities for Forms 8, 9, and 10 of the ASVAB range from .57 to .90 with a median of .79. Reliabilities of the composite scores tend to be somewhat higher. The mean weighted predictive validity for the AFQT composite was estimated by Hartigan and Wigdor (1989) to be about .33, similar to the mean validities for the VG–GATB composites. Validity at this level is considered acceptable for aiding in the prediction of training outcomes and perhaps job performance.

Norms for the ASVAB are based on data gathered in 1980 from a nationally representative sample of 9,173 people (4,550 men and 4,623 women) between the ages of 16 and 23. Certain minority groups were oversampled to provide more accurate estimates of their performance. Using these data, norms were developed separately for males and females in grades 10, 11, and 12 and in postsecondary education.

TABLE 5.2.
ASVAB Subtests

- General Science (GS)
- Work Knowledge (WK)
- Paragraph Comprehension (PC)
- Electronics Information (EI)
- Code Speed (CS)
- Arithmetic Reasoning (AR)
- Mathematics Knowledge (MK)
- Mechanical Comprehension (MC)
- Auto and Shop Information (AS)
- Numerical Operations (NO)

Among the obvious limitations are the datedness of the norms, the restricted access to the test, and the speededness of 2 of the 10 subtests. Additionally, the composite scores are calculated using some of the same tests, resulting in high correlations with each other. In a similar vein, the ASVAB scores tend to load highly on general ability (g). As a result, the test does not yield differential information on multiple aptitudes—information necessary for successfully placing people in different jobs. In a thorough review and critique of the ASVAB, Elmore and Bradley (1994) concluded that the ASVAB and the accompanying career exploration program are recommended "for everyone considering joining the military within two years . . . [and] for those who wish to avail themselves of a free career exploration program. However, until more studies of the ASVAB Career Exploration Program are completed, we would not recommend it for all high school students" (p. 77). Rogers (2001) is more sanguine in his review, stating that "the ASVAB is one of the finest examples available of a multiple-aptitude battery based on its superb psychometrics, extensive norming data, and excellent materials" (p. 99). He does, however, note concerns over the test's predictive validity for civilian occupations and possible bias regarding Hispanic and African American students.

DAT

The *Differential Aptitude Tests* (DAT; Psychological Corp., 1992), first published in 1947, were designed for use with young adults in grades 7 through 12 and with adults for vocational and educational guidance (Psychological Corp., 1992). Additional options available with the DAT include a Career Interest Inventory and a computer adaptive testing version of the DAT. The eight subtests of the DAT, which require a total of 156 minutes of administration time, are displayed in Table 5.3.

TABLE 5.3.
DAT Subtests

- Verbal Reasoning
- Numerical Reasoning
- Abstract Reasoning
- Perceptual Speed and Accuracy
- Mechanical Reasoning
- Space Relations
- Spelling
- Language Usage

The eight constructs measured by DAT subtests were derived rationally, rather than empirically—that is, the subtests represent aptitudes that the DAT authors considered vocationally and educationally important. In addition to scores on the eight subtests, a composite score, Scholastic Aptitude, is obtained from combining the Verbal Reasoning and Numerical Reasoning subtest scores.

A wealth of reliability and validity information is available for the DAT. Internal consistency and alternate forms reliabilities range from the .70s through the .90s for all subtests across all grade-level-by-gender groupings. Abundant concurrent validity information is presented in the DAT manual (Psychological Corp., 1992).

Norms for the DAT are based on 192,000 students from 520 school districts for grades 7 though 12. The amount of normative data is vast, and the norms were developed to be proportionate in terms of geographic region, socio-economic status, residence in rural or urban areas, ethnicity, and attendance at public or nonpublic schools using nationwide school enrollment statistics. However, several of the subtest scores are highly intercorrelated (e.g., Verbal Reasoning correlates .70 with Language Usage), limiting the usefulness of the scores in making differential predictions for different training activities or jobs.

As previously noted, a computer adaptive edition of the DAT is also available. This version is taken and scored by a computer using computer adaptive testing methodology. Through this approach, test items are presented based on the correctness of previous responses, allowing testing time to be markedly abbreviated. Although this version holds promise, its psychometric properties are not adequate for general use (see Wise, 1995). A DAT for Personnel and Career Assessment is another specialized form developed for use with adults in training and employment settings. This version has strengths and limitations that are similar to those of the standard DAT (Willson, 1995; Wing, 1995).

In conclusion, the evidence is generally highly supportive of the DAT, although the relative lack of construct, predictive, and incremental validity information in the manual is problematic (Willson & Stone, 1994). Similarly, Hattrup (1995) stated that "the most serious weakness of the battery continues to be the lack of evidence of differential validity for different criteria, and incremental validity of specific subtests in prediction contexts . . . . Evidence of the DAT's validity as a predictor of job performance is still absent in the latest revision" (p. 304). Wang (2001), echoing these concerns, calls for more information on construct validity, norms for ethnic minorities, and additional criterion-related validity evidence. Finally, Bragger and Becker (2005), while noting its substantial strengths, pointed out that jobs in the U.S. economy have changed markedly since the publication of the latest edition. Professionals using this test must keep this in mind when interpreting the results for clients.

While the DAT is the best established aptitude test commercially available, it embodies limitations that should alert professionals using this instrument to use it cautiously. Counselors interpreting the results for individual clients must keep in mind that no test, including the DAT, provides uniformly accurate information upon which to make vocational predictions.

AE

The *Ability Explorer* (AE: Harrington & Harrington, 1996, 2006) was developed to provide students and adults with information concerning how their abilities relate to the world of work. It has 14 subtests: Artistic, Clerical, Interpersonal, Language, Leadership, Manual, Musical/Dramatic, Numerical/Mathematical, Organizational, Persuasive, Scientific, Social, Spatial, and Technical/Mechanical. Two levels of the AE are machine-scorable only. Level 1 is for grades 6 through 8, while Level 2 is for grades 9 through 12 and adults. These versions have three parts. Part One contains 140 items that ask how good examinees are, or would be, at doing an activity. Part Two has 112 activities with response options of 1 (tried activity and did not do well), 2 (tried activity and did it well), 3 (tried activity and did it very well), and NT (never tried the activity). Part Three lists school subjects, and the examinees indicate their grades for courses they have taken. The AE is untimed but usually takes between 35 and 45 minutes. There also is a hand-scorable version of the AE, which is written at the 8th-grade level and contains the same 140 items that are in Part One described above.

This instrument can be used with groups or individuals. It directly links to career guidance and counseling literature and to resources from the U.S. Department of Labor, particularly the *Occupational Outlook Handbook* (published biennially).

The AE was normed on more than 8,000 people and has been used in many settings. The Cronbach alpha reliabilities for the AE are modest to high, ranging from .55 to .91. Content validity was established by building the test based on the *Guide for Occupational Exploration* (Harrington & O'Shea, 1984). Concurrent validities with the GATB, however, are modest to very low. No predictive validity studies are reported in the manual (Borman, 2001).

Given that the AE bases aptitude estimates on self-ratings, as opposed to objectively tested aptitudes, it should be used with great caution. As discussed previously, self-ratings are subject to considerable error. Basing vocational plans solely on how individuals perceive their aptitudes and abilities may lead to very poor decisions and unnecessary failures. Nonetheless, the AE is a well-constructed instrument that can contribute to the career development of rehabilitation consumers when used with caution by trained professionals in the context of a counseling relationship.

APTICOM

APTICOM (Harris & Danski, 1991) is a computer-based, vocational assessment system intended for adolescents and adults reading at the 4th grade level or above. This instrument contains a multiple aptitude battery as well as an interest test. This review will discuss the aptitude battery, which requires about 45 minutes of administration time.

This instrument is unique in that it is totally contained in a personal computer without a keyboard or monitor. Examinees respond by using 2-foot by 3-foot templates containing several rows and columns of switch ports. They select from multiple alternatives for some subtests or perform manipulative tasks on other subtests by inserting a wired probe into a port. Other manipulative tasks are performed with external devices (e.g., a foot switch) that interface with the computer. The administrator controls the progress of the test by using buttons and switches on the back of the computer.

The APTICOM, designed to measure 10 aptitudes assessed by the GATB, has 11 subtests: Object Identification, Abstract Shape Matching, Clerical Matching, Eye–Hand–Foot Coordination, Pattern Visualization, Computation, Finger Dexterity, Numerical Reasoning, Manual Dexterity, Word Meaning, and Eye–Hand Coordination. The 10 aptitudes assessed by the subtests are General Learning Ability (G), Verbal Aptitude (V), Numerical Aptitude (N), Spatial Aptitude (S), Form Perception (P), Clerical Perception (C), Motor Coordination (K), Finger Dexterity (F), Manual Dexterity (M), and Eye–Hand–Foot Coordination (E).

Information on the reliability and validity is somewhat limited. Test-retest reliabilities with a 1-week interval for 67 trade school students revealed coefficients of .65–.89; reliabilities for Dexterity, Coordination, and Clerical Perception tended to be at the lower end of this range. Similarly, concurrent validity was demonstrated by correlating scores from the APTICOM with those from the GATB for a sample of 417 individuals. The coefficients ranged from the .60s to .80s for General Learning Ability, Verbal Aptitude, Numerical Aptitude, Spatial Aptitude, Form Perception, and Clerical Perception. Lower coefficients were obtained for Motor Coordination, Finger Dexterity, and Manual Dexterity subtests.

Information concerning the norms for the APTICOM has not been clearly reported, which is a significantly negative factor. Similarly, the limited validity and reliability studies are a major concern. Considering the high cost of the APTICOM ($6,000 in 1994) and limited normative, reliability, and validity information, a prospective user would be well-advised to consider another instrument with a more solid psychometric foundation (Green, 1994). The APTICOM is no longer being produced, although refurbished versions are still available (Instructional Technologies, 2006; see http://www.intecinc .net/prod_vri_apticom.htm).

BAB

The *Ball Aptitude Battery* (BAB; Ball Foundation, 1998a, 1998b, 1998c, 1998d) was developed to provide an objective aptitude assessment to assist individuals in career planning. Form M of the BAB has 12 paper and pencil subtests measuring Analytical Reasoning, Associative Memory, Auditory Memory Span, Clerical, Idea Generation, Inductive Reasoning, Numerical Computation, Numerical Reasoning, Paper Folding, Vocabulary, Word Association, and Writing Speed. The 12 subtests in Form M, which take 2 hours and 10 minutes to administer, may be grouped into seven categories: Speed and Accuracy, Memory, Reasoning, Academic, Spatial, Creativity, and Orientation. Five additional subtests not included in Form M may be used to provide extra information; the five subtests are Shape Assembly, Idea Fluency, Finger Dexterity, Grip Strength, and Karma Music Test.

The BAB has two levels. Level 1A is for 9th and 10th grade students and Level 2A is for 11th-grade students, 12th-grade students, and adults. The BAB can be scored only through a machine scoring service; hand scoring or local machine scoring is not available.

Test-retest reliabilities with 2- to 6-week intervals had a median of .79, while test-retest reliabilities over a 4-year period had a median of .50. Internal consistency reliabilities had a median of .80. Concurrent validities of the BAB with the DAT, GATB, and the *Comprehensive Ability Battery* had a median of .63 (Thompson & Patrick, 2001).

The BAB appears to be a well-designed instrument. It should be effective in rehabilitation settings as a counseling tool for individuals who can take traditional paper-and-pencil tests.

CS

The *CareerScope* (CS; Vocational Research Institute, 1998) is a self-administered, computer-based battery that measures both aptitudes and interests. The software can be installed on a single Windows machine or on a network. The CS is available in Spanish or English and has an audio version that provides an orientation, gives test instructions, and reads interest items to the examinee. The interests measured are the 12 interests identified by the U.S. Department of Labor (1979) and include Artistic, Plants/Animals, Mechanical, Business Detail, Accommodating, Lead/Influence, Scientific, Protective, Industrial, Selling, Humanitarian, and Physical Performing interests. This review will focus on the aptitude section, which has subtests measuring General Learning Ability, Verbal Aptitude, Numerical Aptitude, Spatial Aptitude, Form Perception, and Clerical Perception. The battery, which has a 4th-grade reading level, takes about 1 hour to complete. The CE appears to be an update and extension of the APTICOM.

Harris (2001) reported that only a few reliability and validity studies have been completed. Reliabilities ranged from .the .50s to the .80s. Concurrent validity coefficients with the GATB ranged from the .30s to .80s.

In summary, the CS is a computer-based aptitude and interest assessment system that would be useful in rehabilitation settings for individuals with disabilities that do not preclude operating a computer. The technical data are meager. Therefore, the CS should be used with care for counseling and guidance rather than prediction or placement purposes.

CPS

The *Career Planning Survey* (CPS; American College Testing Program, 1997, 1998, 1999) is a comprehensive system whose purpose is to help young adults gain self-awareness, learn about the structure of the world of work, and explore personally relevant vocational options. The CPS contains several components, including the *Unisex Edition of the ACT Interest Inventory* (UNIACT) and the *Inventory of Work-Relevant Abilities* (IWRA). Optional academic ability tests include a reading test and a numerical abilities test. The UNIACT is scored on six career clusters—Business Contact, Business Operations, Technical, Science, Arts, and Social Service. The IWRA has 15 work-related areas on which students rate themselves. The 15 areas are Meeting People, Helping Others, Sales, Leadership (Management), Organization, Clerical, Mechanical, Manual Dexterity, Numerical, Scientific, Creative/Artistic, Creative/Literary, Reading, Language Usage, and Spatial Perception. This review focuses on the IWRA, which requires about 23 minutes of testing time and has norms on more than 16,000 students (Reardon & Vernick, 2001).

Much of the extensive validity information presented for the IWRA is based on correlations between the IWRA and UNIACT. Although the validity data presented for the IWRA are extensive, one must be concerned that much of the supporting information is based on correlations of self-reported interests (UNIACT) with self-rated aptitudes (IWRA). At the beginning of this chapter, serious questions concerning self-ratings of aptitudes were noted. This concern is compounded when self-reported interests are used as a criterion for self-estimated aptitudes. One can speculate that a substantial portion of these correlations may be due to aspects unrelated to the constructs of interests and aptitudes, namely that both instruments use similar subjective ratings of work-related items. Nevertheless, the ACT CPS is a well-constructed battery that can contribute to the career development of middle and high school students when used with caution by trained professionals in the context of a counseling relationship.

OASIS-3

The purpose of the *Occupational Aptitude Survey and Interest Schedule–Third Edition* (OASIS-3; Parker, 2001) is to assist adults and students in Grades 8 through 12 in self-exploration, vocational exploration, and career development. It contains a separate interest inventory (Interest Schedule) and aptitude battery (Aptitude Survey). The Interest Schedule has 12 scales that were developed from the *Guide for Occupational Exploration* (U.S. Department of Labor, 1979): Artistic,

Scientific, Nature, Protective, Mechanical, Industrial, Business Detail, Selling, Accommodating, Humanitarian, Leading–Influencing, and Physical Performing. This review will focus on the Aptitude Survey (AS) component of the OASIS-3.

The AS has five subtests (see Table 5.4), which require 45 minutes to administer. In addition to the five factors listed in Table 5.4, a General Ability composite score is obtained by summing the Vocabulary and Computation raw scores.

The AS manual reports alpha, split-half, alternate forms, and test-retest reliabilities. Reliabilities range from .70 to .94 with a median of .86, suggesting adequate reliability for career exploration. Four types of construct validity are also reported, including evidence from factor analysis, internal consistency, relationships with other tests, and convergent and discriminant validity. Using exploratory factor analysis, Parker (2002) found that 73% of the variance in the 12 GATB subtests was accounted for by five factors, labeled Verbal, Numerical, Spatial, Perceptual, and Manual Dexterity aptitudes. This finding led to the development of the OASIS, which is a much shorter battery consisting of five subtests (instead of 12 used in the GATB) and requiring a 45-minute administration time (versus 150 minutes for the GATB and 156 minutes for the DAT). Correlations between the AS and GATB aptitude factors ranged from .37 to .84, with similar factors correlating .61 to .84. These latter levels of validity coefficients are consistent with *reliability coefficients* typically reported for aptitude batteries. This finding suggests that the AS may be viewed as a reliable, short form of the GATB. Convergent and discriminant validities reported for the AS are supportive, although long-term predictive validity studies have not been done (Blackwell, 2003).

Norms are based on a nationally representative sample of 2,005 adults in postsecondary education and students in Grades 8 through 12. The upward extension of the norms to include adults is a new addition to the OASIS-3. In reviewing the previous edition, Miller and Hollingshead (2001) indicated that the OASIS-2 AS and IS are particularly valuable tools in early career explora-

TABLE 5.4.

Aptitude Factors and Subtests of the OASIS–3 Aptitude Survey

Aptitude Factor	Subtest
Verbal Aptitude	Vocabulary
Numerical Aptitude	Computation
Spatial Aptitude	Spatial Relations
Perceptual Aptitude	Word Comparison
Manual Dexterity	Making Marks

tion for both the general population and early senior high school levels. "These tests could be easily included as a portion of a career exploration unit in either English or Social Studies classes . . . [The OASIS-2] is a well-designed and well-researched [instrument that] . . . should be a valuable tool for vocational exploration and career development activities for students of junior and senior school age" (pp. 154–156).

PESCO

The PESCO 2001 ONLINE (Loch, 1993a, 1993b, 1999; www.pesco.org) was developed to screen individuals from grade 8 through college for jobs and training programs and to use in educational and vocational counseling. It is an online extension of its predecessor, the *System for Assessment and Group Evaluation* (SAGE). The PESCO 2001 contains six tests—the Vocational Aptitude Battery (VAB), Cognitive and Conceptual Abilities Test (C-CAT), Center for Innovative Teaching Experience Learning Styles Inventory (CITE LSI), Work Attitudes Assessment (WAA), Vocational Interest Inventory (VII), and Temperament Factor Assessment (TFA).

The VAB is scored on 11 aptitude factors similar to those found in the GATB that include General, Verbal, Numerical, Form Perception, Color Discrimination, Clerical Perception, Spatial, Motor Coordination, Finger Dexterity, Manual Dexterity, and Eye–Hand–Foot Coordination. The C-CAT subtests are Language, Math, and Reasoning. Test results yield General Educational Development (GED) levels and U.S. Department of Labor Secretary's Commission on Achieving Necessary Skills (SCANS) levels. The CITE LSI measures preferred learning styles in terms of sensory modalities, social preferences, and written or oral expressiveness. The WAA assesses attitudes concerning the world of work and employer expectations. The VII measures the 12 interest factors identified in the *Guide for Occupational Exploration* (U.S. Department of Labor, 1979), as do several of the aforementioned instruments. Finally, the TFA assesses 11 temperament factors related to specific work environments (Rojewski, 2001).

Overall, the PESCO 2001 system is a comprehensive vocational assessment system. Rojewski (2001, p. 163) concluded that "despite some concerns with instrument validity, TFA and VII in particular, professionals in vocational rehabilitation facilities, career assessment centers, and job training/placement services should find PESCO 2001 a valuable assessment tool." The validity and reliability of the VAB, which is the PESCO subtest relevant to the topic of this chapter, was regarded as "generally acceptable" (Rojewski, 2001, p. 162).

Recommendations

In summary, the 10 multiple aptitude batteries meeting criteria of vocational focus, recency, technical adequacy, and availability include three tests (GATB,

ASVAB, and DAT) with longstanding reputations for excellence. Because the GATB and ASVAB are not readily available for purchase, rehabilitation professionals should seriously consider using the DAT when selecting vocational aptitude tests for guidance and counseling with consumers. The other tests (AE, APTICOM, BAB, CS, CPS, OASIS-3, and PESCO) all show promise but should be used with caution.

When a consumer's future plans are at stake, care must be taken in judiciously selecting, administering, and interpreting psychometric instruments. Many rehabilitation professionals use psychological and vocational reports provided by psychologists or other professionals. Special caution must also be exercised in evaluating and using information from professional reports. It is usually not the use, but the *misuse,* of tests that leads to problems. In the next section, several problem areas in aptitude and general test usage are discussed.

Problems in Aptitude Assessment

The use of aptitude tests to assist and evaluate individuals has many problems. Several of the more salient issues are presented here, including (a) interpretation of test results; (b) reliability, validity, and VG; (c) general versus special norms; and (d) clinical versus statistical prediction.

Interpretation of Test Results

A number of technical aids or methods help rehabilitation professionals present testing data cogently to individuals without becoming overly subjective. These aids may be divided into two groups: descriptive and predictive interpretive methods. Norms and test profiles are included in the descriptive category. They present information regarding the individual's standing relative to the performance of other similar individuals. The professional counselor is required to extrapolate, or make educated guesses, to develop statements of what descriptive data mean in terms of the individual's future. Predictive methods, however, allow the professional to use probability statements regarding the success of an individual's future plans. Such predictive approaches include expectancy tables, multiple cutoff procedures, and regression and discriminant equations.

Descriptive Methods

Norms are the most basic kind of interpretative aid at the descriptive level. They allow the professional to describe the individual's level of performance relative to an appropriate comparison group. Raw scores, usually taken as the number of items answered correctly, are totally meaningless in and of themselves. Knowing that an individual answered 50 items correctly on a verbal ability test gives no information whatsoever about the relative level of performance. If, however, it had been previously established that a raw score of 50 on this test was equivalent to the average performance of college graduates, the score would be meaningful.

Tables of norms allow professionals to convert raw scores to more meaningful derived scores, such as percentiles. A percentile score refers to the percentage of people in the standardization sample who obtained lower raw scores. Percentile scores are the most frequently reported and the most easily understood derived scores.

Considerable judgment must be exercised in selecting the proper table of norms when several are available. Rehabilitation personnel often wonder whether to use norms based on general groups or norms based on groups of people with a disability when interpreting the test scores of rehabilitation consumers. This question is discussed in more detail later.

A profile is another method of displaying descriptive information. It is a graphic, comparative representation of test scores in several areas. Profiling test scores can provide individuals with an extremely meaningful picture of their relative performance on a series of scales. However, profiles not meeting the following three basic requirements may be extremely misleading. First, *subtests or scales* reported on a profile must be similar in content and nature. Profiling scores from both aptitude and interest tests side by side, for instance, may confuse both the individual and the professional. Second, the *measurement units* must be the same across the whole profile. The whole profile should be plotted in terms of the same derived score (e.g., percentiles). Third, the *standardization and normative samples* upon which the derived scores are based must be similar (ideally the same) from subtest to subtest. Once these requirements are met, test score profiles are among the most useful tools in the professional's repertoire of interpretive aids (Cronbach, 1990).

Predictive Methods

One of the techniques used to predict success from test scores is the *multiple-cutoff approach*. Test authors, researchers, local institutions, and agencies frequently develop cutoff scores for use in their selection procedures. For example, employers often use cutoff scores on tests of clerical aptitude in the selection of job applicants for clerical positions. To develop cutoff scores, one first determines which measures are most important in the performance of a job or other criterion task. Then, for each of the selected measures, a cutoff score is statistically computed so that there is maximal differentiation between successful and unsuccessful workers. Each cutoff score represents the lowest amount of each important characteristic a person can have to succeed in a particular job or task.

The GATB used the multiple-cutoff procedure. According to research by the USES, three aptitudes are essential for a Counselor II: General Intelligence, Verbal Aptitude, and Clerical Perception. To be minimally equipped to handle the job, an applicant is expected to score at the 60th percentile on each of the three aptitudes. If an applicant scored substantially above the 60th percentile on two aptitudes but fell substantially below the required level on one, the applicant would be regarded as not meeting the minimal aptitude qualifications of the job. The multiple-cutoff approach, then, assumes that a superior aptitude in one area does not compensate for a substandard aptitude in another important area (Anastasi, 1988).

Another technique for predicting success based on test scores is the *expectancy table,* an easily constructed tool. A simple expectancy table depicts the relationship between one predictor variable and a criterion variable—for instance, IQ (predictor) versus grades in college (criterion). Table 5.5 demonstrates the relationship between scores on the College Qualification Tests (CQT) and grade point average (GPA). Inspection of the table reveals that those receiving high CQT scores tended to get A and B grades (39%), while those with low CQT scores tended to obtain D and F grades (80%). For similar samples, one could generalize these results. That is, if a person received a high CQT score, one could estimate that his or her chances of having an A or B average would be approximately 39 out of 100 (Wesman, 1966).

Rehabilitation professionals can readily construct their own tables when they possess both the initial test scores and eventual outcome data for a group of individuals. The first step in constructing an expectancy table is to categorize both the predictor and the criterion variables into meaningful units; for instance, one could categorize verbal reasoning scorers into high, medium, and low groups. The final step is to fill in the cells of the expectancy table with the data that were gathered both in raw frequencies and in percentages. Expectancy tables are like extended versions of norms tables: They show the relationship between the test score and an outcome or criterion variable.

TABLE 5.5.

Relationship Between CQT Total Score and
GPA in a Sample of Men ($N = 1,340$)

CQT Total	GPA			Total (%)
	D and F (%)	C (%)	A and B (%)	
High	16	45	39	100
Middle	43	50	7	100
Low	80	19	2	100

Note. High means the score fell in the 70th–99th percentile range; middle, in the 30th–69th percentile range; and low, in the 0–29th percentile range.

Source. Reprinted with permission from A. Wesman, Double-Entry Expectancy Tables, *Test Service Bulletin,* No. 56, May 1966, of The Psychological Corporation, a Harcourt Assessment Company.

Regression and *discriminant equations* are also used to predict success using test scores. These equations are sophisticated statistical techniques involving multiple linear regression and discriminant analysis. Regression analysis is a method allowing one to compute the importance of predictor variables to a criterion. For instance, this technique could be used to determine weights to be applied to measures of verbal and numerical aptitude in predicting success as an accountant. Regression analysis allows the development of weights so that when each weight is multiplied by its respective predictor score and the products are summed, the result is an estimate of the criterion. For example, if the criterion of success as an accountant were a supervisor's rating of work performance on a 5-point scale, the regression equation would yield a prediction of the supervisor's rating on a scale of 1 to 5.

Discriminant equations are similar in nature, although their ultimate purpose is somewhat different. These equations may be used to determine an individual's similarity to one or more groups using a number of test scores. In contrast to a regression equation, which yields a predicted criterion score, a discriminant equation provides a score that can be compared with discriminant scores of other groups. If an individual receives a discriminant score that is similar to those of a specific group (e.g., successful rehabilitation counselors), this indicates probable membership in that group. The reader may refer to Anastasi and Urbina (1997) and Goldman (1971) for more detailed, nontechnical discussions of regression and discriminant methods.

Reliability, Validity, and VG

Reliability and validity, discussed extensively elsewhere in this *Handbook*, are of paramount importance in test evaluation. Relatively high degrees of both reliability and validity are some of the major distinguishing characteristics of multiple aptitude tests. Comprehensive surveys indicate that the reliabilities for aptitude, achievement, intelligence, and other similar tests tend to cluster in the high .80s and low .90s. In contrast, reliabilities for personality, interest, and attitude measures tend to fall in the high .70s and low .80s. This comprehensive picture supports the assertion that the reliabilities of aptitude and related ability tests tend to be superior to those of other types of tests (Helmstadter, 1964; Siebel, 1968). Lower reliabilities should be regarded with suspicion, particularly for instruments intended for classification or selection of job or program applicants.

When compared with other kinds of tests, the validity of aptitude tests is also generally high. Considering that validity is usually regarded as the single most important aspect of a test, one might expect aptitude tests to also have considerable utility in rehabilitation counseling. To evaluate the general validity of a category of tests (i.e., aptitude tests), researchers usually review the validity indices reported in test manuals and literature. The type of validity index most often used is criterion-related validity, which includes both predictive and concurrent validity. This index is frequently sought because it is readily quantifiable and is approximately comparable from one study to another. Siebel (1968) reported that criterion-related validity coefficients for aptitude tests usually ranged from .30 to .60, although some (particularly concurrent indices) reached .80.

Several investigators have taken a more empirical approach in evaluating the validity of aptitude tests. For example, in 1966 Ghiselli published a landmark study that assessed the general validity of occupational aptitude tests. Professional literature published from 1919 to 1964 was systematically searched. To report the data consistently, Ghiselli grouped tests into those of intellectual abilities, spatial and mechanical abilities, perceptual accuracy, motor abilities, and personality traits. For criteria of occupational success, two broad categories were identified. The first category was training criteria, which included such things as grades in occupational training courses. The second category was job proficiency criteria, which included such things as supervisor's ratings of job performance, measures of productivity, dollar volume of sales, and frequency of accidents. Finally, Ghiselli had to deal with the problem of combining validity coefficients across different studies in a meaningful way. To accomplish this, Fisher's z transformation was employed and validity coefficients were then averaged. Because of the statistical error involved in averaging coefficients of tests with widely varying reliabilities, the average validity coefficients presented were most likely underestimates of the true coefficients.

Ghiselli found that for most occupations, trainability was predicted relatively well. Predictions of job proficiency were more tenuous, with the validity coefficients typically in the .20s and rarely above .30. This conservative conclusion by Ghiselli was subsequently revised. Hunter and Hunter (1984) reanalyzed Ghiselli's lifelong work using a newer methodology, *meta-analysis*. Their conclusions indicated that tests of cognitive ability (intelligence, verbal aptitude, and numerical aptitude) possess an effective range of validity from .32 to .76 for predicting training success and from .29 to .61 for predicting job proficiency. Furthermore, the average validity of cognitive and psychomotor tests combined is .53, with only slight variability across job families.

Hunter and Hunter (1984) did not stop with estimates of validity coefficients; they translated their findings into practical terms. Using utility equations, they were able to estimate the cost in dollars of various selection strategies. Excluding aptitude tests and using other measures instead as predictors for federal entry-level jobs would cost the government from $3.12 billion if job tryouts were substituted to $15.89 billion if age of the applicant was used as the sole selection criterion. Other selection criteria (i.e., biodata) had costs falling between these two figures. In another study, Schmidt and Hunter (1981) estimated that national workforce productivity would be $80 billion per year greater when aptitude and other cognitive ability tests were uniformly used in selection than when they were not used. In other words, failure to use these tests would cost the United States an amount equal to total corporate profits or, alternatively, to 20% of the federal budget at that time.

Despite the foregoing endorsement of multiple aptitude testing, there remained a longstanding concern that validity findings were situation specific and were influenced by undetected differences across different workplaces. This means that each time a test was used in a new setting, it would have to be revalidated for that setting (Aiken, 1998; Hartigan & Wigdor, 1989). Hunter, Schmidt, and colleagues disagreed. They argued that the variability in validity coefficients of a test across situations was the result primarily of sampling error, not deficiencies in the test (Schmidt & Hunter, 2003; Schmidt, Hunter, Pearlman, et al., 1985). Using meta-analysis to combine the findings of small-sample studies, they believed, would demonstrate the stability of validity data for aptitude and other tests of cognitive abilities. This hypothesized stability was referred to as validity generalization (or VG).

Hunter applied this line of thinking on VG to the GATB. First, Hunter showed that the nine factor scores on the GATB are adequately represented by three composites: Cognitive, Perceptual, and Psychomotor (discussed earlier in this chapter). Then, he reduced the more than 12,000 jobs in the U.S. economy into five complexity-based families using the data-people-things classification of the *Dictionary of Occupational Titles* (U.S. Department of Labor Employment and Training Administration, 1991).

The five job families are (1) setup/precision work, (2) feeding/offbearing jobs, (3) synthesize/coordinate jobs (professional and supervisory jobs), (4) analyze/compile/compute jobs (skilled trades and clerical jobs), and (5) copy/compare jobs (semiskilled jobs). Hunter next analyzed 515 GATB validity studies published over 35 years and found that corrected multiple correlations (validity coefficients) of the composites for predicting performance in the job families ranged from .49 to .59, with an average of .53. These findings supported the VG hypothesis and led to the development of the VG-GATB (Bolton, 1994; Hartigan & Wigdor, 1989; Schmidt & Hunter, 2003).

Hunter's VG research, however, was called into serious question. In a thorough and technically sophisticated critique, Hartigan and Wigdor (1989) asserted that (a) Hunter's analysis that led to VG-GATB composite scores was flawed, (b) his categorization of all jobs into five job families failed to usefully advance prediction of job performance, and (c) his corrected validities were inflated because of the inappropriate corrections he used to address anomalies in the data. They concluded from their reanalyses that validities for about 90% of the jobs studied ranged from .20 to .40, considerably lower than Hunter's estimates. Unfortunately, the GATB was a casualty of this debate and the issue of subgroup norming mentioned earlier. The controversy over VG and Hunter's research continues today (Landy, 2003; Murphy, 2003; Schmidt & Hunter, 2003).

General Versus Special Norms

Once test-taking problems associated with disability are identified and accommodated (Ekstrom & Smith, 2002), rehabilitation professionals often wonder whether to use general norms or special norms that compare individuals only to those with similar disabilities. On one side of this issue are those who proclaim that general norms should be used because the individual with a disability will have to compete with the general population in obtaining employment. Those on the other side, however, state emphatically that the use of general norms discriminates unfairly against persons with disabilities.

This issue is most confusing until one analyzes the question in terms of descriptive and predictive interpretive techniques. Descriptive devices, including norms, merely locate the individual's performance within some reference group. By using norms, one might determine that a particular individual scored at the 75th percentile in mechanical aptitude (i.e.,, scored higher than 75% of the comparison group). If the reference group consisted of successful auto mechanics, one might predict that this individual would also be successful as an auto mechanic. However, this kind of prediction involves subjective judgment, assuming there is no research evidence that a score at the 75th percentile ensures a high probability of success in auto mechanics.

However, if all the relevant variables in auto mechanic performance had been identified and a prediction equation (e.g., a regression equation) had been developed, the individual's chances for success in auto mechanics could be directly determined with a specified degree of statistical probability. This latter prediction procedure would require no subjectivity. These two predicting modes are frequently referred to as clinical (or subjective) prediction and statistical (or actuarial) prediction, respectively.

In any particular instance, the same test scores could be used to describe and to make predictions about an individual's behavior. However, rehabilitation personnel frequently fail to make a conceptual separation between descriptions and predictions, and this is a major cause for the confusion surrounding the general versus the special norms controversy. For descriptive purposes, one may easily decide to use either or both special and general norms to ascertain an individual's standing within the selected norm group. It is within the realm of prediction that the issue becomes most confused. Predictions based solely on scores derived from norms involve armchair speculation, or what has been referred to as clinical judgment. A number of authors (e.g., Meehl, 1954) have pointed out the limitations of making clinical judgments. If possible, predictive, statistical methods should be used in making predictions. In this way one can be aware of the chances of making a correct prediction. The general versus special norms issue dissipates when prediction is the goal because norms are descriptive, not predictive, in nature. When one wishes to use norms in a descriptive fashion, there should be no difficulty in selecting either or both general and specific norms, assuming both are available.

Clinical Versus Statistical Prediction

The history of science is replete with examples of human observational and judgmental error. Human error is particularly pervasive in the behavioral sciences (Dunning, 2005). Psychiatric diagnoses, for instance, are subject to tremendous variations. In summarizing six studies, Zubin (1967) found that agreement among psychiatrists on diagnosing patients with mental illness ranged from 38% to 84%. In diagnosing general conditions, such as psychosis, neurosis, or organic brain damage, agreement ranged from 64% to 84%. However, in diagnosing more specific forms of psychiatric disorder, agreement ranged from 38% to 66%. These and similar studies suggest that professional judgments based primarily on experience and intuition are particularly prone to error. Motivated by such concerns, Meehl (1954) sought to determine the relative accuracy of clinical judgment when compared to statistical prediction. Reviewing the literature, he located 19 relevant and unambiguous studies relating to this issue. Of the studies, 10 indicated no difference between the two methods of prediction, and 9 found differences in favor of statistical prediction. In an effort to answer criticisms of Meehl's work by Gough (1962), Holt (1958), and others, Sawyer (1966) sought to replicate and extend Meehl's earlier investigation. Sawyer reviewed 45 studies that allowed for a comparison of the accuracy of clinical and statistical prediction in both data collection and data integration. The results were strongly supportive of Meehl's study; statistical prediction was clearly equal or superior to clinical prediction, regardless of the mode of data collection. Aegisdottir et al. (2006) performed a meta-analysis on studies comparing clinical versus statistical prediction over a 56-year period. Using a subsample of 41 studies that were the most conservative of the total 156 identified studies, they found "an effect size of $-.12$ favoring the accuracy of statistical over clinical methods" (p. 367). Although this effect size is small, it is consistent and reliable and reflects 13% greater accuracy of statistical over clinical predictions.

Similar concerns have affected rehabilitation counseling. Although dated, two studies are particularly interesting. Roehlke (1965) compared statistical prediction to the clinical predictions of rehabilitation counselors regarding the outcome of a sample of people with psychiatric disabilities in various rehabilitation programs. Statistical predictions based on demographic, psychological, and vocational variables yielded an averaged predictive accuracy of about 80%. The most effective counselors reached a 55% level of predictive accuracy, while many others did much worse.

Bolton, Butler, and Wright (1968) compared statistical and counselor clinical assessments of rehabilitation consumers' likelihood for success in a rehabilitation program. As with previous studies, statistical predictions were generally more accurate than clinical predictions. Of 28 counselors who closed at least 35 cases, however, two exceeded the statistical formula in predictive accuracy. Although there was wide variability in counselor predictive accuracy, no relationship was found between accuracy and either education or experience of the counselor. Cook (1980) similarly grappled with the clinical versus statistical prediction issue as it applies to the practicing rehabilitation counselor. His review of the rehabilitation and related literature suggested the superiority of statistical over clinical prediction.

The overall conclusion is that statistical prediction, using what were earlier referred to as predictive interpretive methods, is generally more accurate than the clinical judgments of experienced professionals. These conclusions may place rehabilitation professionals in a quandary because predictive interpretive methods (i.e., statistical modes of prediction) are often unavailable (Strohmer & Arm, 2006). Consequently, professionals must continue to use their intuition in decision making, but in doing so they should be aware of the fallibility of their intuitive judgments. Counselors should keep records of the various judgments they are required to make so that they may determine their accuracy in predicting client outcomes. Through keeping such records, counselors would be able to identify and correct recurrent errors they make (Anastasi & Urbina, 1997).

Conclusion

This chapter began by presenting definitions of aptitude followed by a brief history of the development of aptitude testing. Next, problems in using self-ratings as a substitute for aptitude test scores were discussed. Then, 10 aptitude batteries were described and evaluated (GATB, ASVAB, DAT, AE, APTI-COM, BAB, CS, CPS, OASIS-3, and PESCO). Three tests (GATB, ASVAB, and DAT) have longstanding reputations for excellence. Among the three, the DAT, which is the only current, commercially available test of the three, was recommended for use in rehabilitation settings despite various problems documented in the review. The other seven tests (AE, APTICOM, BAB, CS, CPS, OASIS-3, and PESCO) were noted as showing promise but needing to be used with caution. Finally, several issues in aptitude testing were presented: (a) interpretation of test results; (b) reliability, validity, and VG; (c) general versus special norms; and (d) clinical versus statistical prediction. In spite of these issues, vocational aptitude tests offer consumers and rehabilitation professionals critical information to assist them in educational and vocational guidance, career development, and job placement.

References

Aegisdottir, S., White, M., Spengler, P., Maugherman, A., Anderson, L., Cook, R., et al. (2006). The meta-analysis of Clinical Judgment Project: Fifty-six years of accumulated research on clinical versus statistical prediction. *Counseling Psychologist, 34,* 341–382.

Aiken, L. (1998). *Tests and examinations: Measuring abilities and performance.* New York: Wiley.

Aiken, L. (2003). *Psychological testing and assessment.* Boston: Allyn & Bacon.

American College Testing Program. (1997). *Career planning program.* Iowa City, IA: Author.

American College Testing Program. (1998). *Career planning survey: Technical manual.* Iowa City, IA: Author.

American College Testing Program. (1999). *Career planning survey: Counselor's manual.* Iowa City, IA: Author.

Anastasi, A. (1988). *Psychological testing* (6th ed.). New York: MacMillan.

Anastasi, A., & Urbina, S. (1997). *Psychological testing* (7th ed.). New York: Prentice Hall.

Ball Foundation. (1998a). *Ball career system: Administration manual.* Glen Ellyn, IL: Author.

Ball Foundation. (1998b). *Ball career system: Counselor training manual.* Glen Ellyn, IL: Author.

Ball Foundation. (1998c). *Ball career system: Examiner's manual.* Glen Ellyn, IL: Author.

Ball Foundation. (1998d). *Ball career system: Technical manual.* Glen Ellyn, IL: Author.

Blackwell, T. (2003). [Review of the test *Occupational Aptitude Survey and Interest Schedule–Third Edition*]. *Rehabilitation Counseling Bulletin, 46,* 247–250.

Bolton, B. (1994). USES General Aptitude Test Battery (GATB)/USES Interest Inventory (USES-II). In J. Kapes, M. Mastie, & E. Whitfield (Eds.), *A counselor's guide to career assessment instruments* (3rd ed., pp. 117–123). Alexandria, VA: National Career Development Association.

Bolton, B., Butler, A. J., & Wright, G. N. (1968). *Clinical versus statistical prediction of client feasibility* (Wisconsin Studies in Vocational Rehabilitation, Monograph No. 7). Madison: University of Wisconsin, Regional Rehabilitation Institute.

Borman, C. (1994). *Occupational Aptitude Survey and Interest Schedule–Second Edition* (OASIS-2). In J. Kapes, M. Mastie, & E. Whitfield (Eds.), *A counselor's guide to career assessment instruments* (3rd ed., pp. 106–110). Alexandria, VA: National Career Development Association.

Borman, C. (2001). *Ability Explorer.* In J. Kapes & E. Whitfield (Eds.), *A counselor's guide to career assessment instruments* (4th ed., pp. 76–81). Columbus, OH: National Career Development Association.

Bragger, J., & Becker, A. (2005). [Review of the test *The Differential Aptitude Tests–Fifth Edition*]. In D. Keyser (Ed.), *Test critiques* (Vol. XI, pp. 72–88). Austin, TX: PRO-ED.

Carroll, J. (1985). Second-language abilities. In R. Sternberg (Ed.), *Human abilities: An information processing approach* (pp. 83–102). New York: Freeman.

Carroll, J. (1993). *Human cognitive abilities: A survey of factor-analytic studies.* New York: Cambridge.

Civil Rights Act of 1991 (P.L. 102-166) (1991).

Conoley, J. C., & Impara, J. (Eds.). (1995). *The twelfth mental measurements yearbook.* Lincoln, NE: Buros Institute of Mental Measurements of the University of Nebraska–Lincoln.

Cook, D. (1980). Clinical versus statistical prediction revisited: Issues in building rehabilitation diagnostic capacity. *Rehabilitation Counseling Bulletin, 24*(2), 151–160.

Cronbach, L. (1990). *Essentials of psychological testing* (5th ed.). New York: HarperCollins.

Dawes, R., Faust, D., & Meehl, P. (1993). Statistical prediction versus clinical prediction: Improving what works. In G. Keren & C. Lewis (Eds.), *A handbook for data analysis in the behavioral sciences: Methodological issues* (pp. 351–367). Hillsdale, NJ: Erlbaum.

DuBois, P. (1970). *A history of psychological testing.* Boston: Allyn & Bacon.

Dunning, D. (2005). *Self-insight: Roadblocks and detours on the path of knowing thyself.* New York: Psychology Press.

Ekstrom, R., & Smith, D. (2002). *Assessing individuals with disabilities in educational, employment, and counseling settings.* Washington, DC: American Psychological Association.

Elmore, P., & Bradley, R. (1994). Armed Services Vocational Aptitude Battery (ASVAB) Career Exploration Program. In J. Kapes, M. Mastie, & E. Whitfield (Eds.), *A counselor's guide to career assessment instruments* (3rd ed., pp. 73–77). Alexandria, VA: National Career Development Association.

Galton, F. (1869). *Hereditary genius: An enquiry into its laws and consequences.* London: Collins.

Ghiselli, E. (1966). *The validity of occupational aptitude tests.* New York: Wiley.

Goldman, L. (1971). *Using tests in counseling* (2nd ed.). Englewood Cliffs, NJ: Prentice Hall.

Gough, H. (1962). Clinical vs. statistical prediction in psychology. In L. Postman (Ed.), *Psychology in the making* (pp. 526–584). New York: Knopf.

Green, J. (1994). APTICOM. In J. Kapes, M. Mastie, & E. Whitfield (Eds.), *A counselor's guide to career assessment instruments* (3rd ed., pp. 65–70). Alexandria, VA: National Career Development Association.

Guilford, J. (1967). *The nature of human intelligence*. New York: McGraw-Hill.

Harrington, J., & Harrington, T. (1984). *Ability Explorer*. Indianapolis, IN: JIST Works.

Harrington, J., & Harrington, T. (1996). *Ability Explorer*. Chicago: Riverside.

Harrington, T., & O'Shea, A. (Eds.). (2006). *Guide for occupational exploration* (2nd ed.). Circle Pines, MN: American Guidance Services.

Harris, J. A. (2001). CareerScope assessment and reporting system. In J. Kapes & E. Whitfield (Eds.), *A counselor's guide to career assessment instruments* (4th ed., pp. 116–122). Columbus, OH: National Career Development Association.

Harris, J. A., & Danski, H. (1991). *APTICOM: System technical manual*. Philadelphia: Vocational Research Institute.

Hartigan, J., & Wigdor, A. (1989). *Fairness in employment testing: Validity generalization, minority issues, and the General Aptitude Test Battery*. Washington, DC: National Academy Press.

Hattrup, K. (1995). [Review of the test *Differential Aptitude Tests–Fifth Edition*]. In J.C. Conoley & J. Impara (Eds.), *The twelfth mental measurements yearbook* (pp. 301–304). Lincoln, NE: Buros Institute of Mental Measurements of the University of Nebraska–Lincoln.

Helmstadter, G. (1964). *Principles of psychological measurement*. New York: Appleton-Century-Crofts.

Holland, J., Fritzsche, B., & Powell, A. (1994). *Self-directed search: Technical manual*. Odessa, FL: Psychological Assessment Resources.

Holt, R. (1958). Clinical and statistical prediction: A reformulation and some new data. *Journal of Abnormal and Social Psychology, 56,* 1–12.

Humphreys, L. (1962). The organization of human abilities. *American Psychologist, 17,* 475–483.

Hunter, J., & Hunter, R. (1984). Validity and utility of alternative predictors of job performance. *Psychological Bulletin, 96,* 72–98.

Impara, J., & Plake, B. (Eds.). (1998). *The thirteenth mental measurements yearbook*. Lincoln, NE: Buros Institute of Mental Measurements of the University of Nebraska–Lincoln.

Instructional Technologies. (2006). *VRI's APTICOM*. Retrieved May 24, 2006, from http://www.intecinc.net/prod_vri_apticom.htm

Kapes, J., & Whitfield, E. (Eds.). (2001a). A counselor's guide: Introduction to the fourth edition. In J. Kapes & E. Whitfield (Eds.), *A counselor's guide to career assessment instruments* (4th ed., pp. 1–13). Columbus, OH: National Career Development Association.

Kapes, J., & Whitfield, E. (Eds.). (2001b). *A counselor's guide to career assessment instruments* (4th ed.). Columbus, OH: National Career Development Association.

Kelley, T. (1928). *Crossroads in the mind of man: A study of differentiable mental abilities*. Palo Alto, CA: Stanford University Press.

Kirnan, J. (2005). [Review of the test *General Aptitude Test Battery*]. In D. Keyser (Ed.), *Test critiques* (Vol. XI, pp. 100–108). Austin, TX: PRO-ED.

Landy, F. (2003). Validity generalization: Then and now. In K. Murphy (Ed.), *Validity generalization: A critical review,* (pp. 155–196). Mahwah, NJ: Erlbaum.

Loch, C. (1993a). *The new Cognitive and Conceptual Abilities Test (C-CAT): A preliminary development manual*. Pleasantville, NY: Pesco International.

Loch, C. (1993b). *The new Vocational Interest Inventory (VII): A preliminary development manual*. Pleasantville, NY: Pesco International.

Loch, C. (1999). *A manual of research and norm studies*. Pleasantville, NY: Pesco International.

Mabe, P., & West, S. (1982). Validity of self-evaluation ability: A review and meta-analysis. *Journal of Applied Psychology, 67*, 280–296.

Meehl, P. (1954). *Clinical versus statistical prediction.* Minneapolis: University of Minnesota Press.

Miller, R., & Hollingshead, C. (2001). *Occupational Aptitude Survey and Interest Schedule–Second Edition.* In J. Kapes & E. Whitfield (Eds.), *A counselor's guide to career assessment instruments* (4th ed., pp. 150–157). Columbus, OH: National Career Development Association.

Murphy, K. (Ed.). (2003) *Validity generalization: A critical review.* Mahwah, NJ: Erlbaum.

Parker, R. (1983). *Occupational Aptitude Survey and Interest Schedule: Aptitude Survey examiner's manual.* Austin, TX: PRO-ED.

Parker, R. (1991). *Occupational Aptitude Survey and Interest Schedule–Second Edition: Aptitude Survey examiner's manual.* Austin, TX: PRO-ED.

Parker, R. (2001). *Occupational Aptitude Survey and Interest Schedule–Third Edition: Aptitude Survey examiner's manual.* Austin, TX: PRO-ED.

Parker, R., & Schaller, J. (1994). Relationships among self-rated and psychometrically determined vocational aptitudes and interests. *Educational and Psychological Measurement, 54,* 155–159.

Plake, B., & Impara, J. (Eds.). (2001). *The fourteenth mental measurements yearbook.* Lincoln, NE: Buros Institute of Mental Measurements of the University of Nebraska–Lincoln.

Plake, B., Impara, J., & Spies (Eds.). (2003). *The fifteenth mental measurements yearbook.* Lincoln, NE: Buros Institute of Mental Measurements of the University of Nebraska–Lincoln.

Psychological Corp. (1992). *Differential Aptitude Tests–Fifth Edition: Technical manual.* San Antonio, TX: Author.

Reardon, R., & Vernick, S. (2001). *Career Planning Survey.* In J. Kapes & E. Whitfield (Eds.), *A counselor's guide to career assessment instruments* (4th ed., pp. 109–115). Columbus, OH: National Career Development Association.

Roehlke, H. (1965). *Predicting outcome of rehabilitation of psychiatric patients.* Unpublished doctoral dissertation, University of Missouri, Columbia.

Rogers, J. (2001). *Armed Services Vocational Aptitude Battery Career Exploration Program* (ASVAB). In J. Kapes & E. Whitfield (Eds.), *A counselor's guide to career assessment instruments* (4th ed., pp. 93–101). Columbus, OH: National Career Development Association.

Rojewski, J. (2001). PESCO 2001. In J. Kapes & E. Whitfield (Eds.), *A counselor's guide to career assessment instruments* (4th ed., pp. 158–163). Columbus, OH: National Career Development Association.

Sawyer, J. (1966). Measurement and prediction, clinical and statistical. *Psychological Bulletin, 66,* 178–200.

Schmidt, F., & Hunter, J. (1981). Employment testing: Old theories and new research findings. *American Psychologist, 36,* 1128–1137.

Schmidt, F., & Hunter, J. (2003). History, development, evolution, and impact of validity generalization and meta-analysis. In K. Murphy (Ed.), *Validity generalization: A critical review,* (pp. 31–66). Mahwah, NJ: Erlbaum.

Schmidt, F., Hunter, J., Pearlman, K., Hirsch, H., Sackett, P., Schmitt, N., et al. (1985). Forty questions about validity generalization and meta-analysis with commentaries. *Personnel Psychology, 37,* 407–422.

Siebel, D. (1968). Measurement of aptitude and achievement. In D. Whitla (Ed.), *Handbook of measurement and assessment in behavioral sciences* (pp. 261–314). Reading, MA: Addison-Wesley.

Spies, R., & Plake, B. (Eds.). (2005). *The sixteenth mental measurements yearbook.* Lincoln, NE: Buros Institute of Mental Measurements of the University of Nebraska–Lincoln.

Strohmer, D., & Arm, S. (2006). The more things change, the more they remain the same. *Counseling Psychologist, 34,* 383–390.

Thompson, D., & Patrick, J. (2001). *Ball Aptitude Battery.* In J. Kapes & E. Whitfield (Eds.), *A counselor's guide to career assessment instruments* (4th ed., pp. 102–108). Columbus, OH: National Career Development Association.

Thurstone, L. (1938). Primary mental abilities. *Psychometric Monographs,* No. 1.

Tracey, T., & Hopkins, N. (2001). Correspondence of interests and abilities with occupational choice. *Journal of Counseling Psychology, 48*(2), 178–189.

Urbina, S. (2004). *Essentials of psychological testing.* Hoboken, NJ: Wiley.

U.S. Department of Defense. (1995). *ASVAB 18/19 counselor manual: The ASVAB career exploration program.* North Chicago, IL: U.S. Military Entrance Processing Command.

U.S. Department of Defense. (1999). *Technical manual for the ASVAB 18/19.* North Chicago, IL: U.S. Military Entrance Processing Command.

U.S. Department of Labor. (1970). *Manual for the USES General Aptitude Test Battery, Section III: Development.* Washington, DC: U.S. Government Printing Office.

U.S. Department of Labor. (1979). *Guide for occupational exploration.* Washington, DC: U.S. Government Printing Office.

U.S. Department of Labor. (published biennially). *Occupational outlook handbook.* Washington, DC: U.S. Government Printing Office.

U.S. Department of Labor Employment and Training Administration. (1991). *Dictionary of occupational titles* (4th rev. ed.). Washington, DC: Author.

U.S. Department of Labor Employment and Training Administration. (2002). *O*NET Ability Profiler users guide.* Washington, DC: Author.

Vocational Research Institute. (1998). *User's guide: CareerScope.* Philadelphia: Author.

Wesman, A. (1966). Double-entry expectancy tables. *Test Service Bulletin,* No. 56. New York: Psychology Corp.

Willson, V. (1995). [Review of the *Differential Aptitude Tests for Personnel and Career Assessment*]. In J. C. Conoley & J. Impara (Eds.), *The twelfth mental measurements yearbook* (pp. 305–307). Lincoln, NE: Buros Institute of Mental Measurements of the University of Nebraska–Lincoln.

Willson, V., & Stone, E. (1994). *Differential Aptitude Tests.* In J. Kapes, M. Mastie, & E. Whitfield (Eds.), *A counselor's guide to career assessment instruments* (3rd ed., pp. 93–98). Alexandria, VA: National Career Development Association.

Wing, H. (1995). [Review of the *Differential Aptitude Tests for Personnel and Career Assessment*]. In J. C. Conoley & J. Impara (Eds.), *The twelfth mental measurements yearbook* (pp. 307–308). Lincoln, NE: Buros Institute of Mental Measurements of the University of Nebraska–Lincoln.

Wise, S. (1995). [Review of the *Differential Aptitude Tests: Computerized adaptive edition*]. In J. C. Conoley & J. Impara (Eds.), *The twelfth mental measurements yearbook* (pp. 300–301). Lincoln, NE: Buros Institute of Mental Measurements of the University of Nebraska–Lincoln.

Zubin, J. (1967). Classification of the behavior disorders. *Annual Review of Psychology, 18,* 373–406.

Chapter 6

Assessment of Personality

Samuel E. Krug

n the broadest sense, personality assessment may be defined as the formal process of quantifying influences that explain a person's behavior in a specific situation. The situation may relate to vocational choice; treatment planning; therapeutic intervention; or, more likely, some combination of these and other concerns. The influences to be quantified may be characteristics such as intelligence or cognitive abilities that are shaped by interactions of internal and external factors (R. B. Cattell, 1971); interpersonal processes that explain interactions between people (Wiggins, 1985); or dynamic characteristics such as attitudes, interests, and values that are essential to understanding career choice and adjustment to employment (Bolton & Roessler, 1986). Regardless of choice of model or theoretical point of view, personality assessment is the formal process concerned with measuring such influences.

Personality study has fascinated philosophers, writers, and others since the dawn of recorded history. But, while the analysis of temperament and motivation is penetrating and insightful in Aristotle's *Poetics* and James's *The Turn of the Screw,* these efforts must be viewed as informal precursors of what evolved into a science only in the 20th century.

Today, personality assessment is one of the most technically advanced areas within psychology. The tests that have been developed in recent years are the result of sophisticated psychometric engineering and are uniquely associated with both the science and practice of psychology.

This was not always so. When scientific psychology first emerged in the German laboratories of the 1870s, the primary emphasis was on general laws, like the Weber-Fechner law, which related stimulus to response with formulaic precision and mathematical elegance. For scientists like Wilhelm Wundt, the founder of modern experimental psychology, the deviation of an individual's response from the mean of the group response represented nothing more than measurement error.

But in England at about the same time, Francis Galton recognized that "individual differences," far from being measurement error, represented replicable patterns of behavior that could be systematically measured. These measures, in turn, permitted more precise predictions than had previously been possible by application of general laws of behavior alone. Galton's work laid the foundation for modern personality assessment.

The first psychological tests to be developed assessed general and specific abilities. This focus on abilities arose partly from the emphasis in the early laboratories on discriminative tasks and partly from a practical need to identify students who had special educational needs. Although prototypical personality "tests" existed in such forms as word association tasks, attempts to assess personality remained largely unscientific and unstandardized until the 1919 appearance of Woodworth's *Personal Data Sheet* (Woodworth, 1930) at the time of World War I. The *Personal Data Sheet* contained 116 items that represented a variety of anxiety-related symptoms. Woodworth's pioneering effort led directly to test construction efforts by L.L. Thurstone and indirectly to most clinical scale development that has followed. Woodworth's items were robust. Many can be found relatively unchanged in contemporary clinical inventories.

Since most psychological instruments help explain a person's behavior in a specified situation, they might all in that sense be classified as personality tests. But, as the term is more commonly understood, personality tests represent only a small fraction of that total, being reserved primarily for tests that describe how people *typically* function. This is in contrast to cognitive ability tests, for example, which assess *maximum* performance potential, or achievement tests, which assess how well students have mastered particular skills. Within the personality context, tests can be thought to fall into two broad classes: unstructured and structured. Unstructured tests include projective techniques, such as the *Rorschach* and the *Thematic Apperception Test,* which use relatively ambiguous stimuli and permit a broad range of responses. Structured tests consist of inventories that have a fixed set of items and response options. Some structured tests, such as the *Minnesota Multiphasic Personality Inventory* (MMPI) or the *Clinical Analysis Questionnaire,* focus primarily on clinically relevant content. These are discussed in Chapter 7. The focus of the present chapter is on structured inventories that measure normal-range (i.e., nonclinical) constructs.

Why Assess Personality?

The purpose of assessment is to provide relevant information that can be used to reduce uncertainty and error in making decisions. Just within rehabilitation settings, there are a large number of client decisions that require answers. With clients who abuse substances, for example, a simple history that records onset and length of addiction, type of substances used, and similar issues does not adequately address effective treatment procedures, nor does it provide great insight into probable outcomes. For example, Cloninger (1987) identified two major types of alcoholism. Type I alcoholics are distinguished by high levels of trait anxiety, highly regulated alcohol consumption, and high levels of guilt and shame related to alcohol consumption. Type II alcoholics are characterized by a vastly different motivational pattern of unregulated and impulsive alcohol consumption accompanied by antisocial and criminal behavior. Not only do these two types of alcoholism reflect different personality patterns, they also require different treatment strategies. Additional information about characteristics such as maturity, adjustment, and sensitivity proves to be very helpful in predicting the course of therapy and structuring individual treatment plans. Increased pressure to make treatment more efficient and more cost-effective (Beutler, Goodright, Fisher, & Williams, 1999; Lambert & Lambert, 1999) can only stimulate the need for reliable and early assessment of a patient's strengths and weaknesses.

The assessment of normal-range characteristics plays a significant role in reducing uncertainty related to vocational counseling decisions. It may be true, as some authors (e.g., Hunter, 1986) have argued, that cognitive ability is the most important predictor of job performance. However, cognitive ability alone cannot explain why people who *should* be able to do a job well don't always. First-year turnover among insurance agents, for example, may run as high as 90%. In some positions, job stress seems to take its toll, but there are always those who survive the stress. By helping to determine whether a person is suited for the psychological requirements of a job—requirements that transcend general cognitive ability or specific knowledge—normal-range personality characteristics are very useful to vocational counseling.

Meta-analyses of the research literature have identified consistent personality predictors of job performance across different instruments used to assess those characteristics (Barrick & Mount, 1991; Judge, Heller, & Mount, 2002). Others have found that the level of predictability is substantially increased when instruments are aligned with job analyses and studies are conducted with incumbents who have reasonable tenure in the position (Tett, Jackson, & Rothstein, 1991). Reviews of these data have led still others to the conclusion that well-developed measures of normal-range personality are probably significantly underutilized in decisions about job placement and job performance (Hogan, Hogan, & Roberts, 1996).

Validity and Utility of the Self-Report Method

The charge occasionally arises that self-report measures are of little practical use in predicting behavior. Some of the reasons offered in support of that assertion are that they are too confounded by irrelevant sources of variance (e.g., the social desirability of various answer choices), that they are transparent and too sensitive to deliberate distortion to give real insight into underlying personality dynamics, or that they are simply not valid enough to be of practical use.

While the self-report method has been the primary target of attacks, it is important to emphasize that all assessment modalities are subject to distortion (Krug & Cattell, 1971). Psychologists are typically interested not in the attributes directly assessed by their measures but in the attributes they infer from those measures. Measures of blood pressure or heart rate, for example, are used to infer attributes such as psychological stress, vulnerability to disease, or resilience. Whether the focus is on responses to items in a personality test or recordings of physiological events, the use of any measures to infer some hypothetical construct must be guided by theory. Perhaps the concerns about the accuracy of self-reporting arise simply from the fact that it is by far the most highly researched and critically examined mode of measurement.

The charge that psychological tests simply aren't valid enough to be practically useful has been examined and dismissed (Meyer et al., 2001). The study compared the validity of medical tests, such as the Pap test, with that of typically used psychological tests—structured and unstructured—and found that very often there was little difference between the two. In some cases, psychological tests and medical tests were indistinguishable in their ability to predict the same outcome (e.g., neuropsychological tests and magnetic resonance imaging predictions of dementia).

The response to a questionnaire item, as is any behavior, is multiply determined. Test designers consider various important sources of variance that may influence responses. Then they structure the items and scales to maximize substantive variance and minimize irrelevant factors. The *Jackson Personality Inventory,* which is described more fully later in this chapter, provides an excellent example of this feature of test construction.

With respect to deliberate faking, Hogan and Hogan (1995) have argued that the ability to alter scores on personality measures is a function of social competence and valuable information in itself. Further, they point out that the base rate for faking in the job application process is much lower than might have been thought.

Some people undoubtedly still feel that questionnaires represent an inadequate substitute for more "accurate," in-depth methods of assessment, such as interviews or direct observation methods (i.e., assessment centers). While it is true that personality assessment by questionnaire tends to be much less expensive than these alternatives, it is not clear from the research literature that this type of personality assessment results in significant loss in reliability, validity, or utility. For example, Kleinmuntz (1982, p. 208) has concluded that interviews do not add much to the information obtained by more formal psychometric techniques. There are reliability and validity problems with direct observation and behavior rating methods as well.

In the final analysis, it may be that structured personality inventories represent the best approach currently available to fairly and accurately measure underlying personality characteristics.

The Dimensionality and Structure of Normal-Range Personality

During the late 1960s and the 1970s, much discussion focused on the number of "real" or important personality factors. Interest in this topic greatly exceeded the level of agreement. R. B. Cattell (1973, 1986), Eysenck (1976, 1986), and Guilford (1975) were probably the most vocal because their own structural models and tests were central to the debate. Each argued for a different number of factors that led to different conclusions about the nature of personality. Eysenck, for example, focused at first on two very broad factors, neuroticism and extroversion, then later added a third, psychoticism. Guilford, whose studies began in an attempt to separate hypothesized components of extroversion–introversion, argued for 13 factors. Cattell, in turn, championing an approach to more specific traits of personality, argued for no less than 23 factors and as many as 35 if the full domain of pathology was to be included (R. B. Cattell & Krug, 1986). These debates were lively and unrelenting. Although everyone conceded that differences in factor analytic procedures, variable representation, and subject sampling could lead to differences in interpretation, no one gave in on the number or nature of personality structure.

The focal issue was which level was the "best" at which to investigate personality processes. Broader factors such as Eysenck's neuroticism and extroversion were typically more reliably assessed than lower-order components, and this, theoretically, leads to more valid predictions from the more reliable broad factors. However, the components don't always operate together in predicting real-life outcomes, and this, practically, leads to more valid predictions from the less reliable components.

More recently, the debate has softened considerably with the introduction of the "five-factor" model (Digman, 1990; Wiggins, 1996), which is based on a half-century of factor analytic research on the structure of peer ratings. The model proposes that there are five highly replicable, broad dimensions that account for most of the ways in which we describe others and ourselves. According to one author, these domains represent "the highest level that is still descriptive of behavior with only general evaluation located at a higher and more abstract level" (Goldberg, 1993, p. 27). The five dimensions are identified as Extroversion (or Surgency), Agreeableness (or Friendliness), Conscientiousness (or Will), Emotional Stability (or Neuroticism), and Intellect (or Openness to Experience or Culture). The fact that so many *or*'s are needed to describe these five suggests that consensus is not quite as extensive as some would have us believe, and some authors have argued persuasively that "there are plenty of dimensions of behavior beyond the Big Five" (Ashton, Jackson, Helmes, & Paunonen, 1998, p. 243). However, Wiggins and Trapnell's (1996) thoughtful review of five-factor developments over the past half-century points out that different versions of truth may exist simultaneously without causing chaos.

The five-factor model has played a fundamental role in guiding the development of newer instruments such as the *NEO Personality Inventory* and the *Hogan Personality Inventory.* Even instruments like the *16 Personality Factor Questionnaire,* which were not originally developed within the context of the five-factor model, have attempted to construct a linkage between their underlying personality models and the five-factor model. In short, the five-factor model has enjoyed wide acceptance and has assumed an important, some would say central, role in guiding thinking about the structure of normal-range personality since the 1980s.

It should come as no surprise to anyone that there is some agreement about the structure of personality. This is true in many areas of study. In the cognitive ability area, for example, almost everyone agrees that g (general ability) exists and is important. Beyond that, however, there is considerable diversity of opinion. In the area of human abilities, for example, Spearman's basic model assumed a single, general ability factor. R. B. Cattell (1971) then argued for a refinement by introducing the concepts of fluid (gf) and crystallized (ge) ability. Thurstone and others pursued a more complex primary ability model. More recently, some authors (e.g., Hunter, 1986) have argued that little is to be gained in predicting job performance from ability variables beyond *g*. But on that point, others disagree (Hartigan & Wigdor, 1989).

The situation is no different in personality. As noted earlier, the fact that so many *or's* are needed to name the five dimensions suggests there may be considerable variance in the way the model is implemented in different instruments. Correlations between various measures of the big five are informative in that regard. With regard to scales that purport to measure Emotional Stability, Extroversion, and Conscientiousness, correlations are usually quite high, often .80 or above. With regard to the latter two domains, Agreeableness and Intellect, there is much less agreement across tests. That is, correlations between similarly named scales are much lower, often as low as .20 to .30.

The five-factor model has been useful in helping us understand the natural overlap that exists among many different personality inventories. Marketing literature notwithstanding, there are some "unique features" that are probably not all that unique. But during the past half-century there has been a proliferation of scales and labels to measure a variety of constructs. The five-factor model provides a framework in which to evaluate similarities and differences among various personality measures.

Rather than one best level at which to describe personality, there are several. R. B. Cattell (1973) was articulate in this respect. The scales of his major test, the *16 Personality Factor Questionnaire* (16PF), lay, by his definition, at the "primary" factor level. Above them existed a replicable set of "second-order" factors (e.g., extroversion, anxiety) that were also useful in describing personality (Chernyshenko, Stark, & Chan, 2001). In addition, answers to individual ("critical") test items, which represent a micro level, are also informative in gaining a total personality picture. Others (e.g., Karson, Karson, & O'Dell, 1997) have developed this notion to show how primary and secondary levels interact usefully in describing personality and predicting clinically important outcomes.

The five-factor model, however, tends to emphasize a single level or layer of personality analysis at the cost of ignoring other useful dimensions that lie below or above it. Nevertheless, the best level at which to measure personality is governed by the needs of the assessment context. Reliably measurable differences exist within each of the big five domains. For example, two people may score equally high on the Extroversion scale of the *16 Personality Factor Questionnaire* but differ on the Warmth scale, one of the key contributors to extroversion. The low Warmth extrovert will usually be perceived as more shallow and less sincere than the high Warmth extrovert. As a result, people will respond differently to the two. Perhaps these kinds of differences in expression help explain why even very ardent proponents of the five-factor model have simultaneously pursued the development of scores that break down the five domain scores into narrower subscales or facets (e.g., Costa & McCrae, 1992b; Hogan & Hogan, 1995).

Review of Major Resources

It is difficult to estimate how many structured personality inventories are currently available. Reference sources like the *Mental Measurements Yearbook* and *Tests* list hundreds of such instruments. Many of these have enjoyed rather limited usage or have very specific applications. Others are general-purpose instruments that address a number of relevant concerns within the context of rehabilitation. This section reviews six instruments that have fairly broad applications and are in wide use.

16 Personality Factor Questionnaire

The *16 Personality Factor Questionnaire* (16PF; Cattell, n.d.) is one of the most widely used theory-based instruments for assessing normal-range personality characteristics in adults. Since its first U.S. publication in 1949, the test has been translated into nearly 50 languages. The test is used worldwide to evaluate a set of 16 reasonably independent personality characteristics that predict a wide range of socially significant criteria. Adaptations of the original questionnaire have been developed for assessing personality in younger populations, effectively extending the age range of the test to the early school years.

Raymond B. Cattell and a series of coauthors developed the test over many decades on the basis of extensive research intended to clarify the basic organization of human personality. Cattell was interested primarily in identifying a relatively small set of "source traits" that could be used to explain variations in the much larger set of "surface" characteristics observable in behavior and recorded in language. Cattell looked to language in his search because he was convinced that "all aspects of human personality which are or have been of importance, interest, or utility have already become recorded in the substance of language" (R. B. Cattell, 1943).

Whether or not it is true that the English language exhaustively delimited the personality domain, it is certainly true that the English language extensively described it. At about the time Cattell began his studies, Allport and Odbert (1936) had identified about 18,000 words in an English language dictionary that described distinctive aspects of human behavior. When they eliminated terms that were essentially evaluative (e.g., adorable, evil), were metaphorical (e.g., alive, prolific), or described temporary states (e.g., rejoicing, frantic), 4,504 terms still remained. Cattell began with that list of 4,504 words and conducted a series of analyses to eliminate overlap among them. His analyses encompassed a variety of perspectives (e.g., peer ratings, self-reports), populations (e.g., undergraduates, military personnel, working adults), and methodologies (e.g., cluster analysis, factor analysis). By beginning his search with the universe of trait names and conducting the analyses systematically, Cattell reasoned that the resulting final set must be judged to be "source traits." His undergraduate training as a chemist undoubtedly influenced Cattell's argument. Water, for example, can be conceptualized as a weighted combination of elementary molecules (two parts hydrogen, one part oxygen). Cattell believed that human characteristics such as creativity or depression could be similarly conceptualized as weighted combinations of the source traits that survived his analyses.

The first publication of the 16PF did not occur until more than a decade after Cattell began his studies. Since then the test has undergone several major, and more numerous minor, revisions. The most recent, in 1993, was the last Cattell completed before his death in 1998.

The most widely used U.S. test form (Conn & Riecke, 1994) contains 185 items, requires 35 to 50 minutes to complete, and has a 5th-grade reading level. The test can be scored by hand, but computerized scoring and an extensive array of interpretive reports are also available. The test provides scores for 16 "primary" scales and five "global" factors. The global factors (called "second-order" factors in earlier test editions) result from factor analyses of the 16 primary scales and are conceptualized as major organizing influences behind the primary scales. The average test-retest reliability coefficient is .83 after a few weeks and .72 over a period of 2 months for the primary scales. Corresponding values for the global scales are slightly higher. Internal consistency reliabilities of the primary scales average .75.

The primary scales of the test, which are designated by alphanumeric symbols, are as follows: A–Warmth, B–Reasoning, C–Emotional Stability, E–Dominance, F–Liveliness, G–Rule-Consciousness, H–Social Boldness, I–Sensitivity, L–Vigilance, M–Abstractedness, N–Privateness, O–Apprehension, Q1–Openness to Change, Q2 Self-reliance, Q3–Perfectionism, Q4–Tension. The five global factors (Extroversion, Anxiety, Tough-Mindedness, Independence, and Self-control) assess features similar to those defined by the five-factor model. Besides the primary scales and global factors, the 16PF can be scored for approximately 100 criteria that derive from years of research on 16PF applications in clinical, counseling, and organizational psychology. The 16PF also provides three response style indicators: Impression Management, Infrequency, and Acquiescence. These scales are helpful in identifying unusual response patterns that may affect the validity of the profile.

Three additional comments about the 16PF are pertinent here. First, a special form of the test, Form E, which differs from the other published forms of the test in several important ways, has been extensively used with rehabilitation populations. The test is much shorter, and the reading level of the items has been dramatically reduced. Items are presented in a forced-choice format to simplify responses. Finally, the test has been specifically validated on and norms exist for a variety of special populations, including persons with visual and aural handicaps, clients receiving rehabilitation services, and people who are in prison. Despite some major differences in the nature of the item pool, questionnaire format, and normative data, research has demonstrated that Form E measures the same primary personality dimensions as the other forms that were designed for use with unselected adult populations (Bolton, 1977a; Burdsal & Bolton, 1979; Hughey & Burdsal, 1982).

Second, the 16PF has been a popular instrument in studies of the psychological characteristics of persons with disabilities, and thus, much interpretive data relevant to rehabilitation populations have been accumulated. The interested reader is referred to Roessler and Bolton (1978, Chapter 2) for a detailed summary of the results of 20 investigations. The conclusion to be drawn from a great deal of research on Form E is that it appears to be particularly well-adapted for use with rehabilitation populations (Bolton, 1974, 1977b, 1978; Davis, 1983; Tango & Kolodinsky, 2004).

Third, an adapted version of the test for use with Spanish speakers living in the United States has been developed to facilitate the test's use in a linguistically increasingly diverse society. The item development process reconciled several different translations into a single form understandable to Spanish speakers from a variety of countries and backgrounds, and statistical checks were made to ensure that the test retained its essential structure in translation (H. E. P. Cattell, 2005).

By itself, the 16PF is not well-suited to assess major affective and cognitive disturbances. Although experienced interpreters of the profile have identified certain score patterns suggestive of depression (Karson, Karson, & O'Dell, 1997), such a diagnosis from the 16PF scales alone is usually difficult or impossible for the vast majority of those who work with the test.

The 16PF is also a challenging instrument with which to work. Much of Cattell's extensive research on the instrument was directed toward theoretical and psychometric concerns. He paid less attention to practical issues of profile analysis or clinical interpretation. Fortunately, other authors have developed a variety of interpretive resources that help users understand the meaning of the scales in a variety of contexts (H. B. Cattell, 1989; Karson, Karson, & O'Dell, 1997; Krug, 1981; Lord, 1997, 1999).

The 16PF is an important instrument whose utility has been enhanced by extensive research and by periodic updating. It is theoretically grounded in research on the basic structure of adult personality and represents a significant resource for decision makers in a variety of rehabilitation settings.

California Psychological Inventory

The *California Psychological Inventory* (CPI) was designed by Gough to permit a trained interpreter to develop an informative and recognizable portrait of the test taker. Each scale was developed so as to maximize its relationship to external criteria. The first edition of the test was published in 1957, and the most recent edition, the third, appeared in 1996 (Gough, 2000; Gough & Bradley, 2002).

The CPI consists of 434 true/false items, of which 171 were taken from the MMPI item pool. The items were generally arranged into scales following the method of contrasted groups. Rather than contrast clinical and normal groups as was done with the MMPI, however, Gough contrasted those who were rated high in dominance with those who were rated low in dominance in the development of the Dominance (Do) scale, for example, or women with men in the development of the Femininity/Masculinity (F/M) scale. Again, the development focus was on maximizing the external validity of the scales. The current form has 20 basic scales. Computer reports provide information with respect to additional, special-purpose scales. Since 1987, three higher order constructs, called vectors, which represent three fundamental orientations—toward people, toward the rules and expectations of interpersonal life, and toward self—have also been scored.

The CPI has been extensively researched. Within the rehabilitation context it has been used, for example, to study personality differences between short-term recovered alcoholics and those whose drinking had been controlled for a minimum of 4 years (the latter scored significantly higher on responsibility [Re], tolerance [To], and achievement via independence [Ai]; Kurtines, Ball, & Wood, 1978); psychological precursors of coronary artery disease (Musante, MacDougall, Dembroski, & VanHorn, 1983; Palladino & Motiff, 1981); addiction and substance abuse (Alterman, Renner, & Cacciola, 2000; Alterman, Rutherford, et al., 1998; Cook, 1998; Cook, Young, Taylor, & Bedford, 1998); and career and work adjustment (Briddick, Watkins, & Savickas, 1998; Collins, & Griffin, 1998; Connors et al., 2000; Day, Bedeian, & Conte, 1998; Newman, Gray, & Fuqua, 1999).

In terms of reliability characteristics and normative base, the CPI appears to be well-designed and constructed (Gough & Bradley, 2002). One of its most impressive features is the extensive research base that currently forms the foundation for the test (CPI, 2003; Craig, 1999; McAllister, 1996; Meyer & Davis, 1992). Since its first appearance in 1957, more than 2,500 published articles have appeared covering a broad range of topics related to CPI. This undoubtedly results in part from the fact that its scales address a number of immediately important criteria.

Adult Personality Inventory

The *Adult Personality Inventory* (API; Krug, 2004) provides a technology for assessing major dimensions of adult personality and reporting them in terms that are understandable and relevant to a wide array of decisions. Although the API is a relative newcomer on the test scene, its roots lie deep within an assessment tradition that spans more than half a century.

The test consists of 324 items that were selected to measure the same primary trait dimensions included by Cattell in the 16PF. In the scoring process, these trait scales are transformed into three sets of content scales. Each set of scales, 21 in all, provides a different, theoretically based template for understanding personality and its contribution to predictability in different kinds of situations. The Personal Characteristic scales (Extroverted, Adjusted, Tough-Minded, Independent, Disciplined, Creative, and Enterprising) are very broad dimensions that define a factor space that represents the basic structure of phenotypic personality traits. That is, these scales are thought to be located at the highest level of abstraction that is still descriptive of behavior (John, Hampson, & Goldberg, 1991). As would therefore be expected, these scales show substantial content overlap with the five-factor measures of personality (Costa & McCrae, 1992b; Goldberg, 1981, 1993; Norman, 1963).

Individuals differ in many ways. Within personality study, the interpersonal domain—individual differences in how people behave toward one another—has long been a topic of special interest. The eight Interpersonal scales (Caring, Adapting, Withdrawn, Submissive, Uncaring, Non-Conforming, Sociable, Assertive) were developed to provide a representation of the two-dimensional, circular structure that has been found to represent the basic organization of interpersonal traits (LaForge, 1985; Wiggins, 1985). Thus, the eight scales can be represented in a two-dimensional plane, the major axes of which are the Caring–Uncaring and Withdrawn–Assertive dimensions. Because the scales focus on interpersonal relationships, it is not surprising that the scales have been found to be very useful in understanding the dynamics of successful and unsuccessful relationships (Krug & Ahadi, 1986).

The third set of scales, called the Career scales (Practical, Scientific, Aesthetic, Social, Competitive, Structured) relate to career choice, job satisfaction, and lifestyle preferences. These scales were developed empirically by studying response patterns that differentiated people in a broad sampling of occupations (Krug, 1995) and are functionally similar to the Holland occupational types (Ahadi, 1991).

Four validity scales (Good Impression, Bad Impression, Infrequency, Uncertainty) provide a check on various patterns of distortion that can invalidate a test.

Both gender-specific and gender-neutral norms exist to convert raw scores to standard scores. A short form of the API, using only the first 189 items, takes about half the time of the long form. Nevertheless, short-form scale reliabilities are only about 10% lower, on average, than reliabilities for the full test. The average correlation between short- and long-form scales is .88.

The API cannot be scored by hand. Several scoring services provide different kinds of narrative score reports. In addition, several microcomputer editions (Krug, 1985, 1991) provide on-site test administration, scoring, and reporting for PC users. Although most API reports are for professional use, one API report was specifically designed to be shared with clients. The format of the report provides background and contextual information clients can use in analyzing the test scores and focusing the information they contain on a particular problem or decision.

The test can be given to individuals with a 4th-grade reading level, allowing it to be used in a very broad segment of the population. Since responses are computer scored, scoring reliability is virtually perfect.

Technically, the API has a number of positive features. The median reliability across substantive scales, assessed by both internal consistency and test-retest methods, is approximately .82. Norms are based on a sample of more than 1,000 adults who completed Form A of the 16PF at the same time. This made it possible to scale the norms in such a way as to achieve comparability between the component scales of the two instruments. Since the 16PF standardization was perhaps the most extensive ever undertaken with respect to a personality inventory, the linkage of the two sets of scales considerably enhances the normative basis of the API. Like other personality tests, API validation rests on an expanding fabric of interlocking research that links its scales to predicted outcomes and to external measures of theoretically related constructs. This information appears in a series of publications (Krug, 1985, 1986, 1991, 1995, 1997a, 1997b, 2004) and critical reviews (Drummond, 1987; Lanning, 2001) to which interested readers are referred.

Jackson Personality Inventory

The *Jackson Personality Inventory–Revised* (JPI-R; Jackson, 1997) measures 15 bipolar personality characteristics that have particular value in understanding personality functioning in normal individuals. The current (1997) revision of the instrument results from a thoughtfully designed and well-executed strategy of test development intended to produce homogeneous, well-defined scales free from response bias.

Before any test development began, the author prepared a set of carefully written scale descriptions to guide and focus the writers. The initial item pool consisted of 5–10 times more items than would be used in the final test form. This permitted an unusually high degree of item selection during the several rounds of statistical analyses that led to the final test. These analyses were designed to select items that had high content validity, low response bias, and low correlations with other scales in the test. Each scale has an exact balance of true-keyed and false-keyed items.

The test consists of 300 items. Twenty items measure each of the following 15 scales: Complexity, Breadth of Interest, Innovation, Tolerance, Sociability, Social Confidence, Energy Level, Empathy, Anxiety, Cooperativeness, Social Astuteness, Risk Taking, Organization, Traditional Values, and Responsibility. The 15 primary scales are organized additionally in terms of five higher-order clusters: Analytical, Extroverted, Emotional, Opportunistic, and Dependable.

The typical administration requires 45 minutes. The median internal consistency reliability of the scales is approximately .90–.93. Hand scoring takes a few minutes with the carbonless form answer sheet. Mail-in scoring and reporting services are available, as is computer software for on-site processing.

Studies relating scores on the JPI-R to those on other widely used personality tests show a typical pattern of high correlations between like-named scales (e.g., .80 between the Social Confidence scale and the Exhibition scale of the Personality Research Form). Correlations between the JPI-R and the MMPI-R are typically near zero or moderate. Among the largest is a correlation of −.60 between the Social Confidence scale and MMPI Scale 0 (Social Introversion).

As with other normal-range instruments, studies have attempted to understand the relationship of the test's scales to the five-factor model. Despite a reasonable degree of overlap, some scales (Risk Taking, Energy Level, Value Orthodoxy) appeared to lie outside the dimensionality of the five-factor model (Paunonen & Jackson, 1996).

A significant strength of the JPI is its solid psychometric foundation. Few personality tests are as carefully developed. A practical by-product of the elimination of variance related to social desirability responding at the item level during test development is that no validity scales are needed in the final test form.

There is still much to learn about the JPI scales. Despite evidence related to the convergent and divergent validity of the scales reported in the technical manual (Jackson, 1994), validity data are still incomplete. However, the use of the JPI appears to be growing, and it is reasonable to expect that additional validity evidence will be forthcoming.

Hogan Personality Inventory

The *Hogan Personality Inventory* (HPI; Hogan, 1995) was designed primarily for use in personnel selection, employee development, and career-related decision making. It assesses characteristics that aid in understanding how people get along with others and how they achieve educational and career goals. The entire test can be completed in 15–20 minutes and requires about a 4th-grade reading level.

The authors relied explicitly on the five-factor model in the test development process but adjusted the final form to the structure suggested by their own analyses. This involved separating the Extraversion (Surgency) and Intellect (Openness to Experience or Culture) domains into separate components. Consequently, the test is scored for seven major scales: Adjustment, Ambition, Sociability, Interpersonal Sensitivity, Prudence, Inquisitive, and Learning Approach. Six occupational scales (Service Orientation, Stress Tolerance, Reliability, Clerical Potential, Sales Potential, Managerial Potential) provide information directly relevant to career counseling and planning. In addition, the authors identified sets of subthemes within each scale, which they call homogeneous item composites and for which individual scores can also be produced. The test also contains a validity scale that detects careless or random responding.

HPI development relied extensively on samples of employed adults, while most other tests make heavy use of college student respondents. Although personality test developers over the past half-century or more have operated on the assumption that the two populations are interchangeable, there probably are some differences. The HPI benefits from actually having been developed on the populations with which it is used.

The test contains 206 items. The average internal consistency reliability of the scales is .80. Test-retest reliabilities over intervals of 4 weeks or more are somewhat lower (.71, on average).

The test manual (Hogan & Hogan, 1995) provides an interesting summary of validity data that relates HPI scales to peer descriptions and to various aspects of organizational behavior. The former is important to the validity of the test because a primary goal of the authors was to create an instrument that predicted how others would describe a test taker. The latter is refreshing because personality tests are regularly applied, often uncritically, to predict job performances that "sound like" the names of test scales (i.e., employee theft from "integrity," promotion potential from "ambition"). It often works, but it is comforting to see that the test authors can provide documentation, not simply assertions. Meta-analyses of HPI validity data are available in the professional literature (Hogan & Holland, 2003).

The HPI is a relative newcomer compared to tests like the 16PF or the CPI. However, since its introduction at the 1982 Nebraska Symposium, its use has expanded rapidly. The carefully developed validity data that have accumulated so far would seem to predict even wider use for it in years to come.

NEO Personality Inventory

The *NEO Personality Inventory* (NEO PI-R; Costa & McCrae, 1992a), most recently revised in 1995, was specifically developed to assess the five-factor model. "NEO" derives from Neuroticism, Extroversion, and Openness, for which established "facet" scales existed when the test first appeared in 1985. The 1992 revision added facet scales for Agreeableness and Conscientiousness, which were assessed only globally in the first edition.

Two versions of the test exist, one for self-report (Form S) and another for external ratings (Form R). This is an interesting and unusual feature among personality tests, which do not typically provide a parallel instrument for collecting information from outside raters. Each form consists of 240 items to which the test taker responds by selecting one of five responses that range from "strongly disagree" to "strongly agree." In addition to the five domain scores listed above, the test provides scores for 30 facet scales. The test intentionally does not incorporate validity scales per se because the authors believe they may actually detract from the validity of the instrument (McCrae et al., 1989). However, the authors present a series of indicators derived from the performance of a large volunteer sample that provide a check on some common response styles. For example, when the number of "agree" or "strongly agree" responses exceeds 150, the authors suggest a cautious interpretation of the profile because acquiescence may have unduly influenced test results. In addition, the last three questions of the test ask the test taker directly whether he or she has honestly and accurately answered all of the questions and entered the responses correctly. Answers to these questions may be as informative as scores on more sophisticated validity scales.

Internal consistencies for the 48-item domain scales range from .86 to .95. This is unusually, but impressively, high for personality tests, which often appear to be poor cousins of cognitive ability and achievement tests in this respect. Reliabilities for the shorter facet scales are lower (.56 to .90) but still reasonable.

In the 20 years or so since it was first published commercially, an extensive library of research findings has been published (Costa & McCrae, 2003). In addition, given the ubiquity of the five-factor model in contemporary personality research, the NEO PI-R is well-poised to benefit from the accumulation of findings generated by interest in the model itself.

The Role of the Computer in Personality Assessment

With the possible exception of the five-factor model, there is probably nothing else that has had such an impact on applied personality assessment in recent years than the computer. There are three reasons for its involvement. First, it makes the scoring of complicated inventories easy, efficient, and virtually errorless. Second, since Meehl (1954) first presented data to support the argument that statistical prediction is frequently superior to clinical interpretation, it has been repeatedly demonstrated that the computer can outperform the clinician by applying established decision rules uniformly and accurately (Dawes, 1979; Goldberg, 1970; Kleinmuntz, 1963). Finally, the vast outpouring of research results makes it difficult for the unassisted test user to access even a small portion of available test databases reliably and consistently, a task that is easy for the computer. Computer-based test reports can easily represent the accumulated wisdom of many studies and numerous researchers.

Among the earliest attempts to generate electronic reports were those Swenson and Pearson (1964) prepared for the MMPI. The actual program appeared to have been in use for 5 years at the time of their publication. That would make the first computer-based interpretations operational about a decade after computer hardware entered the marketplace and only a few years after programming software developed beyond relatively primitive assemblers.

Other tests soon followed the MMPI lead. At the end of the last millennium, it was difficult to locate a single, important personality instrument that was not supported by computer administration, scoring, and reporting services, many of them Internet-based services.

The first extensive review (Krug, 1984) of the area identified approximately 200 computer-based products and estimated the annual growth rate for such products at 10% to 20%. Less than a decade later, a subsequent review (Krug, 1993) identified a total of 533 such products, with 204 introduced in the 5-year period between 1993 and 1998, which was just about the time Internet testing was beginning to gain interest.

A number of psychologists have voiced concerns about the potential that exists for the misuse of such tools (e.g., Eyde & Kowal, 1984; Matarazzo, 1983; Mitchell, 1984). These concerns relate most often to (a) the technical quality of the products that have been produced so far and the lack of validity information; (b) dangers to the public that could result if these products are allowed to be used by unqualified individuals; and (c) a fear that the computer-based reports may somehow come to replace the professional they were originally created to assist. None of these concerns can be lightly dismissed. A full discussion of the issues involved is beyond the scope of the present chapter. However, it is appropriate to note the following points briefly.

Regarding their technical quality, there has been a gradual improvement in the documentation provided to support the use of many products. This reflects, at least in part, a growing sophistication of users and the increasing availability of better products. That is not to say that adequate documentation exists for every product available. Some seem to have little more substance than the latest self-assessment found in the Sunday supplement.

With regard to the concern about unqualified use, mainline test publishers, at least, appear to control the distribution of these products as carefully as they do the distribution of test materials themselves (Krug, 1993). But controlled access to these products is only a small part of the solution to this problem. Test users need to understand that they need training in such tools just as they need training in the instruments themselves. Failure to use them responsibly can lead to unwanted and serious consequences (Eyde, Robertson, et al., 1993).

As to the fear of professionals' being replaced by technology, one needn't look much further than medicine for some compelling evidence to the contrary. Developments in radiography, advances in pharmacology, and increased reliance on computers in diagnostic testing have not reduced the need for trained professionals; instead, they have dramatically increased their effectiveness.

Conclusion

Normal-range personality inventories provide useful data that contribute to the effectiveness of decisions made in many different rehabilitation settings. Existing instruments incorporate extensive research bases that address a wide variety of relevant issues. Newer instruments, and revisions of well-established instruments, represent increasingly sophisticated products of psychometric knowledge. Greater emphasis on computer applications in test administration, evaluation, and intervention planning appears destined to stimulate further significant advances in applied personality assessment.

References

Ahadi, S. A. (1991). The use of API career factors as Holland occupational types. *Educational and Psychological Measurement, 51,* 167–172.

Allport, G. W., & Odbert, H. S. (1936). Trait-names: A psycholexical study. *Psychological Monographs, 47,* 171.

Alterman, A. I., Renner, B. J., & Cacciola, J. S. (2000). Familial risk for alcoholism and self-reported psychopathology. *Psychology of Addictive Behaviors, 14,* 19–28.

Alterman, A. I., Rutherford, M. J., Cacciola, J. S., McKay, J. R., & Boardman, C. R. (1998). Prediction of seven months methadone maintenance treatment response by four measures of antisociality. *Drug & Alcohol Dependence, 49,* 217–223.

Ashton, M.C., Jackson, D.N., Helmes, E., & Paunonen, S.V. (1998). Joint factor analysis of the Personality Research Form and the Jackson Personality Inventory: Comparisons with the big five. *Journal of Research in Personality, 32,* 243–250.

Barrick, M.R., & Mount, M.K. (1991). The Big-Five personality dimensions in job performance: A meta-analysis. *Personnel Psychology, 44,* 1–26.

Beutler, L.E., Goodrich, G., Fisher, D., & Williams, O.B. (1999). Use of psychological tests/instruments for treatment planning. In M. E. Maruish (Ed.) *The use of psychological testing for treatment planning and outcomes assessment* (2nd ed., pp. 81–114). Mahwah, NJ: Erlbaum.

Bolton, B. (1974). A factor analysis of personal adjustment and vocational measures of client change. *Rehabilitation Counseling Bulletin, 18,* 99–104.

Bolton, B. (1977a). Evidence for the 16PF primary and secondary factors. *Multivariate Experimental Clinical Research, 3,* 1–15.

Bolton, B. (1977b). Rehabilitation client needs and psychopathology. *Rehabilitation Counseling Bulletin, 21,* 7–12.

Bolton, B. (1978). Rehabilitation clients' psychological adjustment: A six-year longitudinal investigation. *Journal of Applied Rehabilitation Counseling, 9,* 133–141.

Bolton, B., & Roessler, R. (1986). *Manual for the Work Personality Profile.* Arkansas: Arkansas Research and Training Center for Vocational Rehabilitation.

Briddick, W.C., Watkins, C.E., Jr., & Savickas, M.L. (1998, March 28–April 1). *Career maturity: A particular type of personal maturity?* Paper presented at the annual meetings of the American Counseling Association, Indianapolis, IN.

Burdsal, C., & Bolton, B. (1979). An item factoring of 16PF-E: Further evidence concerning Cattell's normal personality sphere. *Journal of General Psychology, 100,* 103–109.

Cattell, H.B. (1989). *The 16PF: Personality in depth.* Champaign, IL: Institute for Personality and Ability Testing.

Cattell, H.E.P. (2005). *Spanish-American 16PF fifth edition questionnaire: Technical manual supplement.* Champaign, IL: IPAT.

Cattell, R.B. (1943). The description of personality: Basic traits resolved into clusters. *Journal of Abnormal and Social Psychology, 38,* 476–506.

Cattell, R.B. (1971). *Abilities: Their structure, growth, and action.* Boston: Houghton Mifflin.

Cattell, R.B. (1973). *Personality and mood by questionnaire.* San Francisco: Jossey-Bass.

Cattell, R.B. (1986). The 16PF personality structure and Dr. Eysenck. *Journal of Social Behavior and Personality, 1,* 153–160.

Cattell, R.B. (n.d.). *Sixteen personality factor questionnaire.* San Diego, CA: Educational and Industrial Testing Service.

Cattell, R.B., & Krug, S.E. (1986). The number of factors in the 16PF: A review of the evidence with special emphasis on methodological problems. *Educational and Psychological Measurement, 46,* 509–522.

Chernyshenko, O.S., Stark, S., & Chan, K.Y. (2001). Investigating the hierarchical factor structure of the fifth edition of the 16PF: An application of the Schmid-Leiman orthogonalization procedure. *Educational and Psychological Measurement, 61*(2), 290–302.

Cloninger, C.R. (1987). Neurogenetic adaptive mechanisms in alcoholism. *Science, 236,* 410–416.

Collins, J. M., & Griffin, R. W. (1998). The psychology of counterproductive job performance. In R.W. Griffin & J. M. Collins (Eds.), *Dysfunctional behavior in organizations: Non-violent dysfunctional behavior. Monographs in Organizational Behavior and Relations* (pp. 219–242). Stamford, CT: JAI Press, Inc.

Conn, S.R., & Reicke, M.L. (1994). *The IGPF fifth edition technical manual.* Champaign, IL: Institute for Personality and Ability Testing.

Connors, G. J., DiClemente, C. C., Derman, K. H., Kadden, R. M., Carroll, K. M., & Frone, M. R. (2000). Predicting the therapeutic alliance in alcoholism treatment. *Journal of Studies on Alcohol, 61,* 139–149.

Cook, M., Young, A., Taylor, D., & Bedford, P. (1998). Personality correlates of alcohol consumption. *Personality and Individual Differences, 24,* 641–647.

Cook, T. G. (1998). A typology of antisociality in methadone patients. *Journal of Abnormal Psychology, 107,* 412–422.

Costa, P.T., & McCrae, R.R. (1992a). *NEO personality inventory–Revised.* Odessa, FL: Psychological Assessment Resources.

Costa, P.T., Jr., & McCrae, R.R. (1992b). Normal personality assessment in clinical practice: The NEO personality inventory. *Psychological Assessment, 4,* 5–13.

Costa, P.T., Jr., & McCrae, R.R. (2003). *Bibliography for the Revised NEO Personality Inventory (NEO PI-R) and NEO Five Factor Inventory (NEO-FFI).* Lutz, FL: Psychological Assessment Resources.

CPP, Inc. (2003). *Comprehensive bibliography of the CPI™ assessment: 1948–2002.* Mountain View, CA.

Craig, R.J. (1999). *Interpreting personality tests: A clinical manual for the MMPI-2, MCMI-III, CPI-R, and 16PF.* New York: Wiley.

Davis, A.H. (1983). Motivation: A rational/irrational perspective. *Journal of Applied Rehabilitation Counseling, 14,* 44–51.

Dawes, R.N. (1979). The robust beauty of improper linear models in decision making. *American Psychologist, 34,* 571–582.

Day, D. V., Bedeian, A. G., & Conte, J. M. (1998). Personality as a predictor of work-related outcomes: Test of a mediated structure model. *Journal of Applied Social Psychology, 28,* 2068–2088.

Digman, J.M. (1990). Personality structure: Emergence of the five-factor model. *Annual Review of Psychology, 41,* 417–440.

Drummond, R.J. (1987). Review of the Adult Personality Inventory. In D. J. Keyser & R. C. Sweetland (Eds.), *Test critiques* (Vol. 6, pp. 21–25). Austin: PRO-ED.

Eyde, L.D., & Kowal, D.M. (1984). Ethical and professional concerns regarding computerized test interpretation services and users. *Proceedings of the 92nd Annual Convention of the American Psychological Association.* Washington, DC: American Psychological Association.

Eyde, L.D., Robertson, G., Krug, S.E., Moreland, K.L., Roberston, A.G., Shewan, C.M., et al. (1993). *Responsible test use: Case studies for assessing human behavior.* Washington, DC: American Psychological Association.

Eysenck, H.J. (1976). *The measurement of personality.* Lancaster, England: MTP Press.

Eysenck, H.J. (1986). Can personality study ever be scientific? *Journal of Social Behavior and Personality, 1,* 3–19.

Goldberg, L.R. (1970). Man vs. model of man: A rationale, plus some evidence for a method of improving on clinical inference. *Psychological Bulletin, 73,* 422–432.

Goldberg, L.R. (1981). Language and individual differences: The search for universals in personality lexicons. In L. Wheeler (Ed.), *Review of personality and social psychology* (Vol. 2., pp. 141–165). Beverly Hills, CA: Sage.

Goldberg, L.R. (1993). The structure of phenotypic personality traits. *American Psychologist, 48,* 26–34.

Gough, H. G. (2000). The California Psychological Inventory. In C.E. Watkins & V. L. Campbell (Eds.), *Testing and assessment in counseling practice* (2nd ed., pp. 45–71). Mahwah, NJ: Lawrence Erlbaum Associates.

Gough, H.G., & Bradley, P. (2002). *The California Psychological Inventory manual—Third edition.* Palo Alto, CA: CPP, Inc.

Guilford, J.P. (1975). Factors and factors of personality. *Psychological Bulletin, 82,* 802–814.

Hartigan, J.A., & Wigdor, A.K. (1989). *Fairness in employment testing: Validity generalization, minority issues, and the General Aptitude Test Battery.* Washington, DC: National Academy Press.

Hogan, R. (1995). *Hogan personality inventory.* Tulsa, OK: Hogan Assessment Systems.

Hogan, R., & Hogan, J. (1995). *Hogan Personality Inventory manual—Second edition.* Tulsa, OK: Hogan Assessment Systems.

Hogan, R., Hogan, J., & Roberts, B.W. (1996). Personality measurement and employment decisions. *American Psychologist, 51,* 469–477.

Hogan, J., & Holland, B. (2003). Using theory to evaluate personality and job-performance relations: A socioanalytic perspective. *Journal of Applied Psychology, 88,* 100–112.

Hughey, J., & Burdsal, C. (1982). 16PF-E structure using radial parcels versus items. *Journal of General Psychology, 107,* 107–119.

Hunter, J.E. (1986). Cognitive ability, cognitive aptitudes, job knowledge, and job performance. *Journal of Vocational Behavior, 29,* 340–362.

Jackson, D.N. (1994). *Jackson Personality Inventory manual–Revised.* Port Huron, MI: Sigma Assessment Systems.

Jackson, D.N. (1997). *Jackson personality inventory–Revised.* Port Huron, MI: Sigma Assessment Systems.

John, O. P., Hampson, S. E., & Goldberg, L. R. (1991). The basic level in personality-trait hierarchies: Studies of trait use and accessibility in different contexts. *Journal of Personality and Social Psychology, 60,* 348–361.

Judge, T.A., Heller, D., & Mount, M. K. (2002). Five-Factor Model of personality and job satisfaction: A meta-analysis. *Journal of Applied Psychology, 87,* 530–541.

Karson, M., Karson, S., & O'Dell, J. (1997). *16PF interpretation in clinical practice: A guide to the fifth edition.* Champaign, IL: Institute for Personality & Ability Testing.

Kleinmuntz, B. (1963). MMPI decision rules for the identification of college maladjustment: A digital computer approach. *Psychological Monographs, 77.*

Kleinmuntz, B. (1982). *Personality and psychological assessment.* New York: St. Martin's Press.

Krug, S.E. (1981). *Interpreting 16PF profile patterns.* Champaign, IL: Institute for Personality & Ability Testing.

Krug, S.E. (1984). *Psychware: A reference guide to computer-based products for assessment in psychology, business, and education.* Kansas City, MO: Test Corporation of America.

Krug, S.E. (1985). *TEST PLUS: A microcomputer based system for the Adult Personality Inventory.* Champaign, IL: MetriTech.

Krug, S.E. (1986). Preliminary evidence regarding black-white differences in scores on the Adult Personality Inventory. *Psychological Reports, 58,* 203–206.

Krug, S.E. (1991). *API/Career Profile.* Champaign, IL: MetriTech.

Krug, S.E. (1993). *Psychware Sourcebook: A reference guide to computer-based products for assessment in psychology, business, and education* (4th ed.). Champaign, IL: MetriTech.

Krug, S.E. (1995). Career assessment and the Adult Personality Inventory. *Journal of Career Assessment, 3*(2), 176–187.

Krug, S.E. (1997a). Selection and screening uses of the Adult Personality Inventory in industrial security settings. *Security Journal, 8,* 33–37.

Krug, S.E. (1997b). *Interpretive and technical guide for the Adult Personality Inventory.* Champaign, IL: MetriTech.

Krug, S.E. (2004). The Adult Personality Inventory. In M. E. Maruish (Ed.), *The use of psychological testing for treatment planning and outcomes assessment* (3rd ed., Vol. 3, pp. 679–694). Mahwah, NJ: Erlbaum.

Krug, S.E., & Ahadi, S.A. (1986). Personality patterns among couples participating in a marriage enrichment program. *Multivariate Experimental Clinical Research, 8,* 168–178.

Krug, S.E., & Cattell, R.B. (1971). A test of the trait-view theory of distortion in measurement of personality by questionnaire. *Educational and Psychological Measurement, 31,* 721–734.

Kurtines, W.M., Ball, L.R., & Wood, G.H. (1978). Personality characteristics of long-term recovered alcoholics: A comparative analysis. *Journal of Consulting and Clinical Psychology, 46,* 971–977.

LaForge, R. (1985). The early development of the Freedman-Leary-Coffey interpersonal system. *Journal of Personality Assessment, 49,* 613–621.

Lambert, M.J., & Lambert, J.M. (1999). Use of psychological tests for assessing treatment outcome. In M. E. Maruish (Ed.), *The use of psychological testing for treatment planning and outcomes assessment* (2nd ed., pp. 115–152). Mahwah, NJ: Erlbaum.

Lanning, K. (2001). Review of the Adult Personality Inventory (Revised). In B. S. Plake & J. C. Impara (Eds.), *The fourteenth mental measurements yearbook* (pp. 43–45). Lincoln, NE: Buros Institute of Mental Measurements of the University of Nebraska–Lincoln.

Lord, W. (1997). *16PF5 personality in practice.* Windsor, Berkshire, UK: NFER-Nelson.

Lord, W. (1999). *16PF5 Overcoming Obstacles to Interpretation.* Windsor, Berkshire, UK: NFER Nelson.

Matarazzo, J.D. (1983). Computerized psychological testing. *Science, 221,* 323.

McAllister, L.W. (1996). *A practical guide to CPI interpretation* (3rd ed.). Palo Alto, CA: Consulting Psychologists Press.

McCrae, R.R., Costa, P.T., Jr., Dalhstrom, W.G., Barefoot, J.C., Siegler, I.C., & Williams, R.B., Jr. (1989). A caution on the use of the MMPI K-correction in research on psychosomatic medicine. *Psychosomatic Bulletin, 51,* 58–65.

Meehl, P.E. (1954). *Clinical versus statistical prediction.* Minneapolis, MN: University of Minnesota Press.

Meyer G., Finn S., Eyde L., Kay, G., Moreland, K., Dies, R., et al. (2001). Psychological testing and psychological assessment: A review of evidence and issues. *American Psychologist, 56*(2) 128–165.

Meyer, P., & Davis, S. (1992). *The CPI applications guide.* Palo Alto, CA: Consulting Psychologists Press.

Mitchell, J.V. (1984). Computer-based test interpretation and the public interest. *Proceedings of the 92nd Annual Convention of the American Psychological Association.* Washington, DC: American Psychological Association.

Musante, L., MacDougall, J.M., Dembroski, T.M., & VanHorn, A.E. (1983). Component analysis of the Type A coronary-prone behavior pattern in male and female college students. *Journal of Personality and Social Psychology, 45,* 1104–1117.

Newman, J. L., Gray, E. A., & Fuqua, D. R. (1999). The relation of career indecision to personality dimensions of the California Psychological Inventory. *Journal of Vocational Behavior, 54,* 174–187.

Norman, W.T. (1963). Toward an adequate taxonomy of personality attributes: Replicated factor structure in peer normination personality ratings. *Journal of Abnormal and Social Psychology, 66,* 574–583.

Palladino, J.J., & Motiff, J.P. (1981). Discriminant analysis of Type A/Type B subjects on the California Psychological Inventory. *Journal of Social and Clinical Psychology, 1,* 155–161.

Paunonen, S.V., & Jackson, D.N. (1996). The Jackson Personality Inventory and the five-factor model of personality. *Journal of Research in Personality,* 30, 42–59.

Roessler, R., & Bolton, B. (1978). *Psychosocial adjustment to disability.* Baltimore: University Park Press.

Swenson, W.M., & Pearson, J.S. (1964). Automation techniques in personality assessment: A frontier in behavioral science and medicine. *Methods of Information in Medicine, 3,* 34–36.

Tango, R. A., & Kolodinsky, P. (2004). Investigation of placement outcomes 3 years after a job skills training program for chronically unemployed adults. *Journal of Employment Counseling. 41,* 2, 80–92.

Tett, R.P., Jackson, D.N., & Rothstein, M. (1991). Personality measures as predictors of job performance: A meta-analytic review. *Personnel Psychology, 44,* 703–742.

Wiggins, J.S. (1985). Interpersonal circumplex models: Commentary. *Journal of Personality Assessment, 49,* 626–631.

Wiggins, J.S. (1996). *The five-factor model of personality: Theoretical perspectives.* New York: Guilford.

Wiggins, J.S., & Trapnell, P.D. (1996). A dyadic-interactional perspective on the five-factor model. In J.S. Wiggins (Ed.), *The five-factor model of personality: Theoretical perspectives* (pp. 88–162). New York: Guilford Press.

Woodworth, R. S. (1930). The autobiography of Robert S. Woodworth. In C. Murchison (Ed.), *The history of psychology in autobiography* (Vol. 2, pp. 354–380). Worchester, MA: Clark University Press.

Chapter 7

Assessment of Psychopathology

Rodney L. Lowman and Linda M. Richardson

Assessment of psychopathology or mental disorders in rehabilitation populations has a long history dating back to the post–World War II period. At that time, the rehabilitation population had increased in size and diversity, swelled by the ranks of returning veterans, many of whom had physical and emotional sequelae from the war. This larger and complex population needed to be assessed efficiently, especially given the relative scarcity of trained mental health personnel. In addition, legislation passed in the mid-1940s added persons with behavioral and emotional conditions to the potential rehabilitation population (Brieland, 1971). Rehabilitation psychologists, therefore, expanded their focus from persons with orthopedic and neurological conditions to include people with mental illness and mental retardation (Usdane, 1971). Thus, disabilities addressed by rehabilitation psychologists began to encompass those resulting from birth defects as well as those caused by illness and injury. Assessment techniques to supplement the clinical interview were needed to evaluate the psychological aspects of rehabilitation patients' conditions appropriately and efficiently. These changes in rehabilitation psychology coincided with developments in psychological testing, most notably the publication of the *Minnesota Multiphasic Personality Inventory* (MMPI; Greene, 1991, 1999), now in its second edition (MMPI-2; Butcher, 2000; Butcher, Dahlstrom, Graham, Tellegen, & Kaemmer, 1989; Butcher, Graham, & Ben-Porath, 1995; Greene, 1999). Standardized measures of psychopathology such as the MMPI were less expensive, less time-consuming, and more accurate than interviews and met the need for efficient and effective measures of psychopathology (Eber, 1976). Since then, the psychological assessment of rehabilitation clients has evolved into a complex process determined by the needs of the client as well as the needs of the referral source and the available psychological assessment technology.

Today the assessment of psychopathology is often linked to a more formal diagnostic process since a common referral question is the rather general one entailed in the request for a "diagnostic opinion" about the client's psychological state and health. The primary diagnostic system used by mental health professionals for diagnosing mental disorder is the *Diagnostic and Statistical Manual of Mental Disorders–Fourth Edition* (DSM-IV), published by the American Psychiatric Association (1994). (The next edition of the DSM series, DSM-V, is in development; see, e.g., Schuckit, 2006.) A complete diagnosis consists of assessments on all five dimensions or axes, but only two of the axes, I and II, cover mental disorders. Axis II is limited to personality disorders and mental retardation. Axis III records physical disorders and is often used in the case of rehabilitation clients. Axis IV includes psychosocial and environmental problems, and Axis V consists of a global assessment of the client's current adaptive functioning. The main advantages of DSM-IV are its shorthand, commonly understood, and consensually used language for communicating with other health professionals; its specific diagnostic criteria; and its increasingly empirical emphasis. The disadvantages of this system include the lack of continuity of the diagnoses from one version of the DSM to the next (the list of diagnoses tends to expand, and some of the diagnostic criteria change) and the lack of, or poor quality of, validity data for some of the DSM-IV diagnoses (Neale, Davison, & Haaga,

1996). Although all of the measures to be reviewed in this chapter result in information relevant to generating a diagnosis, some instruments have more explicit links to the DSM diagnostic schema.

Assessing Psychopathology

Goals of Measuring Psychopathology

In contemporary usage, measures of psychopathology with rehabilitation clients have several important goals:

- To identify mental health difficulties in persons experiencing physical disorders or disabilities (This purpose encompasses providing clinical description, differentiating general psychological distress from psychiatric disorder, and differentiating transitory reactions to a disability from a coexisting disorder. It also includes establishing norms for those in the general population and norms for those with a specific disability.)
- To assist in determining how physical conditions or disabilities are best managed or treated (such as in determining how best to treat a patient experiencing chronic back pain that is of both physiological and psychogenic origin)
- To help evaluate the likelihood of a condition's being reported or exaggerated for purposes of secondary gain (e.g., whether a patient with chronic pain is malingering or reporting actual symptoms in an exaggerated or faked manner)
- To evaluate fitness for duty and ability to return to work
- To identify subclinical profiles (i.e., psychological conditions that may influence physical conditions but that may not result in the full criteria for diagnosis of a psychological disorder having been met) that may be associated with physical illness (e.g., Fraguas, Henriques, DeLucia, Iosifescu, Schwartz, Menezes, et al., 2006; Koenig, 2006; Koenig, Vandermeer, Chambers, Burr-Crutchfield, & Johnson, 2006)
- To assist in differentiating psychological conditions causing physical illness versus physical conditions causing medical distress that may appear to be of psychological origin (e.g., Goldstein & Reznikoff, 1972)

Sources of Data and Types of Measures of Psychopathology

Traditionally, measures of psychopathology have been divided into two major types: (1) objective and (2) projective. Objective measures, such as the venerable

MMPI and its successor, MMPI-2 (Butcher et al., 1989; Hathaway & McKinley, 1943), or the much newer *Personality Assessment Inventory* (PAI; Morey, 1991, 1996), attempt to measure psychopathology using a series of forced-choice items to which clients are required to respond. These measures may be further subdivided into (a) omnibus and (b) symptom- or disease-specific measures. Omnibus, or broad-brush, measures of personality cover a number of different types of psychopathology, such as depression, anxiety, and personality disorders. Symptom- or disease-specific measures, in contrast, cover only one disorder, or a limited range of disorders, such as a measure of depression like the *Beck Depression Inventory* (Beck, Ward, Mendelson, Mock, & Erbaugh, 1961), measures of anxiety such as the *State-Trait Anxiety Inventory* (Spielberger, Sydeman, Owen, & Marsh, 1999), or measures of post-traumatic stress disorder (PTSD; e.g., Foa, Cashman, Jaycox, & Perry, 1997).

Projective measures of psychopathology, in contrast, present ambiguous stimuli to which clients are asked to respond. The basic assumption is that the content and structure of an individual's perceptions or responses to such stimuli reflect the person's basic personality style. These measures can be omnibus or more localized. Projective tests are generally not disease or symptom specific. It has been suggested that objective measures are particularly effective in predicting current behavior in specific situations and assessing conscious, behavioral aspects of functioning, while projective measures are especially effective in predicting behavior over time and assessing unconscious, longitudinal, and structural aspects of functioning (Masling, 1997; Stricker & Gold, 1999).

Another method of categorizing measures of psychopathology is on the basis of the extensiveness or breadth of the types of psychopathology assessed. Tests can be grouped into brief screening instruments and more extensive measures of psychopathology. Screening measures such as the *Symptom Checklist-90 Revised* (SCL-90R; Derogatis, 1977, 1994; Derogatis & Savitz, 2000) are short tests used to identify individuals who might be experiencing psychological distress. More extensive measures such as a structured clinical interview or an omnibus objective or projective measure of psychopathology are then given to pinpoint the nature of the client's difficulties as well as to provide a broader understanding of the individual.

Derogatis, Fleming, Sudler, and DellaPetra (1995) suggested the use of screening measures with all patients who are chronically ill followed by the administration of more specific tools for those with positive results on screening. This method would likely result in the identification of some individuals with possible psychopathology that might otherwise go undetected, and it would conserve intensive assessment resources for evaluating those persons with a raised probability of psychiatric disorder.

Typically, clinical assessments of psychopathology have drawn on data from three major sources: the clinical interview (which usually includes historical data and observational data on the client), projective measures, and objective measures. It is generally acknowledged that multiple measures or a test battery are more effective than a single measure in providing information needed to respond to referral questions as a result of the varied methods and sources of data. Selection of measures to use with a specific rehabilitation client will depend on several factors, including the referral question, the functioning of the client (i.e., whether the client has visual, hearing, or physical deficits that might affect his or her ability to complete various measures of psychopathology), and the assessment context. Increasingly, referral sources and third-party payers emphasize cost, speed of feedback, and utility of results when requesting assessment services. Thus, these variables also need to be considered when assembling a psychological test battery. Other significant factors in test selection include the validity, reliability, and utility of the measures under consideration.

Issues in Assessing Psychopathology

When undertaking an assessment of psychopathology, several issues need to be considered, including the background characteristics of the examinee, the setting of the examination, and the likelihood of overreporting or underreporting psychiatric symptoms. Background characteristics of the client are important variables that must be considered in making test selections, in administering the tests, and in interpreting the results. Factors such as ethnicity, culture, and country of origin can have a significant impact in all of these domains (Butcher, 1995). As minority groups continue to grow in the United States, there has been increasing recognition that assessment methodologies developed, standardized, and applied to the majority group may not be suitable to other groups in the population. Dana (1996) urged psychologists to conduct "culturally competent" assessments using culture-specific styles of service delivery, the person's first language, and tests with appropriate cultural norms. He recommended that each person be assessed as a member of a culture prior to initiating testing (Dana, 1996). Likewise, the client's sex and age must be considered. Many psychological tests are normed by gender and sometimes by age as well, reflecting the importance of these variables.

Psychological assessment of rehabilitation clients may take place in a variety of settings, including a hospital (typically a medical–surgical or rehabilitation facility), a long-term care setting (e.g., a skilled nursing facility or rehabilitation center), or an outpatient setting (e.g., the office of the examiner or the rehabilitation counselor). The setting may influence which psychopathology measures can be used. Some settings will offer quiet and privacy, whereas others may be noisy and inappropriate for the administration of certain assessment measures. While an objective measure can be given almost anywhere (although a quiet area is preferable), projective measures require a quiet and private setting, free of interruptions. Clients in some settings may have impairments (e.g., visual impairments, inability to use hands) limiting their ability to complete certain measures on their own or with assistance.

A thorny issue in psychological assessment concerns the possibility that the client may overreport or underreport psychiatric symptoms. Greene (1991,

1999) has suggested that some clients may try to make themselves look more disturbed than they actually are ("fake bad") because they are extremely distressed and want to make sure their distress is noticed. Others may do so because they tend generally to overreact or to experience themselves as traumatized. Others may be trying to look bad for reasons of secondary gain (e.g., their desire to obtain workers' compensation or disability benefits). Rehabilitation clients sometimes may not wish to appear to have restored their functioning if that results in return to work or loss of a financial benefit. Some may want to stop working and may approach the assessment as an opportunity to assist in achieving that goal. It may be easier to make oneself look psychologically disturbed on objective measures of psychopathology than on projective measures since the projective test stimuli are more ambiguous. While it is impossible to prevent clients from malingering on psychological tests, steps can be taken to detect and minimize malingering. Proper preparation of the client for the assessment is essential. In addition, administration of multiple measures of psychopathology, along with a thorough clinical interview and collection of observational data, if possible, is advisable when a comprehensive assessment is possible. If a psychologist does suspect overreporting or malingering, he or she might wish to obtain confirming data from at least two sources (i.e., two psychological measures), including on those tests that include well-validated scales measuring test-taking orientation. Once the clinician is fairly certain that the client has overreported or malingered, he or she should consider counseling with the client and possibly repeating some measures or, as appropriate, making it clear in the assessment report that the results appear not to accurately represent the patient's actual condition.

Although malingering or overreporting is more common, underreporting or trying to minimize psychological symptomatology can also be a potential problem with rehabilitation populations. Clients may underreport mental health concerns because they do not believe they have problems, because they acknowledge having problems but are so accustomed to them that they experience little or no distress, or because they want to look mentally healthy to attain a specific goal (e.g., entry into a specific rehabilitation program). While there is no certain method for preventing underreporting, the clinician can prepare the client for the assessment by stressing the importance of honesty and forthrightness. Clinicians should try to make the client feel comfortable in the assessment situation by establishing rapport and by meeting in a quiet, relaxed setting. Multiple sources of data can be used to support a conclusion that a client's psychopathology was likely underreported. If underreporting is found, the clinician can counsel the client about this issue and consider repeating one or more of the measures.

The amount of time available to conduct an assessment and the budget available for assessment may also be factors in using certain assessment measures with rehabilitation clients. In some cases, only brief screenings may be possible for most rehabilitation patients in a particular setting. Additionally, patients with certain conditions may require nonstandard test administrations. This is because certain physical conditions may slow test administration or because modifications of procedure may be necessary to accommodate specific impairments. Additionally, there is some, if limited, evidence that certain physical conditions (e.g., spinal cord injuries) may be associated with differential results on psychological tests (see, e.g., Rodevich & Wanlass, 1995). Indeed, in certain rehabilitation conditions, sorting out the psychological symptoms that constitute the syndrome or condition itself and whether there is additional psychological impairment that may require its own intervention is an important part of the assessment question.

Specific Measures of Psychopathology

In this section, we will review three major types of measures of psychopathology: structured interviews, objective measures, and projective measures. In each category, many of the most commonly used measures will be discussed. We will cover each test's basic purpose, structure, scoring, interpretation, validity and reliability data, and likely uses with rehabilitation populations.

Structured Interviews

Most clinicians administer an interview when conducting a psychological evaluation. This interview may be individually designed or standardized and have a structured, semistructured, or unstructured format. There are at least three standardized interviews that are widely used in the United States: the *Structured Clinical Interview for DSM-IV* (SCID), the *Diagnostic Interview Schedule* (DIS), and the *Schedule for Affective Disorders and Schizophrenia* (SADS; Groth-Marnat, 1999).

Structured Clinical Interview for DSM-IV

The *Structured Clinical Interview for DSM-IV* (Spitzer, Williams, & Gibbon, 1987; Spitzer, Williams, Gibbon, & First, 1987) is perhaps the most comprehensive of the structured interviews. It was based on the *Research Diagnostic Criteria* (Spitzer, Endicott, & Robins, 1978), which contributed to DSM-III (American Psychiatric Association, 1980). The SCID has been revised several times (in 1983, 1987, and 1995). Although the diagnostic categories of the SCID closely parallel the DSM system and a DSM diagnosis may emerge from the data, the SCID does not cover all DSM diagnostic categories. There are several versions of the instrument, including versions for inpatients, outpatients, nonpatients, Axis I disorders, and Axis II disorders. Additionally, specialized scales have been proposed for this measure, including for the assessment of behavioral disorders in adolescents and dissociative disorders (e.g., Smith, Huber, & Hall, 2005; Steinberg, 2000).

Typically, the SCID is given face-to-face by an examiner, although some forms can be administered on the computer. The instrument has been translated into several languages. Open-ended questions and items that may rule out various conditions provide some flexibility in administration, which usually takes 1 to 2 hours. It is possible to limit the scope of the interview to a specific group of disorders because the questions are clustered in modules of test items by disorder groups. There is also an abbreviated computerized version, the Mini-SCID (First, Gibbon, Williams, & Spitzer, 1995). Because clinical judgment is required to administer this test (because of the open-ended nature of the questions), a trained mental health professional must conduct the interview. Data from sources outside the interview may also be utilized. Research on the SCID indicates that its reliability has been inconsistent and validity research has been quite limited, so more validity and reliability studies are greatly needed (Groth-Marnat, 1999; Segal, 1997).

Potential advantages of using the SCID as a structured interview include its comprehensiveness, its flexibility (given the multiple forms and the test item format), and its compatibility with DSM-IV. Its disadvantages include its length and its somewhat limited validity and reliability data. With rehabilitation populations, it provides a comprehensive assessment of mental disorders and thus may be particularly useful when a mental disorder is suspected but the type of disorder is not known (e.g., Koenig, Vandermeer, Chambers, Burr-Crutchfield, & Johnson, 2006).

In addition, its flexible format allows it to be adapted to the specific disabilities of the client. Note that a new measure—the *Comprehensive Addictions And Psychological Evaluation* (CAAPE; Gallagher, Penn, Brooks, Feldman, & Gallagher, 2006) is a relatively new brief instrument intended to measure some of the same mental health factors as the SCID.

Diagnostic Interview Schedule

The *Diagnostic Interview Schedule* is a highly structured interview that was developed for use in epidemiological research. It was designed to be administered by a nonprofessional interviewer with minimal training (Robins, Helzer, Croughan, & Ratcliff, 1981). It can also be computer administered. This test has undergone several revisions. Its current version is compatible with DSM-IV (Segal, 1997). In the administration of the DIS, as many as 478 ratings are made, requiring 1 to 1.5 hours to complete. The questions are all forced-choice, and a probe flow sheet allows the interviewer to skip areas that are not relevant to the interviewee. No collateral information is sought. The DIS has been translated into several languages. There are 24 primary diagnostic categories generated by the computer-generated data analyses. A version of the instrument has been developed for use with children, adolescents, and parents (Johnson, Barrett, Dadds, Fox, & Shortt 1999).

The record is mixed on the validity and reliability of the DIS. While the reliability appears to be adequate, the validity evidence and test-retest reliability are somewhat problematic (Groth-Marnat, 1999; Hodges, 1994; Segal,

1997; Wells, Burnam, Leake, & Robins, 1988). There has been little research investigating the relationship between the diagnosis generated by the DIS and external diagnostic criteria. Clearly, more research is needed. It has been recommended that mental health professionals avoid using the DIS alone for diagnosis until better validity and reliability data on the instrument are available (Segal, 1997).

The main advantage of the DIS is its ease of administration and scoring, both of which may be done by laypersons or by computer, thus reducing the cost of the assessment (Groth-Marnat, 1999). The DIS may be given by an office assistant with a limited mental health background, saving a clinician's time for follow-up on the data it generates and allowing more clients to be assessed. Its main disadvantage is its potentially problematic validity and reliability.

Schedule of Affective Disorders and Schizophrenia

The *Schedule of Affective Disorders and Schizophrenia* (SADS; Endicott & Spitzer, 1978; Carmer, 1995; Hasin, 1991) is a semi-structured interview developed for use in clinical research. It was intended to provide a standardized method for obtaining homogeneous subject groups by diagnosis, focusing on affective disorders and schizophrenia. It represented one of the earliest systematic efforts to collect diagnostic data (in contrast to the then-typical psychiatric research methods, in which wide variability in information obtained and criteria used to evaluate it was common).

In the SADS, symptoms of psychiatric disorder are rated by the interviewer, and diagnoses are generated using categories gleaned from *Research Diagnostic Criteria,* developed by Spitzer and colleagues (1978). These diagnostic groupings were a forerunner to DSM-III diagnoses and were intended to be an improvement on DSM-II. While the SADS was not created with the intent of generating diagnoses deriving from the *DSM* series, schizophrenic disorders, affective disorders, anxiety disorders, alcohol abuse, and drug abuse are covered by this instrument. Over the years, the SADS has been revised several times, and it has also been translated into multiple languages and used with different populations (e.g., correctional ones; e.g., Rogers, Jackson, Salekin, & Neumann, 2003).

To administer this tool, a trained mental health professional makes ratings on more than 200 items on a Likert-type scale from 1 to 6, assessing symptoms along dimensions of severity of impairment or frequency of occurrence. Data for the ratings are derived from the client interview as well as from any other available source (e.g., records, interviewees' significant others). The test consists of two parts—current symptoms and past problems—which can be given individually or together. When assessing present symptoms, the focus is either the past week or the period of greatest symptom severity during the latest episode. Since clinical judgment is required to make such ratings, the interviewer must be trained in mental health as well as in the use of this instrument. There are several forms of the test that differ primarily with regard to the time period covered. Administration of both parts of the SADS typically takes 1.5 to 2 hours. The SADS items are clustered by diagnostic groups and "rule out" questions precede each section, both facilitating administration and potentially decreasing administration time. Scores are generated on eight Summary Scales—Mood and Ideation, Endogenous Features, Depressive-associated Features, Suicidal Ideation and Behavior, Anxiety, Manic Syndrome, Delusions-Hallucinations, and Formal Thought Disorder—and 24 diagnostic scales. Computer scoring is not currently available.

Of the three structured interview formats discussed in this review, the SADS is probably the most widely used in psychiatric research and has to date the strongest validity and reliability evidence. Its summary scales have very high reliability. The diagnostic scales vary in reliability, although most are high (Segal, 1997). Validity data on the SADS are somewhat weaker, in large part because of the validity of the diagnostic criteria, the *Research Diagnostic Criteria* (Arbisi, 1995). When used with rehabilitation populations, the major advantages of the SADS are its validity and reliability and its symptom severity ratings, while its disadvantages are its length, the necessity of using a trained mental health professional as the test administrator, and its restricted range of covered diagnoses (i.e., PTSD and personality disorders are not included). In addition, since this tool was developed at a time when an earlier version of the DSM was current, the language of some items may not fit contemporary parlance.

Objective Measures

Minnesota Multiphasic Personality Inventory

The *Minnesota Multiphasic Personality Inventory* was originally developed in 1940 and first published in 1942. It is one of the most frequently used measures of psychopathology (Watkins, Campbell, Nieberding, & Hallmark, 1995). Since its introduction, it has been used in a very wide range of clinical and research settings. Its only revision to date, the MMPI-2 (Butcher et al., 1989; Graham, 2006), represents a restandardization of the MMPI. Changes found in the MMPI-2 include the rewording of some items, the creation of a significant number of new items, and the addition of several validity indicators and supplemental scales. Expansion of the normative sample nationally by increasing its size and including minority groups to more accurately represent the current U.S. population was a noteworthy change in the MMPI-2 (Hathaway & McKinley, 1989). The *T* scores (standardizations of the raw scores to facilitate score interpretation) were also revised for all the most commonly used clinical scales (except for the Masculinity–Femininity and Social Introversion scales) and all the content scales, with the result that the scales now have the same range and distribution.

Both the MMPI and MMPI-2 are extremely widely used objective measures of psychopathology. The MMPI-2 is a self-report instrument consisting of

567 true/false items that were obtained from a variety of sources, including the authors' clinical experience and other personality measures. Using an empirical keying method, the items were selected for their ability to differentiate between normal persons and criterion groups representing major psychiatric disorders. Originally, the MMPI clinical scales were intended to identify membership in various diagnostic groups. However, it has been found that because of considerable test item overlap and other test characteristics, the scales may be more effective in describing abnormal personality traits (Groth-Marnat, 1999) rather than as "pure" measures of diagnostic categories.

The MMPI-2 exists in several forms, including the group form, the research form, the audiotape recorded form, and the computer-based form, all with identical item order, and may be given to individuals or groups. It is recommended that the written forms be given only to people age 18 or older with at least an 8th-grade reading level. If the written forms are given to a 16- or 17-year-old person, adolescent norms must be used. Those younger than age 16 should be administered the MMPI-A, the adolescent form of the MMPI. Most adults complete the test in 1 to 1.5 hours. Scoring may be done by hand (using scoring templates) or by computer. Hand scoring of the basic scales can be done fairly rapidly. Scoring by computer yields a profile report, which consists of the client's raw scores and T scores on the basic and additional scales. Interpretive reports can also be generated. Some of the currently available reports include the *Caldwell Report,* the *Minnesota Report,* and the *MMPI-2 Adult Interpretive System.*

Basic scoring of the MMPI consists of computing scores on four validity scales, which assess test-taking attitudes (Cannot Say, Lie, Infrequency, and Correction), and 10 clinical scales, which measure major types of abnormal behavior (Hypochondriasis, Depression, Hysteria, Psychopathic Deviate, Masculinity–Femininity, Paranoia, Psychasthenia, Schizophrenia, Mania, and Social Introversion; Greene, 1991). The basic scales can be scored from the first 370 test items, although it is recommended that the entire test be given, permitting the scoring of many additional specialized scales. Once the raw scores are obtained, they are converted to standard, or T, scores, which are plotted on a profile sheet according to the client's gender. The standardization makes it possible to compare across scales. Once the client's test profile has been reviewed and found to be valid, interpretation of the data focuses on those clinical scales with the highest scores, the elevation of the scores on the various clinical scales, and the overall scale configuration. Based on T scores, low scores are 40 and below, modal scores are 41–55, moderate scores are 56–65, high scores are 66–75, and very high scores are 76 and above (Hathaway & McKinley, 1989). Elevations on isolated test scores are less important than the overall combinations of scales that are elevated. These are often described according to their two highest clinical scale scores that are greater than a T score of 65 on the MMPI-2 (or greater than a T score of 70 on the MMPI) and are referred to as the "two-point code." Since the scores were lower on the MMPI-2 than the MMPI during its development, the T score cutoff was lowered and any score above the cutoff was considered significant. The interpretation of psychopathology is not done on the basis of single-scale elevation, however, but rather by examining the patterns of scales that are elevated.

The MMPI can also be scored on a variety of other scales (see, e.g., Greene, 1999). Supplemental scales include the Anxiety, Repression, and Ego Strength Scale and the *MacAndrew Alcoholism Scale–Revised*. Additional scales include the Overcontrolled Hostility, Dominance, Social Responsibility, College Maladjustment, Gender Role, and Post-Traumatic Stress Disorder scales. There are also 15 content-specific scales, including Fears, Bizarre Mentation, and Work Interference. Critical Items (i.e., those test items thought individually to be of special clinical significance) are also used in interpreting the MMPI. Several versions of these exist, including the Koss-Butcher and Lachar-Wrobel Critical Item sets. There are also subscales such as the Harris-Lingoes subscales, or some of the clinical scales (e.g., Depression, Hysteria, Paranoia). While MMPI and MMPI-2 test data may generate a psychiatric diagnosis that may be compatible with DSM, the scales were not developed to correlate with DSM disorders.

There are extensive data on the validity and reliability of the MMPI (there are thousands of studies), but not all the results have been favorable. There is generally good evidence for the construct validity of the major scales. However, support for the test's temporal stability and internal consistency is only moderate (Butcher et al., 1989; Groth-Marnat, 1999; Hunsley, Hanson, & Parker, 1988).

Nonetheless, there are numerous benefits to using the MMPI in personality assessment. First, since the MMPI is a self-report measure, an examiner is not required. It also demands little examiner time for scoring, whether scoring is done by hand or by computer. Second, the scoring is objective, thus eliminating examiner bias. Third, the data collected can be scored on a variety of scales, and individual responses to critical test items can be assessed as well, providing a large body of information on the individual. Fourth, there is a wealth of clinical and research data available on the MMPI to assist in test interpretation. Fifth, there are considerable data on test-taking orientation including suspected malingering (see, e.g., Bacchiochi & Bagby, 2006; Nelson, Parsons, Grote, Smith, & Sisung, 2006). Sixth, the test permits computerized administration, scoring, and interpretation not only to save examiner time and ensure accuracy and completeness of scoring but also to provide comprehensive interpretive information, minimizing examiner subjectivity (Butcher, 1995; Williams & Weed, 2004).

Despite the ubiquity of their usage, the MMPI/MMPI-2 tests still have potential limitations. First, the test is extremely long, which can easily fatigue certain rehabilitation clients. Even though an abbreviated version of the test (the first 370 items) can be administered, only the basic scales can be scored. There have been several attempts to develop short forms of the MMPI—most notably the *Mini-Mult, Abbreviated MMPI,* and *MMPI-168*—in an effort to address this problem, but the results have been mixed (Greene, 1991). Greene, Gwin, and Staal (1997) advise against the use of short forms at this time because of the low concordance rates and the lack of research validating them. Second, there is considerable overlap of items across scales, resulting in fairly high intercorrelations across the scales. Although recent work to reconstitute the scales is promising (Simms, Casillas, Clark, Watson, & Doebbling, 2006), the commercially available version of the test used in routine clinical practice is still the long one. Third, many of the test items are transparent, perhaps overly so for certain rehabilitation assessment purposes.

Fourth, the number of true items far surpasses the number of false items, which may facilitate attempts at dissimulation. Fifth, the scale names (e.g., Schizophrenia scale) may be misleading because the scales are not necessarily pure measures of the diagnoses for which the scales are named. Finally, computer-generated interpretive reports, while comprehensive and time-efficient, may not always be sufficiently specific, may not fully fit the client, and may seem overly precise scientifically without being clinically meaningful (Butcher, 1995).

Despite these issues, the MMPI-2 and its predecessor are very widely used. The test is well-suited for assessment of special populations and with various ethnic groups (Arbisi, Ben-Porath, & McNulty, 2002; Hall, Bansal, & Lopez, 1999; Butcher, Cheung, & Lim, 2003; Dong & Church, 2003). It has been translated into more than 150 languages for use in more than 50 countries. In addition, there is a videotaped American Sign Language form. However, the translations may not always be completely accurate or culturally sensitive (e.g., Dana, 1996). The test has been used with people with various disabilities and conditions such as anorexia, blindness, chronic pain, deafness, depression, head injuries, schizophrenia, spinal cord injuries, and substance abuse. The test is typically used to describe and classify these populations, to predict treatment success and post-treatment outcome, and to predict satisfaction with treatment—with mixed results (e.g., Belding, Iguchi, Morral, & Husband, 1998; Vendrig, Derksen, & de Mey, 1999). However, since disabled groups are not necessarily homogeneous, it may be overly simplistic to assume that any given disabled group is likely to present in a uniform manner on this or any measure of personality. The MMPI-2 has also been used to describe and predict, with mixed success, who will return to work in a work hardening rehabilitation program (Allen & Webb, 1999). It also has been used extensively in the attempt to identify those who are feigning mental illness for ulterior motives (see, e.g., Bury & Michael, 2002) and in assessment of injured workers and those in rehabilitation (Alexy & Webb, 1999; Colotla, Bowman, & Shercliffe, 2001; Scheibe, Bagby, Miller, & Dorian, 2001).

Personality Assessment Inventory

The *Personality Assessment Inventory,* developed by Morey and first published in 1991 (Morey, 1995), like the MMPI-2, is an omnibus measure of abnormal traits. A self-report instrument, it consists of 344 items that require the subject to choose among four response alternatives: "false, not at all true," "slightly true," "mainly true," and "very true." It is intended for use with adults 18 years of age or older who have a reading level of at least 4th grade. The test takes 50–60 minutes to complete. There is also a short form (see Frazier, Naugle,

& Haggerty, 2006), but its use has generally not been recommended because of the large number of scales and relatively small number of test items (Boyle & Lennon, 1996). Scores are obtained on 22 nonoverlapping scales, including 4 validity scales, 11 clinical scales, 5 treatment scales, and 2 interpersonal scales. In addition, there are subscales on 10 primary scales and a Critical Items Form that contains 27 items from 7 areas that point to behavior or psychopathology that might warrant immediate attention because of the very low frequency of the behavior and its potential for developing into a crisis. Scoring is quite simple because the two-part answer sheet includes a top sheet on which the client responds and a bottom self-carbon sheet on which all the client's responses are scored. In addition to the written form, there is a computerized version of the test. Raw scores are translated into T scores with a mean of 50 and a standard deviation of 10. Scores are then plotted on an Adult Profile Form, which includes a standardization profile and a clinical sample profile. Any score equal to or greater than 70 on the PAI requires further exploration because it suggests a significant deviation from the mean. Interpretation is based on single-scale elevations and the pattern of elevations. The client's profile can also be compared to 10 modal profiles, which were generated by cluster analysis, although it has been noted that the process of assigning a given profile to one of these 10 profile groups is difficult and time-consuming (Kavan, 1995). Computerized interpretive reports are also available. Normative data have been collected on adults residing in the community, college students, clients receiving mental health services, African Americans, and older adults. Few differences have been found by gender or race, but some differences by age have been noted. The PAI has been translated into other languages, including Spanish, Chinese, and Arabic. There is also some evidence of the utility of the dissimulation scales of the PAI (Blanchard, McGrath, Pogge, & Khadivi, 2003).

While much of the research on the PAI suggests that it has value as an assessment instrument, there is some controversy over its construct validity evidence and its factor structure (Boyle, 1995; Conger & Conger, 1996; Deisinger, 1995; Fantoni-Salvador & Rogers, 1997; Morey, 1995; White, 1996). In addition, the validity and reliability data for the Inconsistency and Infrequency scales are weaker than for other scales (Kavan, 1995). Its use by practicing psychologists appears to be limited, although growing, presumably in part because of its relatively recent development and commercial sale. Although not specifically devised to assess DSM disorders, the PAI test data can be used to diagnose some of the disorders.

Advantages of the PAI include its use of contemporary language, its nonoverlapping scale items, and some of its psychometric properties. Its main weaknesses, aside from its lack of widespread usage and the absence to date of an extensive research literature, include the factor analytic data on the test's scales and the relatively large number of scales on the test as compared with the number of test items (Boyle, 1995). Review of the literature on the PAI published to date suggests that the instrument has been used thus far primarily in research on dissimulation, particularly with offender populations (Rogers, Sewell, Morey, & Ustad, 1996). In rehabilitation populations, it has been used most often with patients who abuse drugs or alcohol or patients who are receiving treatment for pain (George & Wagner, 1995; Schinka, 1995; Schinka, Curtiss, & Mulloy, 1994).

Millon Clinical Multiaxial Inventory

The *Millon Clinical Multiaxial Inventory* (MCMI-III; Choca, Shanley & Van Denburg, 1992; Craig, 2005; Jankowski, 2002; Millon, 1994) is an objective personality measure that assesses personality style, emotional adjustment, and test-taking style. In developing this instrument, Millon's goal was to create a personality instrument that would overcome the major liabilities of the MMPI while retaining some of its positive attributes. First published in 1977, the MCMI was revised in 1987 and again in 1994. It is one of the most frequently used objective measures of psychopathology and one of the few that have been widely adopted in general clinical practice in the past 25 years. An objective self-report measure, the MCMI-III consists of 175 true/false items drawn from a large pool of items that were created based on Millon's theories of personality (e.g., Davis, 1999; Millon, 1990, 1996; Millon & Davis, 1996; Widiger, 1999).

The most recent revision, MCMI-III, was updated on the basis of refinements in Millon's theories, data on earlier versions of the instrument, and DSM-IV. Efforts have been made to keep the MCMI consistent with the current version of the DSM. Additions to the MCMI-II incorporated into the MCMI-III include another personality style scale, the Depressive scale, and another clinical syndrome scale, the Post-Traumatic Stress Disorder scale, which was added to reflect the addition of PTSD to the DSM. There were also changes made in the item weighting. Prototype items, which are thought to be of greater importance to the scale, are assigned 2 points and all other items are assigned 1 point (Millon, 1994).

Two forms of the test are now available: one for hand scoring and the other for computer scoring. There is also an audiotaped form, which can be given to clients who are unable to take a written form of the test. Written and audiotaped forms are also available in Spanish. Appropriate clients for this measure are at least 18 years old and have at least an 8th-grade reading level. Typical administration time, according to the test manual, is 20–30 minutes, although we have found that clients often take more time. The test is either hand scored using templates and multiple computations or computer scored by the test publisher. Hand scoring may take a half-hour or more, and the process is complex (and may be unreliable) as a result of the numerous and tedious computations required. The machine scoring is done by mailing the completed answer sheet to a test-scoring service or by automated on-line scoring. The raw data collected from the written form can also be computer scored.

Raw scores from the MCMI-III are generated on 28 scales grouped in five clusters: Modifying Indices (the Validity Index, Disclosure, Desirability, and Debasement scales), Clinical Personality Patterns (the Schizoid, Avoidant, Depressive, Dependent, Histrionic, Narcissistic, Antisocial, Aggressive–Sadistic, Compulsive, Passive–Aggressive, and Self-Defeating scales), Severe Personality Pathology (the Schizotypal, Borderline, and Paranoid scales), Clinical Syndromes (the Anxiety, Somatoform, Bipolar: Manic, Dysthymia, Alcohol Dependence, Drug Dependence, and Post-Traumatic Stress Disorder scales), and the Severe Syndromes (Thought Disorder, Major Depression, and Delusional Disorder scales). These raw scores are then transformed into base rate (BR) scores, which are generated from the frequency with which the particular variable occurs in the population. Finally, depending on the elevation of certain BR scores, adjustments are sometimes made to these scores to obtain the final BR scores. If the Disclosure scale raw score is quite high (greater than 123), scores on several scales will be lowered. Or, if the final BR score on the Anxiety scale is 75 or higher, the scores on several scales will be decreased (Millon, 1994). The final BR scores are then plotted by gender on a profile sheet.

Test interpretation of the MCMI-III involves attention to high point scale scores and profile analysis. These interpretations are made within the context of the subject's test-taking approach. Unlike many tests of psychopathology, the MCMI includes scales assessing both clinical disorders and personality disorders. The Clinical Personality Patterns (Personality Style) scales are thought to reflect the client's enduring psychological functioning, or personality style. The Severe Personality Pathology scales assess psychological disorders of personality. The Clinical Syndromes scales assess distortions of the basic personality style that tend to be transient, are often precipitated by specific events, and represent active psychopathology, with the Clinical Syndromes scales representing moderately severe disorders and the Severe Syndromes scales representing markedly severe disorders (Millon, 1994).

Research on the MCMI indicates that the test has strong internal consistency and generally promising test-retest reliability (Craig, 2005; Jankowski, 2002; Retzlaff, 1998). Data on the validity of the test are more limited than data for some of the long-established measures of psychopathology, although the initial findings are promising (Groth-Marnat, 1999; Hess, 1998). As with most "newer" tests, more research is needed to establish the test's validity for its intended assessment purposes. Part of the difficulty in validating the test is that, in its relatively short existence, it has already been through three rather substantial revisions. It is not clear that the research studies from one version apply to the others.

There are several advantages to using the MCMI-III. First, it is a relatively brief measure, which enhances client cooperation and minimizes fatigue. Second, it includes scales that assess personality style and personality disorders, both of which are important to understanding personality and psychopathology but are rarely included in other measures of psychopathology. Third, it is based on both a theoretical model, which provides a framework for interpreting the test results, and empirical research. Fourth, it has been developed to coordinate with the DSM, which facilitates making diagnoses using that system. Fifth, some of the scales reflect varying levels of symptom severity within a given clinical syndrome (e.g., depression; Millon, 1994).

But the MCMI is not without disadvantages. Tendencies to overpathologize and overdiagnose people and to generate overly negative descriptions in interpretive reports have been reported (Flynn, McCann, & Fairbank, 1995). Since most of the test items are keyed True, those who tend to respond "yes" to items (yea-sayers) are overpathologized (Hess, 1998). The test has been revised often, which can be good, but the frequent revisions complicate research because it is not clear that data collected on one version apply to subsequent versions. There is also considerable item overlap among the scales, resulting in high interscale correlations. Although the BR scale adjustments are made in part to compensate for this characteristic, the high correlations among scales measuring traits (personality scales) and those measuring states (clinical scales) are problematic because personality theory suggests that the opposite would be expected (Groth-Marnat, 1999). Moreover, the use of the BR scores, an interesting new approach to abnormal psychology measurement, needs further research. The instrument is clouded by the fact that epidemiological data for determining BRs for the various scales are lacking (Hess, 1998). Finally, the MCMI has a fairly large number of scales, given the number of test items (Retzlaff, 1998).

The MCMI has been utilized in research with a variety of rehabilitation populations, including persons who abuse substances and persons with bulimia (Craig & Weinberg, 1992; Tisdale, Pendleton, & Marler, 1990). Millon has also developed an assessment tool for individuals with a physical illness and persons who are clients of rehabilitation or behavioral medicine: the *Millon Behavioral Health Inventory* (e.g., Strack, 1999). This self-report measure evaluates health-related psychological coping in adult medical patients. While it may identify persons with problems resulting from a life stressor or a psychological disorder, it was not designed to measure psychopathology. This 150-item true/false test can be given to persons 18 years of age or older with an 8th-grade reading level and requires about 20 minutes to complete. The data are scored on 20 scales that are grouped in four categories: Basic Coping Style, Psychogenic Attitudes, Psychosomatic Correlates, and Prognostic Indicators. While this measure can be very helpful in assessing clients with disabilities, it cannot take the place of a measure of psychopathology.

Clinical Analysis Questionnaire

The *Clinical Analysis Questionnaire* (CAQ; Cattell & Krug, 1985; Cattell & Kameoka, 1985; Krug, 1980), developed by Cattell and his associates, was created both to assess normal personality and to be a quick screen for emotional maladjustment. Its purpose was to expand the utility of the *16 Personality Factor Questionnaire* (16PF; Krug & Johns, 1990), a measure of normal personality, by adding scales measuring psychopathology. Test items were collected from a factor analytic study of clinical symptoms (see Cattell, 1973). The scales of the CAQ are more homogeneous and provide more unique information than those of most other objective personality measures, which were typically developed by empirical keying of contrasting groups, because each item on the CAQ is found on only one primary scale, so the scales are independent from an item perspective (Krug, 1989).

A self-report measure consisting of 272 items, the CAQ in its original form had 128 items that assessed normal personality on 16 scales that constitute a shortened version of the 16PF, whereas the remaining 144 items of the CAQ measure psychopathology. A version of the CAQ is now available that incorporates the full 16PF (4th edition, 187 items). The 16 scales of the 16PF are intended to measure normal personality. The CAQ clinical scales assess six clinical disorders (depression, paranoia, psychopathic deviation, schizophrenia, psychasthenia, and psychological inadequacy) using 12 separate scales. Depression is assessed on seven scales (Hypochondriasis, Suicidal Depression, Agitation, Anxious Depression, Low Energy Depression, Guilt and Resentment, and Boredom and Withdrawal), while the other five disorders are each represented by a single scale. In addition, there is a validity scale that is intended to evaluate the intentional effort to distort one's responses (Himelstein, 1984). Each item has three response options; the middle alternative is an option in between the two extremes. The test can be administered to persons 16 years of age or older with a reading level of 6.7 or more years and is expected to require about 2 hours to complete, although we find that most people finish it in less than 1 hour.

Scoring of the CAQ can be done by hand, using templates, or by computer, by mailing the client's answer sheet to the publisher's test-scoring service. Computer scoring generates a profile of the subject's scale scores along with a narrative report. Hand scoring is straightforward and not overly time-consuming, although it does require a number of computations. Once the raw scores are obtained, they are transformed to *sten,* or standard-ten, scores using the appropriate norm table and graphed on a profile sheet. Several of the scores on the CAQ are adjusted for motivational distortion tendencies. Norms, not recently updated, are available for several groups, including college students, typical adults, clinical diagnostic groups, and offenders. All reported norms include both genders, except for the offender norms, which are reported only for males. Using the 10-point sten scores, a score in the 1–4 range is considered low, 5–7 is moderate or average, and 8–10 is high. The mean is 5.5, and the standard deviation is 2. A series of second-order factors is also computed. Profiles are interpreted according to their individual high and low scale scores and the profile configuration. The test manual provides modal profiles for various diagnostic groups but little guidance on how to use them or how to interpret test profiles more generally (Guthrie, 1985). Test interpretation requires considerable training and experience, and the complicated scale names and abbreviations do not facilitate the process.

Validity and reliability data on the clinical (versus the normal personality, or 16-PF) scales on the CAQ remain quite limited since this portion of the test has been used only in a modest amount of empirical research (Cattell & Krug, 1985). In one study (Krug, 1980), test-retest reliability was demonstrated, but the time interval between test administrations was quite short (1 day). Research on criterion-related and construct validity for the CAQ is minimal. A few studies using external criteria or factor analyses have been reported (e.g., Bellivau & Stoppard, 1995; Boyle, 1987; Carpenter, 1995; Montag & Birenbaum, 1989; Spotts & Shontz, 1991). Also, the rather large number of scales attempting to measure subtle differences of the same underlying construct (e.g., variations of types of depression) argues for the need for considerably more construct validity evidence than what was provided by the test developers or the subsequent research literature. Considerably more research is needed on both the validity and reliability of the CAQ; there has been little literature published to date. Psychometric limitations of the CAQ have also been noted (e.g., Boyle, 1987; Krug, 1989; Zaza & Barke, 1986).

The positive features of the CAQ include the lack of item overlap among the scales; the positive psychometric features of the 16PF portion of the test; the generation of data on both normal personality style and psychopathology; and the use of sten scale scores, which have intended psychological meaning when they are high or low. Disadvantages include the limited availability of validity and normative data specific to clinical and rehabilitation populations, the lack of information on profile interpretation, and the test's apparently infrequent use among clinicians. Krug (1989) has suggested that the utility of the CAQ has been hindered by its 10-point scales, which may be too restrictive to differentiate among various disorders, and stated that the assumption of a normal distribution of the scale scores is not defensible, especially on the pathological scales. Some experts (e.g., Himelstein, 1984) claim that given its state of development, the CAQ cannot now be recommended for use to assess normal and pathological traits and should be used only as a research instrument. The CAQ has inspired limited research in general and even less with rehabilitation populations. Studies with rehabilitation populations included those by Carpenter (1995) and Burns, Kappenberg, McKenna, and Wood (1994).

Symptom Checklist–90 Revised

The *Symptom Checklist–90 Revised,* a brief, objective psychiatric symptom checklist first published in 1975, was developed by Derogatis (1977; Derogatis & Savitz, 2000) to assess specific symptoms and symptom patterns as well as overall symptom severity. The test items, some of which were derived from prior checklists, were written to reflect the content areas to be assessed. The SCL-90R consists of 90 items; the client rates these items on a 5-point scale according to the degree of distress the symptom caused over a specific time period, usually the past week. The checklist takes about 15 minutes to complete, is appropriate for adults, and does not require a high reading level. There is also a shorter version of 53 items called the Brief Symptom Checklist (Derogatis, 1992) and a 27-item version developed for use with patients with chronic pain (Hardt & Gerbershaen, 2001).

The SCL-90R gives scores on global dimensions of functioning (seemingly the best validated use of the test), including the Global Severity Index, Positive Symptom Distress Index, and Positive Symptoms Total. It also attempts to measure nine primary symptom dimensions: Depression, Anxiety, Somatization, Obsessive–Compulsiveness, Hostility, Psychoticism, Phobic Anxiety, Paranoid Ideation, and Interpersonal Sensitivity (Derogatis, 1977). It has been normed by gender.

Although the SCL-90R was never created or designed to generate DSM diagnoses, the test data may be helpful in identifying diagnostic directions to explore further, either by additional tests or by clinical interview. The SCL-90R has been used with a variety of rehabilitation populations, including persons with schizophrenia, other major mental illnesses, alcohol and drug abuse (Choquette, 1994), chronic pain (van der Laan, van Spaendonck, Horstink, & Goris, 1999; Williams, Urban, Keefe, Shutty, & France, 1995), eating disorders (Peveler & Fairburn, 1990; Zubieta, Demitrack, Fenick, & Krahn, 1995), stroke (Woesser, 1996), traumatic brain injury (Hoofien, 2005), spinal cord injury, head injury, heart attack, whiplash, and arthritis, for purposes of description, prediction of treatment completion and outcome, and assessment of treatment effects as well as comparison of the efficacy of various treatment methods and comparison of those who seek treatment and those who do not and the relationship to employment status.

The validity and reliability of the global indices, which indicate the presence and severity of psychopathology, are fairly strong, but the validity and reliability data on the primary symptom dimensions are much weaker (Anastasi & Urbina, 1997). Additionally, the factor structure of the instrument has not been confirmed with all populations and the specific clinical factors generally receive the least confirmation (see, e.g., Rauter, Leonard, Swett, & Chester, 1996). Recent research has attempted to examine the evidence for the measure's utility with racial groups (e.g., Martinez, Martinez Stillerman, & Waldo, 2005) and in various international contexts (e.g., Schmitz, Hartkamp, & Kuise, 2000). These results are promising but mixed and reasonably would be interpreted as not yet conclusive.

The advantages of using the SCL-90R are its brevity, its ease of administration, and its potential use as a rough screen in identifying persons with mental health problems, using the global indices as criteria. Its disadvantages include its transparent test items, which make it highly vulnerable to dissimulation, and the high intercorrelations of the scales (Anastasi & Urbina, 1997). A recent survey of the psychological testing practices of psychologists noted that the advent of managed care has prompted many psychologists to use screening measures such as the SCL-90R and brief symptom-focused measures more frequently than they once did and use measures that require extensive administration and scoring time (e.g., the Rorschach) less often (Piotrowski, Belter, & Keller, 1998; Watkins et al., 1995).

Brief Symptom- or Syndrome-Specific Assessment Measures

An extensive review of symptom-focused measures of psychopathology is beyond the scope of this chapter. However, it should be noted that two types of these measures are in common use. The first group includes measures developed to assess a specific disorder or symptom cluster, such as the *Beck Depression*

Inventory (Beck, Steer, & Garbin, 1988; Beck, Ward, Mendelson, Mock, & Erbaugh, 1961). The second category includes scales that have been derived from broad-based instruments (e.g., MMPI-2 or the SCID) to measure specific disorders or symptom clusters. These include, for instance, the Paranoia scale on the MMPI (Butcher et al., 1989). Such measures have the advantage of brevity and can be useful in determining whether a rehabilitation client is experiencing a particular mental disorder. However, these symptom-focused measures cannot be used to provide a complete psychological profile of the individual.

Projective Measures

Rorschach

The Rorschach is perhaps the most widely used projective measure of personality and psychopathology (Watkins et al., 1995). First published in 1921, it was the first major clinical instrument to be classified as projective (Rabin, 1981). The Rorschach has been the subject of a great deal of clinical and research literature and remains, to this day, the source of considerable controversy. Originally developed to evaluate an individual's modes of perception (assumed to be related to the person's personality and psychopathology), not psychopathology per se, the Rorschach was not based on any particular theory. It was assumed that an individual organizes responses to the famous and widely publicized inkblots in the same way that he or she handles other ambiguous stimuli requiring organization and judgment. The person's perception and interpretation of the stimuli were thought to reflect the basic aspects of the individual's psychological functioning.

Questions of validity and reliability have long plagued the Rorschach (see, e.g., Meyer, 2004; Wood, Nezworski, Lilienfeld, & Garb, 2002). Some research has discouraged the use of the instrument or suggested that other projective inkblots, for example, the Holtzman, have better psychometric and validity characteristics (see, e.g., Meyer, 2004). Numerous Rorschach systems have been developed over the years as a way of organizing and scoring the perceptions generated in response to the inkblots. Five systems have predominated in the United States: those by Beck, Klopfer, Piotrowski, Hertz, and Rapoport (see Exner, 1993, for a review). These systems differ primarily in their emphasis on response content and response characteristics. Because the systems scored the same responses in alternative ways, reliability has been a problem with this test since the research on the measure has been system specific. This problem was addressed in 1974, when Exner first published the *Exner Comprehensive System*. Exner attempted to create a common metric for scoring and interpretation of the test. In the past 25 years, this approach has clearly emerged as the dominant system among practitioners, researchers, and clinical training programs (Hunsley & Bailey, 1999). The *Exner Comprehensive System* (see Exner, 1974, 1993) attempted to combine elements of the five major systems and add new elements with the goal of making the Rorschach more valid and reliable. His system is atheoretical but attempted to identify the best of all of the existing systems of scoring. It is based on, and has generated considerable, empirical research. The system emphasizes response or percept characteristics (e.g., the form quality of the response, the areas of the blot where the content was seen) over response or percept content. The administration and scoring of the *Exner Comprehensive System* were standardized. This helped to generate more valid and reliable data than may have been possible with past systems. Norm tables have been developed for a variety of groups based on age, mental disorder, and other variables, permitting comparison of a given protocol with a variety of populations. Above all, Exner's system has resulted in considerable empirical research from which to guide the use of this measure in practice (e.g., Exner, 1993; Exner & Weiner, 1995).

To administer the Rorschach, a trained examiner, typically a psychologist or psychological examiner, presents, sequentially, 10 inkblots to the client, who is asked to describe what he or she perceives (i.e., "What might this be?"). The client's utterances are recorded verbatim. After all the inkblots have been shown, the examiner reviews with the client each of the responses, one at a time, to obtain information important in scoring the responses. Specifically, the examiner wants to know where the response was seen on the inkblot and what made it look that way (Exner, 1974). The entire procedure is conducted with one highly trained examiner and one adult client and typically takes between 40 and 55 minutes (Exner, Weiner, & Schuyler, 1976). Since the client is not required to be able to read, the client's reading level is not a concern. However, the client must have adequate vision to be able to see the inkblots clearly. The test is not appropriate for use with clients whose cognitive functioning is low.

After the administration has been completed, the examiner scores the client's responses using a complicated scoring scheme. Three major categories scored for each percept are response location (where on the inkblot the percept was seen), determinant (what about the inkblot made it look like that to the client), and content (what is it that was perceived). Some responses may also be scored in additional categories. All scorings are then summarized in terms of frequencies, ratios, percentages, and derivations to form a structural summary, which is then interpreted by the examiner. The quantitative data are categorized into multiple indices (Exner, 1993). These data can be tabulated on a standardized form that summarizes the structural findings and the scores on special indices.

The research literature on the Rorschach is fairly extensive yet fraught with technical problems (Dawes, 1994, 1999). Many of the early studies were poorly designed and executed, and no single Rorschach system was used (Exner, 1974). Until recently, background variables were rarely controlled or even considered to be influential. Nonetheless it seems reasonable to conclude that there is adequate support for the validity of the Rorschach in terms of its general indices. However, at the individual level, a particular protocol is significantly affected by the number of responses. Too low a number of responses can invalidate the profile. Scoring categories vary in their validity; also, the data on the Rorschach's ability to distinguish among various groups is mixed (Viglione, 1999). Two criterion validity meta-analyses on the Rorschach and the MMPI found the results of the tests to be comparable (Atkinson, 1986; Parker, Hanson, & Hunsley, 1988); however, the research is far from fully consistent and cost-utility issues must also be considered.

A potential benefit of using the Rorschach in a test battery includes the possibility of providing a detailed picture of an individual's psychological functioning. It can be effective in identifying underlying psychopathology and presumed patterns of dysfunction. Because it is a difficult measure on which to dissimulate, it is likely that the test data collected provide an accurate picture of the client, although patients may censor the responses they share with the examiner. Its administration is complex, and the scoring criteria are not always easily applied, particularly by neophyte examiners.

Certainly, the *Exner Comprehensive System* has improved the validity and reliability of the Rorschach, but the test continues to have some limitations. Its complexity makes it difficult and time-consuming to learn to use properly, scoring errors (especially in rarely used categories) are common, and problems with protocol interpretation can occur (Groth-Marnat, 1999). Often, several interpretations exist for a given scale or ratio, and these must be considered in the context of the profile as a whole. Norms have been collected on a variety of groups, but there are not yet adequate data on certain cultural and racial groups in the United States (Dana, 1996).

For many years, psychologists and other researchers (e.g., Dawes, 1994; Hunsley & Bailey, 1999) have been very critical of the Rorschach as a result of its questionable psychometric characteristics and the fact that the test has been used in a very idiosyncratic way by many clinicians. The flaws of the instrument have often been identified and its demise predicted (e.g., Jensen, 1965; Meyer, 1999). Nonetheless, surveys of clinical training programs (Durand, Blanchard, & Mindell, 1988) and of practicing clinicians (Watkins et al., 1995) indicate that the measure is still widely used. As research data continue to be collected, many of the past criticisms may be addressed. However, one article (Hunsley & Bailey, 1999) strongly suggested that the Rorschach should be limited to use as a research tool as a result of its small research base, although an alternative view was presented by Viglione (1999).

The Rorschach has been used to describe and classify rehabilitation-related conditions and patient populations and to predict rehabilitation potential, treatment outcome, and post-treatment behavior (e.g., Cruz, Brier, & Reznikoff, 1997). Disabled populations discussed in the Rorschach literature include those with closed head injuries, mental retardation, and substance abuse (e.g., Exner, Colligan, Boll, Stischer, & Hillman, 1996).

Other Projective Measures

Other projective measures of psychopathology include the *Thematic Apperception Test* (TAT; Giesler & Stein, 1999; Holt, 1999), *Draw-a-Person/Human Figure* drawings (Riethmiller & Handler, 1997), incomplete sentences measures (Lah, 1989), the *Hand Test* (Hilsenroth, Fowler, Sivec, & Waehler, 1994), and the *Holtzman Inkblot Test* (Holtzman, 1988; Meyer, 2004). However, these measures are rarely cited in the rehabilitation psychology literature, although one survey of clinical psychologists' test usage practices indicated that the TAT, sentence completion measures, and projective drawings were among the top 10 most frequently used psychological tests, while the *Hand Test* and the *Holtzman Inkblot Test,* both with rather extensive research studies supporting their validity and with some improved psychometric properties over other projectives, were not among the top 38 most commonly used tests (Meyer, 2004; Watkins et al., 1995). Clearly, usage of a given psychological measure is not always related to the psychometric properties or research base of the instrument.

Conclusion

This chapter has discussed the major structured interviews, objective personality measures, and projective personality measures relevant for use with rehabilitation populations. Clearly, there is no perfect measure of psychopathology and the measure of choice to use will depend to a large extent on the specific diagnostic or differential diagnostic question. The amount of time available for screening must be balanced against the validity and reliability of the tests under consideration and, in the case of assessment of rehabilitation clients with medical problems (e.g., brain injury or intellectual deficiencies), the ability of the test to assess psychological conditions that are separate from the medical condition itself. Still, general recommendations for assessment of psychopathology in rehabilitation populations can be made, if not about specific tests, then at least about types of tests for particular assessment tasks.

When the diagnostic question concerns whether a rehabilitation client might be psychologically distressed and time and money issues are significant considerations, then a brief screening measure such as the SCL-90R can help to assess quickly the presence and general nature of the distress. If the results suggest that the person may be experiencing a psychological disturbance needing further assessment, then more extensive psychological assessment is recommended to gain a more in-depth understanding of the individual, to arrive at a mental health diagnosis, and to make suggestions for treatment planning. Should the client present with a documented history of past or current mental illness, then the screening measure could be omitted and the clinician could proceed directly to a more extensive evaluation. An appropriate battery might, in such circumstances, consist of an interview, preferably a structured interview such as the SCID or SADS; an objective measure of personality such as the MMPI-2, the MCMI-III, or the PAI; and possibly a projective measure of personality such as the Rorschach. Such a test battery would provide broad coverage of the individual, would help minimize the overall effects of motivational distortion, and would provide useful information in understanding how to treat the rehabilitation client's psychopathology or distress. A more extensive research literature is also needed to be able to apply these measures with confidence to rehabilitation populations.

References

Alexy, W. D., & Webb, P. M. (1999). Utility of the MMPI-2 in work-hardening rehabilitation. *Rehabilitation Psychology, 44*, 266–273.

American Psychiatric Association. (1980). *Diagnostic and statistical manual of mental disorders* (3rd ed.). Washington, DC: Author.

American Psychiatric Association. (1994). *Diagnostic and statistical manual of mental disorders* (4th ed.). Washington, DC: Author.

Anastasi, A., & Urbina, S. (1997). *Psychological testing.* Upper Saddle River, NJ: Prentice Hall.

Arbisi, P. A. (1995). Review of the Schedule for Affective Disorders and Schizophrenia (3rd ed). In J. C. Conoley & J. C. Impara (Eds.), *The twelfth mental measurements yearbook* (pp. 917–918). Lincoln, NE: University of Nebraska Press.

Arbisi, P. A., Ben-Porath, Y. S., & McNulty, J. (2002). A comparison of MMPI-2 validity in African American and Caucasian psychiatric inpatients. *Psychological Assessment, 14,* 3–15.

Atkinson, L. (1986). The comparative validities of the Rorschach and the MMPI. *Canadian Psychology, 27,* 238–247.

Bacchiochi, J. R., & Bagby, R. M. (2006). Development and validation of the malingering discriminant function index for the MMPI-2. *Journal of Personality Assessment, 87,* 51–61.

Beck, A. T., Steer, R. A., & Garbin, M. (1988). Psychometric properties of the Beck Depression Inventory: Twenty-five years of evaluation. *Clinical Psychology Review, 8,* 77–100.

Beck, A. T., Ward, C. H., Mendelson, M., Mock, J., & Erbaugh, J. (1961). An inventory for measuring depression. *Archives of General Psychiatry, 4,* 561–571.

Belding, M. A., Iguchi, M. Y., Morral, A. R., & Husband, S. D. (1998). MMPI profiles of opiate addicts: Predicting response to treatment. *Journal of Personality Assessment, 70,* 324–339.

Bellivau, J. M., & Stoppard, J. M. (1995). Parental alcohol abuse and gender as predictors of psychopathology in adult children of alcoholics. *Addictive Behaviors, 20,* 619–625.

Blanchard, D. D., McGrath, R. E., Pogge, D. L., & Jhadivi, A. (2003). A comparison of the PAI and MMPI-2 as predictors of faking bad in college students. *Journal of Personality Assessment, 80,* 197–205.

Boyle, G. J. (1987). Psychopathological depression superfactors measured in the Clinical Analysis Questionnaire. *Personality and Individual Differences, 8,* 609–614.

Boyle, G. J. (1995). Review of the Personality Assessment Inventory. In J. C. Conoley & J. C. Impara (Eds.), *The twelfth mental measurements yearbook* (pp. 764–766). Lincoln, NE: University of Nebraska Press.

Boyle, G. J., & Lennon, T. J. (1996). Examination of the reliability and validity of the Personality Assessment Inventory. *Journal of Psychopathology and Behavioral Assessment, 16,* 173–187.

Brieland, D. (1971). Rehabilitation psychologists: Roles and functions. In W. S. Neff (Ed.), *Rehabilitation psychology* (pp. 265–286). Washington, DC: American Psychological Association.

Burns, S., Kappenberg, R., McKenna, A., & Wood, C. (1994). Brain injury: Personality, psychopathology, and neuropsychology. *Brain Injury, 8,* 413–427.

Bury, A. S., & Michael B. R. (2002). The detection of feigned uncoached and coached posttraumatic stress disorder with the MMPI-2 in a sample of workplace accident victims. *Psychological Assessment, 14,* 472–484.

Butcher, J. N. (1995). How to use computer-based reports. In J. N. Butcher (Ed.), *Clinical personality assessment* (pp. 78–94). New York: Oxford Press.

Butcher, J. N. (2002). Revising psychological tests: Lessons learned from the revision of the MMPI. *Psychological Assessment, 12,* 263–271.

Butcher, J. N., Cheung, F. M., & Lim, J. (2003). Use of the MMPI-2 with Asian populations. *Psychological Assessment, 15*, 248–256.

Butcher, J. N., Dahlstrom, W. G., Graham, J. R., Tellegen, A., & Kaemmer, B. (1989). *Manual for administration and scoring: MMPI-2*. Minneapolis, MN: University of Minnesota Press.

Butcher, J. N., Graham, J. R., & Ben-Porath, Y. S. (1995). Methodological problems and issues in MMPI, MMPI–2, and MMPI–A research. *Psychological Assessment, 7*, 320–329.

Carmer, J. C. (1995). Review of the Schedule for Affective Disorders and Schizophrenia (3rd ed.). In J. C. Conoley & J. C. Impara (Eds.), *The twelfth mental measurements yearbook* (pp. 918–919). Lincoln, NE: University of Nebraska Press.

Carpenter, D. R. (1995). Adult children of alcoholics: CAQ profiles. *Alcoholism Treatment Quarterly, 13*, 63–70.

Cattell, R. B. (1973). A check on the 28 factor Clinical Analysis Questionnaire structure on normal and pathological subjects. *Journal of Multivariate Experimental Personality & Clinical Psychology, 1*, 3–12.

Cattell, R. B., & Kameoka, V. A. (1985). Psychological states measured in the Clinical Analysis Questionnaire (CAQ). *Multivariate Experimental Clinical Research, 7*, 69–87.

Cattell, R. B., & Krug, S. E. (1985). The number of factors in the 16PF: A review of the evidence with special emphasis on methodological problems. *Educational and Psychological Measurement, 46*, 509–522.

Choca, J. P., Shanley, L. A., & Van Denburg, E. (1992). *Interpretative guide to the Millon Clinical Multiaxial Inventory*. Washington, DC: American Psychological Association Books.

Choquette, K. A. (1994) Assessing depression in alcoholics with the BJI, SCL-90-R, and DIS criteria. *Journal of Substance Abuse, 6*, 295–304.

Colotla, V. A., Bowman, M. L., & Shercliffe, R. J. (2001). Test–retest stability of injured workers' MMPI–2 profiles. *Psychological Assessment, 13*, 572–576.

Conger, A. J., & Conger, J. C. (1996). Did too, did not! Controversies in the construct validation of the PAI. *Journal of Psychopathology and Behavior Assessment, 18*, 205–212.

Craig, R. J. (Ed) (2005). *New directions in interpreting the Millon™ Clinical Multiaxial Inventory–III*. Hoboken, NJ: Wiley.

Craig, R. J., & Weinberg, D. (1992). Assessing drug abusers with the MCMI: A review. *Journal of Substance Abuse Treatment, 9*, 249–255.

Cruz, E. B., Brier, N. M., & Reznikoff, M. (1997). An examination of the relationship between form level rating on the Rorschach and learning disability status. *Journal of Psychology, 131*, 167–174.

Dana, R. H. (1996). Culturally competent assessment practice in the U.S. *Journal of Personality Assessment, 66*, 472–487.

Davis, R. D. (1999). Millon: Essentials of his science, theory, classification, assessment, and theory. *Journal of Personality Assessment, 72*, 330–352.

Dawes, R. M. (1994). *House of cards: Psychology and psychotherapy built on myth*. New York: Free Press.

Dawes, R. M. (1999). Two methods for studying the incremental validity of a Rorschach variable. *Psychological Assessment, 11*, 297–302.

Deisinger, J. A. (1995). Exploring the factor structure of the Personality Assessment Inventory. *Assessment, 2*, 173–179.

Derogatis, L. R. (1977). *SCL-90 revised version manual I*. Baltimore: Johns Hopkins University School of Medicine.

Derogatis, L. R. (1992). *BSI: Administration, scoring, and procedures manual II* (2nd ed.). Baltimore: Clinical Psychometric Research.

Derogatis, L. R. (1994). *SCL-90-R symptom checklist-90-R: Administration, scoring, and procedures manual*. Minneapolis, MN: National Computer Systems.

Derogatis, L. R., Fleming, M. P., Sudler, N. C., & DellaPetra, L. (1995). Psychological assessment. In P. M. Nicassio & T. W. Smith (Eds.), *Managing chronic illness* (pp. 59–115). Washington, DC: American Psychological Association.

Derogatis, L. R., & Savitz, K. L. (2000). The SCL-90-R and Brief Symptom Inventory (BSI) in primary care. In M. E. Maruish (Ed.), *Handbook of psychological assessment in primary care settings* (pp. 297–334). Mahwah, NJ: Erlbaum.

Dong, Y'L. T., & Church, A. T. (2003). Cross-cultural equivalence and validity of the Vietnamese MMPI-2: Assessing psychological adjustment of Vietnamese refugees. *Psychological Assessment, 15,* 370–377.

Durand, V. M., Blanchard, E. B., & Mindell, J. A. (1988). Training in projective testing: Survey of clinical training directors and internship directors. *Professional Psychology, 19,* 236–238.

Eber, H. W. (1976). Personality and psychopathology inventories. In B. Bolton (Ed.), *Handbook of measurement and evaluation in rehabilitation* (pp. 101–116). Baltimore: University Park Press.

Endicott, J., & Spitzer, R. L. (1978). A diagnostic interview: The Schedule for Affective Disorders and Schizophrenia. *Archives of General Psychiatry, 35,* 837–844.

Exner, J. E. (1974). *The Rorschach: A comprehensive system* (Vol. 1). New York: Wiley.

Exner, J. E. (1993). *The Rorschach: A comprehensive system* (3rd ed., Vol. 1). New York: Wiley.

Exner, J. E., Colligan, S. C., Boll, T. J., Stischer, B., & Hillman, L. (1996). Rorschach findings concerning head injury patients. *Assessment, 3,* 317–326.

Exner, J. E., Jr., & Weiner, I. B. (1995). *Assessment of children and adolescents* (2nd ed., Vol. 3). New York: Wiley.

Exner, J. E., Weiner, I. B., & Schuyler, W. (1976). *A Rorschach workbook for the comprehensive system.* Asheville, NC: Rorschach Workshops.

Fantoni-Salvador, P., & Rogers, R. (1997). Spanish versions of the MMPI-2 and PAI: An investigation of concurrent validity with Hispanic patients. *Assessment, 4,* 29–39.

First, M. B., Gibbon, M., Williams, J. B., & Spitzer, R. L. (1995). *Users manual for the Mini-SCID (for DSM-IV-version 2).* North Tonawanda, NY: Multi-Health Systems/American Psychiatric Association.

Flynn, P. M., McCann, J. T., & Fairbank, J. A. (1995). Issues in the assessment of personality disorder and substance abuse using the Millon Clinical Multiaxial Inventory (MCMI-II). *Journal of Clinical Psychology, 51,* 415–421.

Foa, E. B., Cashman, L., Jaycox, L., & Perry, K. (1997). The validation of a self-report measure of posttraumatic stress disorder: The Posttraumatic Diagnostic Scale. *Psychological Assessment, 9,* 445–451.

Fraguas, R., Jr., Henriques, S. G., Jr., DeLucia, M. S., Iosifescu, D. V., Schwartz, F. H., Menezes, P. R., et al. (2006). The detection of depression in medical setting: A study with PRIME-MD. *Journal of Affective Disorders, 91,* 11–17.

Frazier, T. W., Naugle, R. I., & Haggerty, K. A. (2006). Psychometric adequacy and comparability of the short and full forms of the Personality Assessment Inventory. *Psychological Assessment, 18,* 324–333.

Gallagher, S. M., Penn, P. E., Brooks, A. J., Feldman, J., & Gallagher, S. M. (2006). Comparing the AAPE, a new assessment tool for co-occurring disorders, with the SCID. *Psychiatric Rehabilitation Journal, 30,* 63–65.

Garb, H. N., Wood, J. M., Lilienfeld, S. O., & Nezworski, M. T. (2005). Roots of the *Rorschach* controversy. *Clinical Psychology Review, 25,* 97–118.

George, J. M., & Wagner, E. E. (1995). Correlations between the Hand Test pathology score and Personality Assessment Inventory scales for pain clinic patients. *Perceptual and Motor Skills, 80,* 1377–1378.

Giesler, L., & Stein, M. I. (Eds.). (1999). *Evocative images: The Thematic Apperception Test and the art of projection* (pp. 99–105). Washington, DC: American Psychological Association.

Goldstein, A., & Reznikoff, M. (1972). MMPI performance in chronic medical illness: The use of computer-derived interpretations. *British Journal of Psychiatry, 120,* 157–158.

Graham, J. R. (2006). *MMPI-2: Assessing personality and psychopathology* (4th ed.). New York: Oxford University Press.

Greene, R. L. (1991). *The MMPI-2/MMPI: An interpretive manual.* Boston: Allyn & Bacon.

Greene, R. L. (1999). *The MMPI-2: An interpretive manual.* Boston: Allyn & Bacon.

Greene, R. L., Gwin, R., & Staal, M. (1997). Current status of the MMPI-2 research: A methodologic overview. *Journal of Personality Assessment, 68,* 20–36.

Groth-Marnat, G. (1999). *Handbook of psychological assessment* (3rd ed.). New York: Wiley.

Guthrie, G. (1985). Review of the Clinical Analysis Questionnaire. In J. V. Mitchell, Jr. (Ed.), *The ninth mental measurements yearbook* (Vol. 1, pp. 340–341). Lincoln, NE: University of Nebraska Press.

Hall, G. C. N., Bansal, A., & Lopez, I. R. (1999). Ethnicity and psychopathology: A meta-analytic review of 31 Years of comparative MMPI/MMPI-2 research. *Psychological Assessment, 11,* 186–197.

Hardt, J., & Gerbershaen, H. U. (2001). Cross-validation of the SCL-27: A short psychometric screening instrument for chronic pain patients. *European Journal of Pain, 5,* 187–197.

Hasin, D. S. (1991). Diagnostic interviews for assessment: Background, reliability, validity. *Alcohol Health & Research World, 15,* 293–302.

Hathaway, S. R., & McKinley, J. C. (1943). *Manual for the Minnesota Multiphasic Personality Inventory.* New York: Psychological Corp.

Hathaway, S. R., & McKinley, J. C. (1989). *The MMPI-2: Minnesota Multiphase Manual for administration and scoring.* Minneapolis: University of Minnesota Press.

Hess, A. K. (1998). Review of the Millon Clinical Multiaxial Inventory—III. In J. C. Impala & B. S. Plake (Eds.), *The thirteenth mental measurements yearbook* (pp. 665–667). Lincoln, NE: University of Nebraska Press.

Hilsenroth, M. J., Fowler, C., Sivec, H.J., & Waehler, C.A. (1994). Concurrent and discriminant validity between the Hand Test pathology score and the MMPI-2. *Assessment, 1,* 111–113.

Himelstein, P. (1984). Clinical Analysis Questionnaire. In D.J. Keyser & R.C. Sweetland (Eds.), *Test critiques* (Vol. 1, pp. 202–205). Kansas City, MO: Test Corporation of America.

Hodges, K. (1994). Reply to David Shaffer: Structured interviews for assessing children. *Journal of Child Psychology and Psychiatry, 35,* 785–787.

Holt, R. R. (1999). Empiricism and the Thematic Apperception Test: Validity is the payoff. In L. Gieser & M.I. Stein (Eds.), *Evocative images: The Thematic Apperception Test and the art of projection* (pp. 99–105). Washington, DC: American Psychological Association.

Holtzman, W. H. (1988). Beyond the Rorschach. *Journal of Personality Assessment, 52,* 578–609.

Hoofien, D. (2005). Symptom Checklist-90 Revised scores in persons with traumatic brain injury: Affective reactions or neurobehavioral outcomes of the injury? *Applied Neuropsychology, 12,* 30–39.

Hunsley, J., & Bailey, J. M. (1999). The clinical utility of the Rorschach: Unfulfilled promises and the uncertain future. *Psychological Assessment, 11,* 266–277.

Hunsley, J., Hanson, R. K., & Parker, K. C. H. (1988). A summary of the reliability and stability of MMPI scales. *Journal of Clinical Psychology, 44,* 44–46.

Jankowski, D. (2002). *A beginner's guide to the MCMI-III.* Washington, DC: American Psychological Association Books.

Jensen, A. R. (1965). A review of the Rorschach. In O. K. Buros (Ed.), *The sixth mental measurements yearbook* (pp. 501–509). Highland Park, NJ: Gryphon.

Johnson, S., Barrett, P. M., Dadds, M. R., Fox, T., & Shortt, A. (1999). The diagnostic interview schedule for children, adolescents, and parents: Initial reliability and validity data. *Behaviour Change, 16,* 155–164.

Kavan, C. G. (1995). Review of the Personality Assessment Inventory. In J. C. Conoley & J. C. Impara (Eds.), *The twelfth mental measurements yearbook* (pp. 766–768). Lincoln, NE: University of Nebraska Press.

Kellett, S. C., Beail, N., Newman, D. W., & Mosley, E. (1999). Indexing psychological distress in people with an intellectual disability: Use of the Symptom Checklist-90-R. *Journal of Applied Research in Intellectual Disabilities, 12,* 323–334.

Koenig, H. G. (2006). Differences between depressed patients with heart failure and those with pulmonary disease. *American Journal of Geriatric Psychiatry, 14,* 211–219.

Koenig, H. G., Vandermeer, J., Chambers, A., Burr-Crutchfield, L., & Johnson, J. L. (2006). Comparison of major and minor depression in older medical inpatients with chronic heart and pulmonary disease. *Psychosomatics: Journal of Consultation Liaison Psychiatry, 47,* 296–303.

Krug, S. E. (1980). *The Clinical Analysis Questionnaire manual.* Champaign, IL: IPAT.

Krug, S. E. (1989). Linear T scores norms for the Clinical Analysis Questionnaire. *Multivariate Experimental Clinical Research, 9,* 1–9.

Krug, S. E., & Johns, E. F. (1990). The 16 Personality Factor Questionnaire. In C. E. Watkins, Jr., & V. L. Campbell (Eds.), *Testing in counseling practice. Vocational psychology* (pp. 63–90). Hillsdale, NJ: Lawrence Erlbaum.

Lah, M. I. (1989). Sentence completion measures. In C. S. Newmark (Ed.), *Major psychological assessment instruments* (Vol. 2, pp. 133–163). Needham Heights, MA: Allyn & Bacon.

Martinez, S., Stillerman, L., & Waldo, M. (2005). Reliability and Validity of the SCL-90-R With Hispanic College Students. *Hispanic Journal of Behavioral Sciences, 27,* 254–264.

Masling, J. M. (1997). On the nature and utility of projective tests and objective tests. *Journal of Personality Assessment, 69,* 257–270.

Meyer, G. J. (1999). Introduction to the special series on the utility of the Rorschach for clinical assessment. *Psychological Assessment, 11,* 235–239.

Meyer, G. J. (2004). The reliability and validity of the Rorschach and Thematic Apperception Test (TAT) compared to other psychological and medical procedures: An analysis of systematically gathered evidence. In M. J. Hilsenroth & D. L. Segal (Eds.), *Comprehensive handbook of psychological assessment, Vol. 2: Personality assessment* (pp. 315–342). Hoboken, NJ: Wiley.

Millon, T. (1990). *Toward a new personology: An evolutionary model.* New York: Wiley.

Millon, T. (1994). *MCMI-III Manual.* Minneapolis, MN: National Computer Systems.

Millon, T. (1996). *Personality and psychopathology: Building a clinical science: Selected papers of Theodore Millon.* New York: Wiley and Sons.

Millon, T., & Davis, R. (1996). Conceptions of personality disorders: Historical perspectives, the DSMs, and future directions: An evolutionary theory of personality disorders. In J. F. Clarkin & M. F. Lenzenweger (Eds.), *Major theories of personality disorder* (pp. 221–346). New York: Guilford.

Montag, I., & Birenbaum, M. (1989). On the relationship between the MMPI and Cattell's normal and abnormal personality factors. *Multivariate Experimental Clinical Research, 8,* 275–286.

Morey, L. C. (1991). *The Personality Assessment Inventory professional manual.* Odessa, FL: Psychological Assessment Resources.

Morey, L. C. (1995). Critical issues in construct validation: Comment on Boyle and Lennon (1994). *Journal of Psychopathology and Behavioral Assessment, 17,* 393–401.

Morey, L. C. (1996). *An interpretive guide to the personality assessment inventory (PAI).* Odessa, FL: Psychological Assessment Resources.

Neale, J. M., Davison, G. C., & Haaga, D. A. F. (1996). *Exploring abnormal psychology.* New York: John Wiley.

Nelson, N. W., Parsons, T. D., Grote, C. L., Smith, C. A., & Sisung, J. R., II. (2006). The *MMPI-2* fake bad scale: Concordance and specificity of true and estimated scores. *Journal of Clinical and Experimental Neuropsychology, 28,* 1–12.

Parker, K. C. H., Hanson, R. K., & Hunsley, J. (1988). MMPI, Rorschach, and WAIS: A meta-analytic comparison of reliability, stability, and validity. *Psychological Bulletin, 103,* 367–373.

Peveler, R. C., & Fairburn, C. G. (1990). Measurement of neurotic symptoms by self-report questionnaire: Validity of the SCL-90R. *Psychological Medicine, 20,* 873–879.

Piotrowski, C., Belter, R. W., & Keller, J. W. (1998). The impact of "managed care" on the practice of psychological testing. *Journal of Personality Assessment, 70,* 441–447.

Rabin, A. I. (1981). Projective methods: A historical introduction. In A. I. Rabin (Ed.), *Assessment with projective techniques: A concise introduction.* New York: Springer.

Rauter, U. K., Leonard, C. E., & Swett, C. P. (1996). SCL-90–R factor structure in an acute, involuntary, adult psychiatric inpatient sample. *Journal of Clinical Psychology, 52,* 625–629.

Retzlaff, P. (1998). Review of the Millon Clinical Multiaxial Inventory–III. In J. C. Impara & B. S. Plake (Eds.), *The thirteenth mental measurements yearbook* (pp. 667–668). Lincoln, NE: University of Nebraska Press.

Riethmiller, R. J., & Handler, L. (1997). Problematic methods and unwarranted conclusions in DAP research: Suggestions for improved research procedures. *Journal of Personality Assessment, 69,* 459–475.

Robins, L. N., Helzer, J. E., Croughan, J. L., & Ratcliff, K. S. (1981). National Institute of Mental Health Diagnostic Interview Schedule. *Archives of General Psychiatry, 38,* 381–389.

Rodevich, M. A., & Wanlass, R. L. (1995). The moderating effect of spinal cord injury on MMPI-2 profiles: A clinically derived T score correction procedure. *Rehabilitation Psychology, 40,* 181–190.

Rogers, R., Jackson, R. L., Salekin, K. L., & Neumann, C. S. (2003). Assessing Axis I symptomatology on the SADS-C in two correctional samples: The validation of subscales and a screen for malingered presentations. *Journal of Personality Assessment, 81,* 281–290.

Rogers, R., Sewell, K. W., Morey, L. C., & Ustad, K. L. (1996). Detection of feigned mental disorders on the Personality Assessment Inventory: A discriminant analysis. *Journal of Personality Assessment, 67,* 629–640.

Scheibe, S., Bagby, R. M., Miller, L. S., & Dorian, B. J. (2001). Assessing Posttraumatic Stress Disorder With the MMPI–2 in a Sample of Workplace Accident Victims. *Psychological Assessment, 13,* 369–374.

Schinka, J. A. (1995). PAI profiles in alcohol-dependent patients. *Journal of Personality Assessment, 65,* 35–51.

Schinka, J. A., Curtiss, G., & Mulloy, J. M. (1994). Personality variables and self-medication in substance abuse. *Journal of Personality Assessment, 63,* 413–422.

Schmitz, N., Hartkamp, N., & Kiuse, J. (2000). The Symptom Check List-90-R: A German validation study. *Quality of Life Research: An International Journal of Quality of Life Aspects of Treatment, Care & Rehabilitation, 9,* 185–193.

Schuckit, M. A. (2006). The empirical basis of substance use disorders diagnosis: Research recommendations for the Diagnostic and Statistical Manual of Mental Disorders, fifth edition (*DSM-V*). *Addiction, 10,* 170–173.

Segal, D. I. (1997). Structured interviewing and DSM classification. In S. M. Turner & M. Hersen (Eds.), *Adult psychopathology and diagnosis* (3rd ed., pp. 24–57). New York: John Wiley.

Simms, L. J., Casillas, A., Clark, L. A., Watson, D., & Doebbling, B. N. (2006). Psychometric evaluation of the restructured clinical scales of the *MMPI-2. Psychological Assessment, 17,* 345–358.

Smith, D. C., Huber, D. L., & Hall, J. A. (2005). Psychometric evaluation of the structured clinical interview for DSM-IV childhood diagnoses (KID-SCID). *Journal of Human Behavior in the Social Environment, 11,* 1–21.

Spielberger, C. D., Sydeman, S. J., Owen, A. E., & Marsh, B. J. (1999). Measuring anxiety and anger with the State-Trait Anxiety Inventory (STAI) and the State-Trait Anger Expression Inventory (STAXI). In M. E. Maruish (Ed.), *The use of psychological testing for treatment planning and outcomes assessment* (2nd ed., pp. 993–1021). Mahwah, NJ: Lawrence Erlbaum Associates.

Spitzer, R. L., Endicott, J., & Robins, E. (1978). Research diagnostic criteria: Rationale and reliability. *Archives of General Psychiatry, 31,* 197–203.

Spitzer, R. L., Williams, J. B. W., & Gibbon, M. (1987). *Structured clinical interview for DSM-III-R (SCID).* New York: New York State Psychiatric Institute.

Spitzer, R. L., Williams, J. B. W., Gibbon, M., & First, M. B. (1987). The structured clinical interview for DSM-III-R *(SCID):* I. History, rationale, and description. *Archives of General Psychiatry, 49,* 624–629.

Spotts, J. V., & Shontz, F. C. (1991). Drug misuse and psychopathology: A meta-analysis of 16PF research. *International Journal of the Addictions, 26,* 923–944.

Steinberg, M. (2000). Advances in the clinical assessment of dissociation: The SCID-D-R. *Bulletin of the Menninger Clinic, 64,* 146–163.

Strack, S. (1999). *Essentials of Millon inventories assessment.* New York: Wiley.

Stricker, G., & Gold, J. R. (1999). The Rorschach: Toward a nomothetically based, idiographically applicable configurational model. *Psychological Assessment, 11,* 240–250.

Tisdale, M., Pendleton, L., & Marler, M. R. (1990). MCMI characteristics of DSM-III-R bulimics. *Journal of Personality Assessment, 55,* 466–483.

Usdane, W. M. (1971). The state of the art: Rehabilitation research utilization. In W. S. Neff (Ed.), *Rehabilitation psychology* (pp. 321–326). Washington, DC: American Psychological Association.

van der Laan, L., van Spaendonck, K., Horstink, M. W. I. M., & Goris, R. J. A. (1999). The Symptom Checklist—90 Revised Questionnaire: No psychological profiles in complex regional pain syndrome-dystonia. *Journal of Pain and Symptom Management, 17,* 357–362.

Vendrig, A. A., Derksen, J. J. L., & de Mey, H. R. (1999). Utility of selected MMPI-2 scales in the outcome prediction for patients with chronic back pain. *Psychological Assessment, 11,* 381–385.

Viglione, D. J. (1999). A review of recent research addressing the utility of the Rorschach. *Psychological Assessment, 11,* 251–265.

Watkins, C. E., Jr., Campbell, V. L., Nieberding, R., & Hallmark, R. (1995). Contemporary practice of psychological assessment by clinical psychologists. *Professional Psychology Theory, Research, and Practice, 26,* 54–60.

Wells, K. B., Burnam, M. A., Leake, B., & Robins, L. N. (1988). Agreement between face-to-face and telephone-administered versions of the depression section of the NIMH Diagnostic Interview Schedule. *Journal of Psychiatric Research, 22, 207–220.*

White, L. J. (1996). Review of the Personality Assessment Inventory (PAI-super™): A new psychological test for clinical and forensic assessment. *Australian Psychologist, 31,* 38–40.

Widiger, T. A. (1999). Millon's dimensional polarities. *Journal of Personality Assessment, 72,* 365–389.

Williams, D., Urban, B., Keefe, F. J., Shutty, M. S., & France, R. (1995). Cluster analyses of pain patients' responses to the SCL-R90. *Pain, 61,* 81–91.

Williams, J.E., & Weed, N.C. (2004). Relative User Ratings of MMPI-2 Computer-Based Test Interpretations. *Assessment, 11,* 316–329.

Woesser, R. (1996). Emotional distress following stroke: Interpretive limitations of the SCL-90-R. *Assessment, 3,* 291–305.

Wood, J. M., Nezworski, M. T., Lilienfeld, S. O., & Garb, H. N. (2002). *What's wrong with the Rorschach? Science confronts the controversial inkblot test.* New York: Jossey-Bass/Wiley.

Zaza, A. S., & Barke, C. R. (1986). A review of the Clinical Analysis Questionnaire. *Journal of Counseling and Development, 64,* 413–414.

Zubieta, J. K., Demitrack, M. A., Fenick, A., & Krahn, D. D. (1995). Obsessionality in eating-disordered patients: Relationship to clinical presentation and two year outcome. *Journal of Psychiatric Research, 29,* 333–342.

Chapter 8

Vocational Inventories

Nadya A. Fouad, Melissa K. Smothers,
Neeta Kantamneni, and Amy Guillen

n most rehabilitation programs, including state and federal programs, proprietary rehabilitation agencies, and nonprofit rehabilitation facilities, vocational placement is a major goal. Inclusion in the world of work is viewed as a crucial means of assisting persons with disabilities to achieve the most productive, satisfying lives possible. There have been numerous areas of focus in rehabilitation research, including empowerment of clients with disabilities, integration of people with disabilities into classrooms and workplaces, the impact of the Americans with Disabilities Act and the Individuals with Disabilities Education Act (IDEA), the effect of cultural diversity on the definition of disability, and the influence of technology on the work environment (Fabian & Liesner, 2005; Kosciulek, 1998; Schaller, Parker, & Garcia, 1998). Similarly, there has been a focus on the school-to-work transition (Blustein, 1999; Blustein, Kenna, & Murphy, 2005; Lent & Worthington, 2000; Szymanski, 1997) and how individuals navigate the transition process. The emerging success of school-to-work transition programs has stimulated interest in developing career interventions and programs that help individuals manage barriers and provide skills that help them maximize their career choice (Fabian & Liesner, 2005). This, in turn, has prompted similar research on career concerns for persons with disabilities (Feldman, 2004; Hagner, McGahie, & Cloutier, 2001; Menchetti & Garcia, 2003; Noonan, Gallor, & Hensler-McGinnis, 2004). The rehabilitation counselor is a key component in helping clients with disabilities select, prepare for, and seek appropriate career opportunities and choices. Through the world of work, persons with disabilities are more likely to be able to meet their financial needs as well as gain a greater sense of independence and involvement with mainstream American society.

Uses of Vocational Interest and Attitude Inventories

Rehabilitation counselors have a variety of resources to assist in career counseling and placement for persons with disabilities, including a wide range of psychological assessment tools and computerized career development programs. Vocational interest and value inventories can be of considerable assistance to the counselor in helping the client select potential occupations for further exploration. The complex and rapidly changing nature of the labor market, the variety of occupations, and the many advances in rehabilitation engineering and technology that enable adaptation for even the most severely disabled persons often make occupational selection increasingly difficult for even the most sophisticated counselor.

Occupational selection may seem daunting for the client who may be relatively inexperienced and/or who has limited exposure to the world of work. The difficulty in vocational choice may be compounded for the client who has been impaired or disabled from an early age because the career development sequence may be affected. Children with disabilities often have inadequate career education and may lack exposure to career role models that help the development of vocational exploration (Fabian & Liesener, 2005). Simply asking clients who have had limited exposure to the world outside their immediate context to describe their interests may provide limited information to the counselor.

Vocational inventories give the counselor and the client information to help them begin initial career exploration, which should enable the client to make a better-informed occupational choice. Certainly, a high level of interest alone is not sufficient for success in a given career, but a person with both interest in and abilities suitable for a given occupation will be more likely to do well and to be satisfied in that occupation (Dawis, 2005). In addition, client career search self-efficacy, career decision-making self-efficacy, and career maturity may also play a role in determining career behavior (Fabian & Liesener, 2005).

Thus, vocational inventories are just one component of career planning and placement, and the rehabilitation counselor must understand the need to consider the information gained from these instruments only in combination with data gathered from other modified assessment approaches. These modifications may consist of including more informal interviews and observational techniques in assessment (Power, 2000), having family members or significant others participate in helping the individual identify skills or interests, and relying on more contextual assessment methods (Fabian & Liesener, 2005).

In the past, vocational evaluations were based on a deficit model, emphasizing an individual's inabilities and deficits. However, the perception has shifted over time to focus on barriers within the environment, rather than the individual, thereby enlarging career or employment opportunities with the provision of sufficient supports and resources (Wehman, West, & Kregel, 1999).

Information on Vocational Options

The first purpose of vocational inventories with clients with disabilities is to provide clients with information to increase their vocational options. In this regard, rehabilitation clients generally may be divided into two categories: (1) youths with disabilities who have little or no vocational experience or work exposure, and (2) adults who, because of a disability, are no longer able to pursue their former occupations. In working with the young client, the counselor can select and use several instruments to delineate job fields of possible interest. Career aspirations of youths with disabilities have been demonstrated to be significantly different from those of youths without disabilities. Rojewski (1996, 1999) found that youths with disabilities were more likely to possess lower occupational aspirations than individuals without disabilities. Moreover, the realization of the aspirations of a youth with disabilities may need to be modified in light of his or her disability.

Therefore, the complexities of the world of work may seem daunting to all youths who have had limited opportunities to explore career choices. Vocational assessment may help to expand the range of options youths may consider. After testing, the client can be provided with occupational information; observe various workers in action during site visits; receive work samples and evaluation techniques; and, ultimately, be trained to enter the chosen occupation.

Initially, interest measurement was geared primarily to clients with professional aspirations and goals. More recently, however, instruments have been revised to include more nonprofessional occupations (e.g., the *Strong Interest Inventory*). Instruments also are available for clients who may not possess the intelligence or reading ability to take the more commonly used instruments (e.g., *Reading-Free Vocational Interest Inventory: 2*). Vocational inventories that can be used to meet the needs of a broad range of clients with disabilities are reviewed in subsequent sections of this chapter.

Inventories also can be used to gain an understanding of the level of work orientation and vocational maturity of youths with disabilities. Inventories assess both young people's attitudes toward themselves as workers and their knowledge of the process of career selection, which may have been profoundly influenced by being disabled. It seems likely that parental overprotection of children with disabilities might lead to both a lack of work orientation and a lack of understanding of the choice process and its elements. If constructive attitudes toward work and career choice processes have not been developed, it is a mistake for the rehabilitation counselor to begin to discuss specific vocational choices. Attention first should be devoted to assisting clients in better understanding themselves and the decision-making process. Fortunately, as more and more children with disabilities are being mainstreamed into the general educational system, they will be exposed to more "normal" opportunities, including the numerous computerized systems now available to facilitate career choice and development.

In addition, social cognitive factors such as self-efficacy and outcome expectations related to career decisions may influence career exploration among individuals with disabilities. Ochs and Roessler (2004) found that both career decision self-efficacy and career outcome expectations influenced career exploration among youths with or without learning disabilities. Vocational inventories (e.g., *Career Decision Self-Efficacy Scale*) can be utilized to gain an understanding of these constructs.

Rehabilitation counselors also will find vocational inventories useful in assisting older clients who, because of disease or trauma, can no longer participate in their former occupations. For example, a client who has been oriented primarily toward physically demanding occupations (e.g., logging, trucking) and obtains injuries that result in a loss of physical functioning will be forced to select a new career and will probably have to alter his or her lifestyle drastically. In a classic study, Kunce (1969) examined the relationship between measured vocational interests and rehabilitation outcome and found that, although a major interest in physical activity may pose considerable problems for persons with severe physical disabilities in restructuring their lives to include more sedentary occupations, an interest in physical activity may actually be an asset to other clients. More recently, Rohe and his colleagues (Rohe & Athelstan, 1982,

1985; Rohe & Krause, 1998, 1999) studied the vocational interests of persons with spinal cord injuries. The authors found that the interests of their participants were often incongruent with the physical limitations imposed by their disabilities and suggested that counselors must apply extra ingenuity to assist in identifying vocational alternatives for workers with disabilities. They also found that interests of men with spinal cord injuries were as stable as noninjured men 11 years later, and that middle-aged men have the same unique pattern of vocational interests as their younger peers. Dewitt (1994) concluded that vocational interest inventories can be useful in helping with on-the-job evaluation, helping determine reasonable accommodations at work, and helping explore other work possibilities if a career change is needed following a disability. In addition, vocational interest inventories can help identify strengths rather than deficits, a process that can open potential career avenues and choices (Fabian & Liesener, 2004).

As the age of the U.S. population increases, inventories also may be useful in counseling older persons and in working with clients who may wish to prepare for retirement or who are unable to enter competitive or sheltered employment. Leisure time is increasing for all persons, workers as well as persons who are retired or unable to enter employment. The constructive and pleasurable use of leisure time is important for the satisfaction of individual needs and for the maintenance of a stable and integrated society. Persons with disabilities may have fewer avocational activities to choose from, yet they may need those activities more than nondisabled persons do in order to lead meaningful lives. The rehabilitation counselor should be aware of the work that has been done in avocational interest measurement, particularly that of Overs (1970), who developed a model for avocational counseling and a system for classifying and coding avocational activities, the *Avocational Activities Inventory* (Overs, 1971). More recently, the *Leisure Interests Questionnaire* was created to provide a thorough and comprehensive assessment of leisure interests (Hansen & Scullard, 2002). In addition, most vocational interest inventories may be used to aid in exploring avocational and leisure interests as well.

Client Participation in Counseling Process

Vocational inventories can also be used by rehabilitation counselors to facilitate communication and interaction with clients with disabilities. Although many rehabilitation agencies refer clients to psychologists or to facilities for psychological testing, rehabilitation counselors can administer many of the less complex vocational inventories. Discussion centered on these instruments and their results frequently can be of value in communicating with clients who are nonverbal. Instruments such as the *Reading-Free Vocational Interest Inventory: 2* (Becker, 2000) or the *O★NET Interest Profiler* (U.S. Department of Labor, 2000) may stimulate client participation in the counseling process, and careful observation by the counselor can enhance understanding of the client's needs and thought processes. Frequently, clients who are nonexpressive may be considered "unmotivated" and therefore determined ineligible for rehabilitation services. Some clients may appear to be unmotivated because they have no idea of the options available to them. Exploring the numerous varieties of career opportunities through the use of vocational inventories may increase client involvement in rehabilitation.

In discussing vocational inventories with the client, the counselor must remember that interests, per se, are not predictive of success in a given occupation and that the counselor must help the client distinguish among needs, values, interests, and aptitudes as well as recognize the limitations posed by the client's disability. The rehabilitation counselor must understand what a given instrument actually measures and must clearly convey this to the client.

Preparing Client for Testing Process

Vocational inventories also can be of use to the rehabilitation counselor in preparing the client for taking more complex instruments and understanding the overall psychological assessment process. Many clients with disabilities, particularly older clients (Sinick, 1976), have had limited exposure to psychological evaluation and may be extremely threatened when scheduled or referred for testing. In general, vocational inventories are less threatening to clients than aptitude or personality tests and may be used to acquaint clients with the testing and interpretation process.

Computer Applications

A number of vocational inventories reviewed in this chapter, as well as several aptitude or multidimensional batteries described throughout this *Handbook,* can be used with various computer technologies. DISCOVER, produced by the American College Testing Program, and SIGI3 (System of Interactive Guidance and Information), produced by Valpar, are comprehensive interactive computer systems that permit exploration of interests, values, and occupational and educational information. Botterbusch (1983) evaluated the major computerized job-matching systems used in rehabilitation to compare client characteristics to those of appropriate jobs listed in the *Dictionary of Occupational Titles.* Sampson et al. (1994) reviewed 15 computer-assisted career guidance systems (CACG) used in high school, college employment service, vocational–technical school, library, rehabilitation, correctional, and military settings. CACG is a system of interrelated computer-based components designed to facilitate self-assessment; the generation of occupational and educational alternatives; and the use of occupational, educational, and employment information.

Computerized systems have several advantages over noncomputerized ones (Sampson, Purgar, & Shy, 2003). First, their interactive nature allows users to become more actively involved in the career guidance process. Second, they provide immediate feedback, which helps motivate users. Third, they allow the career exploration process to be individualized. Fourth, the computerized systems make the exploration process more systematic and less biased and give users more flexibility within that process. Last, computerized systems can be linked to large databases of up-to-date information about all sorts of topics, including the most recent version of the instruments. However, there are also disadvantages of computerized systems. Some practitioners are concerned about the systems' cost, about preserving users' confidentiality, about the systems' over-reliance on computers, and that some clients may not have access to computers (Sampson et al., 2003).

Although varied in content, most CACG systems have information on the following topics: (a) occupations; (b) the Armed Services; (c) postsecondary institutions; (d) technical and specialized schools; (e) financial aid; (f) interest, ability, and value inventories; (g) decision-making skills; and (h) job search strategies. It is estimated that as information technology develops, the use of computers in career guidance and counseling will expand. In this arena, the quality of information on the computer and the effective use of the computer to obtain that information are more important than the hardware and software alone. Whiston, Brecheisen, and Stephens (2003) found that computer-guided treatments improved with counselor-guided contact, suggesting that the most critical aspect of CACG is the use of the computerized systems as part of counseling, not as a stand-alone component.

Summary

Vocational inventories can be used by rehabilitation counselors to provide clients who have disabilities with information with which to make broader and more appropriate career choices, to facilitate client participation in the counseling and career development process, and to prepare clients for psychological and vocational assessment in general. Although many rehabilitation counselors may not actually administer these inventories themselves, understanding the variety of instruments available, what they measure, and their limitations can result in more informed and appropriate referrals to psychologists and other testing resources and can enable the rehabilitation counselor to use the data reported in psychological evaluations more effectively.

Criteria for Selecting Vocational Inventories

General Criteria

A full inspection of all testing materials and the accompanying manual should precede the selection and use of a psychological test or inventory. Most publishers will provide a sample of these materials at nominal cost so that the user may critically examine the materials prior to deciding whether to use the instrument. To facilitate test review and selection, the following criteria have been identified and defined. In assessing the appropriateness of using a vocational inventory, counselors should consider some general criteria that must be considered before using a test, regardless of the client population: a clear statement of purpose, reliability, validity, and appropriate norms for the counselor's client population.

First, the test manual should clearly state what the instrument was designed to measure. If the author has not discussed the reason for developing the test and the appropriate use of the test, the purpose of the instrument is not clear; thus, it is impossible to tell whether the inventory will provide the information the user wants or needs. Only on the rare occasions when no other instrument is available should a counselor use an instrument that does not have an explicit purpose. In those circumstances, the counselor should consider the use to be experimental and should plan to continually assess the usefulness of the instrument in that specific situation.

Second, the instrument should possess adequate reliability, which indicates how stable the instrument is. Several kinds of reliability data may be available for the inventory, but test–retest reliability is the most important. Many vocational inventories are used to predict occupational satisfaction, and their stability over time must be demonstrated. Most measures of interests and values have test–retest reliability coefficients of at least .80 over short time periods (Walsh & Betz, 2001). Lower reliability estimates should alert the user to the possibility that the inventory results may contain considerable error. In an ideal situation, the test results also should include some information about the standard error of measurement, presented in either written or graphic form.

Third, it is critical that evidence be presented to indicate how well the test measures what it was designed to measure (i.e., evidence of validity should be available for the instrument). Several types of validity information should be available to present evidence that the instrument measures the construct that it was designed to measure (construct validity). Thus, if an author publishes an instrument designed to measure achievement, that author should be able to demonstrate that the measure is related to other achievement instruments as well as to behaviors logically related to achievement. Construct validity is not indicated by a single index or measure. Rather, construct validity is a process that evaluates the construct being measured (e.g., achievement) as well as the theory that incorporates the construct. One indication of construct validity is evidence of how well a test is linked to present and/or future behavior; this is criterion-related validity. Predictive validity (indication that a test is linked to future behavior) is particularly important since many vocational inventories are used to help make decisions about the future vocational behavior of individuals. Thus, if an inventory purports to measure vocational maturity, evidence should be presented that people who eventually make good vocational adjustments score higher on the inventory than those who do not adjust well. In the same way, if an inventory claims to measure interests for specific occupations, data should be presented that indicate that members of those occupations score high on their own occupational scale. Other ways to measure construct validity include intratest methods (which investigate the internal structure of a test), intertest methods (which study relationships among tests), experimental manipulation of variables that may affect test scores, and a multitrait–multimethod matrix to separate convergent validity (correlations between the same traits measured by different methods) and discriminant validity (correlations between different traits measured by the same methods; Thorndike, 1997).

One type of validity that has begun to receive a great deal of attention is that of cross-cultural validity—how valid an instrument is across cultural groups (Fouad, 1999). Test authors should provide information on the application of their instruments to groups other than the majority (white) culture in the United States. This evidence should take the form of (a) translation validity (if the instrument is translated into another language, it has linguistic equivalence [is the same in both languages]) and (b) cross-cultural norm groups (the test has been normed in other cultural groups).

Fourth, it is important that vocational measures used by rehabilitation counselors have norms that are appropriate for their clients. This does not necessarily mean that there must be specific norms for persons with disabilities; rather, norms should be available for the appropriate age range and educational level of the client. For example, norms based on adolescents generally are not suitable for older workers with disabilities. Occasionally, it will be possible to develop local norms for use with rehabilitation clients that incorporate individuals of the appropriate age, educational level, and/or disability. Counselors should keep in mind, however, that if the inventory is to be used to predict the client's job success and satisfaction, it might be necessary to compare the client to the broad working population. If the rehabilitation goal is competitive employment, comparison of the client with workers in general, or workers in a specific occupation, may be useful. However, if the results are to be used to stimulate discussion and exploration, norms based on specific rehabilitation client populations might prove more helpful. Counselors should be particularly alert to possible sex bias and unfairness in some interest measurement procedures. Readers are referred to Drummond (1996) for a comprehensive discussion of this issue. Test manuals should indicate whether norms are appropriate for men, women, or all people.

Special Criteria

Some criteria for vocational measures apply specifically to their use by rehabilitation counselors. First, the readability level of the instrument is especially important since many rehabilitation clients have limited basic educational skills. These limitations may result from the disability and its treatment; thus, the vocational measures used by rehabilitation counselors must allow the client to explore a full range of possibilities without being restricted by the instrument itself. Too frequently, clients are given tests that they simply cannot read or understand and decisions are based on essentially meaningless data.

Second, for the same reason, it is important that rehabilitation counselors use vocational measures that are suitable for administration to clients with physical limitations. In general, measures without time limits and/or measures that do not necessitate the use of a complex mechanical apparatus are best suited for rehabilitation clients.

A related but separate problem is the third special criterion. Inventories for rehabilitation clients should have validity scales that indicate whether the clients are responding appropriately or merely randomly because of poor abilities or lack of motivation. If possible, the instruments also should have validity scales that indicate consistency of response. These scales are desirable in all vocational inventories but are particularly necessary with rehabilitation clients who may be relatively naive about the world of work and are operating from a somewhat different experiential and motivational framework than the usual client.

Vocational Instruments

To assist rehabilitation counselors in selecting and using vocational inventories, the authors reviewed 18 vocational instruments. Following are comprehensive reviews of six instruments that were judged to be particularly useful for rehabilitation clients:

1. *Strong Interest Inventory* (Donnay, Morris, Schaubhut, & Thompson, 2005)
2. *Kuder Career Search with Person Match* (Zytowski, 2006)
3. *Minnesota Importance Questionnaire* (Gay, Weiss, Hendel, Dawis, & Lofquist, 1981)
4. *Reading-Free Vocational Interest Inventory: 2* (Becker, 2000)
5. *Campbell Interest and Skill Survey* (Campbell, Hyne, & Nilsen, 1992)
6. *Self-Directed Search* (Holland, Fritzsche, & Powell, 1994)

There are brief reviews of these other 12 instruments:

1. *Career Beliefs Inventory* (Krumboltz, 1991)
2. *Career Decision-Making System–Revised* (Harrington & O'Shea, 2000)
3. *Career Development Inventory* (Thompson & Lindeman, 1984)
4. *Career Occupational Preference System Interest Inventory* (Knapp & Knapp, 1983)
5. *Career Planning Survey* (American College Testing Program, 1998)
6. *O*✶*Net Interest Profiler* (U.S. Department of Labor, 2000)
7. *Vocational Preference Inventory* (Holland, 1978)
8. *Super's Work Values Inventory–Revised* (Zytowski, 2001)
9. *Career Decision-Making Difficulties Questionnaire* (Gati, Krausz, & Osipow, 1996)

10. *Career Decision Self-efficacy Scale* (Taylor & Betz, 1983)
11. *Revised Unisex Edition of the ACT Interest Inventory* (American College Testing Program, 1995)
12. *Armed Services Vocational Aptitude Battery* (U.S. Department of Defense, 2005)

Strong Interest Inventory

Form. *T291.*

Purpose. The purpose of this instrument is to give individuals information about themselves and their preferences that will help them make sound career decisions; to provide information to professionals, such as rehabilitation counselors, who assist others in making decisions; and to help in studying groups of individuals.

Description. The *Strong Interest Inventory* (SII) is a 291-item inventory designed to "compare [an individual's] pattern of responses to the pattern of responses of people of different types and in different occupations" (Donnay et al., 2005, p. 2). It is the most recent edition of the interest inventory developed by E.K. Strong, Jr.; the first version of the instrument was published in 1927. The SII, like most interest inventories, was designed to provide information about the world of work and to promote occupational exploration by assessing an individual's pattern of interests. The 291 items in the SII, which are answered on a 5-point continuum from *Strongly Dislike* to *Strongly Like,* are grouped into six categories: Occupations (124 items that are the names of occupations), School Subjects (50 items covering educational situations), Activities (119 items about a wide variety of activities), Leisure Activities (34 items covering preferences for types of leisure activities), Types of People (20 items covering the coworkers with whom one would enjoy working), and Your Characteristics (14 self-descriptive statements to which the respondent indicates on a 5-point scale whether the characteristic is *Strongly Like Me* to *Strongly Unlike Me* (Donnay et al., 2005).

The SII profile is divided into four major sections, each with its unique scale construction and contribution to the exploration of vocational interests: 6 General Occupational Themes based on Holland's (1997) typology, 30 Basic Interest scales, 244 Occupational scales, and 5 Personal Style scales (Work Style, Learning Environment, Risk Taking, Team Orientation, and Leadership Style). In addition, administrative indices show the number of total responses, percentages of the responses in the five different response categories, and a typicality index to indicate inconsistent responding.

The average respondent can complete the inventory in a half-hour. The reading level is about 6th grade. Interest inventories of this type generally have been administered only to persons older than 17 years of age because young respondents may not have stable interest patterns.

Scoring is too complex to be completed by hand; a scoring service must be used. Profiles that relate the General Occupational Themes to the Basic Interest and Occupational scales are the usual output, although some scoring services provide interpretive profiles printed individually by computer.

Norms. The General Occupational Themes and Basic Interest scales have been normed on general reference samples of 1,125 men and 1,125 women collected for the 2005 revision. The mean for both sexes is set at a standard score of 50 and a standard deviation of 10. Because there are sex differences in many of the General Occupational Themes and Basic Interest scales, the profile and interpretive material make it possible to determine how an individual stands on norms for the same sex.

The Occupational scales have been normed on a criterion group of people employed in the occupation. Criterion groups were constructed using the profiles of occupational members who met three basic criteria: (1) experience (in their occupation for at least 3 years), (2) satisfaction with their work, and (3) pursuit of typical occupational tasks. Most occupational groups contained 200 or more members; the size of the groups ranged from 53 to 1,187. The mean and standard deviation for each group are 50 and 10, respectively. The Personal Style scales were also normed on the combined General Reference Sample, with a mean of 50 and a standard deviation of 10. Scores on the General Occupational Themes, Basic Interest scales, and Personal Style scales are shown in comparison to members of the same sex since men and women scored differently on many of the scales.

Reliability. There are 1- to 6-month test-retest correlations for each set of scales. Median correlations for the General Occupational Themes ranged from .82 to .92 and from .74 to .93 for the Basic Interest scales. The Occupational scales ranged from .71 to .93 in four different age group samples. In general, the older the group, the more reliable were the test scores.

Validity. The General Occupational Themes and Basic Interest scales have content validity as a result of their item selection procedure. The General Occupational Themes are related to Holland's Theory of Vocational Personality Types (1997). Each type of scale has concurrent validity (i.e., persons in an occupation score higher on their own scales than other people do). Discussion of predictive validity of the scales is available in the *Manual* (Donnay et al., 2005). The results of the studies indicate that approximately 50% to 75% of individuals tested entered the occupations predicted by their profiles. Cross-cultural validity has been demonstrated for the SII across national groups (Fouad & Dancer, 1992; Fouad & Hansen, 1987; Fouad, Hansen, & Arias-Galicia, 1986, 1989) and racial/ethnic groups in the United States (Fouad, 2002; Fouad & Mohler, 2004). Fouad, Harmon, and Hansen (1994) examined differences among the racial and ethnic groups that were part of the criterion groups for the 1994 revision. Few differences were found at the item level, and even fewer differences were found at the scale or profile level. It is important to note, however, that no research has examined whether interpretations are generalizable across cultures.

Comments. The 2005 revision of the SII has several major advantages for rehabilitation counselors. First, the items were updated for language and sensitivity to culture and gender, and a number of technology-oriented occupations were added. Twenty-four new occupations were added to the Occupational scales, including Chiropractor, Rehabilitation Counselor, Computer Scientist, Computer Systems Analyst, and Network Administrator. The Occupational scales include several nonprofessional occupations, including production worker, operations manager, technical support specialist, and firefighter. The large general reference sample (2,500 individuals included) minimizes chance errors. Ethnic or racial group membership of respondents was collected. Thus, the information that there are few meaningful differences in vocational interests related to racial and ethnic group differences is helpful to counselors using the instrument with various groups. The addition of five additional Basic Interest scales and a Team Orientation Personal Style scale will aid in interpreting interests of individuals across a variety of areas.

Kuder Career Search

Form. *Career Search with Person Match.*

Purpose. The purpose of this instrument is to measure individual preferences and to compare them with those of individuals in a variety of occupations. Rather than comparing the individual to a group of professionals, the inventory gives a pool of individuals whose preferences match those of the test taker. The measure was designed for use with middle and high school students, those who have dropped out of school, first-year college students, or adults in need of career planning or job placement guidance.

Description. The *Kuder Career Search* (KCS) *with Person Match* contains 60 triads of three activities. In each triad, the respondent ranks all three activities, indicating first, second, and third most desirable preferences. Answers are recorded directly on an answer form; scoring may be done on-site using a self-scored paper-and-pencil version, using a computer software program, or using an Internet site. Answer sheets may also be sent to the publisher for scoring. Most individuals can complete the inventory in 30 minutes; for those with mobility impairments, the inventory may be read aloud and responses recorded by another individual. Items are written at the 6th-grade reading level. The KCS yields scores on six occupational cluster scores and 10 activity preference scales. The clusters represent groupings of occupations designed to be congruent with Holland's (1997) hexagonal model. Individuals are compared to a particular individual (person match) rather than to a group of individuals in an occupation. In the person match, individuals are given sketches of seven individuals with whom their interests match in their top two clusters; thus they are compared to 14 individuals and receive information on job sketches in those occupations. The job sketches include the individual's job duties, likes and dislikes, and more specific information on how his or her career fulfills him or her.

Norms. The person match database consists of more than 1,600 individuals representing occupations in each of the clusters; these individuals are employed in 90% of the occupations in the *Occupational Outlook Handbook.* The norm group for the KCS consists of 8,791 individuals. The individuals are balanced in terms of age (middle school, high school, and adults), geographic region, and gender.

Reliability. Reliability of the KCS Activity preference scales ranges from .64 to .75 for internal consistency and from .79 to .92 for 3-week test-retest reliability. Over approximately 3 years, a study involving 93 university engineering students indicated a median reliability coefficient of .80. This type of comparison correlates individual profiles rather than scales.

Validity. Validity has been assessed in terms of accuracy of classification of employed subjects as well as by rank ordering of scores of core group members on their own scales. Concurrent validity, therefore, has been established for the scales. Zytowski (1976) followed more than 1,000 men and women who had been tested on the *Kuder Preference Record,* which contains the same items as the KCS and the *Kuder Occupational Scale,* 12 to 19 years prior to the study. Of those followed, 51% were employed in a job consistent with a Kuder Occupational Interest Scale (KOIS). Since the KCS is matching an individual to particular individuals, predictive validity information is not appropriate to determine, although the manual suggests that exploration validity and substantive validity will be important to evaluate in the future.

Comments. The KCS is using a unique approach to interest measurement, one that may be particularly useful for rehabilitation counselors. It is not known whether any of the individuals in the person match database have a disability, but if this information were available, it would increase the role modeling and applicability of the instrument for clients with disabilities. The use of the activity scales may help counselors explore lifestyle considerations and avocational interests, and the inclusion of career clusters allows counselors to apply Holland's (1997) vocational themes, which has not been possible with previous versions of the Kuder. Finally, this instrument will allow counselors to provide clients with occupational information without depending on a shifting occupational environment. It will be important to ascertain whether this will aid clients in exploring their interests and making good career decisions.

Minnesota Importance Questionnaire

Form. *Paired Comparison and Ranked Form,* 1981.

Purpose. The purpose of this instrument is to assess the vocational needs and values of clients and to help clients assess the correspondence between their needs and reinforcer patterns in various occupations. Need–reinforcer correspondence in a particular occupation indicates the likelihood that a client will be satisfied in that occupation.

Description. The *Minnesota Importance Questionnaire* (MIQ) is a 210-item inventory that measures 20 vocationally relevant needs. Clients are asked to choose the one of a pair of statements that they feel is more important to them in their ideal job. Each of the 20 needs is paired with each other, resulting in 190 pairs of statements. Each pair is listed only once. In the last 20 items, clients are asked to indicate whether or not each item is important (yes or no?). Three types of scores are given: 20 needs, 6 values (beliefs underlying needs), and 6 reinforcer clusters (patterns of reinforcers developed through cluster analysis). In addition, a logically consistent triad (LCT) score is given; the LCT is an indication of the logical consistency with which a client responds to the items. The MIQ is a self-administered inventory and typically takes 30 to 40 minutes to complete. Reading difficulty level is approximately 6th grade. Some previous work experience will help clients identify which needs are most important to them in the ideal job. Spanish and French versions are available.

Norms. The MIQ, unlike most of the other instruments reviewed in this chapter, does not compare an individual's scores with a normative group to obtain a scale score. Rather, the score profile is ipsative. MIQ scale values are calculated by converting an individual's raw score into a scale score based on the individual's own mean score, then adjusting all the other scale values with respect to the individual's personal mean. In other words, a given client may have a greater need to use specific abilities and less need to find a secure job. These needs are interpreted for that client without reference to how important it is to a norm group to use the abilities or to be secure. Scale score norms are available, however, for men and women in three different age groups (18–25, 26–45, and 46–70 years). Counselors may use the norms for scale scores between the 15th and 85th percentiles to assess how typical clients' needs are for their age groups. A client's likelihood for satisfaction in a particular occupation may be assessed by the correspondence between the client's needs and the pattern of reinforcers for the occupation. Ninety benchmark occupations are listed in the standard MIQ report; the client receives an S (predicted satisfied), L (likely satisfied), or N (not predicted satisfied) for each occupation. The 90 occupations are clustered into six groups (reinforcer clusters) with similar reinforcer patterns; the client receives an S, L, or N for the cluster as well as for specific occupations.

Reliability. Test-retest reliability data on the individual MIQ scales are available for a range of time intervals, from immediate (.89 median reliability) to 10 months (.53 median reliability). Profile stability data also range from immediate (.95 median reliability) to 10 months (.87 median reliability). Internal consistency reliability coefficients range from .77 to .81.

Validity. The MIQ scale scores have demonstrated divergent and convergent validity—that is, they have shown a median correlation of .00 with *General Aptitude Test Battery* scales (Weiss, Dawis, Lofquist, & England, 1966) but a canonical correlation of .78 with *Strong Vocational Interest Blank* scores (Thorndike, Weiss, & Dawis, 1968). Thus, the MIQ is *not a* measure of abilities; rather, it is an instrument that measures vocational preferences. Extensive construct validity data are available for the MIQ. For example, the instrument has been shown to differentiate among groups (Gay et al., 1971) and to correlate highly with biographical data (e.g., Meresman, 1975; Rounds, Dawis, & Lofquist, 1979). Most of the construct validity of the MIQ, however, has centered around predicting satisfaction from need–reinforcer correspondence (e.g., Betz, 1969; Elizur & Tziner, 1977; Lichter, 1980; Lofquist & Dawis, 1969; Rounds, 1981; Salazar, 1981). Doering, Rhodes, and Kaspin (1988) investigated the factor structure of MIQ and found that three factors extracted: autonomy–achievement, environmental reinforcement–aggrandizement, and safety. A recent study of the genetic and environmental influences on work values yielded that 40% of the variance in measured work values was related to genetic factors, while about 60% of the variance was associated with environmental factors (Keller, Bouchard, Arvey, & Segal, 1992). Cross-cultural validity also has been demonstrated for the MIQ by Salazar (1981), based on a sample of graduates of a guidance program at the University of the Philippines.

Comments. The MIQ is thoroughly grounded in a theoretical framework; it also has been extensively researched. Counselors may interpret the results with confidence. One drawback to the instrument, the tediousness of the paired comparison format, may be eliminated in the near future, as the authors move toward a triad format. An updated technical manual is being prepared for publication. (See independent reviews by P. Benson in *Test Critiques* [Vol. 2; Keyser & Sweetland, 1984–1985], *The Eleventh Mental Measurements Yearbook* [Kramer & Conoley, 1992], and Brook & Ciechalski, 1994.)

Reading-Free Vocational Interest Inventory: 2

Form. *Revised.*

Purpose. The purpose of this instrument is to provide information about vocational preferences for persons with mental retardation and learning disabilities through the use of pictorial illustrations of individuals engaged in various occupational tasks. It is for people with special needs and provides a wide range of information on unskilled, semiskilled, and skilled occupations.

Description. The *Reading-Free Vocational Interest Inventory: 2* (R–FVII:2) is a vocational interest inventory designed to assess, in a forced-choice format, the vocational preferences of clients (age 12–61) who have limited reading ability. There are 165 neutral, nonspecific, black-and-white sketches representing job tasks. The R–FVII:2 contains 55 sets of three illustrations: each illustration depicts an individual engaged in a task typical of an unskilled, semiskilled, or skilled occupation (e.g., one triad shows a man picking apples, a man mopping a floor, and a man opening a car door). Clients select the picture of the task they would most like to do. The R–FVII:2 provides scores in 11 interest areas for men and women. The average time required to complete the R–FVII:2 is approximately 20 minutes. Each client responds to the inventory directly on the test booklet, reducing the confusion of transferring answers to an answer sheet. The R–FVII:2 is scored by hand.

Norms. There are separate normative tables for females and males and for youths and adults in five categories (mental retardation, learning disability, regular classroom, adult disadvantaged, and adult sheltered work) for all 11 interest areas. For persons with mental retardation, with learning disabilities, and in a regular classroom setting, norms are available for males and females in public and private schools in two different age groups (12 years, 0 months to 15 years, 11 months; and 16 years, 0 months to 21 years, 11 months). Norms also are presented for adult men and women in sheltered workshops and who were categorized as disadvantaged. Each sample was based on about 1,000 clients. The normative data were collected in 1997–1998 from a nationwide sample of 15,564 individuals, with a representative sample from each geographic region and level of socioeconomic status.

Reliability. Test-retest reliabilities of the R–FVII:2 over an interval of 2 weeks are reported; most are .8 or higher. The test-retest estimates ranged from .70 to .97 for small subsamples of the 10 standardization samples (sizes ranged from $N = 41$ for females in a regular classroom setting to $N = 76$ for females with mental retardation). Test-retest reliability over a longer interval than 2 weeks is not given in the manual.

Validity. Content validity data are presented for the R–FVII:2 on the basis of the description of item selection. A search was made to select jobs that were realistic and appropriate for clients with mental retardation and learning disabilities; teams estimated the importance of job tasks, which then were depicted in a drawing. Concurrent validity data are provided through comparison of the R–FVII:2 to the Geist Picture Interest Inventory on relatively small samples (*N*s ranged between 51 and 62). Most correlations were statistically significant. No predictive validity data are presented. Limited construct validity data indicate that workers with mental retardation in the 11 occupational areas scored higher in the occupational interest area in which they were engaged. No cross-cultural validity data are presented.

Comments. At present, the R–FVII:2 seems to be a needed addition to the wide array of vocational interest inventories, and it is especially useful for special populations. As a counseling tool, the usable test booklet, pragmatic pictures, and speed of scoring make the R–FVII:2 a very attractive instrument. In addition, counselors may feel confident in comparing their clients to the large, well-represented norm groups. Yet, problems remain—related to jobs that may be suitable for the target population, gender equity, and lack of cultural diversity—that need to be addressed. There are three concerns: (1) very few of the drawings depict the use of technology; (2) the work activities pictured in the inventory are stereotypical of gender and of the kinds of activities perceived to be appropriate for individuals with special needs; and (3) all of the drawings are narrow culturally and there is no attempt at providing any nondominant culture depiction in any of the pictures. Counselors should be cautious about using the instrument as anything other than a device to explore vocational interests until more research is available on the inventory's stability and validity (see independent reviews in *The Fifteenth Mental Measurements Yearbook* [Gratz & Pope, 2003] for details).

Campbell Interest and Skill Survey

Form. *1992*

Purpose. The purpose of this instrument is to "help individuals understand how their interests and skills map into the occupational world" (Campbell, Hyne, & Nilsen, 1992, p. 1).

Description. The reading level for the *Campbell Interest and Skill Survey* (CISS) is 6th grade. The test items are categorized into two sections: 200 interest items and 120 skill items. The responses have six alternatives ranging from "strongly like" to "strongly dislike." The test report includes seven Orientation Scales (Influencing, Organizing, Helping, Creating, Analyzing, Producing, and Adventuring) that describe orientations to the world of work, with individuals receiving scores on their interests and self-perceived skill in each area. The seven Orientation Scales map to Holland's (1997) typology well, with Adventuring and Producing both corresponding to the Realistic Theme. There are also 29 Basic Scales with scores in both interests and skills and 58 Occupational Scales (with both male and female norms). The test report also includes three special scales with measures of occupational introversion/extroversion, academic focus, and variety of interests, and six procedural checks, which help to identify problems in test administration. It typically takes approximately 30 minutes to complete the CISS. The inventory can be administered individually or in groups. The instrument may be taken via paper or pencil, computer, or Internet. Machine scoring is necessary. The profile report graphically presents the scores on each scale and provides interpretative information.

Norms. The Orientation and Basic Scales on the CISS had a reference group of 1,790 women and 3,435 men to norm the scales, drawn from individuals in the occupational groups; race/ethnicity of the norm group is not mentioned. The criteria for inclusion were that individuals were happily employed and doing typical tasks of the occupation. The raw scores of the two gender groups are combined for conversion to a standard score, with a mean of 50 and standard deviation of 10.

Reliability. The test-retest reliabilities for the Orientation Scales are in the .80s for up to 3-month intervals. The internal consistency reliabilities range from .76 to .93, with median alpha coefficients of .87 for both Interest and Skills. The median Basic Interest internal consistency coefficient was .86; the median Basic Skills internal consistency coefficient was .79. The median test-retest correlation was .87 for the Occupational Interest Scale and .79 for Occupation Skill Scale.

Validity. Construct validity for the CISS is achieved by demonstrating intercorrelation between the skills and interests for each Orientation; these range from .66 to .76. Construct validity is also demonstrated by having correlations with other Orientations low. For example, the Producing skills and interests correlate .73, but Producing skills and Influencing interests correlate only .12. In general, the pattern of intercorrelations supports the construct validity of the CISS. Concurrent validity of the Occupations scales is expressed as the degree to which the scales separate scores of occupational groups from those of the general reference group.

Comments. The CISS potentially is a useful measure for rehabilitation clients, particularly for clients who may express interest in an occupational area but who may not have confidence in their skills in the area. The CISS is oriented toward more professional jobs and offers the Special scales of Academic Focus, Extraversion, and Variety of interests. The profile also comes with an interest/skill pattern worksheet to identify areas to develop (high interest, lower skill confidence), areas to pursue (in which both interests and skills are high), areas to avoid (both are low), and areas to explore (skills are high, interests are low). One of the case studies in the manual is of a client who had a serious accident that interrupted his college studies. The critiques of the CISS generally are quite positive (Pugh, 1998; Roszkowski, 1998). Although the CISS is more geared toward professional jobs, the inclusion of both interests and skills makes it one of the most useful and well-developed inventories for measuring the interests of clients who are nonprofessionally oriented.

Self-Directed Search

Form. *1994*

Form R's 1994 revision is intended for use with high school and college students as well as adults. Form E's 1990 version is intended for junior high school students and adults with limited reading skills. Form CP's version is intended for career planning and is a shorter version of the instrument. The reading level of the items for Form R is estimated to be at the 7th or 8th grade level and at approximately the 4th grade level for Form E. Spanish, French, and Vietnamese versions of SDS are available.

Purpose. The purpose of this instrument is to help students and employees find the occupations that best suit their interests and abilities and to provide a counseling tool that can be used to serve a wider population. The instrument can be used as a structural framework for organizing personal and occupational information and for making satisfactory career decisions. The instrument can be used in a variety of settings for multiple purposes such as career counseling, career education and job placement, classification, and training. A further purpose of this instrument is to provide researchers with a psychometrically sound instrument that can be used to examine the validity of Holland's (1997) typology theory. Form E provides a complete career assessment for individuals with limited reading skills.

Description. The *Self-Directed Search* (SDS) is a self-administered, self-scored, and self-interpreted vocational inventory. It consists of an assessment booklet and an Occupations Finder, which lists more than 1,300 occupational alternatives with work environments that suit the client's work personality. The assessment booklet has five sections: Occupational Daydreams (individuals can fill in up to eight self-identified occupations), Activities (11 items for each of the six personality types), Competencies (11 items for each of the six personality types), Occupations (14 items for each of the six personality types), and Self-Estimates (2 items for each of the six work environments). All the scales except Occupational Daydreams are calculated to yield a total score for each of the six personality types. The highest three summary scores determine a 3-digit personality type. For example, a student with high Investigative, Social, and Enterprising interests would be coded ISE.

The *Self-Directed Search* is based on Holland's theory of vocational interests and choice, which theorizes that there are distinct vocational personality types and occupational environments. A match between an individual's personal character and the occupation's requirements and demands leads to increased career satisfaction. The six personality characteristics of Holland's theory are Realistic, Investigative, Artistic, Social, Enterprising, and Conventional. An extensive listing of occupational codes can be found in Gottfredson, Holland, and Ogawa's (1996) *Dictionary of Holland Occupational Codes*. Individuals completing the SDS obtain a 3-digit personality type that closely resembles their interests, which in turn is matched with occupations that correspond to that that personality type. This summary score is compared with Occupational Daydreams and then used with the Occupations Finder (includes approximately 500 occupations) to locate related occupations. Each occupational subtype is arranged according to the level of general educational development as outlined in the *Dictionary of Occupational Titles* (DOT; U.S. Department of Labor, 1991). DOT codes also are listed. Several changes have been incorporated in the 1996 edition, including simplified scoring procedures, the addition of 50 jobs to the Occupations Finder, changes in suggested readings, and revision of some items to reduce sex differences.

Norms. Norms for the SDS scales and codes are provided in the manual. The reference section is presented in the manual with extensive information about the use of the instrument. The norm group for the 1997 *Self-Directed Search Form R* consisted of 2,602 students and adults, including 1,600 females and 1,002 males, with an age range from 7 to 65 years. The norms groups included individuals from 25 states with a broad range of racial background represented.

Reliability. Internal consistency coefficients ranged from 0.72 to 0.92 for the various scales with coefficients varying from 0.90 to 0.94 for the summary scales. Correlations between two Self-Estimate ratings per scale ranged from 0.37 to 0.84, suggesting that ratings contain shared variance but also contribute some unique variance. Test-retest reliability for a small sample ($N = 73$) over 4 to 12 weeks ranged from 0.76 to 0.89, respectively.

Validity. The SDS has impressive construct validity related to Holland's (1997) theory with scales fitting with theoretical model. Studies examining evidence for concurrent validity suggest that adults enter occupations that match their code types approximately 60% of the time (Hansen, 2005). Concurrent validities for the SDS have ranged from 46.7% to 76.0%. The evidence for predictive validity for SDS scores is variable and often depends on age, length of time between tests, and educational level. Predictive validities for 1 to 7 years have ranged from 39.6% to 79.3%, indicating that between 40% and 80% of college students and adults are pursuing majors and occupations that match their Holland's code first letter.

In assessing cross-cultural validity, Gade, Fugua, and Hurlburt (1984) concluded that the SDS may be an inappropriate instrument for use with Native Americans. However, other studies supported the adequacy of using SDS with other minority groups (Henry, Bardo, & Bryson, 1988; Khan & Alvi, 1991; Miller, Springer, & Wells, 1988). In addition to the studies reported in the technical manual, many studies have examined the psychometric merits of SDS with diverse groups (see *The Thirteenth Mental Measurements Yearbook* [Impara & Plake, 1998] for details).

Comments. The SDS is a strong vocational interest inventory based on a solid theoretical background that can be useful in a variety of settings, including in rehabilitation counseling. The SDS has a long history of use and is attractive for rehabilitation counselors because of its utility with a large number of clients without a great amount of counselor involvement. Beyond being an inventory, the SDS is a career education experience that the counselor and client can integrate with other personal and vocational data to help the client arrive at a satisfactory vocational choice. (See independent review by M. Brown in *The Fourteenth Mental Measurements Yearbook* [Brown, 1998].)

The revised SDS demonstrates Holland's commitment to providing an easy-to-use, inexpensive, self-administered vocational assessment tool to the larger population. Scoring procedures have been simplified since the previous edition. However, the SDS is criticized for using raw scores to determine the total test scores and for its overemphasis on self-administration. It is not appropriate for some clients to totally rely on self-administration. More evidence of criterion-related validity and predictive validity also would be useful. The counselor must be cautious about suggesting this measure to clients without the reading and basic math skills necessary for self-scoring.

Instruments Versus Criteria

All instruments listed above were rated by the authors on the selection criteria. Consensus ratings by the authors on evidence for validity as well as pertinent information on reading level and validity scales are presented in Table 8.1.

The purpose of each inventory was rated as plus (+) if it was stated clearly in the test manual. If the manual did not contain this information, the instrument received a minus (−) rating. Test-retest reliability was assessed for each inventory. Ratings were as follows: plus (+), test-retest reliability coefficients

TABLE 8.1.

Evaluation of Vocational Inventories on Selection Criteria

Instrument	Purpose	Test-/Retest Reliability	Validity			Norms		Readability Level	Validity Scale	Cross-Cultural Validity
			Construct	Concurrent	Predictive	Adolescent	Adult			
Comprehensive Reviews										
Campbell Interest and Skill Survey	+	+	+	+	+		+	6th grade	+	–
Kuder Career Search	+	+	+	+	+	–	+	6th grade	+	–
Minnesota Importance Questionnaire	+	+	+	+	+	–	+	6th grade	+	+
Reading-Free Vocational Interest Inventory:2	+	+	+	+	–	+	+	Nonreading	–	–
Self-Directed Search	+	+	+	+	+	+	+	7th grade	+	+
Strong Interest Inventory	+	+	+	+	+	–	+	6th grade	+	+
Brief Reviews										
Career Beliefs Inventory	+	–	+	+	–	+	+	8th grade	–	+
Career Decision-Making System–Revised	+	+	+	+	+	+	+	8th grade	–	+
Career Development Inventory	+	+	+	+	–	–	–	9th grade	–	+
Career Occupational Preference System Interest Inventory	+	+	+	+	–	–	+	6th grade	–	–

(continues)

TABLE 8.1. *Continued.*

Instrument	Purpose	Test-/Retest Reliability	Validity			Norms		Readability Level	Validity Scale	Cross-Cultural Validity
			Construct	Concurrent	Predictive	Adolescent	Adult			
Brief Reviews (Continued)										
Career Planning Survey	+	+	+	+	+	+	–	6th grade	–	+
O*NET Interest Profiler	+	+	+	+	–	+	+	8th grade	–	–
Vocational Preference Inventory	+	+	+	+	+	–	+	NA	+	–
Super's Work Values Inventory-Revised	+	+	+	+	–	+	–	6th grade	–	–
Career Decision-Making Difficulties Questionnaire	+	+	+	+	–	+		6th grade	–	+
Career Decision Self-Efficacy Scale	+	+	+	+	–	–	+	NA	–	+
Revised Unisex Edition of the ACT Interest Inventory	+	+	+	+	+	+	+	NA	–	+
ASVAB	+	+	+	+	+	+	+	6th grade	–	+

Note. NA = not applicable.

of .69 and above; minus (−), coefficients of lower than .69 or information not available.

Construct, concurrent, and predictive validity was assessed for each instrument. Ratings or construct validity were established as follows: plus (+), factor analytic studies available and/or instrument developed on sound theoretical base; minus (−), construct validity evidence available but limited or information not available. Concurrent validity ratings were as follows: plus (+), evidence indicates significant relationship to existing, well-established instruments such as the SII or Kuder, or to external criteria; minus (−), evidence available but limited or information not available. Predictive validity ratings were as follows: plus (+), adequate evidence of predictive validity; minus (−), evidence available but limited or information not available.

Ratings for appropriate adolescent and adult (age 18 and older) norms were defined as follows: plus (+), available; minus (−), available but limited or no information. For readability level, the recommended minimum reading level is given if available; minus (−) ratings indicate this information was not available. The criterion of appropriate verification scales was rated as plus (+) if a verification scale was described in the test manual. A minus (−) rating indicates that a validity scale is not part of the instrument. Ratings for cross-cultural validity were defined as follows: plus (+), available; minus (−), available but limited or no information.

Conclusion

Vocational interest inventories may be of help to counselors in aiding clients with disabilities with career decisions. However, counselors must be aware of limitations. Although rating each instrument on its appropriateness for various disability groups might be desirable, the vast majority of instruments reviewed posed the same limitations for specific disability groups. All paper-and-pencil inventories necessitate hand and finger dexterity if clients are to take the instruments themselves following standardized directions. Persons with motor paralysis or severe dysfunction cannot complete these instruments unassisted. Persons with severe visual impairments obviously cannot take paper-and-pencil inventories without assistance. The reader is referred to Chapter 16 for information on evaluation of clients who are visually impaired.

The majority of vocational inventories also are inappropriate for persons with mental retardation, persons who are illiterate, and persons with limited reading abilities. The pictorial inventories will offer promise for these clients if further research substantiates their effectiveness; readers are referred to Chapter 18 for more specific information related to clients with mental retardation. Finally, the use of vocational inventories for clients from differing cultural and experiential backgrounds still necessitates additional research and is addressed more fully in Chapter 20. The counselor must exercise caution in administering to these clients instruments that were designed for and standardized on the dominant white culture.

References

Allport, G. W., Vernon, P. E., & Lindzey, G. (1970). *Manual: Study of values.* Boston: Houghton Mifflin.

American College Testing. (1995). *Technical manual: Revised unisex edition of the ACT Interest Inventory (UNIACT).* Iowa City, IA: ACT.

American College Testing Program. (1998). *Career planning survey, technical manual.* Iowa City, IA: Author.

Becker, R. L. (2000). *Reading-Free Vocational Interest Inventory: 2 manual.* Columbus, OH: Elbern.

Betz, E. L. (1969). Need-reinforcer correspondence as a predictor of satisfaction. *Personnel and Guidance Journal, 45,* 878–883.

Blustein, D.L. (1999). Career development theories and the school-to-work transition: A match made in heaven? *Career Development Quarterly, 47,* 348–352.

Blustein, D.L., Kenna, A.C., & Murphy, K.A. (2005). Qualitative research in career development: Exploring the center and margins of discourse about careers and working. *Journal of Career Assessment, 13,* 351–370.

Blustein, D.L., Phillips, S.D., Jobin-Davis, K., Finkelberg, Si., & Roarke, A.E. (1997). A theory-building investigation of the school-to-work transition. *Counseling Psychologist, 25,* 364–402.

Bolton, B. (1985). Review of the USES Interest Inventory. In D.J. Keyser & R.C. Sweetland (Eds.), *Test critiques* (Vol. 3, pp. 673–681). Austin, TX: PRO-ED.

Botterbusch, K.F. (1983). *A comparison of computerized job matching systems.* Menomonie: University of Wisconsin–Stout, Materials Development Center.

Brook, S.L., & Ciechalski, J.C. (1994). Review of Minnesota Importance Questionnaire. In J.T. Kapes, M.M. Mastie, & E.A. Whitfield (Eds.), *A counselor's guide to career assessment instruments* (3rd ed., pp. 220–225). Alexandria, VA: National Career Development Association.

Brown, M. (2001).*The fourteenth mental measurements yearbook.* Lincoln, NE: University of Nebraska Press.

Callahan, M.J., & Garner, J.B. (1997). *Keys to the workplace.* Baltimore: Brookes.

Campbell, D.P., & Holland, J.L. (1972). Applying Holland's theory to Strong's data. *Journal of Vocational Behavior, 2,* 353–376.

Campbell, D.P., Hyne, S.A., & Nilsen, D.L. (1992). *Manual for the Campbell Interest and Skill Survey (CISS).* Minneapolis, MN: National Computer Systems.

Crites, J.O. (1978). *Theory and research handbook: Career Maturity Inventory.* Monterey, CA: McGraw-Hill.

Daniels, M.H. (1994). Self-directed search. In J.T. Kapes, M.M. Mastie, & E.A. Whitfield (Eds.), *A counselor's guide to career assessment instruments* (3rd ed., pp. 208–212). Alexandria, VA: National Career Development Association.

Dawis, R.V. (1996). The theory of work adjustment and person-environment-correspondence counseling. In D. Brown & L. Brooks (Eds.), *Career choice and development* (3rd ed., pp. 75–120). San Francisco: Jossey-Bass.

Dawis, R.V. (2005). The Minnesota theory of work adjustment. In D. Brown & R. Lent (Eds.), *Career development and counseling* (pp. 3–23). Hoboken, NJ: Wiley.

Dewitt, D.W. (1994). Using the Strong with people who have disabilities. In L.W. Harmon, J.C. Hensen, F.H. Borgen, & A.L. Hammer (Eds.), *Strong Interest Inventory: Applications and technical guide* (pp. 281–290). Palo Alto, CA: CPP.

Doering, M., Rhodes, S., & Kaspin, J. (1988). Factor structure comparison of occupational needs and reinforcers. *Journal of Vocational Behavior, 32*(2), 127–138.

Donnay, D. A. C., Morris, M. L., Schaubhut, N. A., & Thompson, R. C. (2005). *Strong Interest Inventory: Manual.* Palo Alto, CA: CPP.

Drummond, R.J. (1996). *Appraisal procedures for counselors and helping professionals* (3rd ed.). Englewood Cliffs, NJ: Merrill.

Elizur, D., & Tziner, A. (1977). Vocational needs, job rewards, and satisfaction: A canonical analysis. *Journal of Vocational Behavior, 10,* 205–211.

Everson, J.M., & Reid, D.H. (1997). Using person-centered planning to determine employment preferences among people with the most severe developmental disabilities. *Journal of Vocational Rehabilitation, 9,* 99–108.

Fabian, E.S. & Liesener, J.L. (2005). Promoting the career potential of youth with disabilities. In S.D. Brown & R.W. Lent (Eds.), *Career development and counseling* (pp. 551–572). Hoboken, NJ: Wiley.

Feldman, D. (2004). The role of physical disabilities in early career: Vocational choice, the school-to-work transition, and becoming established. *Human Resource Management Review, 14,* 247–274.

Fouad, N.A. (1999). Validity evidence for interest inventories. In A. Spokane & M.L. Savickas (Eds.) *Vocational interests* (pp. 193–210). Palo Alto, CA: Davies-Black.

Fouad, N. A. (2002). Cross cultural differences in vocational interests: Between group differences on the Strong Interest Inventory. *Journal of Counseling Psychology, 49,* 283–289.

Fouad, N.A., & Hansen, J.C. (1987). Cross-cultural predictive accuracy of the Strong-Campbell Interest Inventory. *Measurement and Evaluation in Guidance, 20,* 3–10.

Fouad, N.A., Hansen, J.C., & Arias-Galicia, F. (1986). Multiple discriminant analysis of cross-cultural similarity of vocational interests of lawyers and engineers. *Journal of Vocational Behavior, 28,* 85–96.

Fouad, N.A., Hansen, J.C., & Arias-Galicia, F. (1989). Cross-cultural similarity of vocational interests of professional engineers. *Journal of Vocational Behavior, 34,* 88–99.

Fouad, N.A., Harmon, L.W., & Hansen, J.C. (1994). Cross-cultural use of the Strong. In L.W. Harmon, J.C. Hansen, F.W. Borgen, & A.L. Hammer (Eds.), *Strong Interest Inventory: Applications and technical guide* (pp. 255–280). Stanford, CA: Stanford University Press.

Fouad, N. A., & Mohler, C. (2004). Cultural validity of Holland's theory and the Strong Interest Inventory for five racial/ethnic groups. *Journal of Career Assessment, 12,* 423–439.

Gade, E.M., Fugua, D., & Hurlburt, G. (1984). Use of the SDS with Native American high school students. *Journal of Counseling Psychology, 31,* 584–587.

Gati, I., Krausz, M., & Osipow, S. H. (1996). A taxonomy of difficulties in career decision making. *Journal of Counseling Psychology, 43,* 510–526.

Gay, E.G., Weiss, D.J., Hendel, D.D., Dawis, R.V., & Lofquist, L.H. (1981). *Manual for Minnesota Importance Questionnaire. Minnesota Studies in Vocational Rehabilitation* (28). Minneapolis: University of Minnesota.

Geist, H.G. (1975). *Manual for the Geist Picture Interest Inventory: Revised.* Los Angeles: Western Psychological Services.

Gottfredson, G.D., & Holland, J.L. (1975). Vocational choices of men and women: A comparison of predictors from the Self-Directed Search. *Journal of Counseling Psychology, 22,* 28–34.

Gottfredson, G.D., Holland, J.L., & Ogawa, D.K. (1996). *Dictionary of Holland Occupational Codes.* Odessa, FL: Psychology Assessment Resources.

Hagner, D., McGahie, K., & Cloutier, H. (2001). A model career assistance process for individuals with severe disabilities. *Journal of Employment Counseling, 38,* 197–206.

Hansen, J. C. (2005). Assessment of interests. In S. D. Brown & R. W. Lent (Eds.), *Career development and counseling: Putting theory and research to work* (pp. 281–304). Hoboken, NJ: Wiley.

Hansen, J. C. & Scullard, M. G. (2002). Psychometric evidence for the Leisure Interest Questionnaire and analyses of the structure of leisure interests. *Journal of Counseling Psychology, 49,* 331–341.

Harrington, T.F., & O'Shea, A.J. (2000). *Manual: The Career Decision-Making System–Revised.* Circle Pines, MN: American Guidance Service.

Henry, P., Bardo, H., & Bryson, S. (1988). The impact of race and gender on Holland's Self-Directed Search for nontraditional premedical students. *College Student Journal, 22,* 206–212.

Herr, E.L., & Niles, S. (1997). Perspectives on career assessment of work-bound youth. *Journal of Career Assessment, 5,* 137–150.

Holland, J.L. (1978). *Manual for the Vocational Preference Inventory.* Palo Alto, CA: CPP.

Holland, J.L. (1997). *Making vocational choices: A theory of vocational personalities and work environments* (3rd ed.). Odessa, FL: Psychological Assessment Resources.

Holland, J.L., Fritzsche, B.A., & Powell, A.B. (1994). *The Self-Directed Search.* Odessa, FL: Psychological Assessment Resources.

Impara, J.C., & Plake, B.S. (Eds.). (1998). *The thirteenth mental measurements yearbook.* Lincoln, NE: University of Nebraska Press.

Jackson, D.N. (1994). *Jackson Personality Inventory–Revised Test Manual.* Port Huron, MI: Sigma Assessment Systems.

Kapes, J.T., Mastie, M.M., & Whitfield, E.A. (1994). *A counselor's guide to career assessment instruments* (3rd ed.). Alexandria, VA: National Career Development Association.

Keller, L.M., Bouchard, T.J., Arvey, R.D., & Segal, N.L. (1992). Work values: Genetic and environmental influence. *Journal of Applied Psychology, 77*(1), 79–88.

Keyser, D.J., & Sweetland, R.C. (Eds.). (1984–1985). *Test critiques* (Vols. 1–4). Austin, TX: PRO-ED.

Khan, S. B., & Alvi, S. A. (1991). The structure of Holland's typology: A study in nonwestern culture. *Journal of Cross-Cultural Psychology, 22,* 283–292.

Klein, M.L., Wheaton, J.E., & Wilson, K.B. (1997). The career assessment of persons with disabilities: A review. *Journal of Career Assessment, 5,* 203–211.

Knapp, L., & Knapp, R.R. (1983). *Technical manual: Career Occupational Preference System* (Form R). San Diego, CA: Educational and Industrial Testing Service.

Kosciulek, J. (1998). Empowering life choices of people with disabilities through career counseling. In N.C. Gysbers, M.J. Heppner, & J. Johnston (Eds.), *Career counseling: Process, issues, and techniques* (pp. 109–122). Boston: Allyn & Bacon.

Krumboltz, J.D. (1991). *Manual for the Career Beliefs Inventory.* Palo Alto, CA: CPP.

Kunce, J.T. (1969). Vocational interest, disability, and rehabilitation. *Rehabilitation Counseling Bulletin, 12,* 204–210.

Lent, R.W., & Worthington, R.L. (2000). On school-to-work transition, career development theories, and cultural validity. *Career Development Quarterly, 48,* 376–384.

Lichter, D.J. (1980). *The prediction of job satisfaction as an outcome of career counseling.* Unpublished doctoral dissertation, University of Minnesota.

Lofquist, L.H., & Dawis, R.V. (1969). *Adjustment to work.* New York: Appleton-Century-Crofts.

Menchetti, B.M., & Garcia, L.A. (2003). Personal and employment outcomes of person-centered career planning. *Education and Training in Developmental Disabilities, 38,* 145–156.

Meresman, J.F. (1975). *Biographical correlates of vocational needs.* Unpublished doctoral dissertation, University of Minnesota.

Miller, M., Springer, T., & Wells, D. (1988). Which occupational environments do black youths prefer? Extending Holland's typology. *School Counselor, 36,* 103–105.

Noonan, B., Gallor, S., & Hensler-McGinnis, N. (2004). Challenge and success: A qualitative study of the career development of highly achieving women with physical and sensory disabilities. *Journal of Counseling Psychology, 51,* 68–80.

Ochs, L. A., & Roessler, R. T. (2004). Predictors of career exploration intentions: A social cognitive career theory perspective. *Rehabilitation Counseling Bulletin, 47,* 224–233.

Overs, R.P. (1970). A model for avocational counseling. *Journal of Health & Physical Education Recreation, 41,* 36–38.

Overs, R.P. (1971). *Avocational Activities Inventory* (Milwaukee Media for Rehabilitation Research Reports Series, No. 5). Milwaukee, WI: Curative Workshop.

Power, P. (2000). *A guide to vocational assessment* (3rd ed.). Austin, TX: PRO-ED.

Psychological Corp. (1981). *Norms and scale clarity tables: Ohio Vocational Interest Survey.* New York: Author.

Pugh, R. C. (1998). Campbell Interest and Skill Survey. In J.C. Impara & B.S. Plake (Eds.), *The thirteenth mental measurements yearbook.* Lincoln, NE: University of Nebraska Press.

Rohe, D.E., & Athelstan, G.T. (1982). Vocational interest of persons with spinal cord injury. *Journal of Counseling Psychology, 29,* 283–291.

Rohe, D.E., & Athelstan, G.T. (1985). Change in vocational interests after spinal cord injury. *Rehabilitation Psychology, 30,* 131–143.

Rohe, D.E., & Krause, J.S. (1998). Stability of interests after severe physical disability: An 11-year longitudinal study. *Journal of Vocational Behavior, 52,* 45–58.

Rohe, D. E. & Krause, J. S. (1999). Vocational interests of middle-aged men with traumatic spinal cord injury. *Rehabilitation Psychology, 44,* 160–175.

Rojewski, J. W. (1996). Occupational aspirations and early career choice patterns of adolescents with and without learning disabilities. *Learning Disability Quarterly, 19,* 99–116.

Rojewski, J. W. (1999). Occupational and educational aspirations and attainment of young adults with and without LD 2 years after high school completion. *Journal of Learning Disabilities, 32,* 533–552.

Roszkowski, M. J. (1998). *Campbell Interest and Skill Survey.* In J.C. Impara & B.S. Plake (Eds.), *The thirteenth mental measurements yearbook.* Lincoln, NE: University of Nebraska Press.

Rounds, J.B. (1981). *The comparative and combined utility of need and interest data in the prediction of job satisfaction.* Unpublished doctoral dissertation, University of Minnesota.

Rounds, J.B., Dawis, R.V., & Lofquist, L.H. (1979). Life history correlates of vocational needs for a female adult sample. *Journal of Counseling Psychology, 26,* 487–496.

Rounds, J.B., Jr., Henly, G.A., Dawis, R.V., Lofquist, L.H., & Weiss, D.J. (1981). *Manual for the Minnesota Importance Questionnaire: A measure of vocational needs and values.* Minneapolis: University of Minnesota, Center for Interest Measurement Research.

Salazar, R.C. (1981). *The prediction of satisfaction and satisfactoriness for counselor training graduates.* Unpublished doctoral dissertation, University of Minnesota.

Sampson, J. P., Jr., Purgar, M. P., & Shy, J. D. (2003). Computer-based test interpretation in career assessment: Ethical and professional issues. *Journal of Career Assessment, 11,* 22–39.

Sampson, J.P., Jr., Reardon, R.C., Wilde, D.S., Peterson, N.G., Strausberger, S.J., Garis, J.W., et al. (1994). A comparison of the assessment components of fifteen computer-assisted career guidance systems. In J.T. Kapes, M.M. Mastie, & E.A. Whitfield (Eds.), *A counselor's guide to career assessment instruments* (3rd ed., pp. 373–380). Alexandria, VA: National Career Development Association.

Savickas, M.L. (1999). The transition from school to work: A developmental perspective. *Career Development Quarterly, 47,* 326–336.

Schaller, J., Parker, R., & Garcia, S.B. (1998). Moving toward culturally competent rehabilitation counseling services: Issues and practices. *Journal of Applied Rehabilitation Counseling, 29,* 40–48.

Sinick, D. (1976). Counseling older persons: Career change and retirement. *The Vocational Guidance Quarterly, 25,* 18–25.

Steere, D.E., Gregory, S.P., Heiny, R.W., & Butterworth, J., Jr. (1998). Lifestyle planning: Considerations for use with people with disabilities. In D.R. Atkinson & G. Hackett (Eds.), *Counseling diverse populations* (2nd ed., pp. 155–170). Boston: McGraw-Hill.

Super, D.F. (1970). *Manual: Work Values Inventory.* Chicago: Riverside.

Swanson, J.L., & Fouad, N.A. (1999). Applying theories of person-environment fit to the transition from school to work. *Career Development Quarterly, 47,* 337–347.

Szymanski, E.M. (1997). School-to-work transition: Ecological considerations for career development. In J.L. Swartz & W.E. Martin (Eds.), *Applied ecological psychology for schools within communities: Assessment and intervention* (pp. 167–185). Mahwah, NJ: Erlbaum.

Taylor, K.M., & Betz, N.E. (1983). Applications of self-efficacy theory to the understanding and treatment of career indecision. *Journal of Vocational Behavior, 22,* 64–71.

Thompson, A.S., & Lindeman, R.H. (1984). *Career Development Inventory: Technical manual.* Palo Alto, CA: CPP.

Thorndike, R.M. (1997). *Measurement and evaluation in psychology and education.* Upper Saddle River, NJ: Prentice Hall.

U. S. Department of Defense. (2005). *ASVAB career exploration program: Counselor manual.* Retrieved May 8, 2006, from http://www.asvabprogram.com

U.S. Department of Labor. (1991). *Dictionary of occupational titles* (4th ed., rev.). Washington, DC: U.S. Government Printing Office.

U.S. Department of Labor. (2000). O*Net Interest Profiler: User's guide, Version 3.0. Retrieved May 5, 2006, from http://www.onetcenter.org

Walsh, W.B., & Betz, N.E. (2001). *Tests and assessment* (4th ed.). Englewood Cliffs, NJ: Prentice Hall.

Wehman, P., West, M., & Kregel, J. (1999). Supported employment program development and research needs: Looking ahead to the Year 2000. *Education and Training in Mental Retardation and Developmental Disabilities, 34,* 3–19.

Weiss, D.J., Dawis, R.V., Lofquist, L.H., & England, G.W. (1966). *Instrumentation for the theory of work adjustment. Minnesota Studies in Vocational Rehabilitation* (21). Minneapolis: University of Minnesota, Center for Interest Measurement Research.

Whiston, S. C., Brecheisen, B. K., & Stephens, J. (2003). Does treatment modality affect career counseling effectiveness? *Journal of Vocational Behavior, 62,* 390–410.

Worthington, R.L., & Juntenen, C.L. (1997). The vocational development of non-college-bound youth: Counseling psychology and the school-to-work transition movement. *The Counseling Psychologist, 25,* 323–363.

Zunker, V.G. (1998). *Career counseling: Applied concepts of life planning* (5th ed.). Pacific Grove, CA: Brooks-Cole.

Zytowski, D.G. (1976). Predictive validity of the Kuder Occupational Interest Survey: A 12- to 19-year follow-up. *Journal of Counseling Psychology, 3,* 221–233.

Zytowski, D.G. (2001). *Super's Work Values Inventory–Revised: User manual.* Adel, IA: National Computer Assessment Services.

Zytowski, D. G. (2006). *Kuder Career Search with Person Match Technical manual.* Retrieved June 19, 2006, from http://www.kuder.com/PublicWeb/kcs_manual.aspx

PART 3

Applications in Rehabilitation

Chapter 9

Assessment Interviewing

Norman L. Berven

Assessment in rehabilitation settings is designed to provide a sound basis for the planning and provision of rehabilitation services, treatment, and programming and may be conceptualized as including the following components: (a) identification and definition of concerns, problems, and barriers faced by clients; (b) development of goals to be pursued through interventions and services, including career and other life goals; and (c) identification of the interventions and services that appear to hold the greatest potential for accomplishing the goals established and developing a comprehensive service or treatment plan (Berven, 2004). Although assessment is particularly important in the early stages of the rehabilitation process, it occurs throughout the process as service and treatment plans are continuously monitored, refined, and revised. Assessment is based on information that is obtained from a variety of sources, including past client records; interviews; direct observations; medical and related examinations; psychological, vocational, and other assessments conducted by other professionals; formal testing and related standardized assessment procedures; and tryouts in jobs and other criterion situations of interest. The information must then be processed and shared with clients in a collaborative manner in order to achieve the necessary determinations and decisions that will guide the treatment and service process. Clinical judgment is central to assessment in interpreting and integrating the information obtained and translating that information into clinical determinations and decisions.

Types of Interviews Used in Assessment

Psychological and vocational tests and other psychometric procedures are most commonly viewed as the primary tools of assessment. However, the interview is by far the most frequently used assessment procedure in rehabilitation and related medical, mental health, and human service settings (Berven, 2004; Groth-Marnat, 2003). Typical standardized tests use a series of questions, often in a paper-and-pencil format, to elicit responses from clients, and the responses are scored to yield some sort of description of the individual, such as a score (e.g., an IQ score), a diagnostic descriptor (e.g., clinical depression), or a narrative description (e.g., a computer interpretation of responses to a personality inventory). In contrast, interviews use practitioner responses, both verbal and nonverbal, to elicit information from clients, which is then interpreted and integrated by the practitioner with other available information to yield clinical determinations and decisions. In addition to providing a direct source of information and observations, interviews also provide the necessary context for understanding all other test scores and other assessment information, and, according to Groth-Marnat, information from these other sources would be meaningless without the context provided by interviews.

Information obtained through interviews, often combined with information provided by family, associates, and professionals who have had significant involvement with an individual, may be the only assessment method used in the provision of service and treatment with many clients. With other clients, formal standardized testing and related assessment procedures may also be used, which will then be integrated with the information and observations obtained through interviews and other sources. Although assessment is a substantial component of all clinical interviews, there are some types of interviews that are particularly focused on assessment, particularly initial interviews and diagnostic and screening interviews.

Structured, Semistructured, and Unstructured Interviews

One of the major distinguishing characteristics among interviews is the amount of structure followed in conducting the interview, which varies along a continuum from highly structured to unstructured (Beutler, 1995; Groth-Marnat, 2003). Structured interviews are comprised of prescribed questions that are asked in a prescribed sequence, with little if any variation. Semistructured interviews are similar to structured interviews in specifying topics and questions, but they provide much greater flexibility in the sequence in which topics are explored, the extent to which particular client responses are followed up, and the interview techniques and strategies used. Finally, unstructured interviews leave virtually all decisions regarding the conduct of interviews to the judgment of the individual counselor, offering maximum flexibility.

In general, the greater the amount of structure, the more standardized that interview will be and the greater the likelihood that different practitioners would reach similar conclusions when conducting an interview assessment with a particular client. Thus, Beutler (1995) suggests that "it is desirable to impose at least a modest amount of standardization on an interview whenever circumstances will permit" (p. 98). However, less highly structured interviews provide greater flexibility to the practitioner in conducting the interview, responding to the client's unique situation, pursuing topics, and following up on client communications in accordance with the judgment of the counselor. Highly structured interviews may seem more mechanical and less appealing to a client in terms of establishing rapport with the practitioner. However, the style and skills of the counselor in producing facilitative interview behavior, both verbal and nonverbal, may be more important in establishing a positive climate and good working relationship with a client than the amount of structure followed in the interview (Whiston, 2005).

Initial Interviews

Practitioners in rehabilitation settings typically begin the provision of services or treatment with an initial interview. Parker and Bolton (2005) distinguish between intake and initial interviews, with intake interviews described as focusing on the completion of client information forms and the provision of information about the agency or program and services available. In contrast, they describe initial interviews as focusing on "relationship building, attending to client behaviors, and developing a beginning picture of the client's cultural context, circumstances, values, needs, aspirations, and goals" (p. 315). Intake interviews may be conducted by an assistant or the professional practitioner, with the elements of what Parker and Bolton define as intake and initial interviews combined. Three goals can be identified that are typically pursued in initial interviews: (1) providing information to the client regarding the role of the agency or program and the services available, the respective responsibilities of the practitioner and client, and informed consent issues (such as confidentiality and the ways in which information from the client may be used); (2) initiating the assessment process; and (3) establishing rapport as a basis for future treatment and service as well as for the assessment process that begins with the interview (Farley & Rubin, 2006; Koch & Rumrill, 2005; Power, 2006). The initial interview thus sets the stage for whatever may follow as the rehabilitation process unfolds with an individual client.

In initiating the assessment process, initial interviews can provide a wealth of information. Clients typically can provide many important facts related to concerns, problems, and barriers that they are facing, along with information on the surrounding context and relevant history contributing to their current life situations. They can also provide their own perceptions of themselves, including their strengths, limitations, preferences, and needs, and their perceptions of other people who play important parts in their lives. The initial interview also provides an opportunity to observe clients in terms of physical appearance, affect, thought processes, coping behaviors, problem-solving skills, reactions to topics discussed, and interpersonal skills and styles.

The assessment information obtained through initial interviews is relevant to a number of determinations and decisions to be made as treatment or service proceeds (Berven, 2004). One decision concerns selection for treatment or service, which can vary substantially from one setting to another and may be based on such criteria as the presence of particular types of problems or disabilities, financial need, and more complex clinical judgments regarding ability to profit from the services available relative to the costs of providing those services. Another common type of determination or decision concerns the development of vocational or career objectives, determining objectives that are most consistent with the individual's strengths, limitations, and needs, which may hold promise for both employment success and satisfaction. Finally, another set of determinations and decisions requires identification of the treatment strategies and services that hold the greatest promise for addressing the client's concerns, problems, and barriers and for accomplishing the goals of service. Obtaining the information required for such determinations is typically an ultimate goal of all assessment procedures, beginning with the initial interview.

Initial interviews may vary substantially in the degree of structure followed. Agencies and programs differ regarding the types of information that must be obtained during the initial interview, depending on eligibility criteria for service or treatment, fees and financial considerations, types of services provided, and a variety of other factors. There is also considerable variability between settings in terms of the degree of structure expected by the agency or program in conducting initial interviews, varying from highly structured to unstructured. In addition, agencies and programs may use service applications or other forms to collect some information from clients prior to the initial interview, with the practitioner then using the written information as a guide in identifying topics to further explore in the interview.

In addition to initial interview guides developed by individual agencies, programs, and practitioners, many published resources on assessment, interviewing, and counseling provide initial interview guides or listings of topics to explore in initial and personal or case history interviews (e.g., Drummond & Jones, 2006; Groth-Marnat, 2003; Sommers-Flanagan & Sommers-Flanagan, 2003), including some developed specifically for rehabilitation settings. For example, Farley and Rubin (2006) provide an initial interview guide that lists interview topics and questions under the following categories: (a) physical factors, including disability-related factors; (b) psychosocial factors, including adjustment, interpersonal relationships, and social networks of family, friends, and associates; (c) educational–vocational factors, including educational and work history; and (d) economic factors, including income, sources of support, debts, and insurance coverage. In addition, Power (2006) provides an intake interview form, listing a number of types of information, along with a structured format for organizing information obtained through the interview, including aspects of client functioning (e.g., general appearance and behavior, mood and affect, coping resources, energy, strengths, interests, and work history) and approaches to obtaining each aspect of functioning to training or employment. Such interview guides can be used as a basis for structured interviews, pursuing the topics and questions specified in a standardized manner. Alternatively, they can serve as a basis for specifying general directions for a semistructured initial interview in the form of topics that might be helpful to pursue, while leaving considerable flexibility in the hands of the practitioner regarding the specific ways in which those topics are explored.

Diagnostic and Screening Interviews

Other types of interviews focus on a more specific assessment purpose, including diagnostic interview assessments and screening interviews focusing on specific types of problems and needs (Hersen & Turner, 2003; Rogers, 2001). Perhaps the most common types of diagnostic interviews are designed to diagnose psychiatric disorders according to criteria specified in various revisions of the *Diagnostic and Statistical Manual of Mental Disorders–Fourth Edition, Text Revision* (DSM-IV-TR; American Psychiatric Association, 2000). As pointed out by Kaplan and Saccuzzo (2005), the evolution of the DSM, beginning with the first edition in 1952, represents an attempt to improve the reliability of psychiatric diagnoses, which had previously been poorly defined, providing specific categories of disorders, each with specific diagnostic criteria. An example of a diagnostic interview protocol is the *Structured Clinical Interview for DSM-IV Axis I Disorders (SCID-I)—Clinician Version* (First, Spitzer, Gibbon, & Williams, 1997), which provides a structured series of interview questions to achieve diagnoses of Axis I disorders according to DSM-IV criteria. The SCID-I guides the practitioner through a branching decision tree of specific questions and criteria for scoring responses to arrive at diagnoses.

Another common type of diagnostic interview assessment is the mental status examination. As discussed by Groth-Marnat (2003), mental status examinations may focus on both psychopathology and cognitive functioning or may restrict their focus to cognitive functioning only. More specific aspects of functioning related to psychopathology that are assessed may include appearance, affect, delusions, and hallucinations, and specific aspects of cognitive functioning may include orientation, memory, attention, concentration, insight, and judgment. Diagnostic determinations are then based on information and observations obtained from the interview, integrated with other data available in records, including history. Protocols vary from more highly to less highly structured, and one of the most commonly used is the *Mini Mental State Exam,* with 11 items focusing on orientation, registration, attention, calculation, and language (Folstein, Folstein, & McHugh, 1975).

A variety of other types of structured clinical interview protocols are available for a variety of specific diagnostic purposes and settings, and listings, descriptions, and reviews are available in the literature (e.g., Groth-Marnat, 2003; Rogers, 2001; Sommers-Flanagan & Sommers-Flanagan, 2003; Vacc & Juhnke, 1997). The different interview protocols available vary considerably in the training that is required to use them effectively. For example, Beutler (1995) points out that the use of the SCID requires initial training of 20 or more hours, with periodic follow-up training to maintain reliability of diagnostic determinations.

Diagnostic interviews to assess vocational capacity and potential are also used in rehabilitation settings. In addition to their application in facilitating career counseling and the provision of vocational rehabilitation services for people with disabilities, practitioners in rehabilitation may be called upon to formulate vocational opinions in a variety of types of legal proceedings. For example, expert opinions may be provided regarding the employment implications of a disability in personal injury (e.g., automobile crashes, professional malpractice, product liability) and worker's compensation, as well as a variety of other legal proceedings (Choppa & Shafer, 1992; Lynch & Lynch, 1998). As discussed by Lynch and Lynch, such opinions typically require the assessment of vocational strengths and limitations of the individual in relation to the demands of different occupations, both before and after the onset of a disability, to determine lost earning capacity. The assessment typically includes a thorough review of medical and related records; physical capacity and related medical evaluations; standardized testing to assist in assessment of aptitudes, strengths, and limitations; and labor market surveys to determine the availability of potential occupations in a defined geographical area and the earnings associated with those occupations. A vocational diagnostic interview plays a major role in the assessment and is often the first procedure used (Toppino & Boyd, 1996). Structured formats are typically followed for the interview, and the focus includes a history of the disability, treatment, and effects, as perceived by the individual, as well as any other unrelated injuries and medical conditions; the individual's perceptions of his or her strengths, limitations, and goals related to employment; a thorough educational and vocational training history; a complete and detailed work history; and a social history, with an emphasis on strengths and barriers that may have an influence on future employment (Cutler & Ramm, 1992).

Interview protocols and procedures have also been developed to screen for common types of problems that may occur among clients but may not be readily recognized, such as suicide risk and alcohol and other drug use (Hood & Johnson, 2002). Such interview protocols identify indicators that should be the focus of inquiry and observation during the interview, along with procedures for quantifying information and achieving a score indicating risk and recommended actions. A common interview protocol to screen for suicide risk is the *SAD PERSONS Scale* (Patterson, Dohn, & Bird, 1983), which focuses on such risk factors as gender, age, affect, alcohol use, social support, history of past suicide attempts, and presence of an organized plan; scoring criteria are provided to indicate recommended clinical actions such as appropriate referrals. An example of an interview protocol to screen for problems in alcohol use is the CAGE questionnaire (Miller, 1976), which is comprised of just four questions that have been found to distinguish individuals with alcoholism from others, with an affirmative response to any of the four questions indicative of the need for further assessment. In general, interview screening of specific types of problems can be helpful in identifying individuals who should undergo more intensive assessments, and can assist practitioners in identifying potential problems that might otherwise be overlooked.

Psychometric Characteristics of Interviews as an Assessment Tool

Critics of the validity of traditional standardized testing and assessment may advocate the use of interviews as an alternative, along with behavioral observations in a variety of situations related to the purpose of the assessment. However, when interviews are used for assessment purposes, they should be subjected to the same scrutiny as any "test" in terms of the reliability and validity of the information obtained and conclusions drawn from that information (Groth-Marnat, 2003). Although traditional standardized testing may produce scores and related information with less than optimal reliability and validity for various assessment purposes, interviews may have even greater limitations in providing reliable and valid information. A thorough review of research regarding the reliability and validity of assessments conducted by means of interviews is beyond the scope of the present chapter. Rather, a review of some of the basic issues will be provided, along with some general conclusions that may be drawn. More thorough reviews of relevant research are provided by Garb (1998, 2005), who discusses reliability and validity of clinical judgment in the areas of assessment of personality and psychopathology, psychodiagnosis, case formulation, behavioral prediction, treatment decisions, and neuropsychological assessment.

Reliability

Reliability refers to consistency of measurement or, alternatively, freedom from measurement error. Traditional standardized tests are vulnerable to a number of sources of error, primarily as a result of two sets of factors: (1) the behavior of the client being assessed, which may vary across occasions of testing or observation because of a variety of factors, such as fatigue, mood, and clarity of thought; and (2) the situational context where testing or measurement occurs, which may also vary across occasions, affecting the behavior of the client and contributing error to the measurement process. Assessment conducted through interviews is vulnerable to these same sources of measurement error but also to other major sources, contributed primarily by the practitioner and his or behavior during the interview, leading to variation in assessment results across interviewers who might conduct an assessment with the same client.

Given the flexibility of semistructured and unstructured interviews in the content and topics addressed by the practitioner, different practitioners may organize an interview differently, with different topics and different questions, influencing the responses of the client and, thus, the information and observations provided. In addition, even when two different practitioners follow a structured format in asking the same set of questions, the way in which questions are asked, and the various verbal and nonverbal behaviors of the practitioner, may lead the client to be more or less open in responding to questions asked, also influencing information and observations produced. Also, given the subjectivity of typical assessments conducted through interviews, there may be substantial differences between practitioners in clinical judgments and determinations when observing identical client responses and behavior. All of these sources of error can limit the reliability of interview assessments, leading to different assessment results if different practitioners were to conduct interview assessments with the same client at the same time.

Because of the measurement error that may be contributed by the practitioner conducting the interview, the reliability of interview assessment procedures may be most appropriately estimated through interrater (or interinterviewer) agreement. To also consider sources of measurement error resulting from the client and situational context in which interviews are conducted in estimating reliability, interrater and test-retest methods may be combined, with different practitioners interviewing the same clients at different points in time and evaluating the consistency of their observations and conclusions. However, little research of this type has been conducted, with the most common research focusing only on some of the potential sources of measurement error. For example, a sample of practitioners might be asked to view a case vignette, including a video interview conducted with a client. The practitioners would then be asked to provide their judgments about the client (e.g., ratings of personality traits, diagnostic categories that seem most appropriate, most likely explanations of factors contributing to the client's behavior, or treatments or services that appear to be indicated), and the agreement between the practitioners would be evaluated (see Garb, 1998, 2005). Such methodologies would likely provide overestimates of reliability because only one major potential source of error from interviewers is considered—specifically, the clinical judgments of clinicians when provided with the same client information and observations—while other major sources of error are not reflected in the reliability estimates (e.g., the specific questions asked by the interviewers and their other verbal and nonverbal behaviors). Those sources of error contributed by the client and situational context are also not considered.

Given the variability in competence and general interview styles and approaches that might be taken by different practitioners, the reliabilities of information and observations provided through interview assessments across practitioners might be expected to be poor. In general, research suggests that reliabilities vary substantially, with structured interviews producing more reliable judgments (see Garb, 1998, 2005; Groth-Marnat, 2003). Garb (1998) concludes that agreement between practitioners tends to "vary wildly" in rating personality traits; it tends to be "good" in rating psychiatric symptoms and "fair to excellent" in rating likelihood of suicidal and violent behavior. In a review of structured and semistructured clinical interviews, Vacc and Juhnke (1997) found "good to excellent" interrater reliabilities on most categories of DSM-IV diagnoses, with kappa coefficients in the .70s and above, but they varied considerably across specific diagnoses. Groth-Marnat points out that structured clinical interviews tend to yield the highest reliabilities in broader, more global diagnostic determinations (e.g., presence or absence of psychopathology or of psychosis) and lower reliabilities with more specific disorders. Again, given the typical methodologies used in estimating reliability, the estimates found may substantially overestimate the actual consistency of measurement, and information and observations derived from interviews would tend to be less reliable than most traditional standardized tests and assessment procedures.

Validity

Validity refers to the inferences that can be drawn from scores or other information obtained through assessment. To take a relatively simple example, a practitioner may be considering referring a particular client for a job that is currently available and needs to assess the client's employability specific to that particular job. The reliability of an interview for assessing employability could be estimated through examining the consistency in determinations achieved by different practitioners conducting interviews with the same client. The validity of an interview in contributing to determination of the client's employability would depend upon the extent to which the information and judgments made through the interview were actually relevant to the client's "employability" and, thus, predictive of the client's likelihood of success if he or she were to be referred for employment in the job.

Foster and Cone (1995) have discussed two phases in documenting validity in clinical assessment. The first phase is concerned with showing that the scores or other types of information obtained actually represent the construct targeted for assessment, which would be employability in the instance of the above example. Evidence might include positive relationships of the determinations of employability achieved through interviews to other measures, such as established standardized tests measuring employability (i.e., convergent validity, showing what the determinations do represent), along with the lack of relationships to measures of different constructs (i.e., divergent validity, showing what the determinations do not represent). Foster and Cone refer to this initial phase as representational or definitional validity, and it corresponds to what is traditionally defined as construct-related evidence. The second phase is concerned with determining the utility of the test or assessment procedure in making inferences relative to specific assessment purposes, such as understanding behavior, predicting future behavior, or deciding upon intervention procedures or services that might facilitate desired changes in client behavior. Again referring to the example above, evidence regarding the relationships between the assessment of employability and subsequent employment success would provide evidence supporting the utility of interview procedures in assessing employability and predicting success. Foster and Cone refer to this second phase as elaborative validity, and it corresponds to what is traditionally defined as criterion-related evidence.

As previously discussed, there are many potential sources of random measurement error that threaten the reliability of assessment information obtained through interviews and, since reliability is basic to validity, these sources of error can also have detrimental effects on validity. In addition, there are many potential sources of error that are systematic, rather than random, and can contribute bias to the assessment process, threatening validity. Some of these systematic sources of error may result from the behavior of the client, leading to a more or less favorable impression or assessment on the part of the interviewer (Groth-Marnat, 2003). Clients may intentionally distort information communicated in an interview or otherwise modify their behavior in order to create a desired impression. In addition, history taking is often a major component of assessment interviews, and retrospective reports can be less than completely accurate, whether or not an individual is attempting to intentionally distort the information presented. Henry, Moffitt, Caspi, Langley, and Silva (1994) found that retrospective reports may often be in error in reporting factual information, such as frequencies and dates of events, and may be particularly poor in reporting psychosocial information such as history of family conflict and emotional distress and problems. It is also important to note that the behavior of the practitioner in the interview can influence the behavior of the client (e.g., openness in providing information in response to questions), which may in turn influence the comprehensiveness and accuracy of the information provided by a client, along with other aspects of client behavior that may influence interview observations.

Other major sources of systematic error relate to the clinical judgment of practitioners in processing information obtained in interviews. Garb (1998, 2005) identifies three categories of cognitive processes that practitioners use in collecting, interpreting, integrating, and remembering information that can influence the validity of judgments. Cognitive heuristics are simple rules that describe how judgments are made, including representativeness, availability, anchoring-and-adjustment, and past-behavior heuristics, which can lead to errors in judgment (Kahneman, Slovic, & Tversky, 1982); for example, the availability heuristic could lead to misinterpretation of information and observations of client behavior as indicative of alcohol or other drug abuse because information about substance abuse was readily available in the practitioner's mind as a result of a recently completed continuing education program on that topic. Cognitive biases include confirmatory bias, hindsight bias, misestimation of covariance, and the ignoring of base rates or norms; for example, confirmatory bias would occur when practitioners formulate hypotheses early in an interview and then seek only information that supports those hypotheses while ignoring information that is inconsistent (Haverkamp, 1993; Strohmer, Shivy, & Chiodo, 1990). Knowledge structures include knowledge and theory regarding problems, pathology, and behavior that are implicitly held by practitioners, as well as stereotypes, prototypes, and scripts; for example, stereotypes related to race may lead practitioners to misdiagnose psychopathology (Lopez, 1989) or to underestimate the educational or vocational potential of clients (Rosenthal & Berven, 1999). Garb provides a thorough review of these cognitive processes and the errors in clinical judgment that may result.

Given the multiple sources of systematic error or bias that may influence clinical judgment, the validity of interview assessments may be expected to be limited. Based on his extensive review of research on clinical judgment, Garb (1998, 2005) concludes that validity tends to be fair to poor in rating clinical symptoms and tends to be poor in diagnosis of psychopathology, case formulation, prediction of future behavior, and determination of effective treatment plans. In general, more highly structured interviews tend to yield more reliable and valid assessments than unstructured interviews and, particularly with unstructured interviews, reliability and validity will be highly dependent on the skills of the individual practitioner. However, in commenting on the general usefulness of interviews in assessment, Beutler (1995) concludes that the "the typical or 'unstructured' clinical interview is also among the least reliable and potentially the least valid measures used in psychological assessment" (p. 94).

Interview Strategies and Techniques

Two factors can be conceptualized as central to the reliability and validity of assessment information and observations obtained through interviews. First, comprehensive and accurate information that is relevant to the purpose of the assessment, including behavior observations, must be elicited from the client. Second, the practitioner must make valid clinical judgments in interpreting, integrating, and remembering the information elicited and behaviors observed during the interview. Clinical judgment is basic both to decisions made in directing the course of the interview, influencing the information that is elicited, and to processing the information and observations obtained.

Structured interviews are standardized, and the practitioner simply follows the standardized procedures of asking the specified questions verbatim and in the sequence specified. Structured interviews tend to yield more reliable and valid assessment information because of their standardization, but the structure eliminates the flexibility that is one of the main advantages of interviews relative to other methods of assessment. As pointed out by Morrison (1993), computers can easily substitute for professional practitioners in conducting structured interviews, simply posing questions to be answered and processing the responses received; in contrast, a skilled professional who conducts interviews in a less structured, more flexible format is able to "give free reign to the informative (client), to guide the rambling one, to encourage the silent one, and to mollify the hostile one" (p. 2). However, with semistructured or unstructured interviews, reliability and validity depend even more highly on the skills of the individual practitioner in directing the interview and eliciting and processing information and observations obtained.

Elicitation of Information

Many entire textbooks have been written on interviewing and counseling that cover strategies and techniques that are relevant to the use of interviews in conducting assessments. Only a few points will be briefly discussed here, and further elaboration can be found in a variety of other sources (e.g., Chan, Berven, & Thomas, 2004; Cormier & Nurius, 2003; Ivey & Ivey, 2007). Beutler (1995) has conceptualized three major components of interviews used for assessment: (1) the context in which the interview is conducted, including both the environmental and interpersonal context; (2) the content of the interview; and (3) the format and techniques used by the practitioner in conducting the interview.

The context provided by the physical environment of an office or other interview setting can facilitate open disclosure if the client perceives the environment as professional, warm, inviting, attractive, quiet, and safe. Aspects of the physical environment that can affect client perceptions include the general decor, furnishings, seating arrangements, colors, lighting, and items displayed on walls, desks, and shelves. In considering seating arrangements, some clients will feel more comfortable with no barriers between them and the practitioner, while others may feel more comfortable with a corner of a desk between them, and clients may vary in the distance away from an interviewer that will feel most comfortable. A well-organized physical environment may convey the perception of care, organization, and responsibility that will also be followed in dealing with clients and the confidentiality of information. The dress and physical appearance of practitioners, receptionists, and other staff can influence the mindset of clients when they first arrive, and friendly, warm greetings by the practitioner and others can substantially enhance the comfort and openness of clients as they begin an interview. A number of authorities have emphasized that there are substantial cultural differences in the ways in which aspects of the physical and interpersonal environment are perceived by clients and the consequent effects on their interview behavior (e.g., see Cormier & Nurius, 2003; Ivey & Ivey, 2007).

Preliminary statements by the practitioner can enhance the comfort of the client and facilitate open disclosure by providing structure and reducing uncertainty. Purposes of the interview can be explained by the practitioner, along with clarification of client and practitioner roles, the procedures to be followed, the possible uses of information provided by the client, and client expectations. A discussion of confidentiality, including limits on confidentiality, can enhance the feelings of safety and trust in the practitioner, facilitating open communication.

The content or topics that are relevant to the purposes of an interview can be identified in advance for subsequent use in guiding the interview. To the extent that empirical evidence exists that the topics to be addressed are relevant to the purpose, the validity of the information obtained for different assessment purposes will be facilitated; for example, if a purpose of an interview is to assess employability, the topics to be addressed can be based on available research evidence regarding factors that contribute to employment success. Interview guides and protocols, as discussed previously, can provide some guidance in identifying topics to be covered in the interview. In a semistructured interview, the identification of the general topics to be explored can provide a degree of structure, facilitating comprehensiveness and validity of the assessment. However, the practitioner can still exercise judgment and flexibility in the ways in which the topics are explored and the extent to which client responses are followed up to provide greater depth of information. In addition, the order in which topics are explored can vary to facilitate smooth transitions and flow of the interview. Finally, some information may be collected in advance through applications for service or preliminary questionnaires (e.g., a written work history), which can be reviewed by the practitioner prior to the interview, allowing more efficient use of time within the interview to follow up and expand upon the written information provided.

The format and techniques used in the interview will be designed to explore the prespecified general content areas or topics with the client in sufficient breadth and depth to elicit comprehensive and accurate information relevant to the purposes of the assessment. Establishment of a positive relationship or rapport with the client can facilitate open disclosure and depth of exploration, enhancing the validity of information provided. To the extent that the practitioner is perceived by the client as a respected expert, interpersonally attractive, and trustworthy, the credibility and interpersonal influence of the practitioner will be enhanced, and more open communication will result (Goldstein & Higginbotham, 1991; Strong, 1968). Among the behaviors that enhance such perceptions of the practitioner are attentiveness to the client through eye contact and body language, insightful and thought-provoking questions, friendliness, keeping of commitments, openness, honesty, and nondefensiveness (Cormier & Nurius, 2003). In addition, the communication of the facilitative conditions of empathy (efforts to understand the client from his or her frame of reference), respect (positive regard), and genuineness (congruence) also serves as a powerful relationship enhancer, facilitating open disclosure on the part of the client (Rogers, Gendlin, Kiesler, & Truax, 1967).

In conducting an interview for assessment purposes, the practitioner attempts to facilitate open, in-depth, comprehensive, and accurate communication on the part of the client or, alternatively, attempts to help clients "tell their stories" (see Ivey & Ivey, 2007). The practitioner presents topics for exploration and then relinquishes much of the control of communication to the client, seeking primarily to facilitate and guide the client's communication, while listening carefully to the information presented and observing the client's nonverbal behavior. Among the techniques that can be particularly helpful in facilitating client communication are open-ended questions, encouragers, paraphrases, reflections of feeling, and summarizations; most programs designed to train professionals in interviewing focus on developing skills in using these techniques. Ivey and Ivey discuss the "basic listening sequence" in which the practitioner introduces a topic of discussion and then follows up with questions, encouragers, paraphrases, and reflections of feeling to continue the client's communication about the topic in greater depth. When exploration of a topic is concluded, the practitioner can then use a summarization response to wrap up that topic and transition into another topic by means of another open-ended question.

One common barrier to eliciting comprehensive and accurate information from clients is insufficient follow-up to expand upon client responses. For example, the following interaction might occur ("P" is used to designate practitioner and "C" to designate client):

P: "How have you been spending your time?"

C: "Well, I've been really trying hard to find a job, but I haven't been able to find anything."

The practitioner may then conclude that the client has been spending a lot of time in job-seeking activity and then move on to another topic. In contrast, the practitioner might further follow up on the client's last response:

P: "Are you frustrated because nothing you're doing seems to work?"

C: "You've got that right! No matter how hard I try, I just keep banging my head against the wall."

P: "Can you give me an example of what a typical day of job hunting has been like for you? Let's take yesterday . . ."

C: "Well, yesterday was a day like all days. I got up and checked the want ads in the newspaper. Just like always, I didn't see a single thing, so I spent the rest of the day playing pool with a couple of friends. It gets frustrating!"

As a result of the additional follow-up, the practitioner obtained a much more thorough and descriptive picture of the client's approach to job hunting and the ways in which he was currently spending his time, all of which was missed when the topic was not fully explored. To the extent that practitioners can take an inquisitive approach to following up on client statements in a facilitative manner, helping clients explore topics in greater depth, more valid assessment information can be obtained.

Clinical Judgment

Clinical judgment is basic to the entire interview assessment process. Each practitioner response is based on judgments about the client's previous responses, and those judgments are then used to make decisions about the next practitioner response. Thus, clinical judgment is central to eliciting information by means of the interview. In addition to the verbal responses of the client, nonverbal behaviors are also observed as important components of communication (e.g., body language, eye contact, rate of speech, and inflections in voice that accompany specific verbal responses and assist in interpreting their meaning).

Berven (2004) discusses the use of clinical judgment in interpreting and synthesizing assessment information from interviews and other sources in facilitating various clinical determinations and decisions. Items of information and observations are examined on an ongoing basis to identify consistencies, themes, and generalizations, and inferences are formulated regarding hypothetical constructs to describe the themes identified (e.g., motivation, frustration, self-esteem). To make sense of the myriad pieces of information obtained, Berven suggests that it may be helpful to organize all information and observations that are relevant to the purpose of assessment under the headings of client assets, limitations, and preferences, which include both information about the individual and the surrounding environmental context and can provide an information base for clinical determinations.

Classic models have been presented regarding the ways in which practitioners synthesize information (e.g., McArthur, 1954; Pepinsky & Pepinsky, 1954) to form working models of clients and then to use those working models to facilitate clinical determinations and decisions. Inductive reasoning is used to identify consistencies in information obtained. As inconsistencies appear, inferences are revised, continuing to build an increasingly sophisticated working model of the client that can incorporate the information obtained. Deductive reasoning is also used in formulating hypotheses from the working model regarding client characteristics and behavior and testing those hypotheses against other information, continuing to revise and refine the working model to account for new information. The working model can then be used in accomplishing a variety of assessment purposes. For example, the model can be projected into employment situations to predict likely behavior and outcomes, which can assist in determining employability and establishing career and vocational objectives. Similarly, the working model can be projected into treatment or service situations to predict likely behavior in response to those interventions, facilitating treatment and service planning.

As previously discussed, there are many threats to the validity of clinical judgments, which, in turn, threaten the validity of assessments conducted by means of interviews. Garb (1998, 2005) makes a number of recommendations for improving clinical judgment, including the following: (a) Attend to empirical research results, and rely less on clinical experience and more on those empirical results in interpreting assessment information; (b) beware of cultural biases that may arise because of the client's race, social class, gender, and other characteristics, and attempt to counteract those biases; (c) describe client strengths and do not focus only on problems and pathology; (d) be wary of judgment tasks and consider the evidence regarding the poor reliability and validity typically associated with clinical judgment; (e) be systematic and comprehensive when conducting interviews; (f) make use of psychological tests and behavioral assessment methods to improve the reliability and validity of judgments; and (g) use debiasing strategies, such as the consideration of multiple alternative explanations and judgments when interpreting and integrating information.

Eliciting client information by means of standardized tests requires skills that may be relatively easy to master, and various aids are often available to assist in interpretation. In contrast, eliciting information by means of interviews is based on complex skills that require substantial training and supervised experience to master. Further, there appears to be extensive variability among practitioners in their skills in eliciting client information and making clinical judgments. However, it does not appear that degree of skills is related to clinical experience. Based on his review of research, Garb (1998) concludes that no differences in skills in clinical judgment have typically been found between experienced clinicians and graduate students, although differences have been found between advanced and beginning graduate students, suggesting that training may be effective in improving skills in clinical judgment. Further, there is substantial evidence regarding the effectiveness of training in improving basic interview skills (see a review provided by Daniels, Rigazio-DiGilio, & Ivey, 1997).

Computer-Based Assessment Interviews

As discussed by Barak and Buchanan (2004), the Internet provides an alternative to face-to-face communication in providing counseling, including assessment interviewing. Such interviews may be conducted in a text format (e.g., electronic mail); with sound, using microphones and speakers; or with video, using Web cams. Barak and Buchanan point out that advantages of Internet-based assessment interviews are the access provided to individuals who might otherwise not have access to services because of distance or cost considerations and the possibility of easily saving the verbatim interviews for further evaluation.

In addition to practitioner-conducted interviews over the Internet, structured interviews lend themselves to automated computer administration, and computer-administered assessment interviews have been developed for diagnosis and screening of psychiatric disorders, suicide risk, inpatient and outpatient psychiatric admission, and problems with alcohol use (Plutchik & Karasu, 1991). For example, a computer screening version of the SCID, the *SCID Screen Patient Questionnaire–Extended,* provides a computer-administered interview of 30–45 minutes that screens clients on DSM-IV Axis I symptoms (Spitzer, Williams, Gibbon, & First, 1996). A particularly novel computer-administered interview to screen for psychiatric disorders is accessed by means of a telephone call, using a touch-tone phone, with the client responding to computer-read questions by pressing the telephone number keys (Kobak et al., 1997). Computer-administered versions of initial interviews can also be used in rehabilitation settings, either alone or together with traditional face-to-face interviews. As a complement to traditional interviews, some assessment information can be obtained through the computer-administered interview, which can then be expanded upon through follow up in a face-to-face interview with the practitioner, adding the advantages of a structured component to the traditional, less structured interview process.

A number of authors have commented on the potential advantages of computer-administered interviews and have reviewed results of research to evaluate their efficacy (Emmelkamp, 2005; Erdman, Klein, & Greist, 1985; Kobak et al., 1997; Plutchik & Karasu, 1991). Computers can be programmed to always ask the required questions, which practitioners conducting face-to-face interviews may not always ask, and can provide a complete record of client responses without reliance on a practitioner's memory. Computers can also be programmed to use decision rules to ask appropriate follow-up questions depending upon prior client responses. Research suggests that computer-administered interviews can often provide more reliable assessments as compared to practitioners, and clients may be more willing to disclose personal and sensitive information to a computer, further enhancing the validity of assessment results. Further, clients have typically expressed satisfaction with computer-administered interviews. Given the advantages offered by computers in conducting some types of interviews, their use in assessment will likely continue to grow.

Conclusion

Interviews appear to be the most widely used method of assessment in rehabilitation settings. However, textbooks on assessment frequently give only passing mention to interviews, and research on reliability and validity has been much more limited as compared to other methods and tools of assessment. Reliability and validity of assessments conducted by means of interviews should receive the same empirical scrutiny as traditional standardized tests, and research on interview assessment and clinical judgment should have high priority. The existing evidence suggests that reliability and validity of interview assessments tend to be poor relative to standardized tests and related assessment tools. Further, reliability and validity are highly dependent on the skills of individual practitioners in interviewing and clinical judgment, and those skills tend to vary substantially among practitioners. However, evidence suggests that skills in interviewing and clinical judgment can be improved through training. Although graduate training programs may typically provide systematic training in interview skills, the training provided in clinical judgment is probably much less systematic and should be improved, becoming a standard part of graduate instruction in the rehabilitation professions. Interviews offer a great deal of flexibility and potential value in contributing to assessment. Thus, greater attention to both training and research would seem to be clearly indicated because interviews will continue to be widely used in assessment.

References

American Psychiatric Association. (2000). *Diagnostic and statistical manual of mental disorders* (4th ed., text rev.). Washington, DC: Author.

Barak, A., & Buchanan, T. (2004). Internet-based psychological testing and assessment. In R. Kraus, J. Zack, & G. Stricker (Eds.), *Online counseling: A handbook for mental health professionals.* London: Elsevier Academic Press.

Berven, N. L. (2004). Assessment. In T. F. Riggar & D. R. Maki (Eds.), *Handbook of rehabilitation counseling* (pp. 199–217). New York: Springer.

Beutler, L. E. (1995). The clinical interview. In L. E. Beutler & M. R. Berren (Eds.), *Integrative assessment of adult personality* (pp. 94–120). New York: Guilford.

Chan, F., Berven, N. L., & Thomas, K. R. (Eds.). (2004). *Counseling theories and techniques for rehabilitation health professionals.* New York: Springer.

Choppa, A. J., & Shafer, K. (1992). Introduction to personal injury and expert witness work. In J. M. Siefker (Ed.), *Vocational evaluation in private sector rehabilitation* (pp. 135–168). Menomonie: University of Wisconsin–Stout, Stout Vocational Rehabilitation Institute.

Cormier, S., & Nurius, P. S. (2003). *Interviewing and change strategies for helpers: Fundamental skills and cognitive behavior interventions* (5th ed.). Pacific Grove, CA: Brooks/Cole.

Cutler, F., & Ramm, A. (1992). Introduction to the basics of vocational evaluation. In J. M. Siefker (Ed.), *Vocational evaluation in private sector rehabilitation* (pp. 31–66). Menomonie: University of Wisconsin-Stout, Stout Vocational Rehabilitation Institute.

Daniels, T., Rigazio-DiGilio, S., & Ivey, A. (1997). Microcounseling: A training and supervision paradigm. In E. Watkins (Ed.), *Handbook of psychotherapy supervision* (pp. 277–295). New York: Wiley.

Drummond, R. J., & Jones, K. D. (2006). *Assessment procedures for counselors and helping professionals* (6th ed.). Upper Saddle River, NJ: Pearson.

Emmelkamp, P. M. G. (2005). Technological innovations in clinical assessment and psychotherapy. *Psychotherapy and Psychosomatics, 74,* 336–343.

Erdman, H. P., Klein, M. H., & Greist, J. H. (1985). Direct patient computer interviewing. *Journal of Consulting and Clinical Psychology, 53,* 760–773.

Farley, R. C., & Rubin, S. E. (2006). The intake interview. In R. T. Roessler & S. E. Rubin (Eds.), *Case management and rehabilitation counseling: Procedures and techniques* (4th ed., pp. 51–74). Austin, TX: PRO-ED.

First, M. B., Spitzer, R. L., Gibbon, M., & Williams, J. B. W. (1997). *Structured Clinical Interview for DSM-IV Axis I Disorders (SCID-I)-Clinician Version.* Washington, DC: American Psychiatric Press.

Folstein, M. F., Folstein, S. E., & McHugh, P. R. (1975). "Mini-Mental State": A practical method for grading the cognitive state of patients for the clinician. *Journal of Psychiatric Research, 12,* 189–198.

Foster, S. L., & Cone, J. D. (1995). Validity issues in clinical assessment. *Psychological Assessment, 7,* 248–260.

Garb, H. N. (1998). *Studying the clinician: Judgment research and psychological assessment.* Washington, DC: American Psychological Association.

Garb, H. N. (2005). Clinical judgment and decision making. *Annual Review of Clinical Psychology, 1,* 67–89.

Goldstein, A. P., & Higginbotham, H. N. (1991). Relationship-enhancement methods. In F. H. Kanfer & A. P. Goldstein (Eds.), *Helping people change: A textbook of methods* (4th ed.). New York: Pergamon.

Groth-Marnat, G. (2003). *Handbook of psychological assessment* (4th ed.). New York: Wiley.

Haverkamp, B. E. (1993). Confirmatory bias in hypothesis testing for client-identified and counselor self-generated hypotheses. *Journal of Counseling Psychology, 40,* 303–315.

Henry, B., Moffitt, T. E., Caspi, A., Langley, J., & Silva, P. A. (1994). On the "remembrance of things past": A longitudinal evaluation of the retrospective method. *Psychological Assessment, 6,* 92–101.

Hersen, M., & Turner, S. M. (Eds.). (2003). *Diagnostic interviewing* (3rd ed.). New York: Kluwer Academic/Plenum.

Hood, A. B., & Johnson, R. W. (2002). *Assessment in counseling: A guide to the use of psychological assessment procedures* (3rd ed.). Alexandria, VA: American Counseling Association.

Ivey, A. E., & Ivey, M. B. (2007). *Intentional interviewing and counseling: Facilitating client development in a multicultural society* (6th ed.). Pacific Grove, CA: Brooks/Cole.

Kahneman, D., Slovic, P., & Tversky, A. (1982). *Judgment under uncertainty: Heuristics and biases.* New York: Cambridge University Press.

Kaplan, R. M., & Saccuzzo, D. P. (2005). *Psychological testing. Principles, applications, and issues* (6th ed.). Pacific Grove, CA: Brooks/Cole.

Kobak, K. A., Taylor, L. H., Dottl, S. L., Greist, J. H., Jefferson, J. W., Burroughs, D., et al. (1997). Computerized screening for psychiatric disorders in an outpatient community mental health clinic. *Psychiatric Services, 48,* 1048–1057.

Koch, L. C., & Rumrill, P. D. (2005). Interpersonal communication skills for case managers. In F. Chan, M. J. Leahy, & J. L. Saunders (Eds.), *Case management for rehabilitation health professionals* (2nd ed., Vol. 1, pp. 122–143). Osage Beach, MO: Aspen Professional Services.

Lopez, S. R. (1989). Patient variable biases in clinical judgment: Conceptual overview and methodological considerations. *Psychological Bulletin, 106,* 184–203.

Lynch, R. K., & Lynch, R. T. (1998). Rehabilitation counseling in the private sector. In R. M. Parker & E. M. Szymanski (Eds.), *Rehabilitation counseling: Basics and beyond* (3rd ed., pp. 71–105). Austin, TX: PRO-ED.

McArthur, C. (1954). Analyzing the clinical process. *Journal of Counseling Psychology, 1,* 203–208.

Miller, W. R. (1976). Alcoholism scales and objective assessment methods: A review. *Psychological Bulletin, 83,* 649–674.

Morrison, J. (1993). *The first interview. A guide for clinicians.* New York: Guilford.

Parker, R. M., & Bolton, B. (2005). Psychological assessment in rehabilitation. In R. M. Parker, E. M. Szymanski, & J. B. Patterson (Eds.), *Rehabilitation counseling: Basics and beyond* (4th ed., pp. 307–334). Austin, TX: PRO-ED.

Patterson, W. M., Dohn, H. H., & Bird, J. (1983). Evaluation of suicidal patients: The SAD PERSONS scale. *Psychosomatics: Journal of Consultation Liaison Psychiatry, 24,* 343–349.

Pepinsky, H. B., & Pepinsky, P. N. (1954). *Counseling: Theory and practice.* New York: Ronald Press.

Plutchik, R., & Karasu, T. B. (1991). Computers in psychotherapy: An overview. *Computers in Human Behavior, 7,* 33–44.

Power, P. W. (2006). *A guide to vocational assessment* (4th ed.). Austin, TX: PRO-ED.

Rogers, C., Gendlin, E., Kiesler, D., & Truax, C. (1967). *The therapeutic relationship and its impact: A study of psychotherapy with schizophrenics.* Madison: University of Wisconsin Press.

Rogers, R. (2001). *Handbook of diagnostic and structured interviewing.* New York: Guilford.

Rosenthal, D. A., & Berven, N. L. (1999). Effects of client race on clinical judgment. *Rehabilitation Counseling Bulletin, 42,* 243–264.

Sommers-Flanagan, J., & Sommers-Flanagan, R. (2003). *Clinical interviewing* (3rd ed.). Hoboken, NJ: Wiley.

Spitzer, R. L., Williams, J. B. W., Gibbon, M., & First, M. B. (1996). *SCID: Screen patient questionnaire–Extended* [Computer software]. North Tonawanda, NY: Multi-Health Systems.

Strohmer, D. C., Shivy, V. A., & Chiodo, A. L. (1990). Information processing strategies in counselor hypothesis testing: The role of selective memory and expectancy. *Journal of Counseling Psychology, 37,* 465–472.

Strong, S. R. (1968). Counseling: An interpersonal influence process. *Journal of Counseling Psychology, 15,* 215–224.

Toppino, D., & Boyd, D. (1996). Wage loss analysis: Vocational expert foundation and methodology. *American Rehabilitation Economics Association Journal, 1,* 1–12.

Vacc, N. A., & Juhnke, G. A. (1997). The use of structured clinical interviews for assessment in counseling. *Journal of Counseling and Development, 75,* 470–480.

Whiston, S. C. (2005). *Principles and applications of assessment in counseling* (2nd ed.). Belmont, CA: Brooks/Cole.

Chapter 10

Assessment of Independence

Nancy M. Crewe and Darlene A. G. Groomes

This chapter discusses assessment of physical functioning and independence in daily living and in the workplace. At one point in the history of rehabilitation, services were focused almost exclusively on helping individuals learn to become physically independent enough to carry out tasks without assistance from other people. On some outcome measures, extra points were even provided for being able to carry out activities of daily living without needing adaptive equipment! Physical functioning is still important, but we are increasingly recognizing that autonomy, rather than physical capacity itself, is the essence of independence and that independence can only be measured within the context of a particular environment.

Hundreds of useful tests, inventories, and rating scales have been developed over the past few decades to measure physical functioning and other aspects of independence. Systems that have provided a foundation for many of the measuring tools have changed in recent years. In particular, revision of the World Health Organization's *International Classification of Impairments, Disabilities, and Handicaps* (ICIDH) and supplementation to the Department of Labor's *Dictionary of Occupational Titles* (DOT) may lead to major shifts in assessment strategies in the foreseeable future. Vocational measures are discussed in several other chapters, so this one will focus primarily on more global measures of independence.

ICIDH and ICF

The World Health Organization (WHO; 1980) developed a system for classifying impairment, disability, and handicap (ICIDH) that served to clarify terminology and to provide a conceptual framework for thinking about how to assess dimensions of health and disability. Impairments were defined as anatomical or structural abnormalities that typically called for medical assessment and treatment. Disabilities were tasks, skills, or behaviors that were affected by impairments. Functional assessment measures provided the means of recording the individual's capabilities and limitations, and rehabilitation services constituted the appropriate intervention strategy. *Handicap* referred to a disadvantage stemming from the interaction between an individual's impairment and the environment where he or she lived and worked. Assessment of handicap involved recording dimensions of disadvantage, and appropriate interventions included education and changes in social policy.

The ICIDH served to encourage the development of functional assessment strategies, which involve enumeration of behavioral capacities (as opposed to identification of a diagnostic label). The measurement of handicap proved to be more elusive since it required an integration of data regarding physical and other individual characteristics with environmental demands.

The ICIDH and its nomenclature were replaced by the *International Classification of Functioning, Disability, and Health* (ICF) in May 2001. This latest addition to the WHO classification system promotes the use of universal classification of function that complements diagnostic information used in health care service provision (Peterson & Rosenthal, 2005). It organizes information about functioning across several domains: (a) body functions; (b) body structures; (c) activities performed by the individual and participation in life experiences; and (d) environmental factors. The new framework parallels to some degree the old categories of impairment, disability, and handicap, although it uses different terminology. Table 10.1 describes the way in which the four domains relate to assessment and intervention approaches. It also suggests the shift in emphasis within vocational and independent living rehabilitation that seems to have occurred over time.

The ICF attempts to bring together the medical and political views of disability by providing "the lexicon for an increasingly unified global discourse about the health and well being of groups including people with disabilities" (Peterson & Rosenthal, 2005, p. 92). Measures of independence can be made at the level of the body, the person, or participation, but the kind of data obtained would vary in a number of ways. Measurement of bodily structure and function can be very detailed and exclusively concentrated on physical dimensions, but the physical characteristics of activity cannot be so isolated. People carry out their activities as integrated beings, so intellectual, emotional, and sensory capacities will be interwoven with physical ones in these measures. Measures of

TABLE 10.1.

Relevance of ICF Domains to Measurement of Functioning in Vocational Rehabilitation

Assessment/ intervention	Body Functions	Body Structures	Activities and Participation	Environmental Factors
Focus of measurement	Movement, mental and sensory functions, voice and speech	Skin, eyes, ears, nervous system, bones	Tasks, skills, behaviors for community integration	Services, policies, products, natural or human-made changes to the environment
Elements of assessment	Body functions	Body structures	Individual activities and social roles	Attitudes, support, and relationships
Level of specificity	Detailed	Detailed	Intermediate	General
Breadth of measurement	Unidimensional	Unidimensional	Likely multidimensional	Necessarily multidimensional
Intervention	Medical treatment or prevention	Medical treatment or prevention	Rehabilitation services, education	Education, environmental and policy changes

Note. Adapted from Frey (1984) and Peterson and Rosenthal (2005).

environmental factors are likely to be still more general and they will invariably involve components that extend beyond the client's physical functioning.

Purposes of Assessing Independence

Frey (1984) pointed out that there have been cumulative shifts in the focus of rehabilitation assessment since 1920. During the first period, 1920–1940, assessment was concerned with providing a basis for workers' compensation, and accurate measures of physical impairment were most relevant to that need. From 1940 to 1960, another impetus to improved assessment was the desire to provide better services to clients. Vocational rehabilitation services are not likely to change bodily structure or functioning, per se; instead, they are aimed at helping the individual carry out vocational activities more effectively, hence the shift to a disability (or functional activity) focus. Since then, another incentive has been added to the ones already mentioned: the need for improved accountability to society in general and funding sources in particular. The "independent living" movement has made it clear that remediating the impairments and disabilities of individuals is insufficient: Social and environmental barriers must also be removed. As a result, interest has grown in the challenge of measuring functioning at the interface with the environment.

In the context of a volume such as this, it is not necessary to belabor the rationale for careful assessment. Assessment has long been recognized as the first step in an orderly counseling process and the foundation for all client services that follow (Crewe, Athelstan, & Meadows, 1975). In recent years, another reason for structured assessment has become increasingly important, particularly to counselors who work in medical settings; it serves as a baseline against which to measure change. Several specific purposes for assessing functioning can be enumerated briefly:

1. Documentation of a physical impairment helps to determine eligibility for services in many vocational rehabilitation programs. It is not necessarily sufficient since an ensuing vocational disadvantage may also need to be demonstrated.
2. Assessment of physical, cognitive, and other personal characteristics may be compared with occupational and job requirements to help in the selection of appropriate vocational goals.
3. The process may serve to identify problems or to uncover hidden limitations or environmental barriers that could otherwise sabotage the rehabilitation plan.
4. Problems that require medical rehabilitation services may be identified.
5. Collection of data on functioning at the beginning of rehabilitation may provide a basis for evaluating client change, thus providing information about the effectiveness of relevant services.

6. Comprehensive assessment may provide data relevant to policy decisions within agencies and to funding sources.

Process of Assessing Physical Functioning and Independence

Several issues confront the counselor who is choosing an approach to assessment.

Level of Data

As described in the preceding section, data can be collected with regard to body functions, body structures, performance of activities and involvement in life roles, and environmental factors. We have noted that recent years have brought an urgent need for data that will help to meet the demands for professional and program accountability, yet this concern did not eliminate earlier needs. The requirement for good information to contribute to eligibility determination and service planning is just as important as ever. The counselor, then, is likely to want data in all four domains in order to create a complete picture of the client's assets and limitations within the context of his or her social and physical environment. A clear understanding about the distinctions between the four types of measures will help to avoid omissions and ensure that appropriate data are applied to each task.

The case of a client with a spinal cord injury provides a concrete example. Data on body functions and structure would include level of injury, completeness of the lesion, and identification of any concurrent or preexisting injuries. Assessment of activity and participation would include descriptions of the individual's ability to use a wheelchair or to walk, ability to transfer, and the ability to carry out activities of daily living such as feeding and dressing. At the level of environment, the counselor might want to know whether the client has good mobility within the home or whether steps, narrow doorways, or other barriers limit access. Obviously, these examples represent only a small sample of relevant variables.

Source of Data

There are several sources of information regarding independent functioning. One is the physical examination carried out by a physician or other health professional. Another involves behavioral observation of performance, with either simulated tasks such as those presented in psychometric testing or work evaluation, or direct observation of actual work or self-care activities. Interviews or questionnaires are a third source of information. Finally, some functional assessment procedures utilize devices, such as a written log or mechanical counter, to record information about actual performance of behaviors in daily life.

Often, the counselor will not carry out an assessment of physical functioning directly but will rely on reports from physicians, physical therapists, chiropractors, or other health professionals. The counselor then organizes the information, evaluates its vocational relevance, and links the information to services and goals.

Breadth of Assessment

Even for clients with a primary physical disability, it is unlikely that a counselor would restrict assessment to issues of physical functioning. This area is one focus of the present chapter, but a holistic picture of the individual, including sensory, psychological, and intellectual factors at all three levels of body, activities, and participation, is appropriate as a basis for vocational planning. Furthermore, the essence of independence is no longer thought to be the ability to physically carry out tasks without assistance. Instead, independence is determined by a person's ability to make choices and to control the direction of his or her life.

Capacities Versus Usual Behavior

For those aspects of functioning that involve client behavior, the issue of whether the assessment process should focus on maximum capacity or on typical activities is significant. With respect to activities of daily living, for example, an occupational therapist is likely to see the individual in a clinic situation and to elicit a demonstration of maximum capacity. The therapist may then report that the client is able to dress without assistance in 30 minutes. At home, however, the individual may typically rely on a parent for help with that task. Either kind of information could be relevant to the counselor's needs, but the differences in meaning should be recognized. Within the ICF system, *Activities* refers to tasks that a person can carry out in a standardized setting and *Participation* indicates a person's actual functioning in his or her usual environment (Homa & Peterson, 2005).

Choice of Measurement System

Choice of measurement system may represent a major challenge for the counselor. The state of measurement and evaluation in medical rehabilitation has been criticized (Keith, 1984) because of lack of standardization, multidimensional scales, disagreement about methods, poorly conceptualized outcome criteria, and a confounding influence of setting on performance. A particularly troublesome issue has been the tendency of many institutions to develop their own measurement devices, often with little attention to basic standards of test construction. Even within the setting in which they were developed, these ad hoc approaches have questionable validity for client assessment, research, or program evaluation.

Equally serious is the effect that the proliferation of instruments, each including different elements and using different language, has had on the field as a whole. Frey (1984) noted that the consequences have included poor communication, disagreement over rehabilitation goals and outcomes, lack of comparability among substantive research efforts, and frustration among epidemiologists and policymakers concerning the inability of professionals in rehabilitation to provide any consistent and useful aggregate data. Andresen (2000) as well as Hahn and Cella (2003) advocate for appropriate methods to evaluate measurement equivalence across diverse patient groups, especially among medically underserved and vulnerable populations.

There is no way to be certain of the number of devices that are in use for measuring aspects of independence; the total may be in the hundreds. Several publications provide descriptions of assessment tools relevant to vocational and medical rehabilitation (Cushman & Scherer, 1995; Scheer, 1990). The remainder of this chapter is devoted to a description of selected approaches that have been relatively well-standardized and widely used in medical and vocational rehabilitation. The decision regarding the ICF category to which each instrument should be assigned is somewhat arbitrary, partly because some instruments are designed to collect information at multiple levels.

Measures of Independence

Measures of Body Function and Structure

To a substantial degree, measurement of body function and structure is within the domain of physicians and their medical examinations. In addition, psychologists often assess personality, cognition, and other neuropsychological functions with their tests. A review of such examinations is beyond the scope of the present volume. Nevertheless, measures of physical capacity and psychological adjustment to disability may be seen to bridge the territory between body function and measures of activity.

Functional Capacity Testing

Functional capacity testing (FCT) takes many forms, depending upon the needs and circumstances of a given client. Typically, it measures an individual's ability to perform specific tasks such as lifting, carrying, standing, sitting, walking, climbing, stooping, reaching, and handling materials. Physical capacity evaluations are frequently structured according to the categories of physical requirements specified in the *Dictionary of Occupational Titles* so that results can be compared to the demands of selected jobs. Physical therapists, occupational therapists, and work evaluators most often conduct functional capacity testing, and specific skills and knowledge are necessary in order to safely generate accurate results. Wickstrom (1990) provides a thoughtful discussion of the complexities of FCT.

Acceptance of Disability Scale

A measure of psychological functioning that is particularly relevant to rehabilitation is the *Acceptance of Disability Scale* (AD Scale; Linkowski, 1987), a 50-item questionnaire that was designed to measure the global construct of adjustment to a medical or physical disability. It is based upon the theory of acceptance of loss developed by Dembo, Leviton, and Wright (1956), which postulates that four value changes form the basis of positive adjustment to disability: enlargement of the scope of values, subordination of physique relative to other values, containment of disability effects, and transformation of comparative-status values to asset values. The AD Scale probes an individual's values and attitudes regarding his or her physical disability and takes 15–20 minutes to complete. It has been widely used, both nationally and internationally, but norms have not been published (Bolton, 1994). Furthermore, although the theoretical framework has been embraced by rehabilitation psychologists for many years, the concept of disability acceptance as a combination of the four value changes has not yet been empirically tested (Keany & Glueckauf, 1993). As of this writing, empirical testing and revisions have been made to the AD Scale, and validation of the revised scale is under way.

Measures of Activity and Participation

Barthel and *PULSES*

The *Barthel* inventory of self-care skills and mobility skills and the *PULSES* scale of severity of disability were two of the most widely used measures of physical functioning in medical rehabilitation through the 1980s. They are both brief, and because they are complementary in purpose they are often used in tandem. Granger and his colleagues (Granger, 1982; Granger, Albrecht, & Hamilton, 1979) incorporated the two into their *Long Range Evaluation System* (LRES) together with a newer measure of social support, *ESCROW*.

As modified by Granger, the *Barthel* includes nine self-care and six mobility items: drinking from a cup, eating, dressing upper and lower body, putting on brace or artificial limb, grooming, washing or bathing, controlling urination and bowel movements, getting in and out of chair, getting on and off toilet, getting in and out of tub or shower, walking 50 yards on level ground, walking up and down one flight of stairs, and (if not walking) propelling a wheelchair. The patient indicates whether it is possible to do the task alone, with someone's help, or not at all. Varying numbers of points are assigned for independence in the activities, with items related to continence and mobility being weighted most heavily. Possible scores range from a low of 0 up to 100, which indicates complete independence. A score of 60 has been used (Granger, Albrecht, & Hamilton 1979) to indicate very severe limitations.

The *PULSES* profile consists of four-point rating scales in six broad areas of disability as follows:

P—Physical condition

U—Upper limb functions, especially self-care

L—Lower limb functions, especially mobility

S—Sensory components, including sight and communications

E—Excretory functions

S—Support factors, including psychological, family, social, and financial

Scores range from 6, indicating little or no disability, up to 24. A score of 12 or more has been used as a cutoff (Granger, Albrecht, & Hamilton 1979) to identify persons with relatively severe disability and 16 to select those who are very severely disabled. Scoring on the *Barthel* and PULSES is reported to be reliable and sensitive to change in patient status over time. Gresham, Phillips, and Labi (1980) reported high levels of agreement between the *Barthel* and two other self-care measures, the *Katz Index of ADL* and the *Kenny Self-Care Evaluation*. They preferred the *Barthel* to the others because of its completeness, its sensitivity to change, its amenability to statistical manipulation, and its widespread use. Goldberg and his associates (Goldberg, Bernad, & Granger, 1980; Goldberg, Hannon, & Granger, 1977) investigated the relationship between the *Barthel* and *PULSES* and vocational rehabilitation outcomes but found an unambiguous connection between them.

Functional Independence Measure

The *Functional Independence Measure* (FIM) is used as a standard tool for collecting data on functional performance of patients in an inpatient rehabilitation setting (Jette, Warren, & Wirtalla, 2005), and it has been widely used in other settings such as nursing homes and clinics (Crewe & Dijkers, 1995). The FIM contains 18 items, each rated on a seven-level scale. A total score (obtained by adding the 18 items) is derived as two continuous subscale scores for cognitive and motor abilities (Granger, Hamilton, Linacre, Heinemann, & Wright, 1993; Heinemann, Linacre, Wright, Hamilton, & Granger, 1993; Jette, Warren, & Wirtalla, 2005).

Stineman, Shea, Jette, Warren, and Witralla (1997) suggested that the scale could be viewed as multidimensional based on a factor analysis that derived four domains of functioning: activities of daily living, sphincter management, mobility, and executive functioning. A large body of literature supports the reliability and validity of the FIM when used in inpatient rehabilitation settings, although some studies have criticized its lack of sensitivity, especially with respect to cognitive and psychological functioning. It is also more effective when used with individuals who have severe (rather than mild) disabilities. Its limitations are reflective of its brevity and to a degree of subjectivity that is inevitable in any rating scale.

Functional Autonomy Rating Scale

The *Functional Autonomy Rating Scale* (FARS) is a relatively new measure that was developed to measure performance changes resulting from day rehabilitation programs (Grebinger et al., 1997). It consists of 41 single-skill items (e.g., eating, wheelchair mobility, reading comprehension, and nonverbal reasoning) that are recorded on zero-to-seven ordinal scales and a global functional autonomy score. The ratings are made by medical rehabilitation team members. The global score correlates quite highly with the average of the individual items, leading the authors to conclude that the conceptual validity of the scale is supported. The scale seemed to work most effectively for persons with stroke or brain injury and less well for those with spinal cord injury. Further research is needed to determine whether this will be a reliable and valid outcome measure for post-acute rehabilitation programs.

Functional Assessment Inventory and the Personal Capacities Questionnaire

The *Functional Assessment Inventory* (FAI; Crewe & Athelstan, 1984) was developed at the University of Minnesota to provide vocational rehabilitation counselors with a brief, yet comprehensive, framework for organizing and clarifying information about client capacities. It consists of 30 four-point scales of functional limitations, a checklist of 10 special strength areas, and 2 global items calling for counselor judgments of severity of disability and the likelihood of employability. The scales are behaviorally anchored with descriptors selected for their vocational relevance. For each, the first level represents no significant impairment, and the others approximate mild, moderate, and severe degrees of limitation. Aspects of physical functioning are included in the FAI, but the content goes beyond that area, attempting to cover the full range of variables that may affect employability. The inventory has been widely used, especially in the public rehabilitation system, to help counselors make decisions about eligibility and to develop a service plan.

Repeated studies have confirmed the reliability of the instrument (Crewe & Athelstan, 1981, 1984; Crewe, Athelstan, & Meadows, 1975). Factor analyses carried out with several different samples have also shown substantial consistency with respect to the dimensions of function that underlie the inventory (Crewe, 1987). Neath, Bellini, and Bolton (1997) conducted the largest such study to date, using 5,741 applicants to Arkansas Rehabilitation Services. They investigated the dimensionality of the FAI based upon the total sample and also upon five diagnostic subsamples: orthopedic, chronic disability, psychiatric, mental retardation, and learning disability.

The FAI was intended as a method to help counselors seek out and organize a rather comprehensive array of information about a client, based upon interviews, reports, testing, and/or observation. Once this has been done, the FAI itself requires only about 10 minutes to complete.

The *Personal Capacities Questionnaire* (PCQ) is an item-by-item translation of the FAI, designed to be answered by clients themselves. Although it has not been as widely researched as the FAI, it can produce valuable information about physical and other aspects of functioning. The counselor can get an overall view of how the client perceives his or her own problems and may learn about previously unrecognized problem areas. Significant differences between counselor and client perspectives as shown by the FAI and PCQ ratings could also provide the basis for fruitful dialogue in counseling.

Rehabilitation Indicators

Rehabilitation Indicators (RIs) consist of a cluster of instruments that were designed to comprehensively measure the impact of rehabilitation services on recipients and to assist with treatment planning (Diller et al., 1983). They provide descriptive profiles of client functioning at moderate to high levels of detail. They cover a wide range of observable behavior, and they strike a balance between standardization at the item level and flexibility in terms of the particular elements selected for use by a given institution. The items are organized into hierarchical frameworks, so that the rater can probe specific areas when general indicators have been flagged.

Three types of instruments have been developed. *Skill Indicators* (SKIs) are most similar to other measures of functional assessment in that they document behavioral strengths and weaknesses. They cover more than 700 skills in the following 15 areas of functioning: self-care; mobility; cognition; communication; social ADL; household business and housework; childcare; political and community skills; selecting an educational program; attending school; problem solving; vocabulary and other basic skills; seeking employment; selecting and advancing within a career ladder; and vocational skills. Assessment can be based upon observation or interview.

Status Indicators (SIs) consist of 51 Descriptors in six areas of functioning, including vocation, education, income, self-care, family role, and transportation. The respondent indicates whether the person performs the skill independently, with assistance, or not at all. Like demographics, they identify an individual's "position" in the world, but SIs include only characteristics that may be influenced by disability and rehabilitation services.

Activity Pattern Indicators (APIs) are a set of instruments that serve to record a person's participation in activities. Although the data are recorded in the form of specific activities, they are typically analyzed by categories. For example, mobility data may be analyzed in terms of amount of travel time, the percentage of time away from home, and the diversity of activities in which the client is engaged while away. A profile of scores on 15 activity areas can be generated. Various approaches to data collection are possible including activity diaries, observation, interview, or questionnaire.

Instrument forms, training manuals, and other resources are available (Diller et al., 1983). The time required for assessment varies, depending upon the component RIs that are needed for an individual. The APIs can be recorded using a structured list of a week's activities that allows for noting frequency, duration, location, social contact, and functional assistance. Infrequent events can be documented on the *Special Events Form.* In completing the *Skills Indicators,* the interviewer first identifies the skills and areas that are relevant to the individual and then records whether or not the individual performs the skill, and if yes, whether or not assistance is used.

From 1977 through 1982, the staff of the *Rehabilitation Indicators* project implemented more than 50 field tests and demonstrations of the RIs in a variety of rehabilitation and independent living settings (Brown, Gordon, & Diller, 1984). These served to build a base of data relating to the instruments' reliability and validity. The authors indicate that the data are encouraging but still incomplete. As might be expected with such a comprehensive system, the purposes to which it might be put are varied, including case management, program administration and evaluation, and documentation of needs for services in a given population.

Craig Handicap Assessment and Reporting Technique

The Craig Handicap Assessment and Reporting Technique (CHART) was probably the first instrument designed to measure the limitations resulting from an interaction between the disabilities of an individual and the restrictions of the environment (Whiteneck, Charlifue, Gerhart, Overholser, & Richardson, 1992). Designed for use with adults who have physical disabilities and are living in the community, it covers the dimensions of physical independence, mobility, occupation, social integration, and economic self-sufficiency. Physical independence reflects the need for care and assistance in activities of daily living. Mobility indicates the number of hours out of bed each day, days per week out of the house, and accessibility of the home and transportation. Occupation describes productive ways of using time: working, attending school, homemaking, housekeeping, volunteering, and engaging in active recreation or self-improvement activities. Social integration is assessed in terms of who shares the household and the frequency and diversity of other social interaction. Economic self-sufficiency measures adjusted total family income.

The CHART is behaviorally anchored and provides the means to compare the individual being rated with norms for nondisabled individuals in society. Each scale is calibrated to produce a score of 100 for most persons without disabilities; lower scores reflect the discrepancy between what a person with a disability is doing and what would typically be expected of independent adults.

Published research (Dijkers, 1991) provides evidence of good reliability and validity. The CHART can be used either for individual assessment and service planning or for program evaluation purposes.

Personal Opinions Questionnaire

The *Personal Opinions Questionnaire* (POQ; Bolton & Brookings, 1998) was developed to measure intrapersonal empowerment, "the capacity of disenfranchised people to understand and become active participants in matters that affect their lives" (Bolton & Brookings, 1998). Bolton and Brookings began by reviewing the literature and developing a list of 20 characteristics of the empowered person with a disability. They created 25 items for each of the characteristics, and then distilled the total to 240, 6 positive and 6 negatively worded statements for each characteristic. They administered the POQ to a sample of veterans and students with disabilities and subjected the data to factor analysis. The resulting instrument consisted of 64 items that comprised 4 factors as follows:

> *Personal Competence:* Sets challenging goals and works to achieve them, assumes responsibility for one's self, is well-organized and disciplined, and understands and relies on one's self.
>
> *Group Orientation:* Works together with other people, participates willingly in community activities, and assists other people with their problems.
>
> *Self-Determination:* Stands up for one's rights; expresses opinions without hesitation; and makes decisive choices, often preferring creative solutions.
>
> *Positive Identity:* Accepts one's disability realistically, doesn't believe disability dominates one's life, and doesn't use disability as an excuse. (Bolton & Brookings, 1998, pp. 136–137)

The authors then examined the correlations between the POQ subscales and the *16 Personality Factor Questionnaire,* finding logical relationships and indications that better personal adjustment may be a basic characteristic of empowerment. Self-determination was related to the 16 PF scales that define extraversion. Personal competence was significantly correlated with three 16 PF scales: Stable, Confident, and Unfrustrated. One surprising finding was that the 16 PF scale, Group Dependence, correlated with three of the four POQ subscales since empowerment has often been assumed to reflect the ability to stand alone. Normative data have been published on a large sample of vocational rehabilitation clients (Brookings & Bolton, 2000).

Personal Independence Profile

Nosek and Fuhrer (Nosek, Fuhrer, & Howland, 1992) found it ironic that most measures of independence focus on the ability to carry out activities, whereas with the independent living movement it has become increasingly clear that the essence of independence involves the individual's ability to make choices and direct his or her life. They sought to operationalize the concept of independence for persons with disabilities in a manner that included perceived control over one's life, physical and cognitive autonomy, psychological self-reliance, and characteristics of the social and physical environment. Drawing indirectly on Maslow's hierarchy of needs, they discussed the independent living dimensions in terms of a continuum that included basic survival, material well-being, productivity, and self-actualization.

Nosek, Fuhrer, and Howland (1992) developed the *Personal Independence Profile* (PIP) from items taken from varied psychometric instruments, eventually creating four self-report scales. Perceived Control consists of 10 items measuring autonomy in areas such as work, health, and recreation. Psychological Self-Reliance consists of 34 items relating to assertiveness, decision-making, self-confidence, and so on. Physical Functioning (25 items) measures independence in mobility, activities of daily living, social roles, physical activity, and dexterity. Environmental Resources covers housing, employment, education, transportation, and income (Nosek, 1992).

The PIP was administered to 185 persons with disabilities along with a locus of control scale, the CHART, and the 16 PF Questionnaire. The PIP was shown to have an acceptable level of internal consistency and to measure the construct of independence. The authors concluded, however, that independence is a complex construct that is affected by both personal and environmental characteristics.

Measures of Environmental Factors

Craig Hospital Inventory of Environmental Factors

The *Craig Hospital Inventory of Environmental Factors* (CHIEF) is a new instrument designed to quantify five environmental variables that may affect persons with disabilities (Craig Hospital Research Department, 1999). *Accessibility* involves physical access, including architectural barriers, answering the question "Can you get where you want to go?" *Accommodation* concerns services, equipment, or modification to tasks that address the question "Can you do what you want to do?" "Are your special needs met?" is the question answered by the *resource availability* items. *Social support* evaluates the attitudes and prejudices of others that may either facilitate or discourage full community involvement. The subject of the fifth topic, *equality,* is simply "Are you treated equally with others?"

The CHIEF was empirically developed and tested. Twenty-five items describing barriers were created, and participants were asked to indicate how frequently they encountered the barriers and how problematic they were. Results were factor analyzed, and six factors were identified: community barriers, physical barriers, work barriers, policy barriers, surroundings/computer/information barriers, and home barriers. Further studies have demonstrated acceptable reliability as well as construct validity because impairment groups differed from one another in predictable ways on their scores (Whiteneck, Harrison-Felix, Mellick, Brooks, Charlifue, & Gerhart, 2004).

Mobility Participation Survey and the Environmental Barriers and Facilitators List

David Gray is leading a project whose goal is to develop an assessment battery to measure community participation among individuals with mobility impairments in a way that is reliable, is valid, is sensitive to individual and environmental factors, and works effectively with the ICF (Gray, 1999). Focus groups of individuals with varied conditions (e.g., polio, cerebral palsy, and spinal cord injury), of spouses, and of professionals were used to develop item pools for two new instruments. The *Mobility Participation Survey* includes 312 questions about 25 areas of life, including, for example, self-care, money management, socializing, and community activities. Respondents are asked a series of questions about each area as follows:

- How frequently they engage in the activity
- Whether participation is limited in any way
- How much choice they have about engaging in the activity
- How satisfied they are with their level of participation
- How important it is that they engage in the activity
- How much time is required to prepare for the activity
- Whether they need help from another person to engage in the activity, and if yes, who provides assistance.
- How often they use accommodations, adaptations, or special equipment to engage in the activity

The *Environmental Barriers and Facilitators List* (EBFL) is composed of 181 questions about whether and how an individual's participation is affected by the accessibility of buildings, home environments, community environments, work and/or school environments, mobility devices used, accessibility features, social institutions, services, and attitudes of others.

In both the MBS and EBFL, specific questions are probed only in areas that are relevant to the individual respondent, so the two instruments together require about 1 hour to complete. Studies that have been completed to date show satisfactory levels of internal consistency and test-retest reliability. Data indicate that when people have greater choice, they report greater satisfaction with their participation. Those areas that are rated most important generally show more choice and satisfaction than less important activities. Furthermore, satisfaction in participation is reported to be greater by people with no limitations than by those with limitations. The work on this project is continuing with studies to determine whether it will satisfactorily measure outcomes following medical and rehabilitation interventions.

Conclusion

Assessment of independence has received attention for many years in rehabilitation. Many functional assessment instruments have been developed since the 1970s, and currently several promising tools are being created to measure community integration and participation.

References

Andresen, E. (2000). Criteria for assessing the tools of disability outcomes research. *Archives of Physical Medicine and Rehabilitation, 81,* 15–20.

Bolton, B. (1994). Acceptance of Disability Scale. In D. J. Keyser & R. C. Sweetland (Ed.), *Test Critiques* (Vol. 10, pp. 8–12). Austin, TX: PRO-ED.

Bolton, B., & Brookings, J. (1998). Development of a measure of intrapersonal empowerment. *Rehabilitation Psychology, 43,* 131–142.

Brookings, J., & Bolton, B. (2000). Confirmatory factor analysis of a measure of intrapersonal empowerment. *Rehabilitation Psychology, 45.*

Brown, M., Gordon, W. A., & Diller, L. (1984). Rehabilitation Indicators. In A. S. H. M. J. Fuhrer (Ed.), *Functional Assessment in Rehabilitation* (pp. 187–203). Baltimore: Paul H. Brookes Publishing Company.

Craig Hospital Research Department. (1999). *Manual of the Craig Hospital Inventory of Environmental Factors.* Englewood, CO: Craig Hospital.

Crewe, N. M. (1987). Assessment of physical functioning. In B. Bolton (Ed.), *Handbook of measurement and evaluation in rehabilitation* (pp. 235–247). Baltimore: Paul H. Brookes Publishing Company.

Crewe, N. M., & Athelstan, G. T. (1981). Functional assessment in vocational rehabilitation: A systematic approach to diagnosis and goal setting. *Archives of Physical Medicine & Rehabilitation, 62,* 299–305.

Crewe, N. M., & Athelstan, G. T. (1984). *Functional Assessment Inventory manual.* Menomonie, WI: Materials Development Center, University of Wisconsin, Stout.

Crewe, N. M., Athelstan, G. T., & Meadows, G. K. (1975). Vocational diagnosis through assessment of functional limitations. *Archives of Physical Medicine & Rehabilitation, 56,* 513–516.

Crewe, N. M., & Dijkers, M. (1995). Functional Assessment. In L. A. Cushman & M. J. Scherer (Eds.), *Psychological Assessment in Medical Rehabilitation* (pp. 101–144). Washington, DC: American Psychological Association.

Cushman, L. A., & Scherer, M. J. (Eds.). (1995). *Psychological Assessment in Medical Rehabilitation.* Washington, DC: American Psychological Association.

Dembo, T., Leviton, G. L., & Wright, B. A. (1956). Adjustment to misfortune—A problem in social psychological rehabilitation. *Artificial Limbs, 3,* 4–62.

Dijkers, M., with the CHART study group. (1991). Scoring CHART: Survey and sensitivity analysis. *Journal of the American Paraplegia Society, 14,* 85–86.

Diller, L., Fordyce, W., Jacobs, D., Brown, M., Gordon, W., Simmens, S., et al. (1983). *Final report: Rehabilitation Indicators Project (Grant No. G008003039).* New York: New York University Medical Center.

Frey, W. D. (1984). Functional assessment in the '80s. In A. S. Halpern & M. J. Fuhrer (Eds.), *Functional Assessment in Rehabilitation* (pp. 11–43). Baltimore: Paul H. Brookes.

Goldberg, R. T., Bernad, M., & Granger, C. V. (1980). Vocational status: Prediction by the Barthel Index and PULSES Profile. *Archives of Physical Medicine & Rehabilitation, 61,* 580–583.

Goldberg, R. T., Hannon, H., & Granger, C. V. (1977). Vocational and functional assessment of clients reopened for service. *Scandinavian Journal of Rehabilitation Medicine, 9,* 85–90.

Granger, C. V. (1982). Health accounting functional assessment of the long term patient. In G. S. F. J. Kottke, & J. S. Lehmann (Ed.), *Krusen's Handbook of Physical Medicine and Rehabilitation.* Philadelphia: W. B. Saunders.

Granger, C. V., Albrecht, G. L., & Hamilton, B. B. (1979). Outcome of comprehensive medical rehabilitation measurement by PULSES Profile and Barthel Index. *Archives of Physical Medicine & Rehabilitation, 60,* 145–154.

Granger, C. V., Hamilton, B. B., Linacre, J. M., Heinemann, A. W., & Wright, B.D. (1993). Performance profiles of the Functional Independence Measure. *American Journal of Physical Medicine and Rehabilitation, 72,* 84–89.

Gray, D. B. (1999). *A test battery to assess participation and environment with mobility limitations.* Paper presented at the annual conference of the American Public Health Association, Chicago.

Grebinger, E., Fawcett, P., Chmela, J., Baber, K., Watts, J., Cash, S. H., et al. (1997). Validity of the Functional Autonomy Rating Scale. *Journal of Rehabilitation Outcomes Measurement, 1,* 1–13.

Gresham, G. E., Phillips, T. F., & Labi, M. L. C. (1980). ADL status in stroke: Relative merits of three standard indexes. *Archives of Physical Medicine & Rehabilitation, 61,* 355–358.

Hahn, E. A., & Cella, D. (2003). Health outcomes assessment in vulnerable populations: Measurement challenges and recommendations. *Archives of Physical Medicine and Rehabilitation, 84,* 35–42.

Heinemann, A. W., Linacre, J. M., Wright, B. D., Hamilton, B. B., & Granger, C. (1993). Relationships between impairment and physical disability as measured by the Functional Independence Measure. *Archives of Physical Medicine & Rehabilitation, 74,* 566–573.

Homa, D. B., & Peterson, D. B. (2005). Using the International Classification of Functioning, Disability and Health (ICF) in teaching rehabilitation client assessment. *Rehabilitation Education, 19,* 119–128.

Jette, D. U., Warren, R. L., & Wirtalla, C. (2005). Functional independence domains in patients receiving rehabilitation in skills nursing facilities: Evaluation of psychometric properties. *Archives of Physical Medicine and Rehabilitation, 86,* 1089–1094.

Keany, K. C. M.-H., & Glueckauf, R. L. (1993). Disability and value change: An overview and reanalysis of acceptance of loss theory. *Rehabilitation Psychology, 38,* 199–210.

Keith, R. A. (1984). Functional assessment measures in medical rehabilitation: Current status. *Archives of Physical Medicine & Rehabilitation, 64,* 74–78.

Linkowski, D. C. (1987). *The Acceptance of Disability Scale.* Washington, DC: George Washington University, Rehabilitation Research and Training Center.

Neath, J., Bellini, J., & Bolton, B. (1997). Dimensions of the Functional Assessment Inventory for five disability groups. *Rehabilitation Psychology, 42,* 183–207.

Nosek, M. A. (1992). Independent Living. In R. M. Parker & E. M. Szymanski (Eds.), *Rehabilitation Counseling: Basics and Beyond* (pp. 103–133). Austin, TX: PRO-ED.

Nosek, M. A., Fuhrer, M. J., & Howland, C. A. (1992). Independence among people with disabilities: II. Personal Independence Profile. *Rehabilitation Counseling Bulletin, 36,* 21–36.

Peterson, D. B. (2005). The International Classification of Functioning, Disability, and Health (ICF): A primer for rehabilitation educators. *Rehabilitation Counseling Bulletin, 19,* 81–94.

Peterson, D. B., & Rosenthal, D. A. (2005). The International Classification of Functioning, Disability, and Health (IDF): A primer for rehabilitation educators. *Rehabilitation Counseling Bulletin, 19,* 81–94.

Scheer, S. J. (Ed.). (1990). *Multidisciplinary Perspectives in Vocational Assessment of Impaired Workers.* Rockville, MD: Aspen.

Stineman, M. G., Shea, J. A., Jette, D. U., Warren, R. L., & Wirtalla, C. (1997).The Functional Independence Measure: Tests of scaling assumptions, structure and reliability across 20 diverse impairment categories. *Archives of Physical Medicine and Rehabilitation, 77,* 1101–1108.

United States Department of Labor. (1991). *Dictionary of Occupational Titles* (4th ed.). Indianapolis, IN: JIST. Available online at: http://www.wave.net/upg/immigration/dot_index.html.

Whiteneck, G. G., Charlifue, S. W., Gerhart, K. A., Overholser, J. D., & Richardson, G.N. (1992). Quantifying handicap: A new measure of long-term rehabilitation outcomes. *Archives of Physical Medicine & Rehabilitation, 73,* 519–526.

Whiteneck, G. G., Harrison-Felix, C. L., Mellick, D. C., Brooks, C. A., Charlifue, S. B., & Gerhart, K. A. (2004). Quantifying environmental factors: A measure of physical, attitudinal, service, productivity, and policy barriers. *Archives of Physical Medicine and Rehabilitation, 85,* 1324–1335.

Wickstrom, R. J. (1990). Functional Capacity Testing. In S. J. Scheer (Ed.), *Multidisciplinary Perspectives in Vocational Assessment of Impaired Workers* (pp. 73–88). Rockville, MD: Aspen.

World Health Organization. (1980). *International classification of impairments, disabilities, and handicaps: A manual of classification relating to the consequences of disease.* Geneva: World Health Organization.

Chapter 11

Neuropsychological Assessment

Ronald M. Ruff and James C. Schraa

Questions That Need to Be Answered

What Are the Patient's Neurocognitive Abilities?

When patients are initially hospitalized in a rehabilitation unit following a neurological illness, it is frequently necessary to first evaluate the level of *attention and concentration*. Thus, the neuropsychologist's role is to assess the patient's capacity to engage during the various neurobehavioral interventions, such as occupational therapy, physical therapy, and speech therapy, as well as during interventions provided by the nurses. If the patient is sufficiently alert and oriented, then *sustained attention* needs to be evaluated in order to assess during what periods of the day and for what duration the patient is capable of engaging in treatment. *Memory and learning* is a second cognitive domain that the neuropsychologist is asked to evaluate. The acquisition of new information is, of course, pivotal to the success of behavioral treatments. Tests should delineate strengths and limitations for memory encoding, storage and retrieval, and learning. A third area that needs to be evaluated by the neuropsychologist is *executive functioning,* which incorporates problem solving and self-monitoring. Deficits in executive functioning can compromise the patient's capacity to comprehend information, generate solutions to *reason abstractly,* and perform in the correct sequence the necessary steps for problem solving. Since neurological impairments result in new and challenging problems for the patient, the demands on executive functioning are significantly increased. Thus, it is essential that testing determine which executive functioning components are impaired and which are preserved. In this chapter, we will address three major cognitive domains that neuropsychologists evaluate in rehabilitation: (a) attention and concentration, (b) memory and learning, and (c) executive functioning. The chapter discusses theoretical underpinnings and examples of test procedures for each domain.

The assessment of neurocognition also includes the evaluation of verbal capacities and spatial abilities. However, within rehabilitation hospital units, the speech and language therapists usually evaluate language functions, and occupational therapists usually focus on spatial capacities. Sensorimotor functions are also part of a typical neuropsychological evaluation. However, during inpatient rehabilitation, physiatrists and physical therapists will evaluate the sensorimotor functions along with the neuropsychologists.

In the hospital setting, various disciplines are involved in evaluating neurocognitive abilities. It is critical that the rehabilitation team avoid getting splintered into various disciplines, thereby hindering transdisciplinary coordination. As a rule, members of the rehabilitation team are more or less familiar with the various assessment techniques that are used by the different disciplines, and the team's reporting forms are also coordinated. This coordination is referred to as *horizontal integration*—integration of testing across the neurocognitive domains. Indeed, the physical medicine and rehabilitation physicians are especially trained in facilitating transdisciplinary interactions with a focus on the functional capacities of a patient.

How Are the Test Findings Utilized?

In rehabilitation, neuropsychological testing informs both diagnosis and treatment. That is, the results of the testing are communicated to (a) the patient; (b) the rehabilitation team, including the treating physician; (c) the family members; and (d) the insurance providers. Because most patients with neurological problems have brain damage, they often lack the ability to fully understand the extent to which various neurocognitive functions are compromised. Thus, the neurocognitive testing results must be communicated at a level that will allow the patient to slowly adjust and understand his or her strengths and weaknesses. In addition to this neurologically based inability to understand the deficits (i.e., organic denial), a patient can have psychological reasons for denying various cognitive deficits (i.e., psychological denial). Therefore, a psychotherapeutic component is incorporated to provide the patients with sufficient emotional support to understand and gain gradual insight into their cognitive limitations. The neuropsychologist also plays an important role in educating team members about how longstanding personality traits influence the development of insight and coping with brain injury. It should be noted that the physical residua of a brain injury are more readily understood, since they are so obvious to everyone. However, more subtle memory or concentration difficulties are, in the early stages, frequently ignored or denied. Throughout the various stages of recovery, there should be multiple testings to address any gains and provide the patient with feedback encouraging awareness and acceptance of the altered mental status.

In most inpatient rehabilitation units, weekly team conferences address both the diagnostic issues and the specific treatment goals. The neuropsychologist can be an asset to the team, helping ensure horizontal integration and analysis of interactions among different aspects of neurocognitive functioning. Examples of such interactions include short-term memory problems, which are predominantly accounted for by attentional difficulties, or executive functioning that affects the patient's capacity to structure the learning process. Family members also need to be educated about the patient's neurocognitive strengths and limitations to facilitate communication and help them adjust their expectations. Finally, neuropsychological test findings need to be documented and summarized for the insurance providers.

What Neurocognitive Gains Will the Patient Make?

Tests can serve as predictors for outcome. Indeed, it is the goal of the patient, the rehabilitation team, and the family members to achieve an optimal outcome. "Outcome" during hospitalization focuses typically on where and how the patient will live following discharge. Thus, during a relatively short hospital stay, the team needs to predict functioning levels subsequent to discharge. For example, the duration of hospitalization for patients who have had a stroke is typically 2.5 weeks, whereas for patients who have had traumatic brain injury, the length of hospitalization depends on severity, ranging from a few days to a few weeks. The duration of stay for patients with spinal cord injury can be months, particularly if the patient depends on a ventilator for breathing. During this time, all energy is focused on helping the patient achieve as much functional independence as possible. In predicting postdischarge status, the neuropsychologist can evaluate safety concerns (e.g., whether the patient is able to maintain medication compliance or dial 911 in an emergency). Tests can assess whether the patient can live independently (e.g., whether the patient can independently utilize means of transportation or prepare meals). Obviously, these evaluations take into account not only neurocognitive tests but also the available support network and the emotional status of the patient.

Who Was the Patient Before the Neurological Illness?

One of the aims of the neuropsychologist is to determine the patient's premorbid strengths and weaknesses. The focus is typically on the neurocognitive functioning, but it can also include the preexisting psychological status. The physicians typically focus on the preexisting medical history. (For a comprehensive review of estimating the cognitive, emotional, and physical domains, see Ruff, Mueller, and Jurica [1996b].) In the last section of this chapter, we address one particularly problematic domain: preexisting learning disabilities. The interaction between these learning disabilities and an acquired brain injury needs to be carefully delineated by integrating the results of neuropsychological testing with preexisting school records and work history.

The role of the neuropsychologist within rehabilitation is, therefore, complex and multifaceted. The tests that are administered focus primarily on neurocognitive assessment. However, psychodiagnostic testing is also frequently incorporated. To avoid overlap, it is essential that the neuropsychologist be part of a transdisciplinary, horizontally integrated team. In addition to this *horizontal integration,* an integration over time or a *vertical integration* is important to evaluate improvements or declines. Ideally, tests can be administered that can be performed in both the inpatient and outpatient settings. Given the complexity of the neuropsychologist's role within rehabilitation, we have limited the focus of neurocognitive assessment to the three following domains: (1) attention and concentration, (2) memory and learning, and (3) executive functioning.

Neurocognitive Assessment

Attention and Concentration

Although numerous investigators have documented attentional deficits while administering neurocognitive tests, relatively few attempts have been made to more precisely understand the nature of attention deficits (Gronwall & Sampson, 1974; Sohlberg & Mateer, 1989; Van Zomeren & Van den Burg, 1985). Agreement exists that there are different types of potential mechanisms. However, in the neuropsychological literature no consensus has emerged about models that would best explain attentional difficulties. In a review article of the cognitive, neuropsychological, and neurophysiologic literature, Niemann, Ruff, and Kramer (1996) have proposed a framework that separates attention into the following three subdivisions: (1) arousal and alertness; (2) selective attention; and (3) effort, resource allocation, and speed of processing.

Arousal and Alertness

Arousal and alertness refer to the drive state that enhances all behavior. For example, immediately following a stroke or traumatic brain injury, patients frequently are unable to process information from their environment. When patients are emerging from a coma, the rehabilitation psychologist's role is to evaluate daily fluctuations in order to identify phases during which a patient is more responsive to external stimuli. During this stage, the assessment focuses on the patient's orientation to self, place, and time. Assessment also encompasses preferences for sensory input to determine, for example, a reduction in hearing, a partial blindness, or a hemi-neglect. The aim is to identify the patient's optimal input and output modes so that the rehabilitation team can most effectively channel its input throughout the phases of recovery.

Once a patient is conscious, it is essential to assess the ability to store information across time. The inability to lay down memory traces from 1 minute to the next is referred to as posttraumatic amnesia (PTA). Levin, O'Donnell, and Grossman (1979) have developed the *Galveston Orientation and Amnesia Test* (GOAT), which evaluates PTA specifically for patients who have suffered traumatic brain injury. The GOAT can be administered on a daily basis and is composed of standardized questions for orientation and recall. Starting out with 100 points, deductions are made for errors. Research has shown that for a patient with a score of less than 75, psychometric testing is unreliable due to insufficient cognitive processing. Although there are a few measures similar to the GOAT, more detailed and sophisticated systems need to be developed in the future for tracking changes in attention and memory as part of the process of emerging from PTA.

Once patients with traumatic brain injury emerge out of PTA, they typically do not revert back unless they develop secondary neurological complications such as hydrocephalus or a bleed. However, patients following a stroke can present severe fluctuations in their awareness often on a daily basis in the early stages of recovery. This phenomenon is referred to as "sundowning": These patients are reasonably oriented during the day, but toward evening, as fatigue sets in, a state of disorientation, confusion, or even agitation takes over. Rehabilitation psychologists can aid in these observations, helping to identify the optimal time and duration for treatment. In patients who are underaroused, a combination of antidepressants and Ritalin is often introduced, and the rehabilitation psychologist can quantify their behavioral effect.

Within arousal, two physiological states can be distinguished: (a) phasic changes, which occur very fast and are often under voluntary control, and (b) tonic changes, which typically occur slowly and more or less on an involuntary basis. An example of a phasic change would be a quick response to a loud noise or sharp pain. In patients who are underaroused, it is possible that there is a lack of responsiveness to such external stimulation. For example, with the *Glasgow Coma Scale,* the phasic changes of patients with traumatic brain injury are evaluated in the critical care unit to determine patients' state of arousal and also grade the severity of traumatic brain injury (scores between 3 and 8 indicate severe traumatic brain injury, scores between 9 and 12 indicate moderate traumatic brain injury, and scores between 13 and 15 indicate mild traumatic brain injury) (Teasdale & Jennett, 1974).

The tonic changes of alertness affect a patient's capacity on a more subtle level. Typically, metabolic changes, along with other factors, can influence tonic alertness. For example, excessive fatigue, significant depression, or high anxiety states can lead to reduced arousal. Finally, sustained attention—the patient's ability to maintain a state of readiness that allows for detection of environmental stimuli over a prolonged period—can also be considered a part of tonic alertness. The level of sustained attention affects the provision of behavioral rehabilitation treatments.

Selective Attention

Selective attention is the ability to set priorities in information processing (Kornhuber, 1984). Individuals who are neurologically impaired are frequently unable to set priorities, which can lead to inattentiveness. Such patients are far more distracted by background noises such as a key chain rattling or elevator doors opening. Premorbidly, the same individuals could selectively subordinate these background noises. Thus, it is the role of the neuropsychologist to assess the patient's ability to attend to the target stimuli rather than the background stimuli.

Shiffrin and Schneider (1977, 1984) proposed two types of processes involved in selective attention. *Automatic processing* is based on overlearned selection mechanisms that operate without demands and, in most individuals, occur without significant interference. *Controlled processing* demands capacity and requires the patient's attention or conscious awareness. Brain injury can differentially affect these two processing modes. If an English-speaking patient finds himself in a room where other patients and therapists are also communicating in English, the patient may have great difficulty in focusing on his own conversation, since he is overly distracted. This would be a new problem that the patient has in controlled processing. If the concurrent conversations in the room are in languages that the patient does not understand, then the distraction should be reduced. However, if the interference is of a similar magnitude, then this would point toward a difficulty of automatic processing.

A classic measure for evaluating the interference caused by overlearned or automatic processing is the *Stroop Color Word Naming Test* (Lezak, Howieson,

& Loring, 2004). There are multiple versions that evaluate the Stroop-like effect, yet they typically all include one or more of the following three parts. First, Xs or circles are printed in different colors of ink and the patients must name the colors. Second, color names are printed in black ink, and the patient must say the words. Third, names of colors are printed in different colors of ink and the patients are asked to state the color of ink, while ignoring the actual printed color name (e.g., the word "green" is printed in blue ink and the patient is asked to state "blue"). The two interfering stimuli categories must be separated. Thus, the *Stroop Color Word Naming Test* evaluates selective attention and response interference (Kahneman & Treisman, 1984; Neumann, 1984).

A test that is very closely aligned with the Shiffrin and Schneider model is the *Ruff 2 and 7 Selective Attention Test* (Ruff & Allen, 1996). In this cancellation test, the patient is asked to identify the targets 2 and 7, embedded in rows of distracters. In the automatic detection condition, the distracters are made up of alphabetical letters, whereas in the controlled processing condition, the 2 and 7 are embedded among other digits. Identifying 2 and 7 from among other digits is typically slower than identifying 2 and 7 among letters. Because this test takes 5 minutes, it allows for the evaluation of sustained attention. Patients with right-hemispheric damage are more compromised in the area of selective and sustained attention than normal patients and patients with left-hemispheric damage (Ruff, Niemann, Allen, Farrow, & Wylie, 1992).

Effort, Resource Allocation, and Speed of Processing

In rehabilitation, a lack of effort on the patient's part can sabotage behavioral interventions. As a rule, the patient's overall available mental energy varies from day to day, and it can also vary across relatively short time periods. Posner (1975) referred to resources, capacity, and effort as components of mental energy. Most individuals with neurological damage continually struggle with fatigue; thus, a rehabilitation psychologist needs to evaluate, within the context of the various treatment modalities, the patient's available energy levels. In some cases, timed tests can be a strong indicator of the patient's resource capacity. Frequently, subtests of the *Wechsler Memory Scale–Third Edition* (WMS-III) (e.g., the Digit Span subtest or the Digit Symbol subtest) are used (Wechsler, 1997). Particularly for those patients who have no sensorimotor deficits, timed test measures are the most powerful indicators of effort and resource allocation.

One of the most frequently used tools is the *Trails A and B Test* (Lezak, Howieson, & Loring, 2004). In Trail A, sequencing is evaluated; the patient is asked to draw a line connecting circles in sequence according to the numbers contained within each circle (e.g., the patient connects 1 with 2, 2 with 3). The circles are configured more or less randomly on a sheet of paper. In Trail B, the patient is asked to both sequence and alternate by connecting not only numbers but also alphabetical letters in their ascending order. That is, the circle with the number 1 needs to be connected with the circle with the letter A, which is followed by the circle with the number 2 and the circle with the letter B, and so on.

A subtest from the *Cognistat* is particularly helpful in evaluating the effort of lower-level patients (Kiernan, Mueller, Langston, & Van Dyke, 1987). On this subtest, three different objects (e.g., a pen, a piece of paper, and some keys) are placed in front of the patient. The patient is then asked in simple, one-step commands, followed by two-step and three-step commands, to, for example, pick up the paper, point to the floor, and hand the examiner the keys. If a patient can handle only two-step commands, the rehabilitation teams should know to adapt instructions to the patient's capacity as necessary (i.e., avoid instructions of three steps or more).

In the literature, the term "effort" describes the process of monitoring that incorporates feedback as well as the evaluation of outcome. Indeed, Norman and Shallice (1986) postulated a unit called "supervisory attentional system," which has also been incorporated in Baddeley's (1986) model of "working memory." Working memory is information that can be concurrently integrated and processed, without necessarily requiring that all of the information be permanently stored. For example, if a neuropsychologist is writing a report and has all the raw test data and medical records available on her desk, then she is utilizing working memory. If the same rehabilitation psychologist was asked a day later to report the test results to a colleague and she did not have these data in front of her, then many of the details would be lost. Thus, working memory allows concurrent prioritization and processing of large amounts of information. In this manner, efforts and resource allocation depend on the time, context, and complexity of information processing. Norman and Shallice introduced the notion that the supervisory attentional system (SAS) is involved in regulating more complex tasks separating routine from nonroutine modes of selection. As the task becomes more nonroutine, the demands on the SAS increase. A dysfunction in SAS can make it more difficult to deal with novelty (Shallice, 2002).

For a more detailed description of arousal and alertness; selective attention; and effort, resource allocation, and speed of processing, see Niemann et al. (1996).

Memory and Learning

Memory and learning are among the most frequently compromised cognitive functions in patients with neurological damage. In rehabilitation, the evaluation of memory and learning is crucial because it is the basis for neurobehavioral interventions. Thus, to introduce the appropriate treatment modalities, it is essential to determine if, indeed, a patient is capable of remembering information from day to day. Multiple dichotomies for memory are proposed in the literature: short- and long-term memory, recent and remote memory, and declarative and procedural memory. Within the context of rehabilitation, the distinction between declarative and procedural memory is particularly relevant, but we will first address the difference between remote and recent memory.

Remote memory is information from before the neurological illness. As a rule, the older the information, the more crystallized it is and the easier it is to access the information, even for patients who are in the beginning stages of a dementia process. Recent memory is information stored since the neurological onset; it is often more significantly compromised than remote memory. *Short-term memory* and *long-term memory* are other terms used to identify the time parameters involved in memory. Short-term memory is information that an individual is able to remember up to 15 minutes, whereas long-term memory is information that is retained after 15 minutes (for up to years).

The most useful dichotomy within the context of rehabilitation is that proposed by Squire (1987): declarative memory and procedural memory. Declarative memory is information that needs to be specifically recalled or recognized by the patient (therapists' names, times that medications must be taken). In contrast, procedural memory refers to acquisition of motor or mental skills (e.g., learning to use a wheelchair, learning to use the nondominant hand for various tasks such as eating if the dominant hand is paralyzed). Declarative memory is tied to the mesial temporal regions, including the hippocampus, whereas procedural memory is not tied to any specific region in the cortex. Thus, procedural memory is frequently preserved, even in patients who suffer from global amnesia. This distinction clearly affects the gains that can be achieved by the various disciplines because the occupational and physical therapists promote the learning of new motor sequences, which relies on procedural memory skills, whereas the speech therapists introduce more cognitive-based remediation techniques that require declarative memory.

The neuropsychologist also needs to evaluate the patient's ability to process audio–verbal and visuospatial information. Right-handed individuals who have sustained left hemispheric damage are primarily compromised in the learning and storage of verbal information. Conversely, the right hemisphere specializes in the storage and learning of visuospatial information. Thus, professionals should select memory and learning tests that separately assess the audio–verbal and visuospatial modes.

Memory and learning tasks are different. Memory is the retention of information that is presented typically on one occasion and is particularly vulnerable to temporal lobe damage. However, learning—information acquired in multiple trials—typically involves both temporal and prefrontal lobe structures.

We will now discuss the more commonly utilized verbal memory and learning tests. A number of batteries evaluate various aspects of verbal memory, including the WMS-III (Wechsler, 1997). Most commonly, the stories of the WMS-III are used for verbal memory measures. Qualitative analyses of the stories include (a) recency versus latency effect, and (b) storyline preserved versus items recalled without semantic connections. Verbal learning tests typically ask the patient to learn lists of words over multiple trials; common tests include the *Selective Reminding Test* (Buschke & Fuld, 1974), the *California Verbal Learning Test* (Delis, Kramer, Kaplan, & Ober, 1987), and the *Rey Auditory Verbal Learning Test* (Lezak, Howieson, & Loring, 2004). In addition to evaluating the immediate recall for both the stories and word list learning, a delayed recall is assessed. That is, 30 minutes after the initial recall, the patients are asked to recall the stories and words to evaluate long-term memory. For evaluating long-term memory, it is important to distinguish the delayed recall of the short stories from the recall of the words. That is, the decay of a short story can be greater than that of the word list since the patient was exposed to the word list on multiple occasions. In some patients with slow learning across trials, the information does eventually get encoded, and the recall can be preserved. Thus, a patient who was able to learn 12 of the words on the *Selective Reminding Test* (composed of 10 trials) may still be able to freely recall 10 of the 12 words a half-hour later. All of these word tests also have a delayed recognition component, which, as a rule, is intact since the recognition among multiple choices is typically preserved, even in patients with global amnesia. That is, even if a patient cannot freely recall many words after a delay, if given multiple choices, the patient will, as a rule, select the correct choices. The assessment of memory and learning side by side will allow the neuropsychologist to distinguish between encoding difficulties (which can be compromised by attention) and storage and retrieval problems.

The *Rey Complex Figure* is one of the most commonly applied visuospatial memory tests (Lezak, Howieson, & Loring, 2004). The patient is asked to copy a geometric figure, and then, after a 3- and a 30-minute delay, is asked to recall the same figure. Scoring looks at the configuration of the Gestalt in its proportion and dimension and also evaluates the degree to which certain details are retained. The WMS-III also contains a visuospatial memory component. However, constructional apraxia (which can compromise drawing) can interfere with these drawings.

There is a relative paucity of visuospatial learning tests. However, the *Ruff Light Trail Learning Test* (RULIT; Ruff & Allen, 1999) does evaluate visuospatial learning within a paradigm that does not depend upon visual acuity or eye–hand coordination. Within randomly arranged dots connected with multiple lines, a 15-step trail needs to be learned, and 10 opportunities are provided. The examiner has the 15-step trail memorized and teaches it to the patient. Again, a learning curve is established, and there is also a delayed recall component to evaluate long-term memory. The RULIT is sensitive to right frontotemporal damage, whereas comparable left-side brain lesions do not result in significant declines (Ruff & Allen, 1999).

Especially designed for older patients, the *Fuld Object Memory Evaluation* (Fuld, 1980) assesses memory according to multiple modalities. Objects placed in a bag (e.g., a ball, keys, scissors) need to be identified by touch and then pulled out of the bag to provide feedback. After a brief interference delay, the objects need to be recalled across four trials, each followed by reminders for those objects that were not recalled. This measure is typically considered easier than word lists, which lack the tactile encoding aspect.

Executive Functioning

The major goals of rehabilitation neuropsychology are (a) to identify deficits that limit the patient's ability to function independently, (b) to identify deficits that limit rehabilitation potential, and (c) to identify workable compensation techniques. It is well-known that treaters and evaluators can readily become the "frontal lobes of the patient" to the degree that the day-to-day effects of impaired frontal functions are masked. Stuss (1999) has demonstrated that frontal lobe dysfunction results in increased variability in behavior. Informative neuropsychological assessments function as a sieve to separate out other sources of neurobehavioral dysfunction. In rehabilitation neuropsychology, assessment takes into consideration how impairments in abilities such as color vision, left neglect, or auditory comprehension may affect specific test performances. When careful consideration is given to test selection and the rehabilitation psychologist carefully considers the impact of conditions such as aphasia, amnesia, and motor speed, it becomes possible to infer the status of frontal lobe functions (Ruff, Evans, & Marshall, 1986). The adequacy of the match of the available test norms to the specific patient being evaluated always needs to be considered as part of the process of drawing inferences about frontal lobe functions.

The tests generally utilized in rehabilitation neuropsychology are not typically considered to be sensitive to behavioral manifestations of orbital frontal lesions (e.g., Stuss & Benson, 1984). It is frequently noted that orbital frontal involvement is associated with the disinhibition of behavior and personality changes. These personality changes are superimposed on the individual's pre-existing character structure. How compromises of the orbital frontal system influence day-to-day functioning is, in part, a function of the patient's pre-injury level of self-control and sensitivity to the effects of his or her behavior upon others. Stuss (1999) describes how the interconnection of the frontal lobes with the limbic system provides emotional markers, which influence decision making.

The rehabilitation neuropsychologist who can observe the patient's behavior and talk with family members over time can better determine how the patient's pattern of emotional responsiveness has changed. Deciding how much an individual is able to reflect on the alteration of his or her behavior as a result of an impairment of frontal functions is a challenging endeavor that involves the integration of history, test results, and observations of the patient across time. Detailed formulations of the impact of impairment of frontal functions upon interpersonal relationships and style of life require multiple contacts with the patient.

Concept Formation

Neuropsychologists use a number of tests to evaluate concept formation. However, the primary test that is utilized is the *Wisconsin Card Sorting Test*. Before discussing the *Wisconsin Card Sorting Test* in detail, let us identify some alternate measures. Reitan and Wolfson (1993) have, as part of the *Halstead-Reitan*

Battery, developed the *Category Test,* which consists of 208 visually presented items. The first six sets of items are organized according to various principles, followed by a seventh set evaluating the patient's recall of previous sets. Thus, the *Category Test* evaluates the individual's capacity to formulate concepts based on a set of rules that need to be abstracted. For example, in the fifth set, geometric figures are made up of solid and dotted lines for which the proportion in solid lines is the correct concept. Across the 208 items, the score is the number of errors made in concept formation. Another test that can be used to evaluate concept formation is the *Raven's Progressive Matrices* (Raven, 1960). This is a well-known multiple-choice paper-and-pencil test designed to evaluate intellectual functioning in a more or less culturally unbiased fashion. The task, in itself, also relies on concept formation based on geometric designs and rules that need to be abstracted.

The *Wisconsin Card Sorting Test* is probably the best known test related to frontal functioning. It is a card sorting task that requires patients to be able to deduce sorting principles from feedback ("correct" or "incorrect") that is provided after each card sorting response generated by the patient. The individual uses this feedback to shift from one simple problem-solving strategy to another during the course of the test. The Wisconsin Card Sorting Test generates a number of scores. The number of perseverative responses that the patient produces is thought to be the most effective at discriminating frontal from nonfrontal cases (Pendleton & Heaton, 1982).

Before deciding that a performance on the *Wisconsin Card Sorting Test* is related to frontal system functioning, the rehabilitation neuropsychologist must first rule out the impact of a number of variables on the patient's test performance, including color blindness, fatigue, left neglect, and impairment of auditory comprehension. In rehabilitation settings, the neuropsychologist needs to consider whether patients have been exposed to cognitive therapy tasks that have sensitized them to the types of strategies utilized in the *Wisconsin Card Sorting Test.* This exposure would render the *Wisconsin Card Sorting Test* task more "posterior" than frontal. Neuropsychologists should also remember that the *Wisconsin Card Sorting Test* is only novel when administered the first time. The first administration of the test probably is most clearly indicative of frontal system functioning. Careful consideration needs to be given to how retesting with the *Wisconsin Card Sorting Test* should be interpreted.

The utility of the *Wisconsin Card Sorting Test* as a measure of frontal functioning has been the subject of much debate. However, Stuss (1999) convincingly argues that when case selection is very carefully undertaken, the sensitivity of the standard administration of the *Wisconsin Card Sorting Test* to frontal lesions can be demonstrated—except in patients with inferior medial frontal lesions. Given that the first administration of the *Wisconsin Card Sorting Test* is most likely to contribute specific information about frontal system functioning, consideration needs to be given to when this test should be administered during the recovery course of patients in rehabilitation. A clinical neuropsychologist in a rehabilitation setting needs to carefully consider what would be the most important question to answer for this specific patient and then choose the appropriate time for the administration of the *Wisconsin Card Sorting Test* to address this specific question.

Behavioral observations of patients who are completing the *Wisconsin Card Sorting Test* can contribute to the qualitative accuracy of the diagnostic formulation provided by the rehabilitation neuropsychologist. For example, the observation that the patient's behavior on the *Wisconsin Card Sorting Test* is dominated by the rapid production of impulsive responses can lead to specific and useful recommendations for the patient regarding taking more time to respond on cognitive tasks. Some patients will also manifest verbal–behavioral dissociations in which they readily verbalize the principles of the *Wisconsin Card Sorting Test* but fail to accurately apply these principles when completing the test. Observation of this difficulty can lead to the development of specific recommendations to help patients relate their cognitive schemata to their behavioral output.

Individuals who are impaired in terms of the number of perseverative responses they produce on the *Wisconsin Card Sorting Test* frequently display cognitive inflexibility in daily life. Thus, test results from the *Wisconsin Card Sorting Test* can be used to educate family members about the changes in their loved one that they may encounter in the home. Individuals who have impaired performances on the *Wisconsin Card Sorting Test* frequently display a reduced capacity for seeing issues from other people's perspective. Thus, performance on the *Wisconsin Card Sorting Test* can become the basis for ongoing work in psychotherapy and treatment groups.

The *Wisconsin Card Sorting Test* is sometimes discussed along with the *Category Test* as a measure of executive functions. However, the two tests are actually quite different and contribute different information to clinical assessments. The *Wisconsin Card Sorting Test* has been demonstrated to be more accurate in identifying patients with focal frontal involvement than the *Category Test* (Pendelton & Heaton, 1982). This is not surprising in view of the nature of the *Category Test,* which involves logical analysis and new concept formation with visuospatial stimuli. Furthermore, the subtests of the *Category Test* are clearly identified, and the *Category Test* does not require the ability to efficiently shift response sets. The *Wisconsin Card Sorting Test* also yields several different scores that are relevant for treatment planning in rehabilitation. For example, the number of failures to maintain set on the *Wisconsin Card Sorting Test* may indicate difficulty with initiating intended tasks in the real world. This would be very beneficial for the neuropsychologist in helping to inform treatment.

Ideational Fluency

Tests of both verbal and nonverbal ideational fluency require the patient to utilize strategies in order to rapidly produce responses without repetition. They require patients:

- to be able to monitor their efficiency of production so that they can determine when to switch strategies

- to be able to inhibit the production of repetitive or intrusive responses
- to recruit and sustain attention over the duration of the task

Early in the rehabilitative course, patients frequently are not able to sustain and focus attention effectively enough to maximize their performance on fluency tests. However, once patients are consistently aroused and are able to focus their attention, the underlying basis for successful completion of fluency tasks appears to be a function, to a large extent, of the integrity of the frontal lobes (Ruff et al., 1986).

Measures of verbal and figural fluency have been demonstrated to reliably distinguish patients with moderate and severe head injuries from normal controls (Ruff et al., 1986). The same study demonstrated that the more severe the head injury, the greater the degree of impairment on tests of fluency. It was found that fluency tasks were the most sensitive of the tests utilized to detect group differences. This is consistent with clinical experience, which yields the impression that fluency tests are sensitive and dependable measures to utilize when assessing frontal lobe functions. Various researchers have contributed to the database showing that there is a specific dissociation between verbal and nonverbal fluency (e.g., Stuss & Benson, 1984). The double dissociation between verbal and figural fluency and left versus right frontal lobe lesions, respectively, makes it possible to utilize fluency tests to detect lateralized frontal lobe lesions (Ruff, Allen, Farrow, Niemann, & Wylie, 1994).

Nonverbal fluency tasks have a long and broad history in neuropsychology laboratories. In 1977, Jones-Gotman and Milner worked with both right and left frontocentral lesion groups. They demonstrated that the patients with right frontocentral lesions had little or no deficit on word fluency but had profound impairment on design fluency. Their left central group was grossly impaired on word fluency but had little to no deficit on design fluency. Another figural fluency test was developed at the neuropsychology laboratory of Dr. Meier at the University of Minnesota Health Sciences Center. However, the *Ruff Figural Fluency Test* has the advantage of being normed in a manner that takes into consideration the effects of both age and education (Ruff, 1996). It consists of five 1-minute time periods in which the patient generates designs or patterns. During each figure generation trial, the patient works with a specified dot matrix that is printed 35 times in a 5×7 array on a sheet of paper. Each of the five parts of the test is preceded by three practice items. It is essential that all of the instructions of the *Ruff Figural Fluency* tests be given as specified in the manual since variations may influence both productivity and the strategies that the patient utilizes. Ruff and colleagues (1986) demonstrated that even in a group of patients with severe brain injury, motor speed could not fully account for the reduction in figural fluency. This same group of investigators failed to find significant correlations between memory and figural fluency performance. Thus, motor speed and amnesia did not appear to significantly influence fluency. An initial study also demonstrated that the *Ruff Figural Fluency Test* achieved acceptable levels in discriminating right frontal from non–right frontal subjects, with 85% of the subjects being accurately classified (Ruff et al.,

1994). Investigators also demonstrated that patients with right frontal pathology generated significantly fewer designs than those with bifrontal, left posterior, or right posterior lesions. The *Ruff Figural Fluency Test* is a useful measure to assess right (nondominant) prefrontal region functioning. It is useful in demonstrating whether patients can switch strategies and inhibit inappropriate responses in the visuospatial mode. Any observed inflexibility in idea generation can thus be identified as a treatment target in rehabilitation settings. Once compromised right frontal functioning has been identified, the rehabilitation neuropsychologist can consider the impact of inflexibility in processing on issues such as personal decision making, appreciation of humor, and the ability to have a perspective on one's own actions in order to make constructive changes over time.

The *Controlled Word Association Test* (COWAT) requires patients to rapidly generate words beginning with specified letters. There are two forms of the test: one with the letters *c, f,* and *l* and the other with the letters *p, r,* and *w*. The patient generates words beginning with each letter over 1-minute time periods. The two forms of the *Controlled Word Association Test* have been demonstrated to be equivalent (Benton, Hamsher, & Sivan, 1994). The term *Controlled Word Association Test* is specifically utilized to describe this test since the term *word fluency* could be confused with the fluency/nonfluency distinction that is made in aphasia (Ruff, Light, & Parker, 1996a). In 1996 the *Controlled Word Association Test* was renormed on a sample of 360 normal volunteers (Ruff et al., 1996a). The new norms include corrections for education and gender. Having subjects retested on the alternate version of the COWAT 6 months after the initial testing assessed stability over time. The test–retest reliability correlation was impressive at $r = .74$, and there was a minimal increase of three words from the initial testing to the second testing. Normative data in regard to the frequency of perseverative responses were also reported. Ruff, Light, Parker, and Levin (1997) analyzed the same normative data in regard to the psychological construct of word fluency and proposed a distinction between the following conditions: (a) poor word fluency secondary to deficits in verbal attention and word knowledge, and (b) impaired word fluency that is primarily due to left frontal lobe damage.

The literature on verbal fluency tests has consistently yielded data establishing sensitivity to left frontal lobe dysfunction. Ruff and colleagues (1986) studied patients who were nonaphasic with closed brain injury and still found a reduction in *Controlled Word Association Test* performances. Thus, the *Controlled Word Association Test* appears to reflect a decrease in flexibility of processing that cannot simply be attributed to a language disturbance. This same study found no significant correlations between memory and fluency performance. Thus, this study helped to more clearly establish the construct that effective performance on the *Controlled Word Association Test* depends on the intactness of the frontal lobes. The same study also established that the *Controlled Word Association Test* demonstrates sensitivity to severity of injury in that for patients with closed brain injury, greater impairment in test performance was associated with more severe injury. Analysis of covariance also demonstrated that the sensitivity of the *Controlled Word Association Test* could not simply be attributed to overall intellectual differences. When the neuropsychologist takes into consideration education, age, and intactness of verbal attention, the *Controlled Word Association Test* can be used to make accurate inferences about left frontal functioning.

The literature is generally consistent with the specific dissociation between verbal and nonverbal fluency (Stuss & Benson, 1984). The rehabilitation neuropsychologist integrates findings on the *Controlled Word Association Test* and the *Ruff Figural Fluency Test* with findings on other tests. For example, patients with bifrontal involvement and right frontal involvement were demonstrated to produce Block Design performances in the borderline range, whereas patients with left frontal involvement were within the average range (Ruff et al., 1986). By producing an integrated analysis of the behavior displayed on testing, the rehabilitation neuropsychologist can assist the rehabilitation team in recognizing that deficits in specific abilities, such as thinking fluently and flexibly in the visuospatial mode, can impair functioning on a variety of day-to-day tasks (e.g., wiring a stereo, assembling bookshelves, moving a large object through time and space).

Evaluation of Effort, Exaggeration, and Malingering

An important role of the neuropsychologist in rehabilitation settings is to determine whether the patient's symptoms and test results make logical sense. The question of whether the patient's deficits on testing, behavioral presentation, and reported complaints are disproportionately severe for the clinical history is important to consider. In some cases poor performances on testing and during therapies is motivated by some form of secondary gain. The behavioral responses of the patient must be evaluated relative to the literature on outcomes and the neuropsychological data available on similar conditions. Over the past decade there has been an increased emphasis on symptom validity testing (SVT) to identify the presence of suboptimal effort in testing. SVT typically involves the use of forced-choice tests consisting of easy two-choice questions. Poor performances on tests composed of two-choice items are used to statistically classify the test performance as being consistent with a good or suboptimal level of effort. Although symptom validity tests are useful tools, the neuropsychologist is charged with considering the clinical history, the consistency of data generated by the patient over time, the patient's coping style, and the patient's present emotional status before drawing conclusions about whether the level of effort has produced valid or invalid test performances. In addition, the neuropsychologist plays an important role in consulting with the treatment team about how variables related to age, sex, education, and ethnicity may affect whether a particular performance is considered to be impaired.

The National Academy of Neuropsychology has published a position paper on the medical necessity for SVT (Bush, Ruff, et al., 2005). For inpatients, administering an SVT is recommended only for those patients in whom malingering is suspected. However, in the context of a forensic neuropsychological evaluation the "*failure to administer at least one symptom validity test and/or administer tests with internal symptom validity indicators would need to be justified*" (p. 425). Note that suboptimal effort is not always a sign of malingering. Indeed, effort is typically not a constant and can vary to some degree between different days or even over the course of the testing. Thus, poor cooperation and reduced effort do not automatically indicate malingering. According to the *Diagnostic and Statistical Manual of Mental Disorders–Fourth Edition* (American Psychiatric Association, 1994) malingering should be considered only if the evaluation is judged to be (a) invalid, (b) with a definite intentional quality, (c) there exists an incentive, and (d) the incentive is external. Thus, even if the first three conditions exist but no external incentive can be identified, then explanations other than malingering must be explored (e.g., fictitious disorder).

Benefits From the Process of Testing

For many patients, the process of neuropsychological testing is one of the very first steps in rehabilitative treatment. When appropriately accomplished, neuropsychological testing in the rehabilitation setting becomes an important part of the treatment process, with many clinical benefits.

The interviews with the rehabilitation neuropsychologist provide an opportunity for the patient to reflect on his or her own behavior. As part of this early interaction, the neuropsychologist can help to foster an attitude of collaboration and promote the discussion of problems in descriptive terms. This interaction helps to define the patient's problems as something that can be understood and managed. Thus, early neuropsychological evaluation can help the patient to develop a coping-oriented stance that contributes positively to the overall rehabilitation process and outcome.

When the patient's condition and the referral question at hand permit, early neuropsychological testing provides an opportunity to begin informally educating patients about cognitive functions. Thus, the very testing process helps to provide a logical foundation for interventions and safety restrictions that may be necessary early on in the recovery. The informal education that occurs during the testing process can then be readily built upon during feedback discussions with the patient and family.

The rehabilitation neuropsychologist helps patients to feel validated as individuals. Unlike many other busy, hurried professionals that patients see in busy hospital environments, the rehabilitation neuropsychologist provides ample opportunity for the patient to voice concerns about his or her condition and treatment. This clinical interaction builds rapport that can be later utilized to reduce frustrations or deal with crises during the rehabilitation process. Just as the physician takes the responsibility to coordinate the diagnosis and treatment for the patient's physical health, the neuropsychologist should take the same role for the patient's cognitive and emotional health.

Interviews with family members and/or significant others can help to reduce the stress of families by conveying the message that the treatment team is interested in their experiences and difficulties. The fact that the rehabilitation neuropsychologist asks detailed questions that may be novel (e.g., about family history of handedness, about the patient's premorbid coping style) helps to instill confidence that the treatment team is motivated to individualize care.

The feedback session on the initial neuropsychological test results provides an opportunity to help the patient and family create a constructive working model in regard to the neuropsychological problem. The fact that the rehabilitation neuropsychologist can integrate the details of the patient's medical history with aspects of the patient's personal history increases confidence that an individualized treatment plan can be developed and executed. Integrating family observations of the patient's behavior into the discussion of the family history and test findings serves to heighten family investment in the treatment process.

The rehabilitation neuropsychologist has the opportunity to creatively present information to increase the clinical impact of education. For example, in patients with greater left hemisphere involvement, the rehabilitation neuropsychologist may utilize charts, models, or scans that have been marked by radiologists in order to integrate visually processed information along with the summary of the test results. For patients who are more analytically minded or individuals with more years of schooling, a detailed discussion of test scores can help define the patient's problems in terms to which he or she can relate. Thus, early in the rehabilitative process the clinical neuropsychologist can utilize knowledge of the patient's brain functioning in order to optimize education and enhance motivation for participation in rehabilitation.

As an integrator of information, the rehabilitation neuropsychologist can help to define the problems at hand in manageable terms. During early feedback about neuropsychological testing, families are often helped to identify how to most effectively utilize their resources to support the patient. The rehabilitation neuropsychologist can also help the treatment team to more readily discern the nature of family problems and the potential means for addressing them. A benefit of early neuropsychological testing is that it permits the rehabilitation neuropsychologist to assess the patient's reactions to both the strengths and weaknesses that he or she manifests during the testing process. For example, the patient who is aware of and disconcerted by producing an impaired performance on the *Wisconsin Card Sorting Test* may be much more readily counseled in regard to making decisions than a patient who discounts such a problem. The neuropsychologist's observations about how a patient reacts to the manifestations of deficits may be the key factor in determining whether the patient is ready to go home under the supervision of a family member.

Recommendations

The results of neuropsychological evaluations that occur early in the patient's hospital course often yield recommendations to address deficits associated with compromised attention, memory, or executive functioning. The rehabilitation neuropsychologist will often offer recommendations to help control agitation that can occur secondary to confused states and reduced awareness. The first of these recommendations is typically to limit visitors to one or two at a time in order to prevent overstimulation. Similarly, many patients will function better in the postacute multitrauma unit or neurotrauma unit when they do not have roommates because of overstimulation. The results of an early neuropsychological consultation may also yield the recommendation that the patient would benefit from the presence of a one-on-one sitter because of a high level of distractibility, inability to sustain attention, or impulsivity. Typically, the sitters also will need education and direction (e.g., to not watch the patient's television when the patient is already behaving in an agitated manner or to limit the amount of stimulation during meals).

When patients are presenting in confused states with extreme levels of distractibility, the rehabilitation neuropsychologist may also need to recommend the room on the floor that has the least external stimulation. Frequently the nursing staff will benefit from consultation in regard to how to position the bed in the hospital room in view of the patient's visual field cuts. At this early stage in the rehabilitative process, the neuropsychologist may also offer useful recommendations regarding how to design either verbal or nonverbal cues to most effectively set the occasion for appropriate responses from the patient. For example, occasionally there are patients with left hemisphere involvement who benefit from the provision of drawings to remind them to utilize the call light. Typically, patients with neurological conditions benefit from the provision of calendars and orientation signs, but this obvious step frequently is overlooked in busy hospital environments. Patients with ongoing difficulties in consolidating new information into memory or word finding difficulties (i.e., anomia) usually appreciate the provision of a written list of the names of their hospital physicians. Cueing systems for the patient typically help staff members to approach the patient more effectively. Thus, photographs that are posted above the hospital bed and demonstrate how to position the patient for a particular activity can direct staff members and the family. Even in the early postcritical care environments there are patients who benefit from having their routine made as regular as possible. The rehabilitation neuropsychologist can frequently serve to facilitate a dialogue between therapists and nursing staff on how at least a basic routine might be achieved.

Throughout the rehabilitation process, the neuropsychologist can provide education that offers a basis for more effective management when the patient returns home. Thus, early discussions about limiting the number of visitors to reduce stimulation are later followed by discussions about preventing excess stimulation and fatigue in the home. Frequently, families benefit from ongoing and supportive discussions about how best to present stimuli to the patient.

Some patients with acquired dyslexia and their families find the recommendation to utilize their state's talking book library to be extremely helpful. With patients with left neglect, utilizing cues such as a ribbon placed on the left side of the page as a marker to promote visual scanning can be therapeutic. The caregivers of older patients who have numerous medications frequently find consultation about how to develop pill management systems that take into consideration the patient's neuropsychological deficits to be quite beneficial to successfully functioning at home. Caregivers often appreciate discussions about how to cue the person to respond to smoke detectors or carbon monoxide detectors that have gone off or other emergencies that can occur in the home.

Early intervention following mild closed brain trauma is another area in which the timely provision of neuropsychological recommendations is extremely important (Raskin & Mateer, 2000; Varney & Roberts, 1999). Indeed, a recent Consensus Conference sponsored by the National Institutes of Health on Rehabilitation of Persons with Traumatic Brain Injury (1998) concluded that mild traumatic brain injuries are significantly underdiagnosed and that early intervention is often neglected. Thus, early postinjury neuropsychological testing of individuals with mild closed brain injuries with the focus on attention/concentration, speed of information processing, memory, executive functions, and integration with the clinical history can provide a sound and well-directed program for gradual return to preinjury activities. Mittenberg, Tremont, Zielinski, Fichera, and Rayls (1996) provide initial data suggesting that recommendations based upon neuropsychological principles can reduce excess morbidity in this diagnostic group.

The richness of neuropsychological data generated by the rehabilitation neuropsychologist provides a basis for formulating constructive recommendations for enriching occupational and physical therapy. For example, for the uninsightful construction worker with left neglect who wants to return to work immediately, the occupational therapist can be asked to generate activities such as picking up nails that have been spilled on the ground. The practical impact of literally not picking up a substantial portion of the nails can contribute to acceptance of the idea that it is too early to return to work. The physical therapist might be asked to have the same patient carry empty boxes either on rough terrain or through storage areas in order to receive immediate environmental feedback on left neglect. Neuropsychological data on cognitive functions should thus be directly translated into practical interventions that can be accomplished around the hospital environment in order to render therapy meaningful to the individual and to affect insight. An important role of rehabilitation neuropsychology is to work with patients and treatment team members to translate recommendations based upon neuropsychological data into interventions that will ultimately apply to the patient's day-to-day life. For example, memory compensation systems that are utilized with the patient during the middle to the end of the rehabilitative course should be those that the patient is most likely to utilize after discharge (e.g., a day planner).

In the rehabilitation setting, neuropsychological evaluations can yield documentation of persistent problems with underarousal and difficulties in sustaining attention for even brief periods of time. Such data may readily contribute to the recommendation that the patient be evaluated for hydrocephalus or possibly treated with an activating medication. It is not unreasonable to recommend that patients who demonstrate persistent problems with slowed information processing speed and attentional compromise be considered for a trial with a medicine that has activating properties. Treatment based upon such recommendations can result in patient reports of gains in the ability to attend to activities (e.g., lectures) or in their ability to concentrate during the workday.

In the rehabilitation setting it is always important to make sure that cognitive strengths are used to enhance compensation. For example, patients with better preservation of visual memory will tend to profit from reviewing the charts, diagrams, and illustrations in textbooks more than they might have before. Their better preserved visual memories can provide more accessible cues for facilitating recall of the material. Better preserved processing of auditory–verbal information will lead to recommendations that textbooks be recorded for the student (a service that can be accessed in many states) or that recordings of lectures be reviewed rather than just lecture notes.

Neuropsychological test data also need to be carefully considered when generating specific recommendations for making psychotherapy sessions more effective. Some patients will benefit from having one of the products of the therapy session be a written outline of both the content and strategies for problem solving that were discussed during the treatment session. Many patients benefit from marking their day planners to perform activities in conjunction with following up on therapy. Many patients will also benefit from the development of a strategy section in their day planner so that they can access coping or self-control–related strategies when they need to review them.

Neuropsychological Consultation in Regard to Learning Disabilities

In the neuropsychological assessment of learning disabilities, extensive and careful premorbid history taking is extremely important. When considering the possibility of a persisting learning disability in an adult, the neuropsychologist needs to carefully consider the role of variables such as level of intelligence and the impact that the patient's level of motivation has had on his or her functioning over time. Whether success in education was valued and supported in the family of origin needs to be considered. In the course of history taking, the rehabilitation neuropsychologist must be cognizant of the different types of learning disabilities and how they may be manifested during the developmental process. The interviewing neuropsychologist needs to be alert to the fact that a learning disability may be a manifestation of a very specific neuropsychological deficit in the context of average or above-average intellectual abilities. Obtaining school records yields a time-sequenced method of tracking academic achievement relative to other data that may exist. The neuropsychologist needs to consider the economic status of the family in which the patient was raised to determine whether family resources might have helped to mitigate the detrimental impact of the learning disability on functioning in school and society.

The possibility of a history of learning disability should always be considered when assessing the impact of other conditions on individuals. For example, it is not unusual to observe that individuals who are able to effectively compensate for mild dyslexia can no longer do so following moderate to severe closed head trauma. Identifying that the patient had a learning disability for which he or she can no longer effectively compensate may be an extremely important contribution to formulating a rehabilitation plan and keeping the patient invested in the rehabilitation process. Many patients who had been treated for preexisting developmental disabilities of one form or another present as more resistant in rehabilitative treatment because the rehabilitative process reactivates unpleasant memories of failure and feelings of being scrutinized. When assessing patients who are referred for a neuropsychological evaluation of other conditions, the clinician needs to be alert for a premorbid history of difficulties that would point to a preinjury learning disability.

When considering learning disabilities, the neuropsychologist needs to be alert to any history of insults that the patient may have sustained while in utero (e.g., fetal alcohol syndrome, cocaine use by the mother). Interviews discussing when the individual was developmentally ready to go to school, difficulties that arose during the individual's early years of schooling, and other important issues should be completed when possible. How the individual progressed physically within the cultural and athletic milieu in which he or she was raised needs to be considered. Also to be considered are conditions for which the patient was treated by his or her pediatrician and any medications that were utilized chronically during the patient's childhood.

Individuals with residual attention-deficit disorder have neuropsychological test scores that reflect an inability to consistently attend and concentrate. This may cause some variability on tests related to other abilities, but the other abilities will basically remain intact. Failure to attend to and process information may interfere with learning, but once material is learned it tends to be retrievable (Orsini, Van Gorp, & Boone, 1988). The inability to consistently attend that is documented on testing often tends to be logically consistent with the developmental history that is obtained during the interview. Such individuals can benefit from coaching on study skill strategies, cognitive behavioral psychotherapy, and possibly treatment with medications.

The assessment of learning disabilities in adults calls for neuropsychological expertise in comparing performances on achievement tests to performances on tests of other abilities. Neuropsychological assessment calls for detailed pattern analysis of test results and integration with the history provided by the patient and historical records where possible. In the assessment of residual learning disabilities it is not possible to rely on the simple overgeneralization that verbal IQ is always reduced relative to performance IQ (Orsini et al., 1988). There are specific subtypes of learning disabilities that need to be considered, including nonverbal learning disability and phonologic processing disabilities. Rourke (2005) describes nonverbal learning disability as being characterized by well-developed single-word reading and spelling in contrast to arithmetic ability. Socially, nonverbal learning disability includes better processing of verbal than nonverbal input. Phonologic processing disabilities include poorly developed single-word reading and spelling relative to arithmetic. Rourke (2005) describes this group as making better use of nonverbal than verbal information in a social context.

Conclusion

In this chapter we have focused on neuropsychological assessment, with an emphasis on inpatient rehabilitation. The field of neuropsychology in rehabilitation is faced with a number of challenges. First, the ecologic validity of neuropsychometric tests needs to be established in the future. Particularly in the area of attention and executive functioning, it is important that the test scores predict day-to-day functioning. Second, rehabilitation neuropsychology needs to emphasize cognitive remediation. Future research will need to match patterns of deficits with compensation techniques. Again, these cognitive rehabilitation techniques need to be functionally oriented. However, remediation can start out with specific tasks for which bridging tasks for day-to-day activities are developed. Third, the interaction among cognitive, emotional, and physical functioning needs to be carefully established. For example, different pain management treatments that incorporate physical and emotional components need to be developed for patients with brain injury. Fourth, rehabilitation psychologists need to expand their services for patients' family members to help them make adjustments.

References

American Psychiatric Association. (1994). *Diagnostic and statistical manual of mental disorders* (4th ed.). Washington, DC: American Psychiatric Association.

Baddeley, A. (1986). *Working memory.* New York: Oxford University Press.

Benton, A. L., Hamsher, K. de S., & Sivan, A. B. (1994). *Multilingual aphasia examination.* Iowa City, IA: AJA.

Buschke, H., & Fuld, P. (1974). Evaluating storage, retention and retrieval in disordered memory and learning. *Neurology, 11,* 1019–1025.

Bush, S. S., Ruff, R. M., Tröster, A. I., Barth, J. T., Koffler, S. P., Pliskin, N. H., et al. (2005). Symptom validity assessment: Practice issues and medical necessity. (NAN Policy & Planning Committee). *Archives of Clinical Neuropsychology, 20,* 419–426.

Delis, D. C., Kramer, J. H., Kaplan, E., & Ober, B. A. (1987). *California verbal learning test manual.* New York: Psychological Corporation.

Gronwall, D. M. A., & Sampson, H. (1974). *The psychological effects of concussion.* Auckland, New Zealand: Auckland University Press/Oxford University Press.

Jones-Gotman, M., & Milner, B. (1977). Design fluency: The invention of nonsense drawings after focal cortical lesions. *Neuropsychologia, 15,* 653–672.

Kahneman, D., & Treisman, A. (1984). *Changing views of attention and automaticity.* In R. Parasuraman & D.R. Davies (Eds.), *Varieties of attention* (pp. 29–61). Orlando, FL: Academic Press.

Kiernan, F.J., Mueller, J., Langston, J.W., & Van Dyke, C. (1987). The neurobehavioral cognitive status examination. *Annals of Internal Medicine, 107,* 481–485.

Kornhuber, H.H. (1984). Attention, readiness for action, and the stages of voluntary decision: Some electrophysiological correlates in man. In O. Creutzfeldt, R.F. Schmidt, & W.D. Willis (Eds.), *Sensory-Motor Integration in the Nervous System: International symposium held on the occasion of the 80th birthday of Sir John Eccles* (pp. 420–429). New York: Springer-Verlag.

Levin, H.S., O'Donnell, V.M., & Grossman, R.G. (1979). The Galveston Orientation and Amnesia Test: A practical scale to assess cognition after head injury. *Journal of Nervous and Mental Disease, 167,* 675–684.

Lezak, M. (1995). *Neuropsychological assessment* (3rd ed.). New York: Oxford University Press.

Lezak, M., Howieson, D.B., & Loring, D.W. (2004). *Neuropsychological assessment* (4th ed.). New York: Oxford University Press.

Mittenberg, W., Tremont, G., Zielinski, R., Fichera, S., & Rayls, K. (1996). Cognitive-behavioral prevention of postconcussion syndrome. *Archives of Clinical Neuropsychology, 11,* 139–145.

National Institutes of Health. (1998). *NIH Consensus Development Conference on the Rehabilitation of Persons with Traumatic Brain Injury.* Bethesda, MD: Author.

Neumann, O. (1984). Automatic processing: A review of recent findings and a plea for an old theory. In W. Prinz & A.F. Sanders (Eds.), *Cognition and motor processes* (pp. 255–293). Berlin, Germany: Springer-Verlag.

Niemann, H., Ruff, R.M., & Kramer, J.H. (1996). An attempt towards differentiating attentional deficits in traumatic brain injury. *Neuropsychology Review, 6,* 11–46.

Norman, D., & Shallice, T. (1986). *Attention to action: Willed and automatic control of behavior* (Technical Report No. 99). Center for Human Information Processing. Reprinted in revised form in Davidson, R.J., Schwartz, G.E., & Shapiro, D. (Eds.), *Consciousness and self-regulation* (Vol. 4). New York: Plenum Press.

Orsini, D.L., Van Gorp, W.G., & Boone, K.B. (1988). *Adult presentation of learning disorders.* New York: Springer-Verlag.

Pendleton, M., & Heaton, R. (1982). A Comparison of the Wisconsin Card Sorting Test and the Category Test. *Journal of Clinical Psychology, 38,* 392–396.

Posner, M.I. (1975). Psychobiology of attention. In M.S. Gazzaniga & C. Blakemore (Eds.), *Handbook of psychobiology* (pp. 441–811). New York: Academic Press.

Raskin, S.A., &. Mateer, C.A. (2000). *Neuropsychological management of mild traumatic brain injury.* New York: Oxford University Press..

Raven, J.C. (1960). *Guide to the standard progressive matrices.* London: H.K. Lewis.

Reitan, R.M., & Wolfson, D. (1993). *The Halstead-Reitan Neuropsychological Test Battery: Theory and clinical interpretation.* Tucson, AZ: Neuropsychology Press.

Rourke, B.P. (2005). Neuropsychology of learning disabilities: Past and future. *Learning Disability Quarterly, 28,* 111–114.

Ruff, R.M. (1996). *Ruff Figural Fluency Test: Professional manual.* Odessa, FL: Psychological Assessment Resources.

Ruff, R.M., & Allen, C. (1996). *Ruff 2 and 7 Selective Attention Test: Professional manual.* Odessa, FL: Psychological Assessment Resources.

Ruff, R.M., & Allen, C. (1999). *Ruff-Light Trail Learning Test: Professional manual.* Odessa, FL: Psychological Assessment Resources.

Ruff, R.M., Allen, C., Farrow, C., Niemann, H., & Wylie, T. (1994). Figural fluency: Differential impairment in patients with left versus right frontal lobe lesions. *Archives of Clinical Neuropsychology, 9,* 41–55.

Ruff, R.M., Evans, R., & Marshall, L. (1986). Impaired verbal and figural fluency after head injury. *Archives of Clinical Neuropsychology, 1,* 87–101.

Ruff, R.M., Light, R.H., & Parker, S.B. (1996a). Benton Controlled Oral Word Association Test: Reliability and updated norms. *Archives of Clinical Neuropsychology, 11,* 329–338.

Ruff, R.M., Light, R.H., Parker, S.B., & Levin, H.S. (1997). The psychological construct of word fluency. *Brain and Language, 57,* 394–405.

Ruff, R.M., Mueller, J., & Jurica, P.J. (1996b). Estimating premorbid functioning levels after traumatic brain injury. *Neurorehabilitation, 7,* 39–53.

Ruff, R.M., Niemann, H., Allen, C., Farrow, C., & Wylie, T. (1992). The Ruff 2 and 7 selective attention test: A neuropsychological application. *Perceptual and Motor Skills, 75,* 1311–1319.

Shallice, T. (2002) Fractionation of the supervisory system. In D.T. Stuss & R.T. Knight (Eds.), *Principles of the frontal lobe* (pp. 261–277). New York: Oxford University Press.

Shiffrin, R.M., & Schneider, W. (1977). Controlled and automatic human information processing: II. Perceptual learning, automatic attending, and a general theory. *Psychological Review, 84,* 127–190.

Shiffrin, R.M., & Schneider, W. (1984). Theoretical note: Automatic and controlled processing revisited. *Psychological Review, 91,* 269–276.

Sohlberg, M.M., & Mateer, C.A. (1989). *Introduction to cognitive rehabilitation: Theory and practice.* New York: Guilford Press.

Squire, L. (1987). *Memory and the brain.* New York: Oxford University Press.

Stuss, D. (1999, February). *Functions of the frontal lobes: A 10-year update.* Paper presented at the International Neuropsychological Society, 25th Annual Conference, Boston.

Stuss, D., & Benson, D.F. (1984). Neuropsychological studies of the frontal lobes. *Psychological Bulletin, 95,* 3–28.

Teasdale, G., & Jennett, B. (1974). Assessment of coma and impaired consciousness: A practical scale. *Lancet, 2,* 81–84.

Van Zomeren, A.H., & Van den Burg, W. (1985). Residual complaints of patients two years after severe head injury. *Journal of Neurology, Neurosurgery, and Psychiatry, 48,* 21–28.

Varney, N.R., & Roberts, R.J. (1999). *Mild head injury: Causes, evaluation and treatment.* Mahwah, New Jersey: L. Erlbaum Associates.

Wechsler, D. (1997). *Wechsler Memory Scale–III Manual.* New York: Psychological Corporation.

Chapter 12

Assessment of Work Behavior

Jeanne B. Patterson

The science of work behavior has been defined as the study of "the interdependence of the social–organizational structure, machine and system design, and worker characteristics" (Landy, 1989, p. 4). With employment the goal of many rehabilitation programs, it is critical for rehabilitation professionals to have knowledge of an individual's work-related strengths and limitations (e.g., stamina, ability to remain on task, ability to follow directions, ability to perform the tasks of a job). The results of work behavior assessments are most often used to predict an individual's ability to work successfully in one or more jobs and to identify rehabilitation services that may address work-related deficiencies.

The work behavior assessments addressed in this chapter vary in terms of the interdependence described by Landy (1989). For example, an assessment may indicate that an individual possesses the personal characteristics needed to maintain a job (e.g., acceptance of supervision, on-task behavior) but is unable to perform the task at the required speed due to the design of a machine. This, of course, highlights the importance of assistive technology and job accommodation/redesign, as well as the fact that an individual must develop competence in using any assistive devices prior to completing an assessment. Alternatively, an assessment may indicate that the individual possesses the requisite worker characteristics and can perform the job, but the assessment may not reflect the influence of the social–organizational structure of the work environment. This may be critical information for determining whether individuals with some types of disabilities (e.g., psychiatric disabilities, learning disabilities, mental retardation, or traumatic brain injuries) will succeed in a job. Landy (1989) identified three additional problems that must be considered: (a) compromised reliability due to insufficient time periods to observe variations in the target behaviors; (b) inability of the assessment to reflect the changing nature of some jobs; and (c) limitations on good objective measures for evaluating performance, although the job analysis forms the foundation for most objective measures of job performance. Many of these problems can be addressed by adhering to the principles recommended by the Commission on Vocational Evaluation and Work Adjustment (2006), which encompass the position statement of the Interdisciplinary Council on Vocational Evaluation and Assessment (Table 12.1; Smith et al., 1994). For example, an assessment of work behaviors should include behavioral observations as well as other tools and approaches with the information verified through alternative methods.

The approaches taken in assessing work behaviors vary with the type of disability, the functions impaired, and the purpose of the assessment. This chapter describes a broad spectrum of assessments ranging from behavioral checklists to on-the-job evaluations, all of which focus on work-related behaviors. Each of the assessments should be evaluated in terms of the interdependence and the problems noted by Landy (1989).

TABLE 12.1.
Guiding Principles

The following seven principles serve as guides to best practice across settings.

1. A variety of methods, tools, and approaches should be used to provide accurate vocational evaluation and assessments. A broad range of questions must be posed to determine what makes an individual, as well as his/her abilities and needs, unique. Separating an individual's attributes into categories, such as interest, aptitude, or learning style preferences, helps organize assessment.

2. Vocational evaluation and assessment information should be verified using different methods, tools, and approaches. Using alternative methods or approaches to validate findings can usually be achieved by the following:

    (a) Observing an individual's demonstrated or manifested behaviors, such as performances on actual work;

    (b) Using an individual's self-report or expressed statements; and/or

    (c) Administering some type of survey, inventory, structured interview, or test.

3. Behavioral observation is essential in any vocational assessment process. Behavioral observation (e.g., observing physical performance, social characteristics, interactions with people, and other aspects of the environment) occurs throughout the assessment process. The observation process:

    (a) can be informal or formal,

    (b) can occur in a variety of environments,

    (c) can be made by a variety of people, and

    (d) should be documented and presented in an objective, non-biased manner.

4. Vocational evaluation and assessment may be an ongoing and developmental process in career development. However, individuals, especially those with disabilities, may need evaluations/assessments of varying degrees given at different junctures over their career lifespan.

5. Vocational evaluation and assessment should be an integral part of larger service delivery systems. Vocational evaluation and assessment should be the basis for planning needed services, resources, and support. Therefore, it can be an integral part of the total service delivery system. Vocational evaluation and assessment information should be interpreted and conveyed to the consumer as well as others within the system.

6. Vocational evaluation and assessment requires the collection of input from a variety of individuals and requires an understanding of how to use the results of the assessment process. An interdisciplinary team approach allows for the effective use of information that can be translated into effective planning, implementation activities (e.g. placements, support service, counseling), and fulfilled vocational development for consumers.

7. Vocational evaluation and assessment should be current, valid, and relevant. Vocational evaluation and assessment is grounded in career, vocational, and work contexts.

Functional, Behavioral, and Physical Capacities Assessments

Terms such as *functional assessment, behavioral assessment, physical capacities assessment,* and *functional capacities assessment* have been used to describe the assessment of work behaviors. Although used interchangeably, each of these terms can have a different meaning depending on the context in which it is used or the professional group using the term. In addition to the use of different tests, Roberts (2005) noted that both the focus and number of domains included in a functional assessment vary by profession. For example, functional behavior assessments have been part of the Individuals with Disabilities Education Act (IDEA) and were included in the 2004 reauthorization of IDEA. In the context of special education, a "functional behavioral assessment" is an examination of problem behaviors within their environment in order to develop behavior intervention plans (Scott & Caron, 2005). In contrast, Geisser, Robinson, Miller, and Blade (2003) described a functional capacity evaluation in terms of a person's work ability as it relates to determining medical impairment ratings and restrictions on work-related activities. Halpern and Fuhrer (1984) defined functional assessment as "the measurement of purposeful behavior in interaction with the environment, which is interpreted according to the assessment's intended uses" (p. 3). Functional or behavioral assessments are often used in conjunction with traditional assessment approaches (e.g., interest and intelligence tests) to provide a more comprehensive view of an individual.

Behavior assessments, which can measure general or specific behaviors, include "checklists, rating scales, and surveys that measure observer's interpretations of behavior in relation to adaptive or social skills, functional skills, and appropriateness or dysfunction within settings/situations" (Buros Institute on Mental Measurements, 2006, p. 1). Advantages to using behavior assessments include that they are easy to use and they do not take a long time to complete. However, most behavior assessments require that the evaluator have some familiarity with the individual being evaluated. Most behavior rating scales attempt to link behaviors to specific social and situational or environmental settings, which is particularly important in identifying interventions that may be needed for transition planning or supported employment. An example of a functional capacity checklist is the *Functional Capacity Skill Checklist,* which is used for transition planning. It is used to assess a student's abilities in seven major areas: mobility (use of public transportation), communication (use of receptive written language), interpersonal skills (accepts supervision), self-direction (follows work rules), self-care (performs basic activities of daily living), work tolerance (has physical tolerance for the job), and work skills (can perform job duties). Each of the 36 items is rated on a 4-point scale ranging from *independent* to *inability to perform with accommodations or supports.* If accommodations or supports are required for any area of functional capacity, they are identified in a comments section. The checklist is part of the Transition Tool Box, available online (http://www.vesid.nysed.gov/specialed/transition/toolbox/home.html).

Power (2006) noted reliability, subjective item scoring, and limited transferability of ratings (i.e., "limited to the conditions under which a person functions") as major concerns with rating scales (p. 258). Examples of standardized measures that have been used to evaluate behavior and functional capacities include the *Minnesota Satisfactoriness Scales,* the *Becker Work Adjustment Profile,* the *Work Personality Profile–Professional Form,* the *Functional Assessment Inventory,* the *Preliminary Diagnostic Questionnaire,* and the *Joule Functional Capacity Evaluation System.*

Minnesota Satisfactoriness Scales

Developed at the University of Minnesota in 1960 and revised in 1966 and 1970, the *Minnesota Satisfactoriness Scales* (MSS; Gibson, Weiss, Dawis, & Lofquist, 1970) is an observer rating system based on the Minnesota Theory of Work Adjustment, a theory of vocational adjustment for people with disabilities (Szymanski, Enright, Hershenson, & Ettinger, 2003). Consisting of 28 items, the MSS is completed by the employer, who compares the worker with coworkers on a three-point scale (3 = *better than,* 2 = *about the same as,* 1 = *not as good as*). The MSS, which can be completed in about 5 minutes, has the following four subscales: Performance (e.g., quantity and quality of work output), Conformance (e.g., ability to follow rules), Personal Adjustment (e.g., degree to which personal problems may interfere with job performance), and Dependability (e.g., motivation and work habits). The last item on the MSS addresses the individual's overall competence in job performance by comparing the worker to other workers by quartile category (e.g., top fourth of the workers, bottom fourth of the workers). The authors report intercorrelations among the subscales, internal consistency reliabilities, and test-retest stability coefficients, all of which suggest that the MSS is a useful measure of satisfactoriness. Although norms are provided for four occupational groups, as well as a "workers-in-general" group, only those for the latter group should be used since the norms are more than 20 years old (Bolton, 1986).

The MSS is an excellent vocational counseling tool. For example, using the MSS to identify a worker's deficiencies can provide a starting point for future counseling sessions. Alternatively, the worker's self-assessment can be compared with the employer's or evaluator's assessment, with counseling sessions focusing on differences in ratings. The MSS is available from Vocational Psychology Research, N657 Elliott Hall, University of Minnesota, Minneapolis, MN 55455-0344; e-mail: vpr@tc.umn.edu.

Becker Work Adjustment Profile

The *Becker Work Adjustment Profile* (BWAP), developed by Ralph Becker in 1989, is a 63-item rating scale to identify work behavior deficits in persons with physical, mental, or emotional disabilities (Bolton, 1991; Li & Tsang, 2002). The BWAP, which takes 20–25 minutes to complete, uses a 5-point rating scale for each of the items. The four subscales of the BWAP are Work Habits and Attitudes, Interpersonal Relations, Cognitive Skills, and Work Performance Skills. The sum of the four subscales produces a total score (Broad Work Adjustment). The raw scores can be converted to percentile equivalents, normalized *T*-scores, and stanines, using the standardization samples (i.e., mental retardation, physical disabilities, emotional disabilities, and learning disabilities). Favorable reliability and validity data are available for the BWAP. In his review of the BWAP, Bolton (1991) recommended disregarding the placement levels (e.g., competitive, transitional, sheltered) associated with various scores. Also, he discouraged use of the 32-item short form since it saves minimal time and half of the items for vocational competency are omitted. The BWAP is available from Elbern Publications, PO Box 9497, Columbus, OH 43209; telephone: (614) 235-2643.

Work Personality Profile

The *Work Personality Profile–Professional Form* (WPP-PF; Neath & Bolton, 2008) is an observational rating scale consisting of 58 work-related behaviors that represent specific job maintenance tasks (e.g., "asks for further instructions if task is not clear," "assumes assigned role in group tasks," "controls temper"). Designed for use in situational assessments after an individual has completed 1 week or 20 hours, the WPP-PF identifies deficiencies that if left unaddressed could be barriers to an individual gaining and sustaining employment. A 5–point scale is used to evaluate each of the work-related behaviors: 4 = *a definite strength, an employability asset;* 3 = *adequate performance, not a particular strength;* 2 = *performance inconsistent, potentially an employability problem;* 1 = *a problem area, will definitely limit the person's chance for employment;* and X = *no opportunity to observe the behavior.* The items reflect an individual's functioning on 11 rationally derived scales (e.g., amount of supervision required, work tolerance, social communication skills) and five factor scales (task orientation, social skills, work motivation, work conformance, and personal presentation). Scoring consists of adding the items within each of the 16 scales and averaging them, which produces a number from 1 to 4 for each of the scales. The WPP-PF is efficient; it takes 5–10 minutes to complete.

A companion version of the WPP-PF (i.e., *Self-Report Version,* WPP-SR), which can be completed by the individual at the same time the WPP-PF is completed by the evaluator, was introduced in 1992 to facilitate consumer involvement in the evaluation and planning process. Consisting of the same 58 items, the WPP-SR can be used as (a) a discussion tool with the consumer (e.g., discussing similarities and differences in the evaluator's scores and the consumer's scores) and (b) as an educational tool to sensitize consumers to critical work behaviors. Because the WPP-SR requires a 7th-grade reading level, an audiotape version must be used with individuals who read at a 6th-grade level or below (Neath & Bolton, 2008).

New features of the WPP-PF and WPP-SR include the *Work Personality Profile and Computer Report* (WPP-CR; Neath & Bolton, 2008), which scores both the WPP-PF and WPP-SR on the 16 scales and compares the individual's work behaviors with the normative group, the behaviors of the job under consideration, and the evaluator and individual's ratings. Also, it includes a job matching feature that identifies 18 entry-level positions that are consistent with the individual's work behaviors. If the individual does not demonstrate the required work behaviors, both behavioral and environmental interventions are provided.

The normative samples for the WPP-PF included 243 individuals at three rehabilitation centers and 181 individuals from another rehabilitation center. Information on the reliability and validity of the WPP-PF is included in the manual. The *Work Personality Profile and Computer Report* is available from PRO-ED, Inc., 8700 Shoal Creek Boulevard, Austin, TX 78757-6897 (http://www.proedinc.com).

Functional Assessment Inventory

The purpose of the *Functional Assessment Inventory* (FAI) is to assist counselors in obtaining a comprehensive view of an individual with a disability prior to initiating rehabilitation planning. The FAI consists of 30 behavioral items ranging from physical capacities to work history and work habits. Each of the items is rated on a 4-point scale, ranging from 0 = *no significant impairment* to 4 = *severe impairment* as determined by the item. For example, a 4 related to "learning ability" indicates that the individual "is capable of learning only very simple tasks and then only with time and repetition," whereas a 4 rating in "endurance" would indicate that the individual is "unable to work for more than one or two hours a day (15 hours or less per week)" (Crewe & Athelstan, 1984, pp. 7, 17).

In addition to the 30 items, the FAI includes 10 items related to potential vocational strengths the individual possesses (e.g., "possesses a vocational skill that is in great demand") and two summary questions related to an overall assessment of severity of disability and likelihood that the individual can get and hold a job. The former is rated on a scale of 1 = *slightly* to 7 = *very severely,* whereas the last question is rated on a 4-point quartile scale (e.g., 1 = *poor,* 0–25%). The *Personal Capacities Questionnaire* (PCQ), a companion instrument to the FAI, has parallel items and is completed by the individual with a disability.

There are many advantages to using one or both of the instruments. First, the counselor must look beyond the presenting disability. Second, because of the parallel format, the counselor and individual can compare their results and discuss differences in ratings. Third, the items include more than physical functioning. As the authors note, "because employability depends on more than an individual's personal characteristics, the inventory also includes a number of social and environmental items" (e.g., the individual's desire to work, his or her ability to get along with supervisors and coworkers, and the amount of encouragement he or she receives from family and friends; Crewe & Athelstan, 1984, p. 6). In an investigation of the predictive ability of counselors' assessments of applicants' functional limitations on the rehabilitation services that were provided, Bellini, Bolton, and Neath (1998) significantly predicted all services, except counseling. The FAI and PCQ are available from the Stout

Vocational Rehabilitation Institute, PO Box 790, Menomonie, WI 54751-0790 (http://www.svri.uwstout.edu or fryer@uwstout.edu).

Preliminary Diagnostic Questionnaire

The *Preliminary Diagnostic Questionnaire* (PDQ), which combines elements of an interview with psychometric testing, provides information on an individual's functioning in five areas: (1) physical condition; (2) mental ability; (3) emotional condition; (4) attitude and motivation; and (5) social, economic, and personal condition (Moriarity, 1981). The PDQ takes about an hour to complete and includes the following eight sections, in addition to six demographic items that correlate with employment outcome:

1. Work Information: measures an individual's general knowledge about work through true/false items
2. Preliminary Estimate of Learning: provides an indication of the individual's intellectual ability
3. Psychomotor Skills: measures gross and fine motor abilities
4. Reading Ability: provides a measure of the individual's reading ability through a brief, orally administered test
5. Work Importance: measures an individual's attitudes toward work
6. Personal Independence: measures through self-report the individual's activities of daily living
7. Internality: measures the person's locus of control (internal or external)
8. Emotional Functioning: provides an indication of psychological pathology

In his review of the PDQ, Bolton (1992) indicated that the PDQ was adequately reliable and valid for its purpose. Among the noteworthy features identified by Bolton are administration and interpretation by the counselor and the provision of both clinical and psychometric information to the counselor. Although no longer in print, the PDQ is now available from the National Clearinghouse of Rehabilitation Training Materials (NCRTM), 6524 Old Main Hill, Utah State University, Logan, UT 84322 (http://ncrtm.ed.usu.edu/).

Physical Capacities Assessment

Physical capacities can be assessed through self-report or behavioral observation. If an employer requires the assessment prior to hiring an individual, behavioral observation usually is required. Depending on the nature of the job, the individual may be required to perform the essential duties of the job (e.g., moving objects weighing 40 pounds) in an evaluation setting.

There are alternative ways for evaluating physical capacities. For example, Ludlow (1990) described a Physical Capacities Assessment based on the 20 physical capacities (also referred to as physical demands) that are part of any job analysis (i.e., strength, climbing, balancing, stooping, kneeling, crouching, crawling, reaching, handling, fingering, feeling, talking, hearing, tasting/smelling, near vision acuity, far vision acuity, depth perception, accommodation, color vision, and field of vision). Ludlow (1990) identified assessment methods for each of these capacities; for instance, handling can be assessed through the *Bennett Hand-Tool Dexterity Test* (Bennett, 1965), and fingering can be assessed with the *Purdue Pegboard* (Tiffin, 1968). When the evaluation question relates to an individual's ability to tolerate a workday, Costello (1991) recommended observing and documenting fatigue at least three times a day but cautioned that the task, interest level, and time of day should always be noted since individuals may have more energy late in the day if they are involved with an interesting task. Also, he recommended recording the amount of time the individual stands and sits. The primary rule in performing a physical capacities assessment is this: "If there is any doubt at all regarding the subject's ability to perform [the assessment tasks,] then the tasks should not be undertaken" (Ludlow, 1990, p. 61). Even with the number of standardized measures that are now available, there is often a risk of reinjury or exacerbation of an existing condition in performing a physical capacities assessment.

Another example of a physical capacities assessment is the *Functional Capacity Checklist* (FCC; Elliott & Fitzpatrick, 2006). The FCC is a self-report instrument consisting of 165 items that correspond to the physical demands noted in the *Dictionary of Occupational Titles* (DOT) and *Classification of Jobs,* as well as items related to self-care. The primary purpose of the FCC is for use in forensic rehabilitation or Social Security hearings since the individual compares functioning preinjury and postinjury on a 6-point scale (e.g., 0 = *I don't know,* 1 = *No Change* to 4 = *very difficult to do* and 5 = *impossible to do or can do only with great pain*). Using hand or computer scoring, the FCC can be used to (a) identify items by function (e.g., walking); (b) level of difficulty, ranging from 5 (impossible) to 1 (no change); or (c) level of difficulty within each of the functions (e.g., screwing a lid off a jar versus changing a light bulb in a ceiling fixture). The FCC and companion software are available from E & F Incorporated, 1135 Cedar Shoals Drive, Athens, GA 30605 (http://www.elliottfitzpatrick.com/).

The other end of the continuum in terms of physical capacities assessment is represented by the *Joule Functional Capacity Evaluation* (FCE) *System* (VALPAR, 2006d), which was introduced in 1999. Managed by Windows-based software, the Joule System includes 10 mandatory protocols (core lifts, unilateral carry, bilateral carry, push/pull, grip, squatting, balance, stair climbing, sustained midlevel reach, and sustained elevated reach) and 11 optional protocols (custom lifts, ladder climb, sit, stand, walk, kneel, crawl, crouch, pinch, repetitive foot motion, and hand coordination). The Joule System uses racks that can be adjusted based on the height of an individual's waist, mid-shin, and eyes. The FCE can be completed in one 4-hour day or more days, depending on the needs of the consumer. Scoring is based on the observable behaviors as well as the consumer's reports. The individual responds to questions related to symptoms, perceived exertion, and perceived safety at several points during each of the protocols. The evaluator classifies the subjective reports into one of three classifications: (1) meaningful—the reporting of specific, timely information, which is consistent with the individual's diagnosis, the activity, and the individual's body mechanics; (2) relevant—although the information is considered valid, it is less specific and may not be timely, which results in the information being viewed as adjunct information; and (3) extraneous—the information is considered "useless," because of its lack of specificity or lack of correspondence to the diagnosis or the activity, and may contradict the objective performance. When the information is viewed as extraneous, it is not used in determining the individual's functional capacities (VALPAR, 2006d).

The Joule System was designed to address a number of deficiencies that exist in other types of functional capacity evaluations (e.g., psychophysical, kinesiophysical), such as who controls the test, the use of objective or subjective information, fatigue factors in terms of sequencing of tests, and safety considerations. The software has a "task logic sequence," which the evaluator can use in designing a protocol for a particular job, as well as the ability to automatically produce customized reports. The Joule System combines these elements by utilizing both the evaluator's and consumer's observations. Some follow-up studies with high interrater reliability have been completed; however, additional research is planned (VALPAR, 2006d). Cost will be a primary factor for organizations that are considering the Joule System. Joule is available from the corporate office of VALPAR International, PO Box 5767, Tucson, AZ 85703 (http://www.valparint.com).

Transferable Skill Assessments/ Job Matching

Transferable skills are those skills that have been used on one job and can be applied to alternative jobs. Therefore, the use of transferable skills for job matching purposes is most applicable to individuals who have a work history. Many of the programs that are termed *job matching* use a transferable skills approach in identifying possible jobs. One of the challenges in using transferable skills has been the decision to no longer update DOT job analyses and move to O★NET. This means balancing the limited number and type of job analyses included in the O★NET (see Chapter 13) with the lack of updated information in the DOT. The Social Security Disability Determination process, as well as some insurance companies and state workers' compensation programs, use the DOT or the *Enhanced Dictionary of Occupational Titles* (eDOT) to address transferable skills (Economic Research Institute, 2006; Truthan & Karman, 2003).

There are advantages and disadvantages to a transferable skills analysis. According to Dunn (2004), "because it is based upon observable, objective work histories, the results are less likely to be skewed by cultural biases, test anxiety, or effects of disability than work samples or psychometric tests" (p. 49). Disadvantages include the quality of the information, inability to identify alternate talents, and the possibility of misinterpreting an individual's work history (Dunn, 2004). Three transferable skills assessment programs are described: *Vocational Diagnosis and Assessment of Residual Employability,* the *Occupational Access System,* and Job Browser Pro and SkillTRAN online services.

Vocational Diagnosis and Assessment of Residual Employability

The *Vocational Diagnosis and Assessment of Residual Employability* (VDARE) system was developed to identify residual employability potential (e.g., transferable skills). Although the VDARE was originally developed for use in providing expert testimony in disability adjudication cases, it can be used as a tool for vocational counseling (Havranek, Field, & Grimes, 2005). The VDARE process includes the following steps:

- Listing the relevant jobs held by an individual
- Identifying the DOT codes for each job
- Recording the worker trait factors and identifying a Work Field code
- Generating the Pre-Vocational Profile by recording "the worker trait code which reflects the highest level of functioning for each trait respectively, across the total work history" (Havranek, Field, & Grimes, 2005, p. 9)
- Identifying the Residual Functional Capacity Profile by determining the changes in functioning that result from the disability
- Reviewing similar or related jobs by (a) maintaining the same first digit of the DOT code and same Work Field code and (b) identifying only jobs that involve no more than the worker trait requirements of the Residual Functional Capacity Profile
- Evaluating the availability of the potential jobs within the local labor market

When VDARE is used in vocational planning, the counselor and individual may identify alternative jobs, including previously performed jobs or jobs in which the individual has expressed an interest. Or, the results may indicate types of rehabilitation services that are needed for the individual to return to work.

The validity and reliability of the VDARE approach is based on (a) the accuracy of the database (Sax, 1979), (b) the accuracy of job-specific information provided by the individual, and (c) the skills of the counselor in determining the functional changes resulting from the disability and/or identifying whether additional information is needed and how to acquire that information. McCroskey et al. (1979) indicated that individuals skilled in using the VDARE process worksheet should be able to complete the assessment in 30–45 minutes or less. The *Transferability of Work Skills Worksheet* used in the VDARE process is available from E & F Publishing, 1135 Cedar Shoals Drive, Athens, GA 30605 (http://www.elliottfitzpatrick.com/).

Occupational Access System

The *Occupational Access System* (OASYS; Brown, McDaniel, & Couch, 1994) is a computerized approach to the transferable skills assessment described in the VDARE process. All of the required databases are part of the program. The process begins when an individual's work history is entered. (If the individual has no work history, test data can be used to build the file on the individual.) One of the advantages to having the OASYS databases is that the counselor does not need to know the DOT codes and job titles because he or she can view a list of similar jobs from the DOT or look at job titles by industry to select the appropriate title. After all of the jobs have been entered, the individual's profile is available. This is comparable to viewing the Pre-Vocational Profile of the VDARE. In the next step, the counselor can make any adjustments. The initial screen for adjusting the profile allows the counselor to view the screen in an abbreviated (coded) format or with a full narrative description, which is very helpful for individuals who are learning to use the transferable skills approach and who have not learned all of the coding used in describing physical demands, specific vocational preparation, educational skills, environmental conditions, work situations, work activities, aptitudes, and data-people-things work functions.

The next step involves a job search based on four different types of skill transfer. The Primary Skill Transfer approach searches the DOT database for jobs that have the identical Work Fields and Materials, Products, Subject Matter and Services (MPSMS) codes. The codes for Work Fields address the Machines, Tools, Equipment, and Work Aids (MTEWA) or the socioeconomic purpose of the work. The Secondary Skill Transfer searches the DOT database for jobs with similar MTEWA and MPSMS codes, whereas the Composite search includes all of the jobs from the Primary and Secondary Skill transfer. The final search, the Extended Worker Trait, searches the entire DOT database of job titles on other factors but ignores the MTEWA and MPSMS codes. OASYS has a Focused Search option that allows one to conduct DOT searches by job families. The Employer Job Bank, an optional item available for an additional cost, allows the counselor to use the Focused Search Option to search by Standard Industrial Classification codes, ZIP codes, or wage ranges.

Although computerized systems are much more expensive than noncomputerized systems, the four databases available with OASYS are a particularly attractive feature of this program. For example, the DOT database includes the DOT title, code number, occupational group arrangement, occupational aptitude patterns, work fields (MTEWA), MPSMS, industry codes, Guide for Occupational Exploration (GOE) codes, Census codes, Standard Occupational

Classification codes, Holland codes, Specific Vocational Preparation, aptitudes, General Educational Development (GED) levels, 14 environmental factors, 20 physical demands, situation codes, and data–people–things codes.

In the database of national and state wage estimates and employment projections and postsecondary training, any additions, deletions, or changes in job analysis are updated at least annually. New 2006 additions to the OASYS include three job search web crawlers (i.e., by right clicking on any job title, one can select "open jobs" and search for job ads on the web for any specified geographic area (B. Chapman, personal communication, May 29, 2007). Comprehensiveness and versatility are major strengths of the OASYS (Brown, MDaniel, & Couch, 1994). The OASYS is available from VERTEK, Inc., 12835 Bel-Red Road, Suite 212, Bellevue, WA 98005 (http://www.vertekinc.com/VERTEKWEB/homepage2.html).

Job Browser Pro and SkillTRAN Online Services

Job Browser Pro was one of the first computerized transferable skills analysis programs that used the DOT database to assess transferability based on MPSMS and MTEWA codes. The initial programs and services were available from a mainframe computer in Spokane, Washington, which allowed them to be accessed by any type of personal computer (Brown et al., 1994). The current version of *Job Browser Pro* is a Windows-compatible software program useful for career counseling, occupational exploration, reference, and "lightweight" transferable skills analyses. In order to adhere to the Social Security definition of transferability, Job Browser Pro uses Work Field, Specific Vocational Preparation (SVP), and MPSMS. Updated via an annual online subscription, *Job Browser Pro* includes the full DOT, all worker characteristics, Department of Labor (DOL) updates through 1998 (the last time DOL updated the DOT), cross-references to all other popular coding systems (including O*NET, SOC, and Census codes), and an extensive array of Labor Market Information (LMI) (i.e., the complete *Occupational Outlook Handbook* [OOH], Census-based national employment numbers and wage data, and Occupational Employment Survey (OES) employment numbers and wages nationally, statewide, and for each reportable Metropolitan/Micropolitan area). *Job Browser Pro* has many easy ways to look up occupations (including by Holland code) and LMI and can generate reports for an occupation for job analysis and career exploration.

SkillTRAN Online Services is the more powerful program, which is changing from a classic text-based format to an easy-to-use, secure, Web-based application accessible via the internet by PC and Macintosh computers. In addition to offering online services for transferable skills analysis, *SkillTRAN Online Services* include searches by interests and industry. *Pre-Injury/Post-Injury Analysis* (PREPOST) conducts 8 transferable skills analysis searches simultaneously to calculate percentage of occupational loss for use in forensic rehabilitation. All SkillTRAN reports can be supplemented with LMI, including long-term employment projections, employment numbers and wages, and 15+ million business listings (updated quarterly) for Labor Market Survey. *SkillTRAN Online Services* also includes access through a common, simple interface to 5.5 million current job openings, aggregated from daily visits to 170,000+ Web sites and job boards. Individuals can purchase a single transferable skills analysis or an annual subscription to the online service.

Job Browser Pro and *SkillTRAN Online Services* are available from Skill-TRAN LLC, 3910 S. Union Court, Spokane Valley, WA 99206 (http://www.skilltran.com).

Work Samples

Work samples tend to be appealing to individuals because the individual "performs actual portions (or simulations) of jobs or training curricula, using the same materials, tools, and equipment that are utilized in the real work or training setting" (Corthell & Griswold, 1987, p. 58). Costello (1991) identified four types of work samples:

1. *Applied job samples:* The machines, equipment, tools, work aids, and materials used in the work sample are the same as those used on the job.
2. *Simulated work samples:* These work samples are more general than applied job samples because they relate to occupational traits rather than specific job requirements.
3. *Single-trait work samples:* These work samples investigate a single trait or characteristic.
4. *Cluster-trait work samples:* Many of the commercial work sample systems utilize this approach, with the work sample containing a number of traits that are related to a job or jobs.

Botterbusch (2005) identified a number of advantages and disadvantages of work samples. One major advantage is that the client's motivation is usually enhanced due to the face validity of the work sample (i.e., the work sample looks like an actual job). Also, performance standards are almost identical to actual jobs. Other advantages include (a) relatively shortened time period to collect occupational information; (b) standardized means of observing behavior and personality; and (c) reduced cultural, literacy, and communication problems associated with other work assessments. Limited studies on reliability, concurrent and predictive validity, and norms are one of the major disadvantages of work samples. Other disadvantages noted by Botterbusch (2005) include the inability of work samples to duplicate environmental, social, customer service, and problem-solving issues. "Fumes, noise, smells, poor lighting, close contacts with co-workers, and the constant presence of supervisors are difficult to simulate" and work samples cannot "measure how a consumer will deal with a misplaced order [or] a request for technical assistance" (p. 294). The cost of commercial work samples can be another disadvantage. To circumvent this problem, some evaluators develop their own work samples that are representative of jobs in their area. However, reliability and validity can still be problematic. The following systems are reviewed in this section: *Microcomputer Evaluation of Careers and Academics* (MECA), *Vocational Interest, Temperament, and Aptitude System* (VITAS), *Talent Assessment Program* (TAP), the *McCarron-Dial Evaluation System,* and systems developed or distributed by VALPAR and Jewish Employment and Vocational Services.

Microcomputer Evaluation of Careers and Academics

The MECA system (MECA, 2006), which is marketed specifically for transition assessments, includes six components, of which one is work samples. These work samples address 20 career areas, such as automotive technology, building maintenance, computer graphics, horticulture, office technology, and health care. There are three levels to each work sample, which represent a range of skill levels from entry level to advanced level. For example, in health care, at entry level an individual may learn to wrap an arm with an elastic bandage, whereas in the advanced level the individual would learn to take a pulse and blood pressure. It takes about 30 minutes to complete each work sample, which uses full video and audio and is available in Spanish and English for both Windows and Macintosh. Using multimedia technology with more than 2,000 video clips contained on a CD, the program includes both an audio option and still text to address the needs of individuals with limited reading skills or hearing impairments. Individuals are provided with appropriate hand tools to accompany the work samples.

In addition to the work samples, the total MECA system includes an interest indicator, learning assessment programs (assesses math, communication, and problem solving), career planners with occupational information, personal responsibility (includes 14 assessments and 60 hours of activities to achieve needed skills), and a success profiler (includes assessment and skills focusing on change, leadership, learning, sensitivity, teamwork, and violence prevention).

The MECA is available from the Conover Company, 2926 Hidden Hollow Road, Oshkosh, WI 54904 (http://www.conovercompany.com/Products/MECA/MECA.htm).

VITAS

The research and development component of Jewish Employment and Vocational Services (JEVS) is the Vocational Research Institute, which has developed a number of work samples and computerized assessments over the years, including the *Vocational Interest, Temperament, and Aptitude System* (VITAS). VITAS, which can be administered in 2.5 days, includes 21 work samples that represent Work Groups in the GOE. Although most of the samples do not require reading, any written material does not exceed the 6th-grade level. The VITAS is useful in comparing work quality and production speed against adult and/or adolescent norms since performance on each work sample is scored according to time to complete the task and number of errors. Examples of the 21 work samples, which range from packing matchbooks to completing laboratory assistant tasks, are provided in Table 12.2.

VITAS may be purchased in "clusters" if the entire system is not needed or a more narrow focus of jobs is to be assessed. Four clusters (Technology Cluster, Clerical-Business Detail, Mechanical Industrial I, and Mechanical Industrial II) are available, with each cluster consisting of 5–10 interrelated samples. For example, the Technology Cluster, which represents four Work Groups (02.04 Lab Technology; 05.03 Engineering Technology; 05.05 Craft Technology; and 06.01 Production Technology), includes the following work samples: Collating Material Samples, Nail and Screw Sorting I, Nail and Screw Sorting II, Pipe Assembly, Lock Assembly, Circuit Board Inspection, Spot Welding, Drafting, and Laboratory Assistant. The time range for completing the clusters is from 3 to 6 hours, depending on the cluster and the individual's work rate. A major limitation of the VITAS is the lack of reliability and validity data (Brown et al., 1994; Kauppi, 1988). Also, Kauppi noted that the VITAS should not be used in isolation since it addresses only 4 of the 12 interest areas in the GOE. VITAS is available from Instructional Technology Inc., PO Box 2056, Easton, MD 21601; 800/274-6832 (http://www.intecinc.net/prod_vri.htm).

Talent Assessment Program

The *Talent Assessment Program* (TAP; 2006) consists of 10 tests, requires no reading, and allows up to 20 individuals to be assessed in 1 day. Instructions can be provided verbally, in writing, signed, or demonstrated. The TAP computer program provides correlation between the individual's demonstrated abilities and jobs in the DOT and the Department of Labor data. The TAP Windows-based software allows for the inclusion of assessment results from other tests.

The 10 TAP tests assess (a) visualization and retention (i.e., form and spatial perception [Test 1], ability to follow flow patterns [Test 9], and retention

TABLE 12.2.
Examples of VITAS Work Samples

- Nuts, bolts, and washers assembly
- Tile sorting and weighing
- Collating material samples
- Pressing linens
- Working as a bank teller

of form and specific details [Test 10]); (b) Discrimination (i.e., fine discrimination [Test 2], color discrimination [Test 3], and tactile discrimination [Test 4]), and (c) Dexterity (i.e., fine motor control [Test 5], manual dexterity [Test 6], quality performance with small tools [Test 7], and ability to use large tools [Test 8]).

Easy to use, TAP is contained in three carrying cases. TAP is available from Talent Assessment Inc., PO Box 5087, Jacksonville, FL 32247-5087 (http://www.talentassessment.com/programs_tap.php).

McCarron-Dial Evaluation System

Originally designed for individuals with neurological disabilities, the *McCarron-Dial Evaluation System* (MDS, 2006) can be used with individuals with most types of disabilities to assess factors that predict an individual's level of community employment/placement. The MDS, which is contained in briefcases, includes a battery of tests to assess five factors: (1) Verbal–Cognitive (language, learning ability, and achievement); (2) Sensory (perceiving and experiencing the environment); (3) Motor (muscle strength, speed and accuracy of movement, balance and coordination); (4) Emotional (response to interpersonal and environmental stress); and (5) Integration–Coping (adaptive behavior). The tests include many commercially available tests, such as the *Peabody Picture Vocabulary Test, Bender Visual Motor Gestalt Test, Emotional Behavior Checklist, Behavior Rating Scale, Observational Emotional Inventory, Haptic Visual Discrimination Test,* and *McCarron Assessment of Neuromuscular Development* (MAND). The MAND includes a hand dynamometer and other components to measure fine and gross motor functions. Other tests that are not included in the system can be used in the assessment process (e.g., the *Wechsler Intelligence Scales, Street Survival Skills,* and other achievement and memory tests). Although the basic battery can be completed in 3 hours, the comprehensive battery may take as long as 5 days since it includes the supplemental tests and a 10–hour observation period.

Only trained personnel are allowed to administer the MDS. Norms are available for most of the instruments that compose the MDS. Brown et al. (1994) identified the construct, concurrent, and predictive validity as a major strength of the MDS, although not all reviewers agree with this assessment (e.g., Solly, 1994). However, both Brown and Solly noted that the MDS is not a true work sample but rather a comprehensive test battery. The MDS is available from McCarron-Dial Systems, Inc., PO Box 45628, Dallas, TX 75245 (http://www.mccarrondial.com).

VALPAR

Founded in 1973 as a provider of vocational evaluation services, VALPAR has developed a number of work samples and computer-based evaluations. Also, VALPAR distributes products manufactured by others (e.g., *Therapists' Por-*

table Assessment Lab). VALPAR uses a criterion-referenced approach to tie its systems to U.S. Department of Labor job standards. Also, VALPAR has analyzed most of its work samples using Methods-Time-Measurement (MTM) standards, which is an approach to analyzing tasks to determine how long it would take an experienced employee to repeatedly perform the exercise over an 8-hour workday (Christopherson, 1995). The work rate allows an individual to compare his or her performance with that of an experienced worker in the applicable work field. As Brown et al. (1994) pointed out, "this should give an excellent indication of the individual's level of performance in reference to what would be expected in the real world of work. It could also be used as a measure of one's progress toward an acceptable performance following additional education, practice, or adjustment training" (p. 55). A rate of work score is obtained by dividing an individual's performance time by the MTM standard. For example, if the MTM standard is 600 seconds and it takes an individual 800 seconds to perform the task, the MTM rate of work score is 75%. To "pass," an individual must achieve at least an 87.5% rate of work score. Because the work score is a comparison of the individual being tested with a well-trained employee and does not address improvement based on experience, VALPAR conducted a series of learning curve studies in the early 1990s. The calculated learning curve provides a means of adjusting the MTM standard so that the more practice the consumer has with the task, the more stringent the adjusted MTM standards become (Christopherson, 1996). However, given the limitations with the learning curve studies, VALPAR encourages evaluators to cross-validate the results of a failed work sample ("especially where the correlation coefficient is modest") before concluding that the individual lacks the necessary potential in a particular area (VALPAR, 1999, p. 1). Information on the products developed and distributed by VALPAR can be obtained at either the corporate office at VALPAR International, PO Box 5767, Tucson, AZ 85703, or at the national sales and training office at 12690 W. North Avenue, Brookfield, WI 53005 (http://www.valparint.com).

VALPAR Component Work Samples

VALPAR defined its 22 component work samples as "generalized work-like tasks" (VALPAR, 2006g, p. 1). The time required to complete each work sample varies with the sample. For example, Small Tools (Mechanical) takes approximately 90 minutes to complete, whereas Numerical Sorting can be completed in 30 minutes. Because each of the work sample/activity units can be administered, scored, and interpreted independently, the system is not a "single, interlocking system" (Brown et al., 1994, p. 49).

A separate manual for each sample includes the purpose of the assessment, special features (e.g., adaptations for individuals with sensory impairments are available for some of the units), and instructions. Each of the work sample manuals includes the factors and factor levels for each work sample (e.g., GED, aptitudes, physical demands), as well as the position in which the work sample can be performed (e.g., sitting, standing, variable). Table 12.3 provides examples of some of the VALPAR component work samples. The Pre-Vocational Readiness Battery and Dynamic Physical Capacities cannot be technically classified as work samples (Botterbusch, 1987; Brown et al., 1994). Brown et al. reported high reliability and good validity for most of the VALPAR components and noted that there were 11 different norm groups.

Pro3000

Pro3000 is the Windows version of System 2000. Seventeen different self-contained modules, each of which can be purchased separately and added at any time, have been developed for the *Pro3000* (VALPAR, 2006e). Examples of some of the available modules include the following:

1. The Career Planner: provides occupational information using occupational clusters for more than 500 Standard Occupational Classification codes
2. COMPASS: a computerized assessment module and work samples that measure GED (language, math, reasoning) and the 11 aptitudes
3. COMPASS Lite: an abbreviated version of COMPASS that assesses academic and cognitive skills but eliminates the work samples
4. Wage and Employment Database

TABLE 12.3.
Examples of VALPAR Component Work Samples

- Small Tools (mechanical) assesses the ability to make precise finger and hand movements and to work with small tools in tight or awkward places.
- Numerical Sorting assesses the ability to perform work tasks involving sorting, categorizing and filing by number arrangement, and using numbers and numerical series.
- Upper Extremity Range of Motion assesses upper extremity range of motion and work tolerance in the upper body.
- Whole Body Range of Motion assesses whole body range of motion, agility, and stamina through gross body movement of the trunk, arms, hands, and legs.
- Eye–Hand–Foot Coordination assesses the ability to move the eyes, hands, and feet in coordination.
- Dynamic Physical Capacities assesses various physical capacities while simulating work of a shipping and receiving clerk.
- Physical Capacities & Mobility Screening evaluation assesses quickly a number of work-related physical capacities.
- Mechanical Reasoning and Machine Tending assesses work skills involving machine tending, positioning and guiding items into a machine or under a needle, and assembling and disassembling using hand tools.

5. DOT Database
6. PET (physical demands, environmental conditions, temperaments) module: a self-report paper-and-pencil questionnaire to evaluate 20 physical demands, 13 environmental conditions, and 11 temperaments
7. Spatial/Nonverbal Module: computerized scoring of the highest level of spatial aptitude and nonverbal reasoning
8. TECO: a test conversion module for converting scores from other tests such as the *General Aptitude Test Battery* (GATB) or the *Wide-Range Achievement Test*
9. Work History: used to develop a composite profile of transferable skills
10. Pictorial Interest Survey: assesses interests through forced choice and ranking using pictures and short descriptions (audio optional)

COMPASS, a criterion-referenced screening assessment, includes 13 computerized subtests, three work samples (Alignment and Driving, Machine Tending, and Wiring), and one paper-and-pencil survey (VALPAR, 2006b). Brown et al. (1994) indicated that the combination of work samples and computerized assessment helps to maintain an individual's interest during the evaluation process. Also, scoring time is reduced since a portion is scored by computer.

VALPAR 300 Series

Used to assess hand and upper extremity functions, the *VALPAR 300* series consists of five compact, portable modules (Small Parts Assembly, Asymmetric Pin Placement, Tool Manipulation, Bi-Manual Coordination, and Angled Pin Placement). Similar to other VALPAR products, the 300 series is criterion-referenced to the Department of Labor standards and MTM standards. The scoring sheets for the modules include space for scoring both standard and non-standard exercises as well as space to record observational ratings of worker characteristics on a 5-point scale (1 = low to 5 = high). Examples of the characteristics include *following instructions* and *physical stamina* (VALPAR, 2006a).

Aviator 3

Aviator 3 is VALPAR's (2006b) aptitude and interest computer-based assessment, which is available in English and Spanish. It consists of a criterion-referenced battery of tests that can be completed in 60 minutes. It measures (a) GED level (Reasoning, Math, and Language); (b) seven aptitudes (General Learning Ability, Verbal, Numerical, Spatial Perception, Form Perception, Clerical Perception, and Color Discrimination); and (c) interests through two Pictorial Interest Surveys that utilize audio in their presentation. The reports generated by *Aviator 3* provide grade levels for Math, Reading, Vocabulary, and Spelling. The academic subtests assess Grades 4–13, although the reading extends to grade 14. Scores are reported in the same format used in the DOT for GED and aptitudes. Also, *Aviator 3* contains two occupational databases, each of which has approximately 1,000 occupations, including projected growth or decline. The Database Manager of Aviator maintains a database of the demographic information and test results of individuals who were tested with the system (VALPAR, 2006b).

Therapists' Portable Assessment Lab

Also distributed by VALPAR (2006f), *Therapists' Portable Assessment Lab* (TPAL) consists of 12 work modules to assess cognitive and psychomotor skills. The modules, which are contained in a single case on wheels for easy transportation in a rehabilitation hospital, take about 2 hours to administer and can be used with a functional capacity evaluation. The TPAL system is linked to the DOT Worker Qualification Profile factors and to MTM industrial performance standards. In addition to the various work modules (e.g., ruler reading, block design, color sort, pipe assembly, alphabetizing), the system includes the Career Assessment Battery, the Learning Styles Inventory, and the Auditory Directions Screen, which is used to assess an individual's ability to follow verbal directions.

Situational Assessments, Job Tryouts, and On-the-Job Evaluations

The terms *situational assessment, community-based situational assessment, job tryouts, on-the-job evaluation,* and *supported employment evaluation* are often used interchangeably. Technically, the terms refer to the systematic observation of individuals in a work setting. When the work setting (e.g., a work station in a psychiatric hospital) is simulated, the term *situational assessment* is more frequently used. If the assessment occurs on an actual job site in the community, the term *on-the-job evaluation* (OJE) may be used. Conversely, situational assessment may occur in any location, with the settings described as "sheltered" or "integrated." The community-based situational assessment is a type of supported employment evaluation that occurs within the community. The purposes of these assessments are twofold: Individuals with disabilities who are not sure what they would like to do have an opportunity to try out different jobs or aspects of jobs in the community, and individuals evaluating the behavior can identify supports that can make future job placements successful, the environments the individual prefers, an individual's learning style, as well as behaviors that may interfere with future job placements. Situational assessments are particularly useful for individuals with mental illness, mental retardation, learning disabilities, and/or traumatic brain injury (Bell, Lysaker, & Bryson, 2003).

There are a number of benefits to a situational assessment or OJE:

- There is less concern with validity and reliability because the individual's ability to perform the job in a manner that satisfies the employer indicates that the person can do the job (Botterbusch, 1978).
- The assessment can "increase self-awareness of strengths and limitations" (Fewell, 1988, p. 192).
- An integrated work setting means that the work is real and the individual may have an opportunity to be hired (Fewell, 1988).
- On-site supervisors can supplement the evaluator's assessment of an individual's behavior (Parker & Bolton, 2005).

Also, there are disadvantages to situational or OJE assessments because they can be "time-consuming, resource intensive, and logistically difficult to arrange" (MacDonald-Wilson, Rogers, & Anthony, 2001, p. 228). For example, in their description of person-centered situational assessment, Abrams, DonAroma, Karan, and Pappanikou indicated that most assessments required "40 hours of on-the-job contact with consumers over a two-week period" (1994, p. 30). Other disadvantages include insurance, wage, and scheduling issues (Kell, 1988).

Power (2006) identified six categories of behaviors that are frequently observed during a situational assessment. These include appearance (e.g., hygiene), attendance (e.g., punctuality), supervisory relationships (e.g., reaction to criticism), perseverance (e.g., distractibility), coworker relationships (e.g., social skills), and generalization of work habits (e.g., production output). A variety of situational assessment instruments has been developed, including individualized behavior checklists. MacDonald-Wilson, Rogers, and Anthony (2001) noted that no single situational assessment instrument has been adopted by a majority of individuals. Examples of instruments used in situational assessments include the *Work Personality Profile–Professional Form* (WPP-PF) previously described, the *Work Behavior Inventory,* the *Work Adjustment Skills Scale* and *Interpersonal Skills Scale,* and the *WorkPlace Mentor.*

Work Adjustment Skills Scale and *Interpersonal Skills Scale*

The *Work Adjustment Skills Scale* (WASS) and the *Interpersonal Skills Scale* (ISS) were developed by Rogers, Sciarappa, and Anthony (1991) to determine the vocational potential of individuals with psychiatric disabilities. These scales were part of a prototype situational assessment process that included a structured interview and identification of an optimal work evaluation environment. Including a "not applicable" category, the 24 items on the WASS are rated from

1 = *Cause to be Fired* to 4 = *Above Acceptable Performance.* The same rating scale is used with the ISS, which contains 14 items. Items include "Recognizes and corrects work errors" (WASS) and "Asks for help when having difficulty with tasks" (ISS).

Raters evaluated the individuals in the situational assessment for 2 hours each day for 10 consecutive days. Rogers and colleagues found good interrater reliability for both instruments. Because few individuals became competitively employed after 1 year, the predictive validity of the tests was lower than anticipated. Rogers and colleagues noted the need for additional studies related to the predictive validity of situational assessment procedures that were normed on individuals with psychiatric disabilities. The WASS and ISS are available from Dr. E. Sally Rogers, Center for Psychiatric Rehabilitation, Boston University, 940 Commonwealth Avenue West, Boston, MA 02215.

WorkPlace Mentor

The *WorkPlace Mentor* model is a computerized approach to supported employment assessment, which encompasses a situational assessment. The first two steps in the *WorkPlace Mentor* include assessing the environment and the individual (e.g., functional demands, worker capabilities, preference and interest factors, and potential supports or accommodations). In Step 3 these assessments are compared to identify the most appropriate job(s) for a situational assessment. The purpose of the fourth step, which includes the collection of observational data on an eight-page form that allows for easy transfer to the computer program, is to evaluate the consumer on a single job and note any accommodations that were used or needed (Vocational Rehabilitation Institute, 2005). The situational assessment focuses on both performance and behavior (e.g., the frequency of specific behaviors and the consumer's interest in carrying out job functions). The four areas that were assessed in both the environmental assessment and the consumer's assessment are evaluated in the situational assessment. These include (1) learning and performing, (2) self-management, (3) critical work behaviors, and (4) social interactions. For example, within learning and performing, the individual may be assessed on learning tasks (e.g., reaches/maintains independent performance within time frame); performing tasks (e.g., uses tools, equipment, and materials properly); academic demands (e.g., meets functional math or reading requirements); and physical demands (e.g., demonstrates stamina). Each of the items within a cluster is evaluated on five rating scales: frequency (1 = *regularly* to 4 = *rarely*), impact of behavior (1 = *significant asset* to 4 = *current liability*), interest (1 = *highly positive* to 4 = *highly negative*), impact of liability (1 = *threatens safety and/or placement* to 3 = *currently not impairing performance*), and behavioral trend (1 = *problem increasing* to 3 = *showing improvement*). Following data input, the fifth step in the process summarizes the data for the five sections, whereas the sixth step allows an individual to use the data collected in Step 5 to develop a consumer's individualized plan. The *WorkPlace Mentor* is available from the Vocational Research Institute, 1528 Walnut Street, Suite 1502, Philadelphia, PA 19102 (http://www.vri.org).

Conclusion

This chapter described four major approaches to assessing work behaviors: functional, behavioral, and physical capacities assessments; transferable skills assessments/job matching; work samples; and situational assessments, job tryouts, and on-the-job evaluations. These approaches can be used singularly or in combination. Because of the wide variations in cost, it is unlikely that most counselors will be able to request a particular system, nor are all evaluators skilled in using all of these systems. Both evaluators and counselors should adhere to the guidelines set forth by the Interdisciplinary Council on Vocational Evaluation and Assessment and remain mindful of the role of norms, validity, and reliability in the assessment of work behaviors.

References

Abrams, K., DonAroma, P., Karan, O.C., & Pappanikou, A. J. (1994). Person-centered situational assessment: A new direction for vocational rehabilitation services. *Journal for Vocational and Special Needs Education, 16*(3), 27–32.

Bell, M.D., Lysaker, P., & Bryson, G. (2003). A behavioral intervention to improve work performance in schizophrenia: Work Behavior Inventory Feedback. *Journal of Vocational Rehabilitation, 18*, 43–50.

Bellini, J., Bolton, B., & Neath, J. (1998). Rehabilitation counselors' assessments of applicants' functional limitations as predictors of rehabilitation services provided. *Rehabilitation Counseling Bulletin, 41*, 242–259.

Bennett, G.K. (1965). *Hand-Tool Dexterity Test.* New York: Psychological Corporation.

Bolton, B. (1986). Minnesota Satisfactoriness Scales. In D.J. Keyser & R.C. Sweetland (Eds.), *Test critiques* (Vol. 4, pp. 434–439). Austin, TX: PRO-ED.

Bolton, B. (1991). Becker Work Adjustment Profile. In J.C. Conoley & J.J. Kramer (Eds.), *The eleventh mental measurements yearbook* (pp. 83–84). Lincoln, NE: University of Nebraska Press.

Bolton, B. (1992). The Preliminary Diagnostic Questionnaire. In D.J. Keyser & R.C. Sweetland (Eds.), *Test critiques* (Vol. 9, pp. 405–410). Austin, TX: PRO-ED.

Botterbusch, K.F. (1978). *A guide to job site evaluation.* Menomonie, WI: University of Wisconsin–Stout, The Rehabilitation Resource.

Botterbusch, K.F. (1987). *Vocational assessment and evaluation systems: A comparison.* Menomonie, WI: University of Wisconsin–Stout, The Rehabilitation Resource.

Botterbusch, K.F. (2005). Work samples. In D.F. Roberts (Ed.), *The review manual for vocational evaluators* (pp. 286–298). Athens, GA: Elliott & Fitzpatrick.

Brown, C., McDaniel, R., & Couch, R. (1994). *Vocational evaluation systems and software: A consumer's guide.* Menomonie, WI: University of Wisconsin–Stout, The Rehabilitation Resource.

Buros Institute on Mental Measurements. (2006). *Behavior assessment*. Retrieved April 14, 2007, from http://www.unl.edu/buros/bimm/html/index19.html.

Christopherson, B.B. (1995). VALPAR and methods-time measurement (MTM). *VALPAR Views and News, 1*(1), 2.

Christopherson, B.B. (1996). VALPAR's learning curve, methods-time measurement, and the worker qualifications profile. *VALPAR Views and News, 1*(2), 2.

Commission on Vocational Evaluation and Work Adjustment. (2006). Guiding principles. Retrieved May 14, 2006, from http://www.ccwaves.org/aboutus/principles.html.

Corthell, D.W., & Griswold, P.P. (1987). *The use of vocational evaluation in VR. Fourteenth Institute on Rehabilitation Issues*. Menomonie, WI: University of Wisconsin–Stout, Research and Training Center.

Costello, J.J. (1991). *Fundamentals of vocational assessment*. Tucson, AZ: RPM Press.

Crewe, N.M., & Athelstan, G.T. (1984). *Functional Assessment Inventory manual*. Menomonie, WI: University of Wisconsin–Stout, Research and Training Center.

Dunn, P. (2004). Understanding transferable skills analysis as a tool in vocational assessment. In C.M. Donnell & Y.V. Edwards (Eds.). *National Association of Multicultural Rehabilitation Concerns eleventh annual summer training conference proceedings*. Retrieved April 14, 2007, from http://www.rcepv.siu.edu/namrc/.

Economic Research Institute. (2006). *Dictionary of occupational titles*. Retrieved April 14, 2007, from http://www.erieri.com/index.cfm?fuseaction=eDOT.Main.

Elliott & Fitzpatrick. (2006). *Functional capacity checklist*. Athens, GA: Author.

Fewell, S. (1988). Situational assessment in an integrated setting for survivors of traumatic brain injury. In R. Fry (Ed.), *The issues papers: Fourth National Forum on Issues in Vocational Assessment* (pp. 187–193). Menomonie, WI: The University of Wisconsin–Stout, The Rehabilitation Resource.

Geisser, M.E., Robinson, M.E., Miller, Q.L., & Blade, S.M. (2003). Psychosocial factors and functional capacity evaluation among persons with chronic pain. *Journal of Occupational Rehabilitation, 13*, 259–276.

Gibson, D.L., Weiss, D.J., Dawis, R.V., & Lofquist, L.H. (1970). *Manual for the Minnesota Satisfactoriness Scales*. Minnesota Studies in Vocational Rehabilitation: XXVII. Minneapolis, MN: University of Minnesota.

Halpern, A., & Fuhrer, M. (1984). *Functional assessment in rehabilitation*. Baltimore: Brookes.

Havranek, J., Field, T., & Grimes, J.W. (2005). *Vocational assessment: Evaluating employment potential* (4th ed.). Athens, GA: Elliott & Fitzpatrick.

Individuals with Disabilities Education Improvement Act of 2004, P.L. 108-446, 118 Stat. 2647.

Kauppi, D.R. (1988). Vocational Interest, Temperament, and Aptitude System. In D.J. Keyser & R.C. Sweetland (Eds.), *Test critiques* (Vol. 7, pp. 623–627). Kansas City, MO: Test Corporation of America.

Kell, P.D. (1988). On-the-job evaluations: Past, present, and future trends. In R. Fry (Ed.), *The issues papers: Fourth National Forum on Issues in Vocational Assessment* (pp. 49–54). Menomonie, WI: University of Wisconsin–Stout, The Rehabilitation Resource.

Landy, F.J. (1989). *Psychology of work behavior* (4th ed.). Pacific Grove, CA: Brooks/Cole.

Li, R.S, & Tsang, H.W. (2002). The Chinese version of the Becker Work Adjustment Profile for use by people with developmental disabilities-BWAP-CV-Becker Work Adjustment Profile. *Journal of Rehabilitation, 68*(4), 52–58.

Ludlow, J. (1990). A practical guide for assessing physical demands requirements and environmental conditions. *Vocational Evaluation and Work Adjustment Bulletin, 23*, 61–64.

MacDonald-Wilson, K., Rogers, E.S., & Anthony, W.A. (2001). Unique issues in assessing work function among individuals with psychiatric disabilities. *Journal of Occupational Rehabilitation, 11*, 217–232.

McCarron-Dial Systems. (2006). Retrieved April 14, 2007, from http://www.mccarrondial.com/index.html.

MECA. (2006). [Online]. http://www.conovercompany.com/Products/meca/meca.htm

Moriarity, J.B. (1981). *Preliminary diagnostic questionnaire.* Dunbar: West Virginia Research and Training Center.

Neath, J., & Bolton, B. (2008). *Work personality profile and computer report.* Austin, TX: PRO-ED.

Parker, R.M., & Bolton, B. (2005). Psychological assessment in rehabilitation. In R.M. Parker, E.M. Szymanski, & J.B. Patterson (Eds.), *Rehabilitation Counseling Basics and Beyond* (pp. 307–334). Austin, TX: PRO-ED.

Power, P. W. (2006). *A guide to vocational assessment* (4th ed.). Austin, TX: PRO-ED.

Roberts, R. (2005). Functional skills assessment. In R. Roberts (Ed). *Test review manual for vocational evaluators* (pp. 38–54). Athens, GA: Elliott & Fitzpatrick.

Rogers, E.S., Sciarappa, K., & Anthony, W.A. (1991). Development and evaluation of situation assessment instruments and procedures for persons with psychiatric disabilities. *Vocational Evaluation and Work Adjustment Bulletin, 24,* 61–67.

Sax, A. (1979). VDARE: The vocational diagnosis and assessment of residual employability. *Vocational Evaluation and Work Adjustment Bulletin, 12*(3), 28–29.

Scott, T.M., & Caron, D.B. (2005). Conceptualizing functional behavior assessment as prevention practice within positive behavior support systems. *Preventing School Failure, 50*(1), 13–20.

SkillTRAN. (1997). Job Browser Pro [Computer software]. Spokane, WA: Author.

Smith, F., Lombard, R., Neubert, D., Leconte, P., Rothenbacher, C., & Sitlington, P. (1994). The position statement of the Interdisciplinary Council on Vocational Evaluation and Assessment Fall 1993. *The Journal for Vocational Special Needs Education, 17*(1), 41–42.

Solly, D.C. (1994). *McCarron-Dial System.* In J.T. Kapes, M.M. Mastie, & E.A. Whitfield (Eds.), *A counselor's guide to career assessment instruments* (pp. 308–314). Alexandria, VA: National Career Development Association.

Szymanski, E.M., Enright, M.S., Hershenson, D.B., & Ettinger, J.M. (2003). Career development theories, constructs, and research: Implications for people with disabilities. In E.M. Szymanski & R.M. Parker (Eds.), *Work and disability: Issues and strategies in career development and job placement* (2nd ed., pp. 91–154). Austin, TX: PRO-ED.

Talent Assessment Inc. (2006). Talent Assessment Program. Jacksonville, FL. Retrieved April 14, 2007, from http://www.talentassessment.com/programs_tap.php.

Tiffin, J. (1968). *Purdue Pegboard Dexterity Test.* Chicago: Science Research Associates.

Truthan, J.A., & Karma, S.E. (2003). Transferable skills analysis and vocational information during a time of transition. *Journal of Forensic Vocational Analysis, 6*(1), 17–25.

VALPAR International Corporation. (1999). *Temporal reliability of selected VALPAR component work samples: Learning curve studies.* Retrieved April 14, 2007, from http://www.valparint.com.

VALPAR International Corporation. (2006a). 300 series. Retrieved April 14, 2007, from http://valparint.com/300_seri.htm.

VALPAR International Corporation. (2006b). *Aviator 3.* Retrieved April 14, 2007, from http://valparint.com.

VALPAR International Corporation. (2006c). *COMPASS.* Retrieved April 14, 2007, from http://valparint.com.

VALPAR International Corporation. (2006d). *Joule, an FCE system by VALPAR.* Retrieved April 14, 2007, from http://www.valparint.com.

VALPAR International Corporation. (2006e). *Pro3000.* Retrieved April 14, 2007, from http://www.valparint.com.

VALPAR International Corporation. (2006f). *TPAL: Therapists' Portable Assessment Lab.* Available online http://www.valparint.com/tpal.htm

VALPAR International Corporation. (2006g). *Work samples.* Retrieved April 14, 2007, from http://www.valparint.com.

Vocational Interest, Temperament and Aptitude System. (2006). Retrieved April 14, 2007, from http://www.intecinc.net/prod_vri_vitas.htm.

Vocational Rehabilitation Institute. (n.d.). Available from http://www.vri.org/

Chapter 13

The O★NET Occupational Information System

Mary Ann Hanson, Leonard N. Matheson,
and Walter C. Borman

Information about the broad array of work demands in the U.S. economy is an essential tool for the rehabilitation professional. To help clients with disabilities perform successfully in the labor market, rehabilitation professionals use occupational information to match clients' abilities, skills, and interests to the world of work. More specifically, rehabilitation professionals use occupational information to: (a) evaluate each client's ability to perform jobs in his or her previous occupation by comparing the client's functional limitations with the demands of the jobs in that occupation; (b) assist clients in developing appropriate vocational goals; (c) combine and interpret information about the client's work history; (d) identify occupations or groups of occupations with a good employment outlook; (e) help clients identify the skills and knowledge they need to develop and appropriate training programs; and (f) facilitate job design, accommodation, and restructuring for safe and optimal productivity as the client prepares to begin a particular job.

For many decades, rehabilitation professionals relied on the *Dictionary of Occupational Titles* (DOT; U.S. Department of Labor, 1991) as their primary source of occupational information, beginning with print versions of the DOT, progressing to mainframe computerized versions that required batch processing, and later moving to microcomputer versions that can be used on an interactive basis. However, the DOT has some limitations (U.S. Department of Labor, 1993) including the following:

I. Job description in the DOT focuses on the tasks performed, rather than the person performing the tasks, and this leads to several limitations:

    A. Information about worker requirements and characteristics (e.g., knowledge, skills, abilities, interests) is derived from the task information and is extremely limited.

    B. Information about the nature and conditions of task performance is also limited. The DOT includes simple information, such as noise, temperature, and work schedule, but fails to include more complex types of information, such as levels of job stress, exposure to hazards, and organizational influences.

    C. For different occupations, these tasks are described in different ways and at different levels of generality. This makes comparisons across occupations difficult.

II. Job descriptive information is collected by analysts and is time consuming and expensive to update.

III. The DOT contains narrative descriptions of occupations. These discrete, qualitative descriptions limit the kinds of analyses that can be conducted.

In the early 1990s, the U.S. Department of Labor (DOL) reevaluated the DOT in light of the nation's occupational information needs and decided to update its approach to collecting and disseminating occupational information.

The result was the *Occupational Information Network* (O★NET): a comprehensive occupational information system intended to replace the DOT and to serve as the nation's primary source of occupational information. The occupational information in the O★NET is designed to (a) help organizations recruit and select workers; (b) help workers choose organizations and jobs and help career counselors and other workforce development professionals provide these workers with career guidance; and (c) help schools and other organizations design and execute training. Potential users of O★NET information include job seekers, career and rehabilitation counselors, training specialists, displaced workers, recruiters, state and federal labor and manpower specialists, and public-sector and private-sector employers. This chapter describes the content and structure of the O★NET, data collection procedures, the present status of the database and related tools, some examples of current applications of the O★NET in rehabilitation, and some further research and development and potential future applications.

The O★NET Content Model

The foundation of the O★NET is a content model that provides a framework for describing jobs. The goal in developing this content model was to identify and include descriptors that can be used to categorize jobs in meaningful ways. The content model is made up of hierarchical taxonomies of descriptors that provide a basis for measuring the similarities and differences observed among occupations. The O★NET content model is based on careful review of relevant theory, research, and previously developed measures. The highest level of the content model hierarchy is shown in Figure 13.1. The O★NET content model is divided into six general groups of content domains. Some of these content domains include information similar to that included in the DOT, and others represent new types of information not previously collected. Each of these domains can be viewed as a different "window" through which we can view the world of work.

The first general group of O★NET descriptors focuses on relatively enduring features of individuals that might influence occupational choice, job performance, or satisfaction. These include abilities, personality characteristics, and interests; and they are referred to as *worker characteristics*. The second broad group of descriptors also describes workers but focuses on characteristics that are developed over time. This category includes skills and knowledge and is referred to as *worker requirements*. The third group, referred to as *experience requirements* or *occupational preparation,* describes the training, experience, and licensure required. A fourth broad group focuses on describing occupations in terms of the activities involved and the context in which these activities occur. These are referred to as *occupational requirements*. Within each of the O★NET content domains, the descriptors are organized into hierarchical taxonomies.

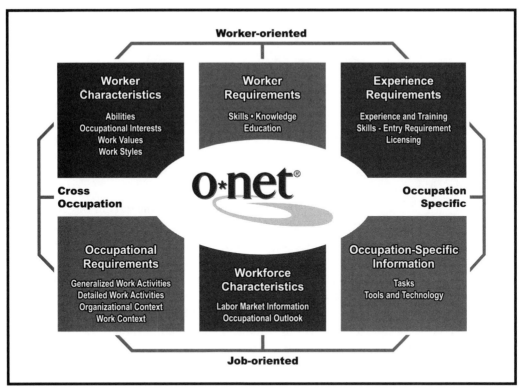

FIGURE 13.1. O★NET content model. *Note.* Available from the O★NET Resource Center online (www.onetcenter.org).

The content domains and descriptors included in each of these four broad groups are described in the sections that follow. The descriptions included here are intended to provide the reader with a sense of the breadth and depth of the O★NET, an overview of the types of descriptors included, and an overview of the justification for each set of descriptors. Complete descriptions of each content model domain, operational definitions of each of the more than 200 descriptors, and a review of the supporting literature can be found in Peterson, Mumford, Borman, Jeanneret, and Fleishman (1995, 1999).

Worker Characteristics

Three domains of worker characteristics are included in the O★NET: (1) abilities, (2) occupational interests and values, and (3) work styles (i.e., personality characteristics). These domains are likely to be particularly useful for applications involving worker placement decisions. Both from the organizations' and the workers' point of view, it is useful to place individuals in occupations in which their personal characteristics are well-matched with the work requirements and rewards.

Abilities

The study of human abilities has a long history, and a number of different models and theories regarding the structure of human abilities have been proposed. Abilities are defined as "relatively enduring attributes of an individual's capability for performing a particular range of different tasks" (Fleishman, Costanza, & Marshall-Mies, 1999, p. 175). Much of our knowledge concerning the nature and structure of human abilities comes from research examining the intercorrelations between performances on a variety of different tasks (within several broad domains of human performance). These intercorrelations are typically factor analyzed to understand the structure of the abilities needed to perform the tasks.

Research on abilities has generally focused on measuring the abilities of individuals (e.g., workers) rather than assessing the ability requirements of jobs. One notable exception is the *Fleishman Job Analysis Survey* (F-JAS; Fleishman, 1975a, 1992). Development of this survey began with the identification of an ability requirements taxonomy. This taxonomy was based on previous models of abilities (e.g., French 1951; Guilford, 1967; Thurstone, 1947) and factor analyses of task performance data. The taxonomy includes a total of 52 different abilities. Behavior summary scales were then developed to evaluate the level of each ability required to perform various jobs and job tasks (Fleishman, 1975b). A great deal of research is now available that supports both the internal and external validity of the F-JAS ability requirement scales. For example, tests and assessments developed on the basis of ability requirements from this system have been shown to have high criterion-related validity (see Fleishman, 1988, for a review).

The F-JAS scales provide a valid and comprehensive assessment of the ability requirements of jobs, so these scales were modified and included in the O★NET. Modifications focused primarily on reducing the reading level and the amount of reading involved and on ensuring that the final scales are appropriate for individuals from a wide variety of cultures and backgrounds. The O★NET contains a total of 52 ability requirement descriptors, ranging from deductive reasoning and originality to trunk strength and peripheral vision (see Fleishman et al., 1999). These ability requirements are organized into a hierarchical taxonomy. Consistent with previous research and theory, O★NET abilities are grouped into four general areas: (1) cognitive, (2) psychomotor, (3) physical, and (4) sensory–perceptual. Within each of these areas, the abilities are further organized into a set of intermediate-level categories. Table 13.1 lists the categories in the ability requirements hierarchy and provides examples of abilities from each category.

Occupational Interests and Values

Occupational interests and values can be described as relatively stable characteristics of individuals based on affective judgments about life events (Dawis, 1991). *Interests* tends to refer to the likes and dislikes of activities, whereas *values* refers to an evaluation of the importance of activities and of other characteristics

TABLE 13.1.
O★NET Ability Requirement Categories and Example Descriptors

Ability Requirement Categories	Examples of Ability Descriptors
I. *Cognitive Abilities*	
Verbal	Oral comprehension; written expression
Idea generation/reasoning	Deductive reasoning; category flexibility
Quantitative	Mathematical reasoning; number facility
Memory	Memorization
Perceptual	Perceptual speed; flexibility of closure
Spatial	Visualization
Attention	Selective attention
II. *Psychomotor Abilities*	
Fine manipulative	Arm–hand steadiness; finger dexterity
Control movement	Multilimb coordination; rate control
Reaction time and speed	Wrist–finger speed
III. *Physical Abilities*	
Physical strength	Static strength; explosive strength
Endurance	Stamina
Flexibility, balance, and coordination	Dynamic flexibility; gross body coordination
IV. *Sensory Abilities*	
Visual	Near vision; night vision; depth perception
Auditory and speech	Hearing sensitivity; speech clarity

of the work environment. Interests and values were included in the O★NET because they are widely believed to be important in understanding motivation, and job performance is a function of ability and motivation. Also, interests have been shown to discriminate among occupations (i.e., "predict" occupational membership), and values have been shown to predict job satisfaction. As with abilities, much of the available information about interests and values involves measuring the characteristics of people (e.g., the *Kuder Occupational Interest Survey* and the *Strong Interest Inventory*) rather than assessing jobs in terms of the interests they involve or the values they can fulfill.

Holland's six-factor taxonomy was used in the O★NET to describe occupations in terms of interests; because an extensive literature supports this taxonomy, it is widely used in career and vocational counseling, and research has shown that this taxonomy can be used to meaningfully describe occupations and individuals. Holland "codes" can be used to describe an occupation in terms of the three possible Holland types that fit that occupation. An occupation's three-point code consists of the first letter of each of the three relevant types (i.e., R = realistic; I = investigative; A = artistic; S = social; E = enterprising; and C = conventional) presented in order of importance.

Regarding occupational values, the *Minnesota Job Description Questionnaire* (MJDQ; Dawis & Lofquist, 1984) was used as the basis for the O★NET values descriptors (see Sager, 1999). The MJDQ assesses the potential of occupations to provide reinforcers that correspond to workers' occupational values. Dawis (1991) has demonstrated that the MJDQ provides reasonably comprehensive coverage of the occupational values domain. An associated instrument, the *Minnesota Importance Questionnaire* (MIQ; Dawis & Lofquist, 1984) asks workers to rank order the same statements included on the MJDQ relative to the importance of these statements for their ideal job. This provides an assessment of workers' values that corresponds to the MJDQ value reinforcing potential assessments for occupations, so individuals can be matched with occupations based on their values. The MJDQ scales were modified substantially for inclusion in the O★NET to reduce administration time. Table 13.2 shows the taxonomy of occupational values included in the O★NET content model and some example descriptors from each category.

Work Styles

The importance of personality traits in the workplace and the links between personality and important organizational outcomes are becoming increasingly recognized. Some would also argue that personality is becoming increasingly important in the workplace as interpersonal and other nontask aspects of work are growing in importance. The O★NET refers to worker characteristics from the personality domain as "work styles" to emphasize that it is the work-related manifestations of personality traits with which the O★NET is concerned (see Borman, Kubisiak, & Schneider, 1999).

Development of the O★NET work style taxonomy was based on the available personality literature, particularly personality taxonomies that have been developed in the context of industrial/organizational psychology and personnel

TABLE 13.2.

O★NET Occupational Value Categories and Example Descriptors

Higher Order Value Categories	Examples of Value Descriptors
Achievement	Ability utilization; achievement
Comfort	Activity; variety; security
Status	Advancement; recognition
Altruism	Coworkers; social values
Safety	Supervision
Autonomy	Creativity; responsibility

selection (e.g., Barrick & Mount, 1991; Guion, 1992; Hogan, 1982; Hough, 1997). One focus in development of the O★NET taxonomy was to include personality constructs that have been empirically demonstrated to correlate with important job behaviors or related criteria to ensure that the work style descriptors included in the O★NET represent aspects of personality that are truly important in the workplace. The work style descriptors are organized into a set of intermediate-level categories. Table 13.3 shows the work style categories and provides examples of descriptors from each category.

Worker Requirements

Job analysis traditionally has focused either on the work to be done (e.g., tasks, work activities) or on relatively stable, enduring characteristics of individuals that affect their capacity to do the work (e.g., abilities, interests). However, as the workplace evolves and changes at a rapid pace, understanding the developed characteristics of individuals that influence job performance has become increasingly important throughout industry, government, and education. The O★NET worker requirements include two different types of developed characteristics: skills and knowledge. Worker requirement descriptors are likely to be of interest to educators, job seekers, and employment counselors. Knowing the skills and knowledge important for various occupations can help individuals prepare for their chosen occupations. This information can also help workers identify occupations that take advantage of the knowledge and skills they already possess.

Basic and Cross-Functional Skills

Much of the available information about the nature of skills comes from cognitive psychology and research on the nature of skilled performance (e.g., Ericsson & Charness, 1994). However, there is less agreement than in the other domains concerning how to define skills and what skills are important in the workplace. Some have described skills in terms of task performance, whereas others define them in terms of educational requirements. For the O★NET, skills have

TABLE 13.3.
O★NET Work Style Categories and Example Descriptors

Higher Order Work Style Categories	Examples of Work Style Descriptors
Achievement orientation	Initiative; persistence
Social influence	Energy; leadership orientation
Interpersonal orientation	Cooperation; concern for others
Adjustment	Self-control; stress tolerance
Conscientiousness	Dependability; attention to detail
Independence	Independence
Practical intelligence	Innovation; analytical thinking

been defined as procedures for acquiring and working with information (see Mumford, Peterson, & Childs, 1999).

The O★NET skills are divided into two broad categories: basic skills and cross-functional skills. Basic skills include the fundamentals that should be provided by any sound educational system (e.g., reading, writing, mathematics, science). They also include skills related to the general strategies, processes, and procedures that facilitate learning (e.g., using multiple strategies, ongoing appraisal of learning progress). Cross-functional skills apply broadly across jobs and fall into several general performance domains, including problem solving, technical, and resource management. Table 13.4 shows the hierarchical structure of the O★NET basic and cross-functional skills and provides examples of skill descriptors from each category.

Knowledge

Another set of developed capacities important in the workplace is knowledge. Knowledge has been defined as a collection of discrete but related facts, information, and principles about a particular domain. Job-relevant knowledge is composed of those facts and structures that are necessary for successful job performance. The 33 knowledge requirement descriptors in the O★NET are grouped into 11 categories, including business and management, engineering and technology, health services, and arts and humanities (see Costanza, Fleishman, & Marshall-Mies, 1999). Examples of some specific knowledge descriptors are

TABLE 13.4.
O★NET Skill Requirement Categories and Example Descriptors

Skill Requirement Categories	Examples of Skill Descriptors
I. Basic Skills	
Content skills	Reading comprehension; speaking; mathematics; science
Process skills	Learning strategies; monitoring
II. Cross-Functional Skills	
Complex problem-solving skills	Problem identification; information gathering; idea evaluation; implementation planning
Social skills	Social perceptiveness; persuasion; instructing
Technical skills	Technology design; installation; operation and control; troubleshooting; programming
Systems skills	Systems perception; identification of key causes; judgment and decision making
Resource management skills	Time management; management of financial resources

food production, building and construction, biology, public safety and security, and transportation.

Occupational Preparation

Another way to describe the developed capacities of individuals important for occupations is to identify the training, education, and work experiences that influence knowledge and skill development. Rather than describing characteristics of the workers, variables in this domain indicate that a person has performed similar work previously or obtained education or training associated with the knowledge or skills required. Descriptors in this area include requirements for job tenure in related jobs and training experiences in a work context, such as apprenticeships, on-site training, and on-the-job training. This domain also includes descriptors of the amount and type of education, licensure, or certification required (Anderson, 1999).

Finally, to summarize the amount of preparation needed for each occupation, analysts have assigned each occupation to one of five job zones (Oswald, Campbell, McCloy, Rivkin, & Lewis, 1999). Occupations in each of these job zones are similar in terms of the amount of experience, education, and on-the-job training needed to do the job.

Occupational Requirements

The O★NET occupational requirements describe the work that is performed and the conditions under which this work is done. As opposed to the domains discussed to this point, focused on the worker, descriptors in this group of domains focus on the work itself. This includes the activities in which workers are engaged (i.e., generalized work activities [GWAs] and occupation-specific tasks) and the context in which these activities are carried out, both the immediate work context and the broader organizational context.

Generalized Work Activities and Tasks

Any job description must consider the work to be done and the tasks people do. However, specific job tasks, such as those used in the DOT, lack the generality needed to formulate a viable set of cross-job descriptors. An alternative to describing jobs in terms of the tasks performed is to describe them in terms of the behaviors of the workers performing these tasks, and this approach was adopted by the O★NET. Work behaviors are not specific to tasks or technologies, so they allow widely divergent occupations or jobs to be studied using a common frame of reference. Analytic techniques can be used to understand relevant similarities and differences across jobs. This approach has been shown to facilitate many applications, including synthetic validity (i.e., estimating predictor validities for jobs where validity data have not or cannot be collected) and the clustering of occupations to identify families of similar jobs (Cunningham, 1996). In fact, many have suggested that understanding the dimensionality of work centers on the question of identifying general job behavior constructs (e.g., Harvey, 1991).

In the O★NET, a GWA is defined as an aggregation of similar job activities/ behaviors that underlies the accomplishment of one or more major work functions (Jeanneret, Borman, Kubisiak, & Hanson, 1999). The O★NET GWAs were identified by examining earlier factor analyses of job task analysis inventories (e.g., Cunningham, 1988, McCormick, Jeanneret, & Mecham, 1972), taxonomies of the underlying dimensions of supervisory or managerial jobs (e.g., Borman & Brush, 1993; Yukl, 1987), and research on previously identified general behavioral dimensions of work (e.g., Dowell & Wexley, 1978; Outerbridge, 1981). The O★NET contains 42 GWA descriptors organized into higher order categories. Table 13.5 shows the GWA hierarchy of descriptors and provides examples of some of the descriptors from each category. The O★NET also includes occupation-specific tasks, which can be useful in specifying training, developing position descriptions, or redesigning jobs.

TABLE 13.5.
O★NET Generalized Work Activity (GWA) Categories and Example Descriptors

GWA Categories	Examples of GWA Descriptors
I. Information Input	
Looking for and receiving job-related information	Getting information; monitoring processes
Identifying and evaluating job-related information	Identifying objects; inspecting equipment
II. Mental Processes	
Information/data processing	Evaluating information; analyzing data
Reasoning/decision making	Making decisions; developing objectives; scheduling work
III. Work Output	
Performing physical and manual work activities	Performing physical work tasks; handling objects; controlling machines
Performing complex/technical activities	Interacting with computers; specifying equipment; repairing (electronic equipment)
IV. Interacting with Others	
Communicating/interacting	Communicating (internal); selling or influencing; working with the public
Coordinating/developing/managing/ advising others	Coordinating others' work; teaching others; providing consultation
Administering	Staffing organizational units; monitoring resources

Work and Organizational Context

Work context variables describe the conditions under which the job activities must be carried out. Social, physical, and organizational contexts can serve as the impetuses for tasks and activities and can greatly affect the worker, job performance, and work outcomes. The work context can also affect employee health and satisfaction. Research relevant to describing the context in which work tasks are performed comes from a variety of disciplines, including medical research, industrial engineering, physiology, organizational theory, organizational development, industrial organizational psychology, and social psychology. Physical aspects of the work context include temperature and noise. Social psychological aspects include time pressure and dependence on others. Table 13.6 shows the structure of the work context domain and provides examples of descriptors from each category (see Strong, Jeanneret, McPhail, Blakley, & D'Egidio, 1999).

Organizational context refers to organization-level aspects of the work context that might interact with the operational environment and affect how people

TABLE 13.6.
O★NET Work Context Categories and Example Descriptors

Work Context Categories	Examples of Work Context Descriptors
I. Interpersonal Relationships	
Communication	Communication method; frequency of job-related social interaction; formality of communication
Types of role relationships	Supervisory roles; service roles; adversarial roles
Responsibility for others	Responsibility for safety; responsibility for work outcomes and results
Conflictual contact with others	Interpersonal conflict; strained interpersonal relations
II. Physical Work Conditions	
Work setting	Types of work settings; privacy of work area
Environmental conditions	Exposure to extreme environmental conditions; possibility of injury from job hazards
Job demands	Body positioning; work attire
III. Structural Job Characteristics	
Criticality of position	Consequences of error; impact of decisions; responsibility/ accountability
Routine versus challenging work	Degree of automation; task clarity; required attention to detail; frustrating circumstances
Pace and scheduling	Frequency and stringency of deadlines; machine-driven work pace

go about doing their work. Variables in the organizational context area include organizational structure (e.g., flat versus hierarchical); industry type; human resource systems and practices; organizational values; individual and organizational goals; and various features of role relationships, including conflict, negotiability, and overload (see Arad, Hanson, & Schneider, 1999). Incumbents in a given occupation are likely to work in a variety of different organizational and industry contexts, so the O★NET can eventually describe not only the typical organizational context but also the variety of different organizational contexts in which an occupation is typically found.

Collecting O★NET Job Description Information

Information concerning the O★NET content model descriptors could be collected from a variety of different sources and by use of a variety of different procedures. Ratings represent the most common technique for obtaining descriptions of occupation characteristics. It is important to obtain job description information from people who have the expertise needed to provide accurate, meaningful assessments of occupational requirements. Some research has shown that incumbents (i.e., people working on the job), supervisors, and occupational analysts provide similar job descriptive information (e.g., Peterson, Owens-Kurtz, Hoffman, Arabian, & Whetzel, 1990). Incumbents may be best suited to provide information across all domains, especially complex or difficult to observe occupation characteristics, such as work styles and some organizational context variables. In addition, large samples of knowledgeable incumbents are available, which should contribute to the reliability of the resulting system. Finally, incumbents base their ratings on the smallest possible unit of analysis: the positions of individual workers. So, incumbent ratings were selected as the primary source for O★NET job description data (see Peterson, Mumford, Levin, Green, & Waksberg, 1999).

The O★NET content model was used to develop a set of prototype job description questionnaires. Information about each descriptor is collected using one or more numerical rating scales, and raters are provided with the operational definition of the descriptor variable. The rating scales used to collect job description information vary somewhat by domain, according to the content of the descriptors. For most domains, multiple types of ratings are obtained for each variable. For example, each GWA descriptor was originally rated in terms of the level of performance required, its importance, and the frequency with which it is performed. After the field test (described in the next section), the frequency scale was dropped, and GWAs are currently described relative to importance and level (see section on current status of the O★NET database). Figure 13.2 shows the rating scale currently being used to collect job analysis information for one GWA descriptor: monitoring processes, materials, or sur-

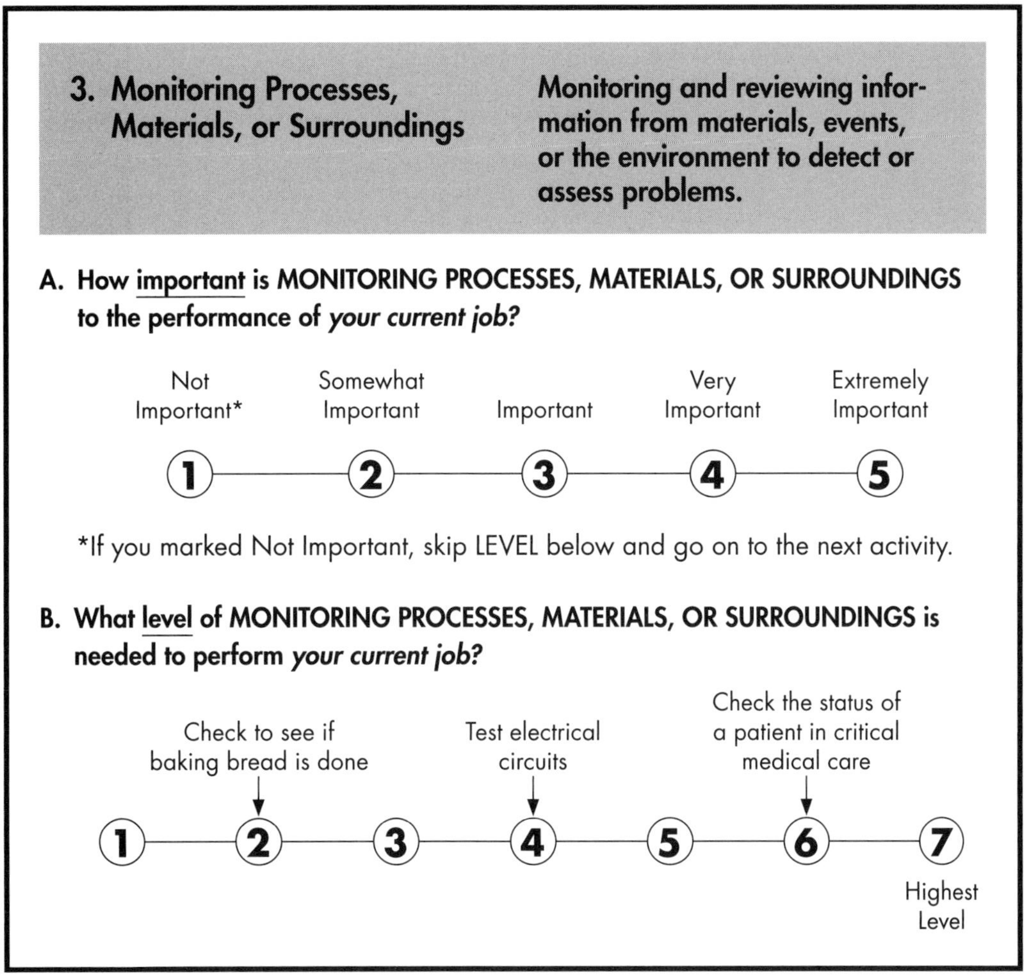

FIGURE 13.2. Example of an O★NET rating scale. *Note.* Available from the O★NET Resource Center online (www.onetcenter.org).

roundings. Note that this rating scale includes behavioral anchors that help define the behaviors and activities represented by various points on the level scale. These are included to minimize differences across raters in terms of how they use these scales and to enhance the interpretability of the resulting job description information.

For two O★NET domains—occupational interests and values—analysts provided the ratings that are included in the O★NET database. Regarding interests, analysts provided ratings for each of Holland's six codes for each occupation (Rounds, Smith, Hubert, Lewis, & Rivkin, 1999). These ratings can be used to generate a numerical profile for each occupation or to select the most descriptive Holland themes. Regarding occupational values, anchor occupations were added to the MJDQ (Dawis & Lofquist, 1984), and these scales were used by analysts to rate the potential of each of the occupations to provide reinforcers that correspond to each of the occupational values (McCloy, Waugh, Medsker, Wall, Rivkin, & Lewis, 1999).

Table 13.7 provides a summary of the more than 200 descriptors in the O★NET content model. This table lists the content domains, the number of descriptors included in each domain, and the types of rating scales used to collect occupational information for each descriptor. The level ratings (e.g., for abilities, skills, and knowledge) include behavioral anchors to help raters use the scales appropriately.

TABLE 13.7.

Summary of O★NET Occupation Descriptors

Content Domain	Number of Descriptors in Prototype	Current Number of Descriptors[a]	Current Rating Scales[a]
Abilities	52	52	Level, Importance
Interests	NA[b]	NA[c]	NA
Work values	21	NA[c]	NA
Work styles	17	16	Importance
Basic and cross-functional skills	46	35	Level, Importance
Knowledge	33	33	Level, Importance, Job Specialty Requirements
Education, Training, Licensure/Certification, and Experience	7	6	Varied (e.g., yes/no, check one, open-ended)
Generalized Work Activities (GWAs)	42	41	Level, Importance
Work context	97	57	Varied (e.g., importance, frequency, exposure, likelihood of injury, etc.)
Organizational context[d]	33	0	Varied (e.g., importance, number, significance, etc.)
Organizational characteristics	NA	NA	Drawn into O★NET by linking to other databases

Note. NA = not applicable.

[a]Since the field test, review and revision has resulted in deleting some items and rating scales (Hubbard et al., 2000).

[b]Codes were derived from the *Dictionary of Holland Occupational Codes* (DHOC; Gottfredson & Holland, 1996) for occupations in the prototype data collection.

[c]Occupational interest and value data are provided by analysts.

[d]Much of the organizational context data was collected from a single organizational representative from each establishment via a telephone interview. The 33 questions referenced on this table were part of the incumbent questionnaire.

Evaluation of the O★NET Prototype Data Collection Procedures

O★NET Field Test

The field test was an initial set of studies to evaluate the prototype O★NET instruments. A complete description of the field-test procedures and results can be found in Peterson, Mumford, Borman, Jeanneret, and Fleishman (1996, 1999). Here we provide a brief summary and some highlights of the results to provide readers with a summary of the information concerning the reliability and validity of O★NET data. The initial goal was to collect complete O★NET data for 80 occupations and to obtain at least 30 incumbent responses for each occupation. The 80 target occupations were sampled carefully to ensure that they were both appropriate and representative. Most of the field test data were provided by incumbents from the target occupations. Each incumbent who participated in the field test rated his or her job on only a subset of the O★NET descriptors, so the initial target for this data collection was more than 7,000 incumbents. However, response rates were much lower than expected, and the field test sample ultimately included only about 30 occupations (a total of about 2,000 incumbents) and fewer incumbents per occupation than anticipated. Occupations were included in the field test analyses if at least four respondents had provided data that survived initial screening.

To assess how well incumbents rating the same occupation agreed, interrater reliabilities were computed for each rating scale for each descriptor (using standard intraclass coefficients; Shrout & Fleiss, 1979). These reliabilities were also used as the basis for estimating what the reliability would have been for 30 raters (using Spearman-Brown corrections) to provide a projection as to what the reliability of the fully developed system would be once the goal of 30 raters was reached for each of the occupations included. Most of the 30-rater interrater reliability estimates for individual descriptors were in the 90s, indicating that the O★NET questionnaires produce reliable results. Reliabilities were lower for some of the occupational value and organizational context descriptors and a few of the work style descriptors. The fact that interrater agreement was generally high means that descriptor score profiles for occupations have meaning in the sense that they are stable representations of these occupations' requirements. For example, when a search is initiated for occupations requiring high levels of one or more particular skills, the answer is likely to be reliable and replicable.

The individual O★NET descriptors may be too detailed for some applications. For example, job seekers may want to start by looking at a more general set of skill descriptors and eliminating some occupations from consideration before moving to more detailed consideration of the remaining occupations. As mentioned previously, each content domain is arranged hierarchically, so ratings made on the descriptors, which are at the lowest level of the hierarchy, can be aggregated to provide more general occupational descriptions. The interrater reliabilities of aggregate scores, computed on the basis of the O★NET's original hierarchical structure, are at about the same level as the reliabilities for individual descriptors, which supports the use of these aggregate descriptors. Factor analyses and correlational analyses conducted for the descriptors within each domain were also consistent with the a priori taxonomies. Another way to assess the construct validity of the descriptors is to determine whether the relationships between descriptors across domains conform to theoretical and rational expectations. Several different analytical approaches were used in such cross-domain analyses, and each provided a somewhat different perspective on the relationships between descriptors from the various O★NET content domains (Hanson, Borman, Kubisiak, & Sager, 1999). A series of a priori hypotheses was generated and tested concerning expected correlations between individual descriptors from different domains. All the tests of these a priori cross-domain hypotheses showed that when strong correlations between O★NET descriptor scores were expected, strong correlations were in fact obtained. To summarize these O★NET cross-domain relationships, composites were also developed within each domain on the basis of the factor analysis results, then intercorrelated across domains. These results also made a great deal of sense. For example, work activities (i.e., GWAs) involving information had strong correlations with many cognitive ability and skill requirements. Achievement (a work style descriptor) and other more cognitively oriented work styles were also strongly related to activities involving information, as well as to cognitive ability and skill requirements. The analyses also showed that O★NET constructs that are conceptually unrelated generally do not correlate. For example, physical and psychomotor ability requirements were not significantly correlated with work activities involving information or people.

Results of the field-test analyses for the O★NET prototype, taken together, show that data collected using the O★NET descriptors and rating scales are generally very reliable and have meaningful underlying structure within each content domain, and that the patterns of correlations between content domains are highly interpretable. These analyses also provided preliminary evidence that the O★NET descriptors discriminate between occupations in a sensible manner.

O★NET Ratings From Occupational Analysts

The O★NET prototype evaluation also included a study to determine whether job descriptions obtained from incumbents—people working on the job—are similar to descriptions obtained from occupational analysts (Peterson, Mumford, Levin, Green, & Waksberg, 1999). The analysts for this study were professional occupational analysts and industrial/organizational psychology graduate students. These analysts provided ratings for a set of 1,122 occupational units (OUs). The OUs are at a level of specificity between the more general Occupational Employment Statistics (OES) taxonomy and the more specific DOT taxonomy and are designed to provide a comprehensive taxonomy of occupations. Each occupation was rated independently by at least five analyst raters, using a subset of the O★NET descriptors: basic and cross-functional skills, GWAs, abilities, knowledges, and some of the work context descriptors. Analyses of these data show that the analyst data share the favorable characteristics of the incumbent data described previously. Further, for the approximately 30 occupations for which incumbent data are also available, the incumbent and analyst data are comparable.

One advantage of the O★NET system is that it can be used to group occupations on the basis of any of a variety of job descriptors, depending on the needs of the particular project or set of users. For example, occupations could be grouped on the basis of their scores on the ability requirement descriptors if the desire is to identify groups of occupations that have similar ability requirements, perhaps for career counseling purposes. The O★NET analyst data provided an opportunity to conduct an initial set of investigations exploring different methodological approaches to clustering occupations and comparing the cluster results obtained using different sets of descriptors (Baughman, Norris, Cooke, Peterson, & Mumford, 1999). These studies provide insight concerning the relative effectiveness of various approaches to clustering occupations and demonstrate that the O★NET can yield highly interpretable clusters of occupations at a variety of different levels of specificity.

O★NET Database Releases and Revisions

As mentioned, the field-test version of the O★NET was a prototype, and this initial set of O★NET instruments was expected to benefit from revision and improvement. An initial round of revisions has already been completed (Hubbard et al., 2000). Many of the revisions involved rewording instructions, descriptor definitions, and scale anchors to make them more understandable and easier to use and to lower the reading level required. The questionnaire format was also revised. For several domains, one or more rating scales were dropped. For example, the frequency scale was dropped for the GWA domain, the job entry requirement scale was dropped for the skills domain, and the level scale was dropped for the work styles domain. In a few cases, descriptors were dropped or collapsed. One descriptor was dropped from the work styles domain and one from the GWAs. For the skills domain, several descriptors were combined to reduce redundancy. Finally, many work context descriptors were combined or dropped. The third column in Table 13.7 shows the current number of descriptors for each content domain. Hubbard et al. (2000) provide detailed information concerning the revisions that were made and the reasons for each set of revisions. These revised instruments were submitted for Office of Management and Budget (OMB) approval and are now being used to collect job description information from incumbents for all occupations. These questionnaires will be used to continually update the database and keep the occupation information current.

As mentioned earlier, the O★NET analyst job description ratings were collected for 1,122 OUs. Since that time, the government released a new set of *Standard Occupational Codes* (SOC 2000), and the O★NET analyst data were restructured to reflect the SOC 2000 occupational structure and released as O★NET 3.0. These same data were further restructured to reflect the revisions to the O★NET descriptors and questionnaires (Hubbard et al., 2000) and released as O★NET 4.0. The DOL is now in a cycle of data collection and database updates. Updates are released twice annually, and each includes comprehensively updated data for an additional 100 occupations. Table 13.8 describes the various database releases to date.

The most recent release, O★NET 11.0, has also been restructured to reflect more recent revisions made to the O★NET-SOC structure (O★NET-SOC 2006). These revisions (summarized in National Center for O★NET Development, 2006a) are part of the O★NET Program's continuous improvement effort, and the main goals were to ensure that future O★NET data are collected at the appropriate level of specificity and reflect changes occurring in the world of work (e.g., due to new technologies, innovative business practices, and the organization of the work). The common SOC structure will greatly facilitate

TABLE 13.8.
Summary of O★NET Database Releases

Release	Release Date	Primary Rating Source	Number of Occupations	Occupational Structure	Structure of Descriptors
O★NET 98	Oct 1998	Analysts	1,122	OUs	Prototype
O★NET 3.0	Aug 2000	Analysts	900+	SOC 2000	Prototype
O★NET 4.0	June 2002	Analysts	900+	SOC 2000	OMB-Approved
O★NET 5.1	Nov 2003	Incumbents	54	SOC 2000	OMB-Approved
O★NET 6.0	July 2004	Incumbents[a]	180[b]	SOC 2000	OMB-Approved
O★NET 7.0	Dec 2004	Incumbents[a]	280[b]	SOC 2000	OMB-Approved
O★NET 8.0	June 2005	Incumbents[a]	380[b]	SOC 2000	OMB-Approved
O★NET 9.0	Dec 2005	Incumbents[a]	480[b]	SOC 2000	OMB-Approved
O★NET 10.0	June 2006	Incumbents[a]	580[b]	SOC 2006	OMB-Approved
O★NET 11.0	Dec 2006	Incumbents[a]	680		

[a]Incumbents are the primary source for more recent data collections, but analysts provide some ratings (e.g., ability requirements).

[b]Number of occupations with comprehensively updated data. The original analyst data are available for the remaining occupations.

linking O★NET data to other available sources of occupational information, such as occupation outlook, wage information, and even specific job openings. A variety of "cross-walks" are also available linking the SOC codes to other codes, such as the DOT codes, the *Military Occupational Classification* (MOC) system, the *Classification of Instructional Programs* (CIP), and the *Registered Apprenticeship Information System* (RAIS). The fact that the O★NET is an electronic database, rather than a book, makes it much easier to continue to update and revise the occupational information, and this will allow the O★NET to evolve and change over time.

To help ensure timely incorporation of additional workforce changes and to remain responsive to user needs, the National Center for O★NET Development (2006b) has also developed a process for identifying and incorporating new and emerging occupations into the O★NET. Briefly, occupations will be added if they involve significantly different work than performed by job incumbents of other occupations and if they are not adequately reflected by the existing O★NET-SOC structure.

Current Status and Newer Features of O★NET

The National Center for O★NET Development is responsible for continually developing and updating the O★NET database and related products for the U.S. DOL Employment and Training Administration (ETA), as well as for providing technical support and customer service to users of O★NET. As already mentioned, the most recent release of the O★NET is version 11.0, which contains detailed, up-to-date information for 680 occupations and some information, mainly from occupational analysts, for the remaining occupations.

The National O★NET Center maintains an Internet Web site to provide up-to-date information concerning the status of O★NET and the release of new products (http://www.onetcenter.org). This Web site also provides access to a variety of tools and supplemental materials that have been developed by the DOL team. This includes a set of career exploration tools that allow users to assess their own interests, work-related values, and abilities and to use this information as they search the O★NET database for occupations. There is also a "code connector" designed to help workforce professionals identify O★NET job codes by searching the O★NET titles, lay titles, job descriptions, and so on for a title, phrase, or word entered by the user. This allows users to easily determine an appropriate occupational code to use in classifying job seekers or job orders. In addition to the various O★NET releases mentioned in the previous section, there is also a Spanish version of the O★NET 4.0 release.

The O★NET Center has also developed a variety of supplemental data files, which can be accessed from their Web site. One of these files, the Detailed Work Activities (DWAs), was developed to fill the gap between the GWAs and the occupation-specific tasks. The GWAs allow for cross-occupation comparisons, while the tasks are useful for differentiating nuances within and between occupations. The DWAs are at in intermediate level of specificity that allows for some cross-occupational comparisons and matching while preserving differentiation. They provide a common language for comparing jobs, and because they cut across occupations, they can be particularly useful for identifying transferable skills and skill gaps, generating job descriptions, and writing resumes. Other supplemental files include Emerging Tasks (derived from open-ended responses on O★NET data collection instruments), Lay Titles (alternate occupation titles linked to the O★NET-SOC classification system), and Tools and Technology (information on machines, equipment, tools, and software that workers use, with a focus on cutting-edge technology and emerging workplace practices). Details concerning these and other supplemental data files can be found at http://www.onetcenter.org.

The DOL has also released an on-line version of O★NET with a Web-based interface (http://online.onetcenter.org). This Web-based application provides user-friendly access to the O★NET occupational information. It is intended that users will also develop additional, specific interfaces for their particular applications, and the DOL provides downloadable databases and Data Dictionaries to facilitate these applications; even an O★NET graphic is provided. The National O★NET Center has also developed two additional Web sites to provide other types of support for O★NET users. The first, http://www.onetknowledgesite.com, provides information about O★NET use and training and allows users to share information with peers and join an online community of O★NET users. The second, http://www.onteacademy.com, provides online O★NET training, including self-paced courses and tutorials and live "webinars."

O★NET Applications and Implications for Rehabilitation Professionals

Taken together, the O★NET descriptors provide a comprehensive, detailed picture of each occupation in the U.S. economy. In addition, because much of this information is collected using a standardized set of descriptors, it is ideal for making systematic comparisons across occupations and for matching workers with appropriate occupations. O★NET job description information may also be more accessible to clients than the DOT information. Recall that behavioral anchors are included on all of the descriptor level rating scales. In addition to helping the incumbents who provide job analysis ratings to use these scales consistently, these scales can also be provided to O★NET users to enhance the interpretability of the numerical ratings in the O★NET database. Via the SOC, the O★NET job descriptions have been linked to much of the other available occupational information, including wages, video clips of occupations, occupational outlook, incumbents' educational levels, and even specific job postings.

The O★NET represents a major shift in the approach taken by the DOL to collect occupational information and is designed to replace the DOT as the nation's primary source of occupational information. It will necessarily take time for communities of DOT users, including the rehabilitation community, to fully embrace the new system and take advantage of all of its capabilities. While the O★NET is already beginning to be found useful in a variety of rehabilitation-related contexts and for a variety of purposes, application is still somewhat limited and many rehabilitation professionals continue to rely on DOT-based occupational information. This section describes some of the current uses of the O★NET database and tools, ongoing research and development related to O★NET, and a few possible applications for the future.

The current and future applications of the O★NET in occupational rehabilitation necessarily take place in the context of the evolving profession. New service delivery models are emerging that represent a subtle but important shift from traditional vocational rehabilitation as practiced by many vocational rehabilitation counselors and industrial rehabilitation and physical therapists. These new approaches to occupational rehabilitation are led by rehabilitation psychologists and occupational therapists. Philosophically, the shift is away from vocational rehabilitation to occupational rehabilitation. This is a broadening of perspective, including all significant meaningful occupation roles in which the client participates, rather than focusing exclusively on the client's vocation. As a key occupational role, the client's vocation continues to be an important reference, but other roles outside the workplace are also important. Occupational rehabilitation professionals consider the client's participation based on person abilities rather than job demands, which is exactly the change in emphasis from the DOT to the O★NET. Thus, the broader O★NET perspective on occupation, even if it is intended to be focused on a job in the workplace, coincides with the evolving and broadening rehabilitation perspectives on occupation.

A Case Study of O★NET in Rehabilitation

The Occupational Performance Center (OPC) in The Rehabilitation Institute of St. Louis, Missouri (a joint project of the Program in Occupational Therapy at the Washington University School of Medicine and the HealthSouth Corporation) and the Employment Potential Improvement Corporation (EPIC) in St. Charles, Missouri, use O★NET in their practices for a variety of purposes. Several of these applications are described here briefly to highlight the ways in which one group of rehabilitation professionals have found O★NET useful and to provide potential users with a variety of ideas for O★NET applications. Additional information about other applications of O★NET in rehabilitation, as well as in other contexts, can be found at the National O★NET Center Web site (http://www.onetcenter.org).

Career Exploration

One of the primary purposes of the O★NET is to serve as an information resource for career exploration. For many years, the information from the DOT was at the heart of most computerized career information delivery systems, and the O★NET information will likely replace the DOT in most of these systems. In addition, the Internet application "O★NET OnLine"—which was developed by the DOL to provide user-friendly access to the O★NET occupational information—can be used by rehabilitation professionals and their clients as a career exploration tool. The National O★NET Center is continually working to enhance O★NET OnLine, and current features include the ability to focus on high growth, in-demand occupations or to search for occupations based on specific descriptors (e.g., to look for all jobs that require high levels of one or more specific abilities).

At the OPC, occupational therapists orient clients to O★NET OnLine using an online computer workstation and encourage clients to explore the O★NET information independently, both at the OPC and at home. Increasingly, online computer use and the availability of online computers at public facilities such as libraries extend the efficacy of therapists providing occupational rehabilitation services beyond the confines of the occupational rehabilitation clinic. The experience at OPC has been that O★NET OnLine is sufficiently user-friendly so that a substantial proportion of persons with disability, even those with cognitive demands such as many OPC clients, are able to navigate through the system and independently explore. The video clips of various occupations have been found especially useful, as well as the data concerning earnings and job availability in various regions of the country.

With younger clients who have not yet developed a career path and with adult clients whose functional limitations appear to preclude return to the original career path, OPC vocational exploration employs the Holland system, typically within the context of the *Career Assessment Inventory* (CAI; Johansson, 1986). Using both the Career and the Vocational versions of the CAI, the occupational therapists work with the clients to identify alternate occupational goals. The fact that the O★NET also uses the Holland method of organizing vocational interests (Holland, 1966, 1973) facilitates this vocational exploration.

Identification of Transferable Skills

The O★NET makes it possible to efficiently and accurately identify clusters of occupations that require similar skills, abilities, and other worker requirements, even when the actual tasks performed by workers differ. The same O★NET descriptors were used to describe all occupations to facilitate such cross-occupation comparisons. Workers typically develop a variety of job-related skills and knowledge in the course of working in a particular job. The O★NET can help them determine how to take advantage of the skills and knowledge they have already developed when searching for a new occupation.

At the OPC, the O★NET descriptors have also been found helpful in working with clients to understand their employment histories. Adult clients are typically referred to OPC several weeks after experiencing an acquired brain injury through trauma, stroke, or spinal cord injury. Many persons with acquired brain injury have problems with cognition that interfere with their ability to be optimal historians, including difficulties with providing information about their previous work duties. Additionally, many of these clients have problems with executive function that interfere with, among other things, appropriate goal setting and planning. The O★NET is used at OPC to help the occupational therapist and client communicate with each other so that the client can provide good information about previous job tasks as well as necessary skills and abilities. Based on the title of each client's previous occupation, a questionnaire is generated that is populated with the relevant O★NET occupational task factors and used by the therapist to facilitate collecting employment history information.

Ability Assessment and Disability Determination

At EPIC, the O★NET is used in work capacity evaluation and occupational disability determination. As a tool for work capacity evaluation, the O★NET is used to identify the ability constructs most important in a client's current occupation. The O★NET is a portal to information used by the vocational evaluator to match the person's residual functional capacity to the job. Matching based on the cognitive and interpersonal domains is much better with O★NET than with the DOT aptitude, temperament, interests, and educational development scales (issues related to physical abilities are discussed in the next section). At EPIC, a review of the O★NET description of each client's previous occupation is used to develop an initial focus for the constructs to be addressed in the work capacity evaluation.

For example, the registered nurse with a traumatic brain injury who is attempting to return to work will need to be assessed with instruments that are sensitive to the tasks in her job. Rather than attempt to perform a complete and comprehensive assessment of her ability to perform all job tasks, the O★NET information is used to focus on those abilities that are both pertinent to her job and in which she has some significant limitations. After review and identification of the core tasks, the O★NET is queried in the abilities domain by the vocational evaluator, often assisted by the client to identify the most important abilities with which she has difficulty in her job's core tasks. Because clients often have difficulty understanding the definitions of the ability constructs, the vocational evaluator undertakes this in concert with the client. This is sometimes facilitated through the use of the *Fleischman Job Analysis Survey* (FJAS; Fleishman & Reilly, 1992)—which provides information comparing and contrasting the various ability constructs as well as behavior-anchored rating scales associated with each ability factor (on which the O★NET Abilities domain is based)—to provide a better understanding of the ability constructs.

After the task and ability constructs that are most pertinent to the particular client have been identified, the vocational evaluator selects standardized psychological and vocational tests to assess the client's status. Although there is not a simple cross-reference between O★NET tasks or abilities and most standardized tests, an experienced vocational evaluator should be sufficiently conversant with task and ability constructs so that test selection is not encumbered. After test administration, the vocational evaluator must interpret test results and translate these results in terms of each of the pertinent constructs and how the client's scores relate to his or her occupation. For many tests, direct comparison to normative test scores for the client's occupational group is not readily available. For most standardized tests, normative data have been collected and published for only a few occupations, with the exception of a few instruments such as the *Wonderlic Personnel Test* (Wonderlic Personnel Test, Inc., 1998). Although normative interpretation is performed optimally when there are closely matched occupational groups, appropriate interpretation can be accomplished through cross-walking within the O★NET from occupations for which normative data have been collected to the client's target occupation.

Regarding disability determination, EPIC cross-walks the O★NET ability constructs to the *Functional Assessment Constructs* (FAC) taxonomy (Gaudino, Matheson, & Mael, 2001; Matheson, Kaskutas, McCowan, Shaw, & Webb, 2001). The latter is used to organize information about the client's functional limitations, with this information coming from medical records, client self-report, performance testing, and collateral reports. Information from these various sources is collected and synthesized so that ratings of functional limitations within the FAC taxonomy are obtained. The ratings range from "slightly limited" to "unable" along a 4-point scale. The determination of the client's disability in terms of the usual and customary occupation is completed through comparison of the functional limitations to the task demands and core abilities identified through the use of O★NET.

Development of Occupation-Related Goals

Another application of O★NET is in goal development and vocational planning. The OPC is a strongly goal-directed return-to-work program, and the O★NET is used to facilitate an intervention goal setting procedure based on the *Canadian Occupational Performance Measure* (Law et al., 1998). OPC professionals have developed a *Work Performance Questionnaire* (Kaskutas, 2006) that is focused on necessary skills and abilities identified through the use of the O★NET. The occupational therapist uses this questionnaire to work with the client to select meaningful goals and set performance targets that will subsequently guide intervention. This early focus facilitates subsequent return to work because the interventions are designed to develop occupational performance tailored to the development of skills and abilities that the client has helped to select. Using this procedure to set goals for each skill and ability and measure progress toward these goals helps to maintain a client-centered focus, which facilitates empowerment of the client. This approach seems to help deal with especially sticky problems with motivation and frustration as the client participates in the program and encounters barriers or difficulties in progressing at a rate that is personally acceptable.

Development of Realistic Work Simulations

The OPC philosophical orientation emphasizes the importance of general occupational performance, recognizing the interplay between the person with the occupation and the environment. For this reason, work simulation is a key method to both evaluate the client and provide opportunities for development of the client's work skills and abilities. The O★NET has been a key reference in the development of Structured Work Activity Groups (SWAGs), a type of structured work simulation pioneered at the OPC. The SWAG approach uses low-fidelity virtual reality as a context for graded demand work simulations. These are similar to the job component work samples developed by the Materials Development Center (MDC) at the University of Wisconsin-Stout and the structured work simulations developed by the Employment and Rehabilitation Institute of California (ERIC). In the SWAG approach, a "virtual employer" is the context for a variety of jobs that involve the impaired skills and abilities of the OPC clientele. These skills and abilities are challenged on a progressive demand basis through the involvement of clients in job tasks that are graded to begin with the client's current ability and extend up to a competitive employment standard.

For example, SWAG #1 is the Saint Francis International Library, a virtual employer in the suburbs of Denver, Colorado. Job tasks include answering the telephone and recording messages accurately, scheduling the two library conference rooms for community organizations, bookkeeping for the overdue books and videos, planning for purchasing of replacement books and videos, maintaining the patron database and mailing list, and mailing tasks. The O★NET was used as one of two key references in the development of this SWAG and the other subsequent SWAG simulations in two ways. The first was to develop a description of the task content within a job cluster that could be found within a single employer. Rather than focus on one job, such as in the MDC or ERIC approach, multiple job tasks naturally occurring within one employer setting were identified.

This is a more current approach than the earlier models, which focused on a particular job with the assumption that clients' work tasks would be similarly structured in an insular manner rather than require clients to work across strict job boundaries in cooperation with other workers. A second use of O★NET in the development of the SWAG activities has been to research the frequency of occurrence of jobs and the likely job growth. Although the development of the SWAG activities has been organic from the point of view that they must be developed to serve OPC clients, there was also a concern that the SWAG activities anticipate future employment trends.

Additional Research and Development to Support Future Applications

In the future, O★NET users will benefit a great deal from additional research and development and new (or improved) applications that further tailor the O★NET data to their needs. Development of new applications that take advantage of the inherent strengths in the O★NET design can also facilitate acceptance in the rehabilitation community. Because of its consistent design across domains, the O★NET is extremely amenable to the development of new applications by front-line professionals.

Assessment of Physical Abilities

The O★NET includes nine physical ability descriptors (e.g., static strength, stamina), 10 perceptual ability descriptors (e.g., night vision, hearing sensitivity), and 10 psychomotor ability descriptors (e.g., manual dexterity, reaction time). The greater number of O★NET descriptors in these ability areas provides greater specificity than the DOT information, with the potential to help match persons with disabilities to appropriate jobs. The O★NET includes ratings of the importance of each of these descriptors and the ability level required for each occupation.

One particularly critical linkage for rehabilitation professionals will be between the O★NET physical ability descriptors and the assessments of physical functioning used in rehabilitation. Most or all of the currently available functional capacity evaluation standardized test batteries have been designed to provide information to match the DOT factors (Dusik, Menard, Cooke, Fairburn, & Beach, 1993; Fishbain et al., 1994; Hart, Iserhagen, & Matheson, 1993; Isernhagen, Hart, & Matheson, 1999), and there is not a simple cross-walk from O★NET factors to DOT factors. This is especially problematic in the DOT physical demand areas: The physical ability factors from the O★NET are conceptualized in terms of person abilities, and the DOT focuses on job demands. For example, a key part of job analysis using the DOT model is to examine the lifting demands of the job. The performance targets for these tests are based on the job demands that have been observed by the job analyst, typically measured in terms of amount of the load and frequency and vertical range of the lift. This information is used in a functional capacity evaluation by the occupational rehabilitation professional who administers tests in which the evaluee performs lifting (Gross, Battie, & Cassidy, 2004; Kuijer et al., 2006; Matheson, 1986; Matheson, Isernhagen, & Hart, 2002). No simple analog is available in the O★NET model.

To begin to address this issue, Johnson, Carter, and Dorsey (2002) conducted analyses to determine whether linear combinations of scores on O★NET descriptor variables could be used to accurately reflect/predict occupational strength demands. They conducted this analysis using 43 O★NET variables/descriptors and 387 occupations that could be cross-walked from the O★NET to the DOT. Using discriminant analysis, they selected those variables that best classified O★NET occupations into four DOT strength categories: Sedentary, Light, Medium, and Heavy/Very Heavy. (The Heavy and Very Heavy Categories were combined because there were so few occupations in the latter.) The O★NET variables that contributed most to the discriminant analysis were Static Strength, Standing, and Controlling Machines and Processes. Using these and several other O★NET variables, approximately 84% of the occupations could be correctly classified. These researchers suggest that it may be both useful and desirable to use these equations to directly classify O★NET occupations in terms of a DOT-like strength category. This may hold promise for occupational rehabilitation professionals.

Assessment of Cognitive Abilities

Another promising line of research that has potential to help rehabilitation professionals is the translation of O★NET ability dimensions to aptitude scales in a standardized aptitude test battery. A project in which the *Ball Aptitude Battery* (BAB; Ball Foundation, 1995) was linked to the occupational ability domain in the O★NET to facilitate person–occupation fit (Converse, Oswald, Gillespie, Field, & Bizot, 2002) indicates that this is a reasonable area of development. Using expert raters' judgments and previous research findings to establish rational and empirical links between the BAB scales and the O★NET abilities factors, these researchers used a hierarchical model of cognitive ability to provide a theoretical framework and filter to develop a method to cross-walk from aptitude scales to the O★NET ability requirement ratings. Based on this model, a set of scoring algorithms that allowed comparison of profile levels and shapes, based on a person's aptitudes and the occupation's ability requirements, was developed.

These early successful efforts to cross-walk the O★NET to established systems should encourage test developers and purveyors to undertake similar projects so that occupational rehabilitation professionals (and others) can have the tools available to assess the client's performance. To the degree that this occurs, O★NET will be increasingly valued in the occupational rehabilitation community. The benefit of this type of translational research is important for the practice of occupational rehabilitation and will hopefully be undertaken more broadly.

Understanding the Work Environment

Another potential area of promise for occupational rehabilitation professionals that O★NET presents is the possibility of better understanding the work environment. An exploratory factor analysis of O★NET has been conducted (Hadden, Kravets, & Muntaner, 2004) that identified four environmental factors in the O★NET database: Substantial Complexity, People Versus Things, Physical Demands, and Bureaucracy. These researchers suggest that the O★NET variables can be used to provide "relatively objective and up-to-date assessments of work environments." As occupational rehabilitation professionals integrate environmental demands of the client's occupation into assessment and intervention, the ability to use O★NET variables in this manner will be more appreciated and adoption of O★NET in practice will likely occur more broadly.

Conclusion

The O★NET provides a carefully developed framework for describing jobs that is based on state-of-the-art research in each of the O★NET content domains.

It is intended to provide a truly comprehensive descriptive system that allows users to view occupations from a variety of different perspectives. Each content domain can be regarded as a "window" through which an occupation can be viewed. These multiple windows provide different insights concerning the nature of the work and the people doing the work.

The O★NET content model includes more than 200 common, cross-job descriptors. Complete updated information for all of these descriptors is currently available for about 580 occupations, and this information will be available for all occupations in the *Standard Occupational Code* (SOC) classification system (more than 800) by late 2007. In the meantime, a database populated by analyst (rather than incumbent) ratings is available for the remaining occupations and a subset of the O★NET descriptors. Once incumbent data are available for all occupations, this database will replace the analyst database and contain information for the entire set of O★NET descriptors for all occupations. Analyses to date indicate that the O★NET descriptors and data collection procedures provide high-quality data. Both the analyst and incumbent ratings showed good reliability and meaningful interrelationships, both within and across content domains.

The O★NET OnLine has been put to use by many rehabilitation professionals. It is an excellent information resource for career exploration, and once introduced to this system, many clients are able to explore independently. The use of the Holland codes provides ready links to many available interest measures. The O★NET can also be used to obtain information about the ability requirements and tasks involved in clients' previous occupations, and along with information about their current limitations, this can provide an excellent starting point for work capacity evaluation. Also, the O★NET occupational information can be used to help clients set performance goals that focus on the skills and abilities directly related to their occupational objectives, which can empower clients and help keep them motivated. Another current use of the O★NET database is in the development of work simulations that are both realistic and focused on occupations that occur frequently and/or are likely to grow.

The O★NET has enormous potential for helping rehabilitation professionals, and the applications described here are just a beginning. Additional research and development are needed before the O★NET can realize its full potential for rehabilitation professionals. Research described in this chapter provides a good start, including work to link the O★NET physical abilities to the DOT strength factors (and, by extension, to many of the available assessments of physical functioning; Johnson et al., 2002) and to develop links between O★NET ability level requirements and a currently available standardized aptitude battery (Converse et al., 2002). After cross-walks have been developed, careful attention also needs to be paid to the most appropriate ways of linking scores on worker assessment tools with level requirements on the O★NET descriptors, and Oswald et al. (1999) provide an example of person–occupation matching that takes into account both the level and the shape of the person and occupation ability profiles. The O★NET is designed to provide a comprehensive, flexible source of occupational information. This chapter has highlighted several possible applications of O★NET for rehabilitation professionals, but a wide variety of other applications will also be possible with additional research and development.

References

Anderson, L. E. (1999). Occupational preparation: Education, training, experience, and licensure/certification. In N. G. Peterson, M. D. Mumford, W. C. Borman, P. R. Jeanneret, & E. A. Fleishman (Eds.), *An occupational information system for the 21st century: The development of O★NET* (pp. 91–104). Washington, DC: American Psychological Association.

Arad, S., Hanson, M. A., & Schneider, R. J. (1999). Organizational context. In N. G. Peterson, M. D. Mumford, W. C. Borman, P. R. Jeanneret, & E. A. Fleishman (Eds.), *An occupational information system for the 21st century: The development of O★NET* (pp. 147–174). Washington, DC: American Psychological Association.

Ball Foundation. (1995). *Technical manual for the Ball Aptitude Battery* (3rd ed.). Glen Ellyn, IL: Author.

Barrick, M. R., & Mount, M. K. (1991). The big five personality dimensions and job performance: A meta-analysis. *Personnel Psychology, 44,* 1–26.

Baughman, W. A., Norris, D. G., Cooke, A. E., Peterson, N. G., & Mumford, M. D. (1999). Occupation classification: Using basic and cross-functional skills and generalized work activities to create job families. In N. G. Peterson, M. D. Mumford, W. C. Borman, P. R. Jeanneret, & E. A. Fleishman (Eds.), *An occupational information system for the 21st century: The development of O★NET* (pp. 259–271). Washington, DC: American Psychological Association.

Borman, W. C., & Brush, D. H. (1993). More progress toward a taxonomy of managerial performance requirements. *Human Performance, 6,* 1–21.

Borman, W. C., Kubisiak, U. C., & Schneider, R. J. (1999). Work styles. In N. G. Peterson, M. D. Mumford, W. C. Borman, P. R. Jeanneret, & E. A. Fleishman (Eds.), *An occupational information system for the 21st century: The development of O★NET* (pp. 213–226). Washington, DC: American Psychological Association.

Converse, P., Oswald, F., Gillespie, M., Field, K., & Bizot, E. (2002). *Beyond gut instinct: Exploring careers using aptitudes and O★NET.* Paper presented at the 17th Annual Conference of the Society for Industrial and Organizational Psychology, Toronto, Ontario, Canada.

Costanza, D. P., Fleishman, E. A., & Marshall-Mies, J. C. (1999). Knowledges. In N. G. Peterson, M. D. Mumford, W. C. Borman, P. R. Jeanneret, & E. A. Fleishman (Eds.), *An occupational information system for the 21st century: The development of O★NET* (pp. 71–90). Washington, DC: American Psychological Association.

Cunningham, J. W. (1988). Occupation analysis inventory. In S. Gael (Ed.), *The job analysis handbook for business, industry, and government* (Vol. 2, pp. 975–990). New York: Wiley.

Cunningham, J. W. (1996). Generic job descriptors: A likely direction in occupational analysis. *Military Psychology, 8*(3), 247–262.

Daubert, William et al v. Merrell Dow Pharmaceuticals, Inc, No. 92-102. (1993). *Supreme Court Reporter, 113,* 2786–2800.

Dawis, R. V. (1991). Vocational interests, values, and preferences. In M. D. Dunnette & L. M. Hough (Eds.), *Handbook of industrial and organizational psychology* (Vol. 2, 2nd ed., pp. 833–872). Palo Alto, CA: CPP.

Dawis, R. V., & Lofquist, L. H. (1984). *A psychological theory of work adjustment: An individual-differences model and its applications.* Minneapolis, MN: University of Minnesota Press.

Dowell, B.E., & Wexley, K. N. (1978). Development of a work behavior taxonomy for first-line supervisors. *Journal of Applied Psychology, 63,* 563–572.

Drucker, P. (1994). Jobs and employment in a global economy. *Atlantic Monthly, 1,* 132–136.

Dusik, L. A., Menard, M. R., Cooke, C., Fairburn, S. M., & Beach, G. N. (1993). Concurrent validity of the ERGOS work simulator versus conventional functional capacity evaluation techniques in a workers' compensation population. *Journal of Occupational Medicine, 35*(8), 759–767.

Ericsson, K. A., & Charness, N. (1994). Expert performance: Its structure and acquisition. *American Psychologist, 49*(8), 725–747.

Fishbain, D., Abdel-Moty, E., Cutler, R., Khalil, T., Sadek, S., Rosomoff, R., et al. (1994). Measuring residual functional capacity in chronic low back pain patients based on the Dictionary of Occupational Titles. *Spine, 19*(8), 872–880.

Fleishman, E. A. (1975a). *Manual for ability requirement scales (MARS).* Bethesda, MD: Management Research Institute.

Fleishman, E. A. (1975b). *Physical abilities analysis manual.* Bethesda, MD: Management Research Institute.

Fleishman, E. A. (1988). Some new frontiers in personnel selection research. *Personnel Psychology, 41,* 679–701.

Fleishman, E. A. (1992). *Fleishman-Job Analysis Survey.* Bethesda, MD: Management Research Institute.

Fleishman, E. A., Costanza, D. P., & Marshall-Mies, J. C. (1999). Abilities. In N. G. Peterson, M. D. Mumford, W. C. Borman, P. R. Jeanneret, & E. A. Fleishman (Eds.), *An occupational information system for the 21st century: The development of O*★*NET.* Washington, DC: American Psychological Association.

Fleishman, E., & Reilly, M. (1992). *Administrator's guide: Fleishman job analysis survey.* Palo Alto, CA: CPP.

French, J. W. (1951). The description of aptitude and achievement tests in terms of rotated factors. *Psychometric Monographs, No. 5.*

Gaudino, E., Matheson, L., & Mael, F. (2001). Development of the Functional Assessment Taxonomy. *Journal of Occupational Rehabilitation, 11*(3), 155–175.

Gottefredson, G. D., & Holland, J. L. (1996). *Dictionary of Holland occupational codes* (3rd ed.). Odessa, FL: Psychological Assessment Resources.

Gross, D. P., Battie, M. C., & Cassidy, J. D. (2004). The prognostic value of functional capacity evaluation in patients with chronic low back pain: Part 1. Timely return to work. *Spine, 29*(8), 914–919.

Guilford, J. P. (1967). *The nature of human intelligence.* New York: McGraw-Hill.

Guion, R. M. (1992, April) Matching position requirements and personality. In L. M. Hough (Chair), *Industrial and Organizational Psychology.* Symposium conducted at the 7th annual meeting of the Society for Industrial and Organizational Psychology, Montreal, Canada.

Hadden, W., Kravets, N., & Muntaner, C. (2004). Descriptive dimensions of U.S. occupations with data from the O★NET. *Social Science Research, 33*(1), 64–78.

Hanson, M. A., Borman, W. C., Kubisiak, U. C., & Sager, C. E. (1999). Cross-domain analyses. In N. G. Peterson, M. D. Mumford, W. C. Borman, P. R. Jeanneret, & E. A. Fleishman (Eds.), *An occupational information system for the 21st century: The development of O*★*NET* (pp. 247–258). Washington, DC: American Psychological Association.

Hart, D., Iserhagen, S., & Matheson, L. (1993). Guidelines for functional capacity evaluation of people with medical conditions. *Journal of Orthopedic and Sports Physical Therapy, 18*(6), 682–686.

Harvey, R. J. (1991). Job analysis. In M. D. Dunnette & L. M. Hough (Eds.), *Handbook of industrial and organizational psychology* (2nd ed., Vol. 2, pp. 71–163). Palo Alto, CA: CPP.

Hogan, R. (1982). Socioanalytic theory of personality. In M. M. Page (Ed.), *1982 Nebraska symposium on motivation: Personality-current theory and research* (pp. 55–89). Lincoln, NE: University of Nebraska Press.

Holland, J. (1966). *The psychology of vocational choice: A theory of personality types and model environments.* Waltham, MA: Blaisdell.

Holland, J. (1973). *Making vocational choices: A theory of careers.* Englewood Cliffs, NJ: Prentice Hall.

Hough, L. M. (1997). Personality at work: Issues and evidence. In M. Hakel (Ed.), *Beyond multiple choice: Evaluating alternatives to traditional testing for selection* (pp. 131–166). Hillsdale, NJ: Erlbaum.

Hubbard, M., McCloy, R., Campbell, J., Levine, J., Nottingham, J., Lewis, P., & Rivkin, D. (2000). *Revision of O★NET data collection instruments.* Raleigh, NC: National Center for O★NET Development, Employment Security Commission.

Innes, E., & Straker, L. (1999). Validity of work-related assessments. *Work, 13,* 125–152.

Isernhagen, S., Hart, D., & Matheson, L. (1999). Reliability of independent observer judgments of level of lift effort in a kinesiophysical functional capacity evaluation. *Work, 12,* 145–150.

Jeanneret, P. R., Borman, W. C., Kubisiak, U. C., & Hanson, M. A. (1999). Generalized work activities. In N. G. Peterson, M. D. Mumford, W. C. Borman, P. R. Jeanneret, & E. A. Fleishman (Eds.), *An occupational information system for the 21st century: The development of O★NET.* Washington, DC: American Psychological Association.

Johansson, C. B. (1986). *Career Assessment Inventory.* Minneapolis, MN: National Computer Systems.

Johnson, J., Carter, G., & Dorsey, D. (2002). *Development of an occupational strength requirement measure from O★NET descriptors.* Paper presented at the 17th Annual Conference of the Society for Industrial and Organizational Psychology, Toronto, Ontario, Canada.

Kaskutas, V. (2006). *Work Performance Questionnaire.* St. Louis, MO: Washington University School of Medicine Program in Occupational Therapy.

Kuijer, W., Brouwer, S., Reneman, M., Dijkstra, P., Groothoff, J., Schellekens, J., et al. (2006). Matching FCE activities and work demands: An explorative study. In *Journal of Occupational Rehabilitation Online* (pp. 1–15). The Netherlands: Springer.

Law, M., Baptiste, S., Carswell, A., McColl, M., Polatajko, H., & Pollock, N. (1998). *Canadian Occupational Performance Measure.* Ottawa, Ontario, Canada: CAOT Publications.

Matheson, L. (1986). Evaluation of lifting and lowering capacity. *Vocational Evaluation and Work Adjustment Bulletin, 19*(4), 107–111.

Matheson, L., Isernhagen, S., & Hart, D. (2002). Relationship between lifting ability and grip force and return to work. *Physical Therapy, 82,* 249–256.

Matheson, L., Kaskutas, V., McCowan, S., Shaw, H., & Webb, C. (2001). Development of a database of functional assessment measures related to work disability. *Journal of Occupational Rehabilitation, 11*(3), 177–199.

McCloy, R., Waugh, G., Medsker, G., Wall, J., Rivkin, D., & Lewis, P. (1999). *Determining the occupational reinforcer patterns for O★NET occupational units.* Raleigh, NC: National Center for O★NET Development, Employment Security Commission.

McCormick, E. J., Jeanneret, P. R., & Mecham, R. C. (1972). A study of job characteristics and job dimensions as based on the Position Analysis Questionnaire (PAQ). *Journal of Applied Psychology Monograph, 56,* 347–368.

Mumford, M. D., Peterson, N. G., & Childs, R. A. (1999). Basic and cross-functional skills. In N. G. Peterson, M. D. Mumford, W. C. Borman, P. R. Jeanneret, & E. A. Fleishman

(Eds.), *An occupational information system for the 21st century: The development of O*NET.* (pp. 49–69). Washington, DC: American Psychological Association.

National Center for O*NET Development. (2006a). *Updating the O*NET-SOC taxonomy: Summary and implementation.* Raleigh, NC: Author.

National Center for O*NET Development. (2006b). *New and emerging (N&E) occupations: Methodology development report.* Raleigh, NC: Author.

Oswald, F., Campbell J., McCloy R., Rivkin D., & Lewis P. (1999). *Stratifying occupational units by specific vocational preparation (SVP).* Raleigh, NC: National Center for O*NET Development, Employment Security Commission.

Outerbridge, A. N. (1981). *The development of generalizable work behavior categories for a synthetic validity model.* Washington, DC: U.S. Office of Personnel Management, Personnel Research and Development Center.

Peterson, N. G., Mumford, M. D., Borman, W. C., Jeanneret, P. R., & Fleishman, E. A. (Eds.). (1995). *Development of prototype occupational information network (O*NET) content model* (Vols. 1 & 2). Salt Lake City: Utah Department of Employment Security.

Peterson, N. G., Mumford, M. D., Borman, W. C., Jeanneret, P. R., & Fleishman, E. A. (Eds.). (1996). *O*NET final technical report.* Salt Lake City: Utah Department of Employment Security.

Peterson, N. G., Mumford, M. D., Borman, W. C., Jeanneret, P. R., & Fleishman, E. A. (Eds.). (1999). *An occupational information system for the 21st century: The development of O*NET.* Washington, DC: American Psychological Association.

Peterson, N. G., Mumford, M. D., Levin, K. Y., Green, J., & Waksberg, J. (1999). Research method: Development and field testing of the content model. In N. G. Peterson, M. D. Mumford, W. C. Borman, P. R. Jeanneret, & E. A. Fleishman (Eds.), *An occupational information system for the 21st century: The development of O*NET* (pp. 31–47). Washington, DC: American Psychological Association.

Peterson, N. G., Owens-Kurtz, C., Hoffman, R. G., Arabian, J. M., & Whetzel, D. C. (1990). *Army synthetic validation project.* Alexandria, VA: U.S. Army Research Institute for the Behavioral Sciences.

Rounds, J., Smith, T., Hubert, L., Lewis, P., & Rivkin, D. (1999). *Development of occupational interest profiles for 0 *NET.* Raleigh, NC: National Center for O*NET Development, Employment Security Commission.

Sager, C. E. (1999). Occupational interests and values. In N. G. Peterson, M. D. Mumford, W. C. Borman, P. R. Jeanneret, & E. A. Fleishman (Eds.), *An occupational information system for the 21st century: The development of O*NET* (pp. 197–211). Washington, DC: American Psychological Association.

Shrout, P. E., & Fleiss, J. L. (1979). Intraclass correlations: Uses in assessing rater reliability. *Psychological Bulletin, 86*(2), 420–428.

Strong, M. H., Jeanneret, P. R., McPhail, S. M., Blakley, B. R., & D'Egidio, E. L. (1999). Work context: Taxonomy and measurement of the work environment. In N. G. Peterson, M. D. Mumford, W. C. Borman, P. R. Jeanneret, & E. A. Fleishman (Eds.), *An occupational information system for the 21st century: The development of O*NET* (pp. 127–145). Washington, DC: American Psychological Association.

Thurstone, L.L. (1947). *Multiple factor analysis: A development and expansion of the vectors of mind.* Chicago: University of Chicago Press.

U.S. Department of Labor. (1991). *Dictionary of occupational titles* (4th ed., rev.). Washington, DC: U.S. Government Printing Office.

U.S. Department of Labor. (1993). *The new DOT: A database of occupational titles for the twenty-first century.* Washington, DC: U.S. Government Printing Office.

Wonderlic Personnel Test, Inc. (1998). *Wonderlic Personnel Test & Scholastic Level Exam User's Manual.* Libertyville, IL: Author.

Yukl, G. A. (1987, October). *A new taxonomy for integrating diverse perspectives on managerial behavior.* Paper presented at the annual meeting of the American Psychological Association, New York.

Chapter 14

Measurement of Consumer Outcomes in Rehabilitation

Richard T. Walls

An "outcome" is an effect. An outcome may be traceable to a cause. A desirable or undesirable outcome in rehabilitation is an end-product eventuality that may have a complex complement and sequence of causal influence. An outcome may be thought to be a consequence of an input or intervention but, indeed, be only a corollary. Neither the cause nor the effect of rehabilitation is unidimensional. The outcome of rehabilitation is a rich blend of functional–ability, employment, and independence variables. Similarly, the input-intervention process includes a myriad of person–place–event influences of varying quality and quantity. Rehabilitation is not a simple thing.

In 2007 the governing legislation is the Workforce Investment Act of 1998, which included the Rehabilitation Act Amendments of 1998 as Title IV. Thus, Title IV of the Workforce Investment Act of 1998 defined the policy for vocational rehabilitation services, including (a) eligibility for services; (b) individualized plan for employment (IPE); (c) services to facilitate vocational rehabilitation; and (d) operational definitions of clientele, needs, interventions, and outcomes. "Individuals with disabilities, including individuals with the most significant disabilities, are generally presumed to be capable of engaging in gainful employment and the provision of individualized vocational rehabilitation services can improve their ability to become gainfully employed" (Workforce Investment Act of 1998, p. 182). The purposes are as follows:

> (1) to empower individuals with disabilities to maximize employment, economic self-sufficiency, independence, and inclusion and integration into society . . . [and] (2) to ensure that the Federal Government plays a leadership role in promoting the employment of individuals with disabilities, especially individuals with significant disabilities, and in assisting States and providers of services in fulfilling the aspirations of such individuals with disabilities for meaningful and gainful employment and independent living. (Workforce Investment Act of 1998, p. 161)

This legislation lays the groundwork for continuance of the Federal-State Vocational Rehabilitation "VR" program.

Input-Intervention-Output Model

Rehabilitation may be conceptualized as an Input-Intervention-Output paradigm. Regardless of the rehabilitation agent or agency, input must be gained at the Intake Phase, intervention must occur at the Process Phase, and output must occur at the Outcome Phase. State rehabilitation agencies, rehabilitation hospitals, rehabilitation companies, and rehabilitation counselors in private practice use the Input-Intervention-Output paradigm. If individuals with disability are to be rehabilitated to increased levels of self-sufficiency and employment, it is essential that the rehabilitation–service agent facilitate worthy transitions from the input state (Intake Phase) to the output state (Outcome Phase) by providing or arranging beneficial interventions (Process Phase).

Intake Phase (Input)

In the Intake Phase (Input), assessment for determining eligibility and vocational rehabilitation or independent living needs for each case is to include a review of existing data and, to the extent necessary, the provision of appropriate assessment to obtain necessary additional data to make such determination. State rehabilitation programs are authorized by the Workforce Investment Act of 1998 to serve persons with a physical or mental impairment that constitutes or results in a substantial impediment to employment who can benefit from vocational rehabilitation services in terms of an employment outcome. Also, state rehabilitation programs are authorized to serve persons (a) with a physical or mental impairment that substantially limits one or more major life activities (b) who can benefit from services in terms of an independent living outcome.

In the Intake Phase, inputs may include functional capacities, interests, interpersonal skills, intelligence, educational achievements, adjustments, personality, vocational aptitudes, and work experience as well as other pertinent vocational, educational, medical, psychiatric, psychological, cultural, social, recreational, and environmental factors that affect the employment and rehabilitation needs of the individual. Required inputs include age, gender, ethnicity, education, category of impairment, severity of disability, and work status and earnings (if any) at the time of application for rehabilitation services. These assessments in the Intake Phase enable determination of eligibility for services and, if the individual is eligible, projection of the vocational rehabilitation services needed for acquisition of occupational skills and "development of work attitudes, work habits, work tolerance, and social and behavior patterns necessary for successful job performance" (Workforce Investment Act of 1998, p. 164).

A Policy Directive for State Vocational Rehabilitation Agencies (General and Blind) from the Rehabilitation Services Administration (2005) uses the three-part definition for "significant disability" as originally stated in the Workforce Investment Act of 1998. An individual with a significant disability is determined through the assessment (a) to have a severe physical or mental impairment that seriously limits functional capacities "such as mobility, communication, self-care, self-direction, interpersonal skills, work tolerance, or work skills"; (b) to likely require multiple vocational rehabilitation services over an extended period of time; and (c) to have one or more physical or mental disabilities resulting from amputation; arthritis; autism; blindness; burn injury; cancer; cerebral palsy; cystic fibrosis; deafness; head injury; heart disease; hemiplegia; hemophilia; respiratory or pulmonary dysfunction; mental retardation; mental illness; multiple sclerosis; muscular dystrophy; musculoskeletal disorders; neurological disorders (including stroke and epilepsy); paraplegia, quadriplegia, and other spinal cord conditions; sickle cell anemia; specific learning disability;

end-state renal disease; or another disability or combination of disabilities determined on the basis of an assessment for determining eligibility and vocational rehabilitation needs (Workforce Investment Act of 1998, p. 171).

Such assessment may lead to projection of the need for independent living services or supported employment. Supported employment is defined in the law as competitive work in integrated work settings, or employment in integrated work settings in which individuals are working toward competitive work, consistent with strengths, resources, priorities, concerns, abilities, capabilities, interests, and informed choice of the individuals, for individuals with the most significant disabilities (Workforce Investment Act of 1998, p. 74).

No matter whether vocational rehabilitation and independent living services are administered by the designated state agency or an alternate rehabilitation provider, the intake (input) variables listed in Table 14.1 are useful in determining (a) eligibility for services and (b) needs for guiding the rehabilitation process. Various organizations (e.g., Goodwill Industries) and programs (e.g., Social Security Administration's Ticket-to-Work program) are instrumental in the rehabilitation of many individuals with disabilities. The most extensive system, however, is the Federal-State Vocational Rehabilitation Program, under the auspices of the Rehabilitation Services Administration. Current as of 2007, the Vocational Rehabilitation (VR) client (consumer) moves through a series of steps (each designated as a "Status") in the VR process. The flow of a case is depicted in Figure 14.1.

In the Intake Phase of the Vocational Rehabilitation program, Referral (Status 00) designates the point at which an individual is referred for services. This referral can come from physician, hospital, human-service program, family, friend, the individual with the disability, or other sources. Applicant (Status 02) is the juncture at which the potential client applies for services, meets with a rehabilitation counselor, and provides input information during a diagnostic interview. While in the applicant status, the individual's eligibility for vocational rehabilitation services is determined. Records are obtained from various sources as necessary, and evaluations of the individual's disabling condition or conditions, experiences, strengths, and abilities assist in this eligibility determination. In addition to discussions, test results, and past records, a "trial work experience" in an integrated setting and under supervision by community rehabilitation personnel may assist as part of the eligibility-determination process (Workforce Investment Act, 1998). Multiple trial work experiences may assist in assessing an applicant's attitude toward work, work tolerance, skills, interests, and needs. Because of limited resources, a state rehabilitation agency may not be able to provide services to all persons determined to be eligible. If the person is found to be eligible for services but cannot receive them at this time because of not meeting the agency's order-of-selection priorities, he or she is placed on the waiting list for services, Pre-service Listing (Status 04).

The "input" gained at the Intake Phase sets the context for "interventions" in the Process Phase. As noted, in all sorts of rehabilitation programs, not just the state agencies under the Rehabilitation Services Administration, input about the penchants, talents, and needs of the person form the corpus of

TABLE 14.1.
Intake (Input) Variables, Process (Intervention) Variables,
and Outcome (Output) Variables in Rehabilitation

Intake Phase (Input)	*Process Phase (Intervention)*
Category of impairment	Counseling and guidance
Severity of disability	Corrective surgery
Functional capacities	Physical & occupational therapy
Age, gender, ethnicity	Speech & hearing therapy
Education history	Prosthetics & orthotics
Medical history	Eyeglasses & visual services
Environmental factors	Special services (e.g., dialysis)
Interests	Treatment for mental disorders
Interpersonal skills	Treatment for emotional disorders
Adjustment	Maintenance
Personality	Transportation
Intellectual aptitudes	Interpreter & reader services
Vocational aptitudes	Rehabilitation teaching & education
Results from trial work experience	Vocational & other training
Work experience	Licenses, tools, equipment, & supplies
Current work status	Tech assistance for self-employment
	Rehabilitation technology
	Transition services
	Services to the family
	Referral to other agencies
	Supported employment services
	Job search & placement
	On-the-job training
	Employment follow-up & follow-along

Outcome Phase (Output)

Vocational and Economic Outcomes

Economic independence (financial dependency, self-sufficiency, primary source)
Work status at case closure (follow-up, rehabilitated, not rehabilitated)
Work attitudes (work importance)
Work information (interview skills, vocational knowledge)
Occupation (occupational level)
Barriers to employment (barrier reduction or removal)
Speed of placement (difficulty finding work)
Salary (wage rate, money management)
Hours worked per week
Employment benefits (health insurance, retirement)
Advancement (training available)

(continues)

TABLE 14.1. *Continued.*

Vocational and Economic Outcomes (Continued)

Work adjustment (problems, self-control, social skills, cooperativeness, communication)

Work motivation (dependability, initiative, punctuality, self-direction)

Work performance (knowledge, skills, following directions, quantity, quality, safety)

Work tolerance (work capacity, physical demands, endurance)

Work functional limitations (accommodations, reduction, safety)

Work transportation (private, public)

Work support (community workshop, supported employment)

Employment retention (1 year, 2 years)

Satisfaction (employee, employer, family, friends, program services, life)

Public cash or in-kind benefits (discontinuation, reduction)

Savings to workers' compensation

Tax benefits for businesses

Cost of rehabilitation services

Time for service

Changes from intake (input) phase (gains, losses)

Medical, Independent Living, and Psychosocial Outcomes

Physical function (mobility, psychomotor, strength, coordination, balance, parallel-bar walking, pain, use of assistance, energy reserves, object manipulation, personal independence, driving)

Emotional function (emotional episodes, self-esteem, disruptiveness, behavior problems, eye contact, perception of disability, depression, internal–external orientation, psychological status, anxiety, coping, life satisfaction)

Cognitive function (problem solving, vocabulary, reading, functional academic skills, self-direction, alertness, communication, education status)

Daily-living function (food acquisition and preparation, eating, toileting, home maintenance, home safety, self-care, living arrangement)

Role and social function (interpersonal skills, social contacts, role functioning, family role, parenting, time spent in activities, time management, community integration)

Global-health function (health status, health satisfaction, discharge to long-term care, discharge to community, cost of services, time for services, days in the community, recidivism, drug and alcohol use, morbidity, mortality)

Changes from intake (input) phase (gains, losses)

information necessary to determine eligibility for services and plan for effective intervention. The Intake Phase of a case drives subsequent thinking and action.

Process Phase (Intervention)

If determined to be eligible for services, the individual becomes a client. In the Process Phase (Intervention), an individualized plan for services is developed

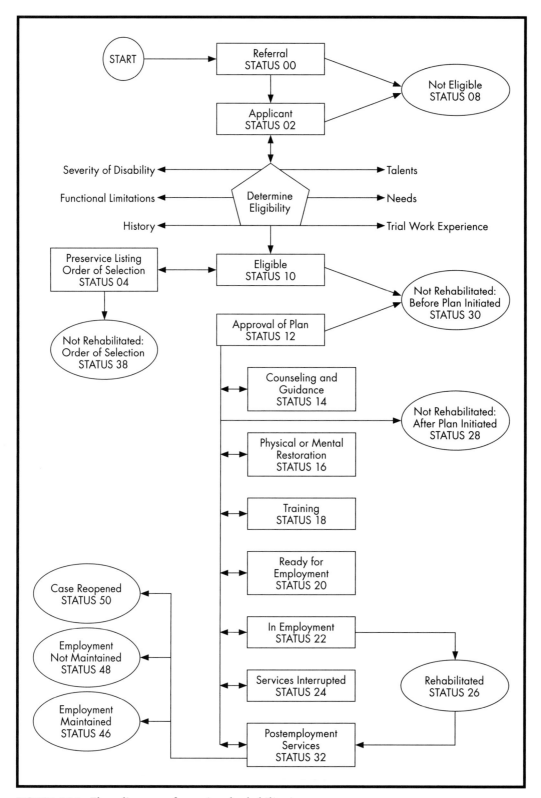

FIGURE 14.1. Flow diagram of vocational rehabilitation cases.

jointly by the client and his or her counselor. This plan can be for independent living services or vocational rehabilitation services, depending on the outcome intended. The Workforce Investment Act of 1998 indicates that

> an individualized plan for employment . . . will be developed and implemented in a timely manner for an individual subsequent to the determination of the eligibility of the individual for services . . . The State plan shall include an assurance that such services will be provided in accordance with the provisions of the individualized plan for employment. (p. 191)

State rehabilitation agencies traditionally use the terms *Individualized Plan for Employment* (IPE) and *Independent Living Plan* (ILP) when referring to the written agreement between client and counselor.

After the client is found to be Eligible (Status 10), development of the written rehabilitation plan begins. Table 14.1 indicates services that often are given, and Figure 14.1 depicts the case-status arrangements for interventions in this Process Phase. In the Federal-State Vocational Rehabilitation system, Approval of Plan (Status 12) indicates that a written plan has been developed jointly by client and counselor, has been approved, and is ready to be implemented. Counseling and Guidance Only (Status 14) connotes a major service of greater depth and longer duration than the ongoing counseling and guidance provided to every client in the course of his or her rehabilitation.

Given the individualization needed for effective casework, it is not necessary that the statuses within the Process Phase be followed in sequence. For example, a client leaving intensive Counseling and Guidance Only (Status 14) might move into Rehabilitation Training (Status 18) or Ready for Employment (Status 20) and then back to Counseling and Guidance Only (Status 14). Physical or Mental Restoration (Status 16) may be required, such as surgery, psychiatric treatment, therapy, or artificial appliance fitting. If Rehabilitation Training (Status 18) will be of benefit, the client's individualized plan may call for academic, business, vocational, personal-adjustment, or any other type of training from a college or university, community college, business or commercial school, rehabilitation facility, tutor, distance-education course, or an on-the-job setting. A case is moved into Ready for Employment (Status 20) when the client has completed the services specified in the written rehabilitation plan and is ready to accept a job but has not been placed or has not yet begun working. When services have been completed and the client is working, the case is classified as In Employment (Status 22). A minimum of 90 days in this status is required. If services are interrupted, the case is moved to Services Interrupted (Status 24). A final Process Phase denotation can be Post-Employment Services (Status 32) in which the client may be receiving additional service, such as supported employment, in order to maintain vocational participation.

"Intensity" of vocational rehabilitation and independent living rehabilitation has been operationalized in terms of the total number of services received by the client (e.g., prosthetics, training, interpreters), duration of services (from the written rehabilitation plan to case closure), and service costs (for purchased services). Bellini, Bolton, and Neath (1998) suggested that service intensity (process) is an appropriate measure of functional limitation and can more fully describe the level of severity of disability. Thus, in line with federal regulations, severity of disability may be defined in terms of a combination of (a) functional limitations in key life areas (mobility, communication, self-care, self-direction, interpersonal skills, work tolerance, work skills) as an input (intake) variable in league with (b) the need for multiple services over extended time as an intervention (process) variable (Neath, Bellini, & Bolton, 1997).

Physical, mental, and even environmental circumstances may constitute or contribute to functional limitations. Examples of environmental considerations are the disincentives associated with the receipt of cash and in-kind benefits, which may have dramatic effects on an individual's enthusiasm for entering the workforce (e.g., Walls, 1982; Walls, Dowler, & Fullmer, 1990). Walls and Dowler (1987) demonstrated an anchoring effect in which the level of public benefits received by the client that might be jeopardized by substantial gainful employment dictates the level of earnings that would be necessary for the person to give up those benefits and go to work. Legislative attempts to reduce those disincentives, education programs to advise consumers and counselors of optimal strategies, and findings from research emphasize the importance of this powerful disincentives variable that has more than a correlational relationship with employment outcomes (Ernst & Day, 1998; Moore & Powell, 1990).

As noted previously, the law encourages Vocational Rehabilitation counselors to work with clients who have significant disabilities rather than "skimming" the easy cases (give them teeth or glasses and close the case). Substantial services can include physical and mental restoration (e.g., corrective surgery, prosthetics, occupational therapy, treatment for emotional disorder, rehabilitation technology, visual and hearing services), training (e.g., college, vocational–technical, on-the-job, independence skills), job search and placement, supported employment, and post-employment services. The Intake Phase (Input) and the Process Phase (Intervention) are necessary prerequisites that set the stage for measurement of gains and accomplishments resulting from the rehabilitation process.

Outcome Phase (Output)

How do we want a rehabilitation case to end? At the Outcome Phase (Output), the fervent desire of rehabilitation agents and their clients is that substantial progress through counseling, restoration, and training should be manifested in independence and economic self-sufficiency. Table 14.1 lists possible outcomes. Cooperative agent–client mutuality and substantial rehabilitation services can result in medical improvement or recovery, increased skills for independent living, and/or competitive employment (Majumder, Walls, & Fullmer, 1999). Unfortunately, as illustrated in Figure 14.1, not rehabilitated is also a possible outcome.

Figure 14.1 shows that clients may exit the process in any of several outcome statuses. Not Eligible (Status 08) means that the individual was determined to be ineligible for vocational rehabilitation or independent living services and therefore was not accepted for services. Not Rehabilitated: Before Plan Initiated (Status 30) indicates that although the person was determined eligible and was accepted for services, he or she dropped out, died, or for some reason did not progress to the point that services actually were initiated. Not Rehabilitated: After Plan Initiated (Status 28) requires that at least one of the services specified in the individualized plan for employment or the independent living plan must have been initiated. The client, however, dropped out or died or for some other reason did not continue in the rehabilitation process. Rehabilitated (Status 26) is, of course, a coveted outcome. For a rehabilitated outcome, the person with a disability (a) is declared eligible for services; (b) receives appropriate assessment; (c) has a plan of vocational rehabilitation or independent living services formulated; (d) completes that program of services, including counseling; and, (e) for a vocational rehabilitation case, is suitably employed for a minimum of 90 days. Independent living cases must achieve the independent living plan goal for a minimum of 60 days.

For clients who do not need postemployment services, Rehabilitated (Status 26) signifies the final designation of success. If, however, the case is moved into Post-Employment Services (Status 32) to provide extended support, it can exit with Employment Maintained (Status 46), Employment Not Maintained (Status 48), or Case Reopened (Status 50). The only other exit condition is Not Rehabilitated: Order of Selection (Status 38) because the rehabilitation agency did not have sufficient resources available to provide services to a person on the waiting list.

Desirable outcomes of independent living services could be improved physical functioning as well as adaptive cognitive and social functioning. With respect to employment outcomes, the Workforce Investment Act refers to an individual "entering or retaining full-time or, if appropriate, part-time competitive employment in the integrated labor market . . . satisfying the vocational outcome of supported employment; or . . . satisfying the vocational outcome of self-employment, telecommuting, or business ownership" (p. 166). State rehabilitation programs are required to report "the number who ended their participation in the program . . . the number who achieved employment outcomes after receiving vocational rehabilitation services . . . the number . . . who were employed 6 months and 12 months after securing or regaining employment . . . the number who earned the minimum wage rate . . . or another wage level set by the Commissioner, during such employment . . . [and] the number who received employment benefits from an employer during such employment" (Workforce Investment Act, p. 192). States also are required to report the reasons for individuals' terminating participation in the program without achieving an employment outcome (p. 193). In 2005, there were 206,695 clients (33.5%) who were "rehabilitated" and 410,184 clients (66.5%) who were "not rehabilitated" (RSA Data Archive, 2005). The Rehabilitation Services

Administration (2005) Policy Directive specifies the reasons for unsuccessful case closure:

- Unable to locate or contact the client
- Disability too significant to benefit from VR services
- Refused services or further services
- Death
- Individual in institution
- Transferred to another agency
- Failure to cooperate
- No disabling condition
- No impediment to employment
- Transportation not feasible or available
- Does not require VR services
- Extended services not available
- All other reasons

An analysis of the year 2005 Rehabilitation Services Administration data for all Vocational Rehabilitation cases in the United States indicated that the top three reasons for unsuccessful cases were as follows:

- Client Refused Services or Further Services, $n = 105,302$ clients
- Unable to Contact the Client, $n = 96,436$ clients
- Client Failure to Cooperate, $n = 85,863$ clients

Workforce development performance measures (U.S. Department of Labor, 1998) have been developed to assess effects of activities legislated by the Workforce Investment Act of 1998. These measures are summarized in Table 14.2. There are nine Key Indicators of Success (Core), nine Other Measures of Success (Non-core), and six Developmental Measures (Non-core). These measures of success as might be applied to One-Stop Centers, Vocational Rehabilitation, or other programs are difficult to document accurately. Thus, the state Workforce Investment Boards have, in some cases, appealed for a "waiver" to allow a simpler, more appropriate set of "Common Measures" that would be used in their workforce investment programs. For example, in one state, the 2006 set of Common Measures for adults was (a) earnings increase, (b) entered employment, and (c) employment retention. Another state uses those three Common Measures plus a fourth one (expenditures divided by total number of individuals served). These are, obviously, less demanding than the full set of Workforce Development Performance Measures listed in Table 14.2. But, those measures provide excellent guidance for responsible program evaluation.

Measuring Outcomes

Outcomes in rehabilitation are by no means unidimensional. Centers for Independent Living increase consumer control, self-help, empowerment,

TABLE 14.2.
Workforce Development Performance Measures

Key Indicators of Success (CORE)

1. *Entered Employment Rate:* The percent of people who got a job during or the quarter after receiving workforce development services excluding people who are in training or education services who did not get a job and people who maintain their current job.

2. *Annual Earnings Gains:* The 12-month earnings of people who got a job as a result of receiving workforce development services, minus any earnings they may have had during the 12 months before receiving workforce development services.

3. *Employment Retention:* The percent of people who got a job and remained employed up to 1 year as a result of receiving workforce development services.

4. *Postemployment Ratio of Self-Sufficiency:* The 12-month earnings of a person who got a job after receiving workforce development services compared to the average annual cost of living for a family of three who live in the same area.

5. *Basic Skills Attainment:* The percent of people 16 and older who complete basic skills training that leads to or includes graduating from high school or getting a GED as a result of their participation in workforce development services.

6. *Occupational Skill Attainment:* The percent of people 16 and older who get a college degree, complete an occupational or advanced job skill training program, or enter an apprenticeship program as a result of their participation in workforce development services.

7. *Transition Success Rate:* The percent of people who complete basic or occupational skill training and go on to employment or an advanced level of education/training or both as a result of their participation in workforce development services.

8. *Job Opening Fill Rate:* The percent of workforce development system job openings filled by workforce development system applicants.

9. *Customer Satisfaction:* The degree to which customers are satisfied with the services provided by the workforce development system.

Other Measures of Success (NON-CORE)

10. *Employment Rate:* The percent of people who received any workforce development service during the quarter who got or kept a job.

11. *Starting Wage at Entered Employment:* The average starting hourly wage of people who were seeking first, new, or better jobs and got a job during or after receiving workforce development services.

12. *Reduction or Closure of TANF Grant:* The percent of people whose welfare payments are reduced or cases closed as a result of getting a job through assistance from the workforce development system.

13. *Reduction of Benefit Duration:* The average length of time people who receive additional workforce development services continue to receive unemployment insurance benefits compared to everyone who receives unemployment insurance benefits.

14. *Participation Equity Rate:* Percent of people in target groups such as unemployed workers, people receiving welfare, African Americans, Hispanics, older workers, recipients of unemployment insurance, people with disabilities, etc., who receive workforce development services in a given area.

15. *Diversity of Occupations:* To what degree job openings listed and occupations of job seekers in the local workforce development system reflect the entire range of jobs and occupations in the local job market.

(continues)

TABLE 14.2. *Continued.*

Other Measures of Success (NON-CORE) (Continued)

16. *Information/Service Access Compared to Community:* The number and type of workforce development services available through a local one-stop center compared to all workforce development services available in the community.

17. *Information/Services Access/Received by Job Seeker + Customers:* The number of people looking for a job or training who access information or services by each of the following methods: (a) from computers, (b) at a one-stop center without any help from staff, or (c) one-on-one or in a group setting with the help of staff.

18. *Cycle Time to First Service:* The number of days it takes for a person to receive service from the day a person first identifies a need for service to workforce development staff.

Developmental Measures (NON-CORE)

19. *Information/Service Access Compared to Fixed Federal List:* The number of programs and services available at a one-stop center compared to a list of the major federal workforce development programs and services.

20. *Employers Using WDS:* The percent of employers using workforce development services at least once and the percent using workforce development services more than once.

21. *Administrative Data Shared Among Agencies:* The percent of individual agencies and programs in a state's workforce development system that can access each other's program data by computer.

22. *Return on Investment:* The total annual increase in earnings and decrease in welfare for all people who received a workforce development service divided by the total cost of the program.

23. *Time to Positive Outcome by Service Cluster:* The amount of time it takes people to get a job, achieve self-sufficiency, obtain basic or advanced skills, or go on to a higher level of skills training/education from the time they completed or left workforce development services.

24. *System Penetration Rate:* The percent of people who need a specific workforce development service who actually receive it.

Note. From Workforce Development Performance Measures (http://nortec.org/cb/onestop/wdpm_menu .html), 1998, by U.S. Department of Labor.

productivity, and full inclusion in the mainstream of society (O'Day, Wilson, Killeen, & Ficke, 2004). Hundreds of independent–living skills might be taught and learned to maintain or improve ability to live independently. Six examples of such independent–living competencies from the *Independent Living Behavior Checklist* (Walls, Zane, & Thvedt, 1979) are the following:

- PINCER GRASP

    CONDITION: Given a needle, pin, piece of 6–inch thread, button, pencil, and container.

    BEHAVIOR: Client picks up each item and puts it in the container.

    STANDARD: Behavior within 30 seconds. All items must be picked up with a pincer grasp (between thumb and index finger) and placed in the container.

- DRYER

    CONDITION: Given a load of clean wet clothes, ready to be dried, and a coin-operated or home automatic dryer.

    BEHAVIOR: Client places the clothes in the dryer and operates the machine.

    STANDARD: Behavior within 10 minutes (for starting the machine). The clothes must be added and the machine operated according to the laundromat's or the machine manufacturer's instructions. When the clothes are removed, they must be dry to the touch.

- CLIMATE CONSERVATION

    CONDITION: Given a heater or air conditioner in operation.

    BEHAVIOR: Client closes all windows and exterior doors or leaves them closed.

    STANDARD: Behavior within 10 minutes. All windows and exterior doors must remain closed during operation of the heater or air conditioner.

- SHOPPING

    CONDITION: Given a grocery list of at least 10 different foods, a grocery store, and a cart.

    BEHAVIOR: Client locates the foods on the list and places them in the cart.

    STANDARD: Behavior within 1 hour. All food on the list must be found (unless out of stock). No food must be damaged (e.g., eggs broken, bread mashed).

- PHONE NUMBER

    CONDITION: Given a telephone book (white or yellow pages), a telephone (home or pay), and the name of a person or business to call.

    BEHAVIOR: Client locates the phone number.

    STANDARD: Behavior within 5 minutes. The desired number must be found.

- CHECK

    CONDITION: Given specific item(s) to be purchased at a cash register (e.g., food, clothes), a personal checkbook, and identification.

    BEHAVIOR: Client writes a check to purchase the item(s).

STANDARD: Behavior within 10 minutes. If requested, proper identification must be shown so that the transaction is completed.
The check must not be returned due to insufficient funds. The
check number, date, amount, and recipient must be written in
the checkbook and a new balance computed.

The State–Federal VR program serves clients with independent-living
goals, either through direct services or as contracted through a center for independent living. The independent-living movement traditionally provided
advocacy service, information and referral services, peer counseling, and
independent-living skills training, but more recently, employment-related collaboration and training services have become an organizational goal (Stoddard &
Premo, 2004). One of the successful outcomes in the State–Federal VR program
since its beginning in 1920 has been "homemaker" (Rubin & Roessler, 2001).
In one study of consumers in the VR program who were legally blind, those
placed in "competitive employment" were younger (average of about age 42),
but those placed as a "homemaker" were older (average of about age 62) (Warren,
Cavenaugh, & Glesen, 2004).

Employment outcomes may be with or without "supports" in an integrated
setting. Many community rehabilitation programs have shifted emphasis from
predominantly segregated work in sheltered settings to supported employment
in integrated work settings (Brooks-Lane, Hutcheson, & Revell, 2005). In the
State–Federal VR program, supported employment may be full-time or part-
time and may be above, at, or below the minimum wage (Rehabilitation Services Administration, 2005). Wehman, Revell, and Brooke (2003) proposed
that "quality indicators" of supported-employment programs include (a) wages
and benefits commensurate with those of nondisabled coworkers; (b) consumer
satisfaction with their program of services (supports), the quality/quantity of
their work, and community integration; and (c) for people with intermittent
work history, disability profile, functional capacities, and other barriers to employment, keeping them working consistently at 30 or more hours per week.
Outpatients with schizophrenia participated in a work rehabilitation program (up
to 20 hours per week) and were rated on five scales of the *Work Behavior Inventory*
(Bryson, Greig, & Bell, 2003). During the 6 months of work activity, most participants showed improvement in at least one work domain: (a) Cooperativeness,
(b) Work Quality, (c) Work Habits, (d) Personal Presentation, and (e) Social
Skills. The only dependent variable, in a study of vocational rehabilitation of
persons with orthopedic disabilities, was whether or not the clients achieved
competitive employment as the outcome (Chan, Cheing, Chan, Rosenthal,
& Chronister, 2006).

Rehabilitation outcomes have been defined by Furher (1987) as changes produced by rehabilitation services in the lives of service recipients and their environment. He argued that causal relations between interventions and such
changes are difficult to document. For example, improvement on measures of
impairment, disability, or handicap may be due to remission of the underlying

disease process or attention and social stimulation rather than the rehabilitation services provided. Additionally, failure to document the impact of aging for both elderly persons (advancing age) and children (developmental processes) confounds input–process–outcome interpretations (Wagner, 1987). Fuhrer proposed that outcome analyses deal with either effectiveness or efficiency. Rehabilitation is effective when the process for a given input yields expected short-term or long-term positive output. Rehabilitation is efficient when the degree of short-term or long-term output justifies the extent of investment in the process for a given input (cost-benefit). A potential measurement problem is that for a given input and process, multiple outcomes may be inextricably intertwined, as in the case of achievement of competitive employment, increased income, reduction in receipt of public cash and in-kind benefits, and reduction in responsibilities of other family members. A second potential difficulty is that outcomes should be measured long enough after the intervention to assess genuine and lasting effects but soon enough to allow reasonable inference (Wagner, 1987). A third potential shortcoming is the lack of appropriate norms, either nationally or locally, for determining how high is high and how good is good. Although outcomes for an individual are always the primary concern in rehabilitation, establishment of intervention or program effectiveness and efficiency for multiple recipients is a goal of humanitarian science. Poor descriptions of the inputs, inadequate measurements of the processes, and inappropriate outcome data collection pose threats to accurate and appropriate input–process–outcome assessment for the individual and the science.

Assessment of the vocational, economic, and/or psychosocial characteristics of rehabilitation clients may involve a variety of measures. These measures can be used (a) at one point in time to assess *status* or (b) at two or more points in time to assess *change*. When a rehabilitation intervention such as therapeutic counseling, medical restoration, or vocational skills training is given, the desire is that such intervention will produce positive change (e.g., reduced anxiety, improved mobility, or increased production on the job). Change from one juncture to another has always been a scientific credo. Gain or loss is demonstrated by accurate measures of the same phenomenon at two or more points in time. Although client adjustment continues across time, change from Time 1 (e.g., intake into a rehabilitation program or onset of disability) to Time 2 (e.g., outcome of the rehabilitation or at 1-year follow-up) might include such changes as those noted in Table 14.3.

Although measurement of a client's vocational, economic, and/or psychosocial status early in the rehabilitation process and reassessment to determine gains after rehabilitation intervention has scientific merit, this pre–post measurement approach usually is not the norm for casework. Rather, preliminary assessment usually is used to establish status for (a) determining eligibility for services and (b) determining an appropriate individualized plan for services. If the client completes this rehabilitation plan and gains employment, reassessment with the same instruments usually is forgone in favor of such macro criteria as hours worked per week, earnings, and relative self-sufficiency. When the client

TABLE 14.3.

Examples of Potential Positive Changes in Vocational Rehabilitation

1. Change *from* unemployed *to* employed.

2. Change *from* unemployed and not seeking employment *to* unemployed and seeking employment.

3. Change *from* not wanting to be employed *to* wanting to be employed.

4. Change *from* part-time employment *to* full-time employment.

5. Change *from* fewer hours worked *to* more hours worked.

6. Change *from* lower wage per time worked *to* higher wage per time worked.

7. Change *from* one type of job (e.g., cashier) *to* another type of job (e.g., medical secretary).

8. Change *from* no medical insurance available (or provided) in employment *to* medical insurance available (or provided) in employment.

9. Change *from* no retirement benefits available (or provided) in employment *to* retirement benefits available (or provided) in employment.

10. Change *from* the individual's lower satisfaction (psychosocial adjustment) with the work activity *to* higher satisfaction (psychosocial adjustment) with the work activity.

11. Change *from* an employer's lower evaluation of the satisfactoriness of the employee's performance *to* higher evaluation of the satisfactoriness of the employee's performance.

12. Change *from* not having a particular job skill (e.g., not able to change the oil in the fryers or in Chevrolets) *to* having that particular job skill.

13. Change *from* more functional limitations in employment *to* fewer functional limitations in employment.

14. Change *from* more reliance on public cash or in-kind benefits *to* less reliance on public cash or in-kind benefits.

Note. Change can also be in a negative direction, which would be represented by the opposite (vice versa) of many of the changes listed.

had an independent-living goal rather than an employment goal, a pre–post gain assessment using the same instruments is more likely, but again, a macro achievement may take precedence over reassessment to determine change.

Vocational, Economic, and Psychosocial Functioning

The *raison d'etre* (reason for being) of the publicly supported rehabilitation effort is vocational accomplishment. The measures of vocational outcomes are the grist of evaluation studies and justifications for the public expenditures. Citizens and their legislative representatives want to know that their money was well-spent. The most obvious criteria of good investment in vocational rehabilitation services are getting a job and keeping a job. Less obvious, but nonetheless valid, criteria of productive rehabilitation services additionally contribute to judging genuine value and facilitating accurate understanding.

It is naïve to expect that every individual with a disability who receives any sort of vocational rehabilitation services will achieve and retain substantial gainful employment. Understandings of relationships among intake (input), process (intervention), and outcome (output) have been gained, and elusive relationships, not yet described, remain to be explicated through rigorous research. "Outcome expectations" related to employment and careers have been shown to be positively correlated with career-exploratory intentions and career-decision self-efficacy for students with disabilities or without disabilities (Ochs & Roessler, 2004). It is difficult, however, to have high self-efficacy and outcome expectations in the employment domain if the individual is plagued by chronic illness and disability. When appropriate therapies and rehabilitation services can help the person deal with seemingly overwhelming complexities and incomprehensible chaos, coping skills may be built and may allow adaptive outcomes to gain focus (Livneh & Parker, 2005).

Functional capacity measures that had been reviewed by the Tenth Institute on Rehabilitation Issues were described by Walls and Tseng (1987). Functional capacities and status indicators assessed by these measures may be grouped into emotional functioning, cognitive and educational functioning, social functioning, self-care and mobility functioning, and vocational functioning. Topics related to functional assessment in the area of *emotional functioning* include psychological history, present psychological status, and internal–external orientation. Topics related to functional assessment in the area of *cognitive and educational functioning* include educational history, present educational status, selecting education, cognition, learning aptitude, vocabulary, reading, basic skills, functional academic skills, problem solving, and time management. Topics related to functional assessment in the area of *social functioning* include social history, social contact, social activities, social and communication skills, interpersonal/social relationships, and political/community activities. Topics related to functional assessment in the area of *self-care and mobility functioning* include history of self-care, present activities of daily living, home maintenance and safety skills, food skills, in-the-home activities, outside-the-home activities, family role, time spent in various activities, personal independence, psychomotor abilities, mobility, object manipulation, energy reserves, and use of assistance. Topics related to functional assessment in the area of *vocational functioning* include vocational history, employment seeking, work status, work information, work importance, prevocational skills, job-seeking skills, interview skills, job-related skills, work-performance skills, on-the-job social skills, union-financial-security skills, self-direction, physical demands, work capacity, income, type of employment, advancement, supported employment, community workshop activity, and transportation.

These topics are neither discrete nor exhaustive. Social contact and interpersonal/social activities, for instance, might be measuring some of the same competencies, and examination of the constructs and skills included in these 11 functional-assessment instruments as well as all the other instruments would be necessary to gain an exhaustive list. Some instruments use a rating by the client, family member, counselor, employer, or other person. Some instruments use direct observation to certify that the client can or cannot do behaviors such as reading a passage or responding correctly to an employer's question in a job interview. For instance, seven examples of vocational competencies from the *Vocational Behavior Checklist* (Walls, Zane, & Werner, 1978) are the following:

- GLASS PACKING

  CONDITION: Given a cardboard carton, newspaper, and 10 drinking glasses.

  BEHAVIOR: Client will wrap the glasses in newspaper and pack them in the carton, using crumpled newspaper.

  STANDARD: Behavior within 15 minutes on three of four occasions. Each glass must be completely wrapped in newspaper, and crumpled newspaper should be stuffed in the carton so that the glasses will not move if the carton is tilted.

- SOURCES

  CONDITION: Given only the verbal instruction, "Name seven places to find out about job openings."

  BEHAVIOR: Client will name seven sources of job opening information.

  STANDARD: Behavior within 5 minutes on three of four occasions. The sources named must be seven of the following: employers, relatives, friends, newspaper, radio, television, Department of Human Resources (or similar health or welfare agency), or employment agency.

- CLIENT INTERESTS

  CONDITION: Given a simulated job interview.

  BEHAVIOR: Client will ask a minimum of three questions about the job related to tools, clothes, equipment, skill needed, or location of work station.

  STANDARD: Behavior during four consecutive interviews. Answers for all of the questions must be stated clearly by the client and must be in agreement with those given by the interviewer.

- ENTRANCES

  CONDITION: Given specified entrance(s) and exit(s) at the client's place of work.

  BEHAVIOR: Client will enter and exit through the appropriate doors.

  STANDARD: Behavior on 20 consecutive work days. Only the specified entrances and exits must be used by the client each day.

- TASK ORDER

    CONDITION: Given two different job assignments or tasks.

    BEHAVIOR: Client will perform the two job assignments or tasks in order.

    STANDARD: Behavior must occur until there is a new instruction or the job is completed. Both jobs or tasks must be performed correctly and in the order assigned, and the rate of work must be acceptable, as defined by the supervisor.

- CONVERSATION

    CONDITION: Given a specific job assignment or task that involves a minimum of one other worker.

    BEHAVIOR: Client will verbally interact with coworker(s) without disrupting or interfering with their job assignments.

    STANDARD: Behavior during a 20-day work period. The frequency of the client's verbal interactions must be appropriate, as defined by the agreement of all coworkers interviewed at the end of the 20-day period. (Coworkers must be asked, "Did the client ever talk to you so much that you couldn't do your work?")

- JOB TITLE

    CONDITION: Given the client's official job title and hours worked.

    BEHAVIOR: Client will state the job title and the hours worked.

    STANDARD: Behavior within 1 minute on four consecutive occasions. The job title and hours stated must be correct.

Measures of economic, vocational, and psychosocial status or outcomes were described by Bolton (1987). These measures were selected because of their comprehensiveness, parsimony, and practicality. In a later chapter, Bolton (2004) gave a list of the following 22 instruments useful for rehabilitation outcome measurement:

1. *Acceptance of Disability Scale* (ADS; Linkowski, 1987)
2. *Becker Work Adjustment Profile* (BWAP; Becker, 1989)
3. *California Psychological Inventory* (CPI; Gough, 1987)
4. *Disability Factor Scales–General* (DFS-G; Siller, 1970)
5. *Employability Maturity Interview Computer Report* (EMICR; Neath & Bolton, 1997)
6. *Functional Assessment Inventory* (FAI; Crewe & Athelstan, 1984)
7. *Handicap Problems Inventory* (HPI; Wright & Remmers, 1960)
8. *Independent Living Behavior Checklist* (ILBC; Walls, Zane, & Thvedt, 1979)

9. *Minnesota Satisfaction Questionnaire* (MSQ; Weiss, Dawis, England, & Lofquist, 1967)
10. *Minnesota Satisfactoriness Scales* (MSS; Gibson, Weiss, Dawis, & Lofquist, 1970)
11. *Minnesota Survey of Employment Experiences* (MSEE; Tinsley, Warnken, Weiss, Dawis, & Lofquist, 1969)
12. *Personal Independence Profile* (PIP; Nosek, Fuhrer, & Howland, 1992)
13. *Preliminary Diagnostic Questionnaire* (PDQ; Moriarty, 1981)
14. *Personal Opinions Questionnaire* (POQ; Bolton & Brookings, 1998)
15. *Psychiatric Diagnostic Interview–Revised* (PDI-R; Othmer, Penick, Powell, Read, & Othmer, 1989)
16. *Rehabilitation Gain Scale* (RGS; Reagles, Wright, & Butler, 1970)
17. *Rehabilitation Indicators* (RIs; Brown, Diller, Fordyce, Jacobs, & Gordon, 1980)
18. *Service Outcome Measurement Form* (SOMF; Westerheide, Lenhart, & Miller, 1975)
19. *16 Personality Factor Questionnaire–Form E* (16PF-E; Institute for Personality and Ability Testing, 1985)
20. *Vocational Behavior Checklist* (VBC; Walls, Zane, & Werner, 1978)
21. *Work Adjustment Rating Form* (WARF; Bitter & Bolanovich, 1970)
22. *Work Personality Profile* (WPP; Bolton & Roessler, 1986)

Of these 22 measures of status (if administered once) or change (if administered multiple times), the data for 12 of them are gained from self-reports by the client. Of the remainder, three are based on counselor ratings, one on employer ratings, and six on observation of the behaviors of the client. The numbers of items to be rated or behaviors to be observed range from 8 to 854, with a mean of 141.

Reliability and Validity

Some of these 22 instruments have been reported to have reliability and validity of measurement based on the following:

- *Internal consistency reliability.* High internal consistency indicates that the items in the instrument (or each subscale separately) correlate highly with each other. People who score low on one item of the measure tend to also score low on other items, and vice versa.
- *Stability reliability.* High stability indicates that the first administration scores and the second administration scores (test-retest) for the same individuals correlate highly. These two administrations of the instrument should be separated by about 2 weeks, a time period during which there is no intervention that would affect the scores.
- *Interobserver agreement reliability.* High interobserver agreement (interscorer or interrater) indicates that two (or more) independent scorers

have a high percentage of agreement in recording (1) whether or not the client exhibited a particular behavior, (2) how many times the behavior occurred, or (3) how well (accurately or effectively) the behavior was performed.

- *Criterion-related validity.* High criterion-related validity indicates that client performance on the measuring instrument is highly correlated with a real-world outcome. For example, the criterion of independent travel in the community might be correlated with performance on Instrument One (purported to be a measure of independent living potential) given that same week (concurrent validity). A second example would be that the criterion of achieving competitive employment might be correlated with performance on Instrument Two (purported to be a measure of employability) given a year previously at the beginning of vocational rehabilitation services (predictive validity).
- *Construct validity.* High construct validity indicates that client performance on the measuring instrument correlates as it should with other related, but not identical, instruments. Understanding the magnitude of positive and negative correlations with other instruments helps to clarify the nature of the construct being measured by this instrument.
- *Content validity.* All of the 22 instruments appear to possess or have been reported to have high content validity. Content validity is not evidenced by a correlation coefficient. Rather, it is evidence that the domain of concern (e.g., employability) has been fairly sampled and represented in the items of the measuring instrument.

Outcomes Reported in Research

Depending on the input variables and the process variables, the outcomes measured have differed. Depending on the point of intervention and the level of reduction or granularity, the outcomes measured have differed. Depending on the service agency mandates and the service providers' intents, the outcomes measured have differed.

Vocational Rehabilitation

The Workforce Investment Act of 1998 called for a longitudinal study of vocational rehabilitation applicants:

> To assess the linkages between vocational rehabilitation services and economic and noneconomic outcomes, the Secretary shall continue to conduct a longitudinal study of a national sample of applicants for the services . . . The study shall address factors related to attrition and completion of

the program through which services are provided and factors within and outside the program affecting results. Appropriate comparisons shall be used to contrast the experiences of similar persons who do not obtain the services . . . The study shall be planned to cover the period beginning on the application of individuals with disabilities for the services, through the eligibility determination and provision of services for the individuals, and a further period of not less than 2 years after the termination of services . . . The Commissioner shall identify and disseminate information on exemplary practices concerning vocational rehabilitation. (Workforce Investment Act of 1998, p. 177)

Initiated in 1992, this longitudinal study of the public vocational rehabilitation program was commissioned by the Rehabilitation Services Administration and mandated by Congress in the 1992 Rehabilitation Act Amendments. Data collection for a national sample of 8,500 cases began in 1994 and continues under the Workforce Investment Act of 1998. In a report of findings, Research Triangle Institute (1998) indicated that two thirds of the sample had exited from services and one third of the clients were still receiving services. This report included data only for those consumers who achieved an employment outcome (either competitive employment or noncompetitive employment such as homemaker, unpaid family worker, self-employment, or sheltered employment). Former clients of the public vocational rehabilitation service program who achieved competitive employment more often (a) had a nonsevere disability; (b) had an orthopedic or hearing impairment; (c) were male; (d) were younger; (e) had higher reading and math achievement levels; (f) had a current work history at the time of application for rehabilitation services; (g) had work experience in competitive employment; (h) had work experience with higher wages; and (i) received counseling, education, training, and placement services. Of those former vocational rehabilitation clients who achieved competitive employment, they worked an average of 35 hours per week, and they earned an average of $7.35 per hour. More than 60% made $7.00 or less in jobs that were less likely to provide medical benefits. As might be expected, those with lower levels of education as well as lower reading and math skills occupied the lowest paying jobs (Research Triangle Institute, 1998).

Other studies also have used outcomes in the public vocational rehabilitation program as dependent variables. For example, Bellini, Neath, and Bolton (1995a) used measures of client disadvantage as predictor (independent) variables (employment status at referral, educational level, financial assistance, family income, marital status, age, severity of disability, primary disability, and secondary disability). Achievement of competitive employment versus no such achievement was their criterion (dependent) variable. Strongest predictors of competitive employment versus not were (a) employment status at referral, (b) assistance (benefits) at referral, (c) type and severity of disability, and (d) education level. Further validation of their *Scale of Social Disadvantage* yielded similar results (Bellini, Neath, & Bolton, 1995b).

Another example of an investigation examining outcomes in the public vocational rehabilitation program as dependent measures involved 148,188 rehabilitation cases (Majumder, Walls, Fullmer, & Misra, 1997). Those authors examined 19 disabling conditions (e.g., mental illness, hearing impairment) crossed with 15 contributing factors (e.g., severity of disability, education, Social Security Disability Insurance) to create 285 subsets. Probabilities of competitive employment ranged from quite low (e.g., 0.31 for persons with diabetes who received Supplemental Security Income) to near 1.0 (e.g., 0.99 for high school graduates with a substance-abuse disability). For those who had been rehabilitated versus those who had not been rehabilitated, Walls, Misra, and Majumder (2002) documented changes across 20 years (1978, 1988, 1998) in the VR consumer Intake Variables (e.g., increase in percent receiving public benefits at intake), Process Variables (e.g., decrease in percent receiving restoration services), and Outcome Variables (e.g., increase in percent achieving competitive employment).

In their investigation of a possible relationship between VR consumer outcomes and rehabilitation counselor multicultural counseling competencies, Matrone and Leahy (2005) used the outcome measure of successful case closure (rehabilitated) versus unsuccessful case closure (not rehabilitated). The authors of a study in which successful versus unsuccessful employment outcome was the criterion variable suggested that counselor training should take a strong employment-outcomes focus (Fraser, Vandergoot, Thomas, & Wagner, 2004). A study of vocational rehabilitation services for persons with epilepsy yielded findings related to outcomes of (a) achievement of successful employment, (b) increased personal income, and (c) decreased reliance on government support (Mount, Johnstone, White, & Sherman, 2005). In research examining best practices in vocational services for mental health consumers, the target outcome was not just employment in the competitive job market; it also was the consumer's own vocational goal (Akabas, Oran-Sabia, & Gates, 2006). In a study with a similar disability group, a special program of psychiatric vocational rehabilitation compared to the State–Federal VR program yielded no differences between the two programs when the outcomes were assessed on (a) reduced psychiatric symptoms, (b) increased quality of life, (c) increased self-esteem, (d) increased earnings, and (e) increased rate of competitive or supported work (Rogers, Anthony, Lyass, & Penk, 2006). The *Canadian Occupational Performance Measure* assesses self-perceptions of the individual's most important problems with occupational performance related to self-care, leisure, and productivity in employment (Dedding, Cardol, Eyssen, Dekker, & Beelen, 2004). The prime outcome targeted by Social Security Administration's Ticket to Work and Self-Sufficiency Program is, once again, competitive employment, particularly for Supplemental Security Income and Social Security Disability Insurance recipients and persons with severe disabling conditions (e.g., MR/DD; Wehman & Revell, 2005). The key outcomes were (a) employment status (at one point in time) and (b) long-term vocational outcome in a review of recent literature on predictive variables in six disability groups (spinal cord injury, traumatic brain injury, amputation, chronic pain, myocardial infarction or coronary bypass, and severe mental illness; Crisp, 2005).

In an evaluation of consumer choice demonstration projects, Stoddard, Hanson, and Temkin (1999) presented a review of such projects and promising practices. The outcomes described were presumably in relation to consumer discretion, decision making, and choice during rehabilitation intervention (Process Phase). Outcomes were as follows:

- The numbers of participants successfully rehabilitated versus not rehabilitated
- Cost of purchased services
- Length of the case
- Wage
- Type of employment
- Full-time versus part-time employment
- Satisfaction of the consumers with access, staff, services, and communications

More worksite involvement (employers, coworkers, job coaches) earlier in the rehabilitation process has yielded promising results (Lougheed, 1998; Shrey & Mital, 1994). Various research reports suggest the relationships of the following:

- Collaborative problem solving *to* vocational outcomes (Morton, Gibbs, & Ragland, 1997)
- Workplace accommodations *to* functional limitations and job performance (Michaels & Risucci, 1993)
- Assistive technologies *to* employment opportunities (Sowers, 1991)
- Corporate employment initiative *to* employment and tax benefits for businesses (Zivolich & Weiner-Zivolich, 1997)
- Mutually beneficial model with employers *to* successful school-to-work experience (Donovan & Tilson, 1998)
- Job matching and development efforts *to* supported employment (Callahan, 1991)
- Early referral of injured workers *to* savings for workers' compensation and employers through return to work (Gardner, 1991)
- Costs of the rehabilitation program *to* benefits for participants and society (Zivolich, Shueman, & Weiner, 1997)
- Amount of case-service money spent *to* vocational rehabilitation outcomes (Taheri-Araghi & Hendren, 1994)
- Comprehensive vocational evaluation *to* employment outcomes (Peters, Scalia, & Fried, 1993)
- Ratings made by vocational instructors during training *to* work performance (Bolton & Brookings, 1993)

Vocational outcomes have been investigated for consumers with mental retardation, cerebral palsy, epilepsy, psychiatric disability, substance abuse, traumatic brain injury, arthritis, hearing impairment, visual impairment, cancer, spinal cord injury, coronary heart disease, spina bifida, multiple sclerosis, learning disabilities, and autism (Allaire, Anderson, & Meenan, 1997; Ashley, Persel, Clark, & Krych, 1997; Blankertz & Robinson, 1996; Burt, Fuller, & Lewis, 1991; Butterworth, Gilmore, & Shalock, 1998; Cook & Rosenberg, 1994; Depoy, 1992; Deren & Randell, 1990; Fabiano & Crewe, 1995; Kirchner, Johnson, & Harkins, 1997; Lehman, 1995; Michaels & Risucci, 1993; Schriner, Roessler, & Johnson, 1993; Rumrill, Roessler, & Cook, 1998; Shrey & Mital, 1994; West, Revell, & Wehman, 1992). For example, along with employment as an outcome, abstinence from illicit drugs and criminal involvement is used in substance-abuse cases as a criterion of treatment outcome (Platt, 1995). As a second example, Kilmer (1999) surveyed 1,047 persons with neuromuscular disease and reported that 225 used lower extremity orthoses (braces). Of those who used bracing, 76% reported that the braces allowed them to do things they wanted to do, and 66% said the equipment made them feel more independent.

Findings in vocational rehabilitation of consumers with psychiatric disabilities were reviewed by Cook and Pickett (1994), including the following findings:

- Situational assessment may be more indicative of employment outcome and hourly salary than are work-sample batteries.
- Hospitalization histories and diagnoses as schizophrenic or psychotic were associated with poorer vocational outcomes.
- Higher levels of severity of symptoms such as withdrawal or blunt affect were predictive of poorer work skills.
- Feelings of self-esteem, life satisfaction, and coping mastery were higher among those who had experienced positive changes in employment, such as becoming employed or moving to a better job.
- Satisfaction was higher among clients who were placed in employment more quickly.

As is true with other disabling conditions and rehabilitation programs, Farkas and Anthony (1987) noted that outcome studies in psychiatric rehabilitation have been complicated by the varied definitions of rehabilitation and the resultant differences in what was considered appropriate outcome (p. 43). The investigations have focused on (a) skill-training interventions, which teach skills for success; (b) drug-therapy interventions, which reduce symptoms and prevent relapse; and (c) community-support interventions, which improve functioning in community settings. Outcomes measured have been primarily (a) vocational (competitive, transitional, part-time, full-time, earnings, satisfaction with work, productivity, reduction of public benefits) and (b) living status (total days in the community, social adjustment, number of friends and activities, degree of independent living, satisfaction with community adjustment, social skills, role functioning). Behavior frequency counts, behavior ratings, questionnaires, and psychometrically developed scales are used to measure such behaviors and constructs as anxiety, eye contact, behavior problems, tool use, grasping instructions, work initiative, use of public transportation, money management, dressing, satisfaction with services, and recidivism.

Other investigators have included vocational and economic outcomes such as type of occupation, satisfaction with salary, financial status, benefits provided by the job, satisfaction with the benefits, potential for training opportunities and career development, satisfaction with personal life after job placement, barrier reduction or removal, quality of work performance, quantity of work performance, problems on the job (production, supervision, coworkers), job retention, attendance, work attitude, dependability, self-control, following directions, safety practices, amounts of cash and in-kind public benefits, adjustment to supported work environments, difficulty locating a job, optimism about finding a job, interview skills, support from family and friends, and counselor causal performance. These outcomes have been reported in a variety of investigations (Bolton, 1987, 1990; Bolton & Akridge, 1995; Dedding et al., 2004; Dijkers, 1997; Dowler & Walls, 1996; Evans & Ruff, 1992; Gilbride, Thomas, & Stensrud, 1998; Martin, 1999; Roessler & Rumrill, 1995; Sales & McAllen, 1999; Szymanski & Danek, 1992; Walls, 1982; Walls & Batiste, 1996; Walls & Dowler, 1987; Walls, Dowler, & Fullmer, 1990; Walls, Dowler, & Fullmer, 1989; Walls & Fullmer, 1996, 1997; Walls, Fullmer, & Dowler, 1996; Wilgosh, Mueller, & Rowat, 1994; Wood-Dauphinee, 1998). Thus, a number of vocational and economic outcomes (ranging from subjective to objective) have contributed to understanding effects of rehabilitation input and process. Table 14.1 provided a summary.

Real and simulated work activities can be instrumental in helping the consumer gain an accurate picture of what is involved (e.g., pain, risk factors, posture ergonomics, and work practices) in a particular type of job (Goodman, 2005). The complex interactions among input (intake) variables (e.g., age, functional capacities/limitations, and work experience) and process (intervention) variables (e.g., counseling, restoration, training/education, availability of a desired job or another employment opportunity) give extra texture to the prime outcome of "competitive employment." What occupations dominate the vocational spectrum of competitive employment in rehabilitation? The top two-digit *Dictionary of Occupational Titles* (DOT) categories for the 2005 state–federal vocational rehabilitation consumers whose cases were closed in "competitive employment" are listed in Table 14.4. These two-digit DOT codes are not as specific as three-digit codes (e.g., gas welders, trailer-truck drivers, and dieticians) but more specific than one-digit DOT codes (e.g., clerical and sales occupations, service occupations, and benchwork occupations). Table 14.4 shows the top-20 occupational categories for the 206,733 competitive-employment rehabilitants in 2005.

Medical Rehabilitation and Independent Living

Medical rehabilitation concerns severe, long-enduring impairment and disability, and it incorporates multiple interventions designed to improve the indepen-

TABLE 14.4.

The Top-20 Occupation Categories (Two-Digit DOT)
for State–Federal Vocational Rehabilitation Consumers
(Competitive-Employment Rehabilitants) in 2005

Occupation Category	Number of Rehabilitants
1. Food & Beverage Preparation & Service	19,609
2. Misc. Sales	11,654
3. Building & Related Service	10,622
4. Misc. Personal Service	10,497
5. Stenography, Typing, Filing, & Related	9,523
6. Computing & Account Recording	8,677
7. Packaging & Materials Handling	8,051
8. Medicine & Health	7,239
9. Transportation, NEC	6,595
10. Education	6,457
11. Processing, NEC	6,450
12. Managers & Officials	5,752
13. Construction, NEC	5,562
14. Administrative Specializations	4,742
15. Misc. Professional, Technical, & Managerial	4,369
16. Motor Freight	4,110
17. Information & Message Distribution	4,047
18. Production & Stock Clerks & Related	3,784
19. Lodging & Related Service	3,445
20. Barbering, Cosmetology, & Related Service	3,154

Note. NEC = not elsewhere classified.

dence and quality of life of the patient (Johnston, Stineman, & Velozo, 1997). Outcomes may be changes or sustained impacts as a result of rehabilitation strategies and treatments. The research attempts to link outcomes to treatment processes (e.g., medication, nursing, physical therapy, family support, patient motivation) and biologic factors (structural impairment, functional impairment, cellular or molecular pathology, disease). Although randomized studies involving denial of treatment are unethical, substantial variations in rehabilitative practices across different regions, programs, or insurance systems make effectiveness comparison of interventions possible. The authors contended that large databases (e.g., as prompted by the Rehabilitation Accreditation Commission) typically do not contain the depth of measurement necessary to understand crucial relationships among severity of the illness or impairment, medical or therapeutic intervention, and changes or other outcomes. Even the large-scale longitudinal databases for spinal cord injury and traumatic brain injury have yielded only modest gains in tying outcomes to initial case severity, treatments, and cost effectiveness. For the most part, the clinical theories and approaches have not been subject to rigorous scrutiny to determine sustained improvements and separate effects of medical rehabilitation from effects of natural healing. Some clinical experiments, however, have demonstrated relationships of interventions with particular patient groups to (a) the patients' functional limitations, (b) mortality, (c) long-term cost or other cost outcomes, (d) activities of daily living, (e) frequency of discharge to long-term care institutions, (f) loss or gain of functional capacity at 1-year follow-up, and (g) patient satisfaction (Johnston, Stineman, & Velozo, 1997).

Effects of acute medical care in the initial stage give way to effects of therapy and training in the intermediate stage, which in turn, give way to effects of the follow-up services in the final stage. Thus, transition across the spectrum of medical rehabilitation and independent living may require measurement of disease or trauma indicators at one point, progress in regaining strength indicated by parallel-bar walking at another point, and reduction of handicap in activities of daily living, community functioning, or vocational participation at another point (Wagner, 1987).

Jette and Jette (1997) decried the unwarranted separation and independent development of functional assessment in rehabilitation and assessment of health status in general medicine. Outcome indicators in medicine to evaluate effects of treatment and care allow finer-grained analyses than grosser measures of mortality and morbidity. Health status can be thought of in terms of biologic, physical, psychological, and social components and may contribute to a *comprehensive taxonomy of outcomes* in medical, independent living, and vocational rehabilitation.

The health-status instruments discussed by Jette and Jette (1997) included content areas such as physical function (e.g., mobility); social function (e.g., parenting); emotional function (e.g., self-esteem); mental function (e.g., alertness); instrumental function (e.g., work); daily-living function (e.g., food preparation); and global-health function (e.g., health satisfaction). The eight health-status instruments ranged from 9 to 136 items with a mean of 54 items, ranged in administration time from 10 to 30 minutes with a mean of 15 minutes, and were all self-report measures. The scores derived may reflect response to a single item, a subscale composed of several items, or a composite. The instruments have been used with a variety of groups of patients (e.g., hip arthroplasty, postpolio, asthma, coronary artery bypass, peptic ulcer, low-back impairment, cervical impairment). Changes from one juncture to another represent gains or losses (e.g., admission, discharge, periodic outpatient checks, rehabilitation activities, community reintegration). Rather than a single measure at a single time, a profile of health-status metrics across time may present the most valuable findings for improved theory and practice. When repeated assessments of health status, using instruments with reasonable psychometric properties, reveal objective relations among input, process, and outcome, the feedback loop can facilitate appropriate interventions (e.g., home-health aide for a particular service) in subsequent cases (Jette & Jette, 1997).

Independent living is a rehabilitation goal for which training, medical, and counseling services are instrumental more in psychosocial gains than in vocational gains. Consumers with severe disabling conditions increase personal self-determination and minimize unnecessary dependence on others (Nosek, 1987). Services usually include housing assistance, attendant care, readers or interpreters, peer counseling, financial and legal advocacy, community awareness, barrier removal, equipment maintenance, recreation, and independent-living-skills training. The training addresses such areas as attendant management, financial management, consumer affairs, mobility, educational–vocational opportunities, medical needs, living arrangements, social skills, time management, sexuality, and activities of daily living. As Nosek recommended, focus on outcomes for individual people must take precedence over general program outcomes. Further, measures need to be fine-grained enough to be instructive (e.g., more detailed than a yes or no to whether the individual can cook) and yet not so abstruse as to mask relatively straightforward needs (e.g., accessible, affordable housing).

For consumers with mental impairment, instructional programs frequently target domains of academic, independent living, social, and vocational outcomes. Halpern (1987) described issues characterized as (a) multilevel definition of outcomes, (b) multidimensional definition of outcomes, and (c) societal versus client perspectives. Regarding the first issue, for an individual with severe disability, a successful outcome might be semi-independent living or employment with ongoing support. For a person with a less severe disability, however, only complete independence or competitive employment might be considered a successful outcome. Regarding the second issue, a plethora of potential outcome measures involve functional abilities, independence, community integration, and employment. In the absence of wherewithal to measure them all, what are the most crucial ones to assess (Bolton, 1987)? Values also impinge on the third issue noted by Halpern (1987): Is the client perspective or the agency/societal perspective more relevant in operational definition of desirable outcomes (Bolton, 1987)? For instance, work that is interesting and fulfilling to the individual versus employment for high pay may be differentially valued by the client and the Social Security Administration.

Outcome measures have ranged from specific (e.g., strength of an extremity or range of motion) to general (e.g., living arrangement or physical independence). The more specific outcome measures often are appropriate for one disabling condition but not another. For instance, (a) brain-injury rehabilitation might be evidenced by parenting, driving, and financial management; (b) bowel and bladder problems might have an objective of continence or independence in self-management; (c) musculoskeletal impairments may seek results in terms of coordination, balance, and endurance; and (d) emotional-syndrome-rehabilitation treatments could show efficacy through counts of episodes and ratings of disruptiveness. A summary of medical, independent living, and psychosocial outcomes is presented in Table 14.1. As noted by Jette and Jette (1997), a number of instruments have been developed to measure health status based on concepts of pathology, impairment, disability, functional limitations, and subjective well-being. Johnston et al. (1997) indicated that the instruments vary considerably in properties of psychometric rigor. They argued for controlled causal research methods rather than correlational models that may lead to spurious conclusions. They called for both discipline-related theories (e.g., specific to exercise physiology or pharmacology) and systems-related theories (e.g., biologic and social interventions orchestrated by a rehabilitation team). Treatment protocols used in the private sector often are oriented toward cost savings and rapid patient processing, and, as such, they may have limited contribution to rehabilitation theory and long-term gains. Nevertheless, valid links from interventions to both short-term and sustained gains are to be valued. Both contribute to inductive theory building and deductive theory testing. Both contribute to integrated understanding of consumer-sensitive inputs, processes, and outcomes.

Conclusion

The number and variety of outcomes and outcome measures noted in this chapter give a hint to the complexity of the extant concerns and nomenclature. Rehabilitation service providers, government agents, and consumers with disabilities want fair, accurate, and complete measures of accomplishment. Outcomes cannot be considered in a vacuum. Client outcomes in rehabilitation necessarily interact with input and process variables, and those inputs, processes, and outcomes differ across disciplines of medical rehabilitation, independent-living rehabilitation, and vocational rehabilitation. Outcome measures are designed by programs of rehabilitation services as well as independent investigators in attempts to emulate legislated definitions, justify expenditures, evaluate programs, and—of premier importance—facilitate optimal intervention on behalf of individuals with disability. Adequate reliabilities (e.g., internal consistency, stability, interobserver) and validities (e.g., content, construct, concurrent, predictive) have sometimes been demonstrated and sometimes not. Valuable outcome measures can range from self-report questionnaires to reliable observation of behavior. The public vocational rehabilitation program requires 90 days in employment before declaring a successful vocational outcome for a client. An independent living program may consider any substantial reduction in dependence or move toward community integration a significant outcome for a client. A medical program may employ a rigorous measure of disease arrest or a loose measure of consumer satisfaction. All seek to answer the defining question for rehabilitation: (a) What clients, consumers, or patients, (b) with what disabling conditions, abilities, and environmental circumstances, (c) receive what rehabilitation counseling, restoration, training, or other services, (d) with what results or outcomes? If a single, comprehensive system of measures to answer this question was a simple thing to make, someone or some organization would have made it already. The needs and interests may be too diverse to accomplish a unitary system. Perhaps this is as it should be. People are individuals, and success in rehabilitation depends on individualization. But, if we are not to fool ourselves and others, then relevant and trustworthy measures of outcomes as they relate to input variables and rehabilitation processes are necessary.

Author's Note

This work was supported, in part, by the International Center for Disability Information at West Virginia University. Appreciation is expressed to Gina Luci for manuscript preparation.

References

Akabas, S. H., Gates, L. B., & Oran-Sabia, V. (2006). Work opportunities for rewarding careers (WORC): Insights from implementation of a best practice approach toward vocational services for mental health consumers. *Journal of Rehabilitation, 72*(1), 19–26.

Allaire, S., Anderson, J., & Meenan, R. (1997). Outcomes from the Job-Raising Program, a self-improvement model for vocational rehabilitation, among persons with arthritis. *Journal of Applied Rehabilitation Counseling, 28*(2), 26–31.

Ashley, M. J., Persel, C. S., Clark, M. C., & Krych, D. K. (1997). Long-term follow-up of post-acute traumatic brain injury rehabilitation: A statistical analysis to test for stability and predictability of outcome. *Brain Injury, 11*(9), 677–690.

Becker, R. L. (1989). *Becker Work Adjustment Profile: Evaluators manual.* Columbus, OH: Elbern.

Bellini, J., Bolton, B., & Neath, J. (1998). Operationalizing multiple services over extended time as a measure of service intensity. *Journal of Rehabilitation, 22,* 47–64.

Bellini, J., Neath, J., & Bolton, B. (1995a). Development of a scale of social disadvantage for vocational rehabilitation. *Journal of Rehabilitation Administration, 19,* 107–118.

Bellini, J., Neath, J., & Bolton, B. (1995b). A comparison of linear multiple regression and a simplified approach in the prediction of rehabilitation outcomes. *Rehabilitation Counseling Bulletin, 39,* 151–160.

Bitter, J. A., & Bolanovich, D. J. (1970). WARF: A scale for measuring job-readiness behaviors. *American Journal of Mental Deficiency, 74,* 616–621.

Blankertz, L., & Robinson, S. (1996). Adding a vocational focus to mental health rehabilitation. *Psychiatric Services, 47,* 1216–1222.

Bolton, B. (1987). Outcome analysis in vocational rehabilitation. In M. J. Fuhrer (Ed.), *Rehabilitation outcomes: Analysis and measurement* (pp. 57–69). Baltimore: Brookes.

Bolton, B. (1990). Research methodology for investigating the relationship between rehabilitation counselor education and client outcomes. *Rehabilitation Education, 4,* 70–81.

Bolton, B. (2004). Counseling and rehabilitation outcomes. In F. Chan, N. L. Berven, & K. R. Thomas (Eds.), *Counseling theories and techniques for rehabilitation health professionals* (pp. 444–465). New York: Springer.

Bolton, B., & Akridge, R. L. (1995). A meta-analysis of skills training programs for rehabilitation clients. *Rehabilitation Counseling Bulletin, 38,* 262–273.

Bolton, B., & Brookings, J. B. (1993). Prediction of job satisfactoriness for workers with severe handicaps from aptitudes, personality, and training ratings. *Journal of Business and Psychology, 7*(3), 359–366.

Bolton, B., & Brookings, J. (1998). Development of a measure of intrapersonal empowerment. *Rehabilitation Psychology, 43*, 131–142.

Bolton, B., & Roessler, R. (1986). *Manual for the Work Personality Profile.* Fayetteville, AR: Arkansas RRTC.

Brooks-Lane, N., Hutchenson, S., & Revell, G. (2005). Supporting consumer directed employment outcomes. *Journal of Vocational Rehabilitation, 23*, 123–134.

Brown, M., Diller, L., Fordyce, W., Jacobs, D., & Gordon, W. (1980). Rehabilitation Indicators: Their nature and uses for assessment. In B. Bolton & D. Cook (Eds.), *Rehabilitation client assessment* (pp. 102–117). Baltimore: University Park Press.

Bryson, G., Greig, T., & Bell, M. D. (2003). Domain specific work performance change for people with schizophrenia. *Journal of Vocational Rehabilitation, 19*, 167–172.

Burt, D. B., Fuller, S. P., & Lewis, K. R. (1991). Competitive employment of adults with autism. *Journal of Autism and Developmental Disorders, 21* (2), 237–242.

Butterworth, J., Gilmore, D., & Shalock, R. (1998). Rates of vocational rehabilitation system closure into competitive employment. *Mental Retardation, 36* (4), 336–337.

Callahan, M. (1991). Common sense and quality: Meaningful employment outcomes for persons with severe physical disabilities. *Journal of Vocational Rehabilitation, 1*(2), 21–28.

Chan, F., Cheing, G., Chan, J. Y. C., Rosenthal, D. A., & Chronister, J. (2006). Predicting employment outcomes of rehabilitation clients with orthopedic disabilities: A CHAID analysis. *Disability and Rehabilitation, 28*(5), 257–270.

Cook, J. A., & Pickett, S. A. (1994). Recent trends in vocational rehabilitation for people with psychiatric disability. *American Rehabilitation, 20*(4), 2–12.

Cook, J. A., & Rosenberg, H. (1994). Predicting community employment among persons with psychiatric disability. *Journal of Rehabilitation Administration, 18*(1), 6–22.

Crewe, N. M., & Athelstan, G. T. (1984). *Functional Assessment Inventory manual.* Menomonie, WI: University of Wisconsin–Stout.

Crisp, R. (2005). Key factors related to vocational outcome: Trends for six disability groups. *Journal of Rehabilitation, 71* (4), 30–37.

Dedding, C., Cardol, M., Eyssen, I., Dekker, J., & Beelen, A. (2004). Validity of the Canadian Occupational Performance Measure: A client-centred outcome measurement. *Clinical Rehabilitation, 18*, 660–667.

Depoy, E. (1992). A comparison of standardized and observational assessment. *Journal of Cognitive Rehabilitation, 10* (1), 30–33.

Deren, S., & Randell, J. (1990). The vocational rehabilitation of substance abusers. *Journal of Applied Rehabilitation Counseling, 21* (2), 4–6.

Dijkers, M. (1997). Measuring the long-term outcomes of traumatic brain injury: A review of the Community Integration Questionnaire. *Journal of Head Trauma Rehabilitation, 12* (6), 74–91.

Donovan, M. R., & Tilson, G. P., Jr. (1998). The Marriott Foundations Bridges: From school to work program: A framework for successful employment outcomes for people with disabilities. *Journal of Vocational Rehabilitation, 10* (1), 15–21.

Dowler, D. L., & Walls, R. T. (1996). Accommodating specific job functions for people with hearing impairments. *Journal of Rehabilitation, 62*, 35–43.

Ernst, J. L., & Day, E. H. (1998). Reducing the penalties of long-term employment: Alternatives in vocational rehabilitation and spinal cord injury. *Journal of Vocational Rehabilitation, 10*(2), 133–139.

Evans, R. W., & Ruff, R. M. (1992). Outcome and value: A perspective on rehabilitation outcomes achieved in acquired brain injury. *Journal of Head Trauma Rehabilitation, 7*(4), 24–36.

Fabiano, R. J., & Crewe, N. (1995). Variables associated with employment following severe traumatic brain injury. *Rehabilitation Psychology, 40*(3), 223–231.

Farkas, M., & Anthony, W. A. (1987). Outcome analysis in psychiatric rehabilitation. In M. J. Fuhrer (Ed.), *Rehabilitation outcomes: Analysis and measurement* (pp. 43–56). Baltimore: Paul H. Brookes.

Fraser, R. T., Vandergoot, D., Thomas, D., & Wagner, C. C. (2004). Employment outcomes research in vocational rehabilitation: Implications for Rehabilitation Counselor (RC) training. *Journal of Vocational Rehabilitation, 20*, 135–142.

Fuhrer, M. J. (1987). Overview of outcome analysis in rehabilitation. In M.J. Fuhrer (Ed.), *Rehabilitation outcomes: Analysis and measurement* (pp. 1–15). Baltimore: Brookes.

Gardner, J. (1991). Early referral and other factors affecting vocational rehabilitation outcome for the workers compensation client. *Rehabilitation Counseling Bulletin, 34* (3), 197–209.

Gibson, D. L., Weiss, D. J., Dawis, R. V., & Lofquist, L. H. (1970). *Manual for the Minnesota Satisfactoriness Scales* (Minnesota Studies in Vocational Rehabilitation: 27). Minneapolis: University of Minnesota.

Gilbride, D. D., Thomas, J. R., & Stensrud, R. (1998). Beyond Status Code 26: Development of an instrument to measure the quality of placements in the state-federal program. *Journal of Applied Rehabilitation Counseling, 29* (1), 3–7.

Goodman, G. (2005). Work occupations and outcomes internationally and across the lifespan. *Work: Journal of Prevention, Assessment, and Rehabilitation, 24* (1), 1–2.

Gough, H. G. (1987). *California Psychological Inventory administrator's guide.* Palo Alto, CA: Consulting Psychologist Press.

Halpern, A. S. (1987). Outcome analysis for persons with mental retardation. In M.J. Fuhrer (Ed.), *Rehabilitation outcomes: Analysis and measurement* (pp. 29–41). Baltimore: Brookes.

Institute for Personality and Ability Testing. (1985). *Manual for Form E of the 16 PF.* Champaign, IL: Author.

Jette, A. M., & Jette, D. U. (1997). Assessing health status outcomes in rehabilitation. In M. J. Fuhrer (Ed.), *Assessing medical rehabilitation practices: The promise of outcomes research* (pp. 181–207). Baltimore: Brookes.

Johnston, M. V., Stineman, M., & Velozo, C. A. (1997). Outcomes research in medical rehabilitation. In M.J. Fuhrer (Ed.), *Assessing medical rehabilitation practices: The promise of outcomes research* (pp. 1–41). Baltimore: Brookes.

Kilmer, D. D. (1999). Outcome of lower limb orthotic intervention in hereditary and acquired NMD. In Research and Training Center in Neuromuscular Diseases (Eds.), *Rehab info network for neuromuscular diseases.* Davis, CA: University of California.

Kirchner, C., Johnson, G., & Harkins, D. (1997). Research to improve vocational rehabilitation: Employment barriers and strategies for clients who are blind or visually impaired. *Journal of Visual Impairment and Blindness, 91* (4), 377–392.

Lehman, A. F. (1995). Vocational rehabilitation in schizophrenia. *Schizophrenia Bulletin, 21*(4), 645–656.

Linkowski, D. C. (1987). *The Acceptance of Disability Scale.* Washington, DC: George Washington University.

Livneh, H., & Parker, R. M. (2005). Psychological adaptation to disability: Perspectives from chaos and complexity theory. *Rehabilitation Counseling Bulletin, 49* (1), 17–28.

Lougheed, V. (1998). Employer-based rehabilitation. *Canadian Journal of Rehabilitation, 12*(1), 33–37.

Majumder, R. K., Walls, R. T., & Fullmer, S. L. (1998). Rehabilitation client involvement in employment decisions. *Rehabilitation Counseling Bulletin, 42,* 162–173.

Majumder, R. K., Walls, R. T., Fullmer, S. L., & Misra, S. (1997). What works. In F. E. Menz, J. Eggers, P. Wehman, & V. Brooke (Eds.), *Lessons for improving employment of people with disabilities from vocational rehabilitation research* (pp. 263–282). Menomonie, WI: Stout Vocational Rehabilitation Institute.

Martin, T. J. (1999). Evaluation: The image of effective implementation of human resource development principles in rehabilitation. *Rehabilitation Education, 13*(1), 69–77.

Matrone, K. F., & Leahy, M. J. (2005). The relationship between vocational rehabilitation client outcomes and rehabilitation counselor multicultural counseling competencies. *Rehabilitation Counseling Bulletin, 48* (4), 233–244.

Michaels, C. A., & Risucci, D. A. (1993). Employer and counselor perceptions of workplace accommodations for persons with traumatic brain injury. *Journal of Applied Rehabilitation Counseling, 24* (1), 38–46.

Moore, S. C., & Powell, T. H. (1990). Benefits and benefits protection for persons with severe disabilities entering supported employment: A guide for vocational rehabilitation counselors. *Journal of Applied Rehabilitation Counseling, 21* (4), 31–35.

Moriarty, J. B. (1981). *Preliminary Diagnostic Questionnaire.* Morgantown, WV: West Virginia RRTC.

Morton, M. V., Gibbs, R. L., & Ragland, M. (1997). The rehabilitation counselor-employment specialist relationship: A collaborative approach. *Journal of Vocational Rehabilitation, 9* (2), 153–157.

Mount, D., Johnstone, B., White, C., & Sherman, A. (2005). Vocational outcomes: VR service determinants for persons with epilepsy. *Journal of Vocational Rehabilitation, 23* (1), 11–20.

Neath, J., Bellini, J., & Bolton, B. (1997). Dimensions of the Functional Assessment Inventory for five disability groups. *Rehabilitation Psychology, 42,* 183–207.

Neath, J., & Bolton, B. (1997). *Manual for the Employability Maturity Interview Computer Report.* Fayetteville, AR: Arkansas RRTC.

Nosek, M. A. (1987). Outcome analysis in independent living. In M. J. Fuhrer (Ed.), *Rehabilitation outcomes: Analysis and measurement* (pp. 71–83). Baltimore: Brookes.

Nosek, M. A., Fuhrer, M. J., & Howland, C. A. (1992). Independence among people with disabilities: II. Personal Independence Profile. *Rehabilitation Counseling Bulletin, 36,* 21–36.

Ochs, L. A., & Roessler, R. T. (2004). Predictors of career exploration intentions: A social cognitive career theory perspective. *Rehabilitation Counseling Bulletin, 47* (4), 224–233.

O'Day, B., Wilson, J., Killeen, M., & Ficke, R. (2004). Consumer outcomes of centers for independent living program. *Journal of Vocational Rehabilitation, 20,* 83–89.

Othmer, E., Penick, E., Powell, B., Read, M., & Othmer, S. (1989). *Manual for the Psychiatric Diagnostic Interview, Revised (PDI-R).* Los Angeles: Western Psychological Services.

Peters, R. H., Scalia, V. A., & Fried, J. H. (1993). The effectiveness of vocational evaluation program recommendations and successful outcome by disability type. *Vocational Evaluation and Work Adjustment Bulletin, 26* (2), 47–52.

Platt, J. J. (1995). Vocational rehabilitation of drug abusers. *Psychological Bulletin, 117* (3), 416–433.

Reagles, K. W., Wright, G. N., & Butler, A. J. (1970). A scale of rehabilitation gain for clients of an expanded vocational rehabilitation program. *Wisconsin Studies in Vocational Rehabilitation,* No. 13. Madison: University of Wisconsin.

Rehabilitation Act of 1973, 29 U.S.C. § 701 *et seq.* (1973) (amended 1998).

Rehabilitation Services Administration. (2005). *Policy Directive PD-06-01: RSA 911 Case Service Report for State Vocational Rehabilitation Agencies (General and Blind).* Washington, DC: U.S. Dept. of Education, Office of Special Education and Rehabilitative Services.

Research Triangle Institute. (1998). *A longitudinal study of the vocational rehabilitation service program: Characteristics and outcomes of former VR consumers with an employment outcome.* Washington, DC: Rehabilitation Services Administration, ED Contract No. HR92-022-001.

Roessler, R. T., & Rumrill, P.D., Jr. (1995). Promoting reasonable accommodations: An essential postemployment service. *Journal of Applied Rehabilitation Counseling, 26* (4), 3–7.

Rogers, E. S., Anthony, W. A., Lyass, A., & Penk, W. E. (2006). A randomized clinical trial of vocational rehabilitation for people with psychiatric disabilities. *Rehabilitation Counseling Bulletin, 49* (3), 143–156.

RSA Data Archive. (2005). *Vocational rehabilitation case records: RSA Form 911.* Washington, DC: Rehabilitation Services Administration.

Rubin, S. E., & Roessler, R. T. (2001). *Foundations of the vocational rehabilitation process* (5th ed.). Austin, TX: PRO-ED.

Rumrill, P. D., Roessler, R. T., & Cook, B. G. (1998). Improving career re-entry outcomes for people with multiple sclerosis: A comparison of two approaches. *Journal of Vocational Rehabilitation, 10* (3), 241–252.

Sales, A., & McAllan, L. (1999). Evaluation of a continuing education model for delivering a rehabilitation counseling degree: Preliminary findings. *Rehabilitation Education, 13* (1), 61–68.

Schriner, K. F., Roessler, R. T., & Johnson, P. (1993). Identifying the employment concerns of people with spina bifida. *Journal of Applied Rehabilitation Counseling, 24* (2), 32–37.

Shrey, D. E., & Mital, A. (1994). Disability management and the cardiac rehabilitation patient: Job simulation and transitional work strategies. *Journal of Occupational Rehabilitation, 4* (1), 39–53.

Siller, J. (1970). Generality of attitudes toward the physically disabled. *Proceedings of the 78th Annual Convention of the American Psychological Association, 5,* 697–698.

Sowers, J. (1991). Employment for persons with physical disabilities and related technology. *Journal of Vocational Rehabilitation, 1* (2), 55–64.

Stoddard, S., Hanson, S., & Temkin, T. (1999). *An evaluation of choice demonstration projects.* Report to Rehabilitation Services Administration, Contract HR95034001. Berkeley, CA: InfoUse.

Stoddard, S., & Premo, B. (2004). Expanding employment opportunities: Independent living center employment services and collaboration with vocational rehabilitation. *Journal of Vocational Rehabilitation, 20,* 45–52.

Szymanski, E. M., & Danek, M. M. (1992). The relationship of rehabilitation counselor education to rehabilitation client outcome: A replication and extension. *Journal of Rehabilitation, 58* (1), 49–56.

Taheri-Araghi, M., & Hendren, G. (1994). Successful vocational rehabilitation of clients with retinitis pigmentosa. *Journal of Visual Impairment and Blindness, 88* (2), 128–131.

Tinsley, H. E. A., Warnken, R. G., Weiss, D. J., Dawis, R. V., & Lofquist, L. H. (1969). *A follow-up survey of former clients of the Minnesota Division of Vocational Rehabilitation* (Minnesota Studies in Vocational Rehabilitation: 26). Minneapolis: University of Minnesota.

U.S. Department of Labor (1998). Workforce development performance measures. [Online]. Retrieved September 1, 1999, from http://nortec.org/cb/onestop/wdpm_menu.html.

Wagner, K. A. (1987). Outcome analysis in comprehensive medical rehabilitation. In M. J. Fuhrer (Ed.), *Rehabilitation outcomes: Analysis and measurement* (pp. 19–28). Baltimore: Paul H. Brookes.

Walls, R. T. (1982). Disincentives in vocational rehabilitation: Cash and inkind benefits from other programs. *Rehabilitation Counseling Bulletin, 26,* 3746.

Walls, R. T., & Batiste, L. (1996). Job accommodations for fatigue in the workplace. *Technology and Disability, 5,* 335–343.

Walls, R. T., & Dowler, D. L. (1987). Benefits versus earnings for vocational rehabilitation clients: The anchoring effect. *Journal of Behavioral Economics, 16*, 5567.

Walls, R. T., Dowler, D. L., & Fullmer, S. L. (1989). Cash and inkind benefits: Incentives rather than disincentives for vocational rehabilitation. *Rehabilitation Counseling Bulletin, 33*, 118126.

Walls, R. T., Dowler, D. L., & Fullmer, S. L. (1990). Incentives and disincentives to supported employment. In F. R. Rusch (Ed.), *Supported employment: Models, methods, and issues* (pp. 251–269). Sycamore, IL: Sycamore Publishing.

Walls, R. T., & Fullmer, S. L. (1996). Comparing rehabilitated workers to the U.S. workforce. *Rehabilitation Counseling Bulletin, 40*, 153–164.

Walls, R. T., & Fullmer, S. L. (1997). Competitive employment: Occupations after vocational rehabilitation. *Rehabilitation Counseling Bulletin, 41*, 15–25.

Walls, R. T., Fullmer, S. L., & Dowler, D. L. (1996). Functional vocational cognition: Dimensions of real-world accuracy. *The Career Development Quarterly, 44*, 224–233.

Walls, R. T., Misra, S., & Majumder, R. K. (2002). Trends in vocational rehabilitation: 1978, 1988, 1998. *Journal of Rehabilitation, 68* (3), 4–10.

Walls, R. T., & Tseng, M. S. (1987). Measurement of client outcomes in rehabilitation. In B. Bolton (Ed.), *Handbook of measurement and evaluation in rehabilitation* (2nd ed., pp. 183–201). Baltimore: Brookes.

Walls, R. T., Werner, T. J., Bacon, A., & Zane, T. (1977). Behavior checklists. In J. D. Cone & R. P. Hawkins (Eds.), *Behavioral assessment: New directions in clinical psychology* (pp. 77–146). New York: Bruner & Mazel.

Walls, R. T., Zane, T., & Thvedt, J. E. (1979). *The Independent Living Behavior Checklist.* Morgantown, WV: West Virginia RRTC.

Walls, R. T., Zane, T., & Werner, T. J. (1978). *The Vocational Behavior Checklist.* Morgantown, WV: West Virginia RRTC.

Warren, P. R., Giesen, J. M., & Cavenaugh, B. S. (2004). Effects of race, gender, and other characteristics of legally blind consumers on homemaker closure. *Journal of Rehabilitation, 70* (4), 16–21.

Wehman, P., & Revell, G. (2005). Lessons learned from the provision of funding of employment services for the MR/DD population. *Journal of Disability Policy Studies, 16* (2), 84–101.

Wehman, P., Revell, W. G., & Brooke, V. (2003). Competitive employment: Has it become the "First Choice" yet? *Journal of Disability Policy Studies, 14* (3), 163–173.

Weiss, D. J., Dawis, R. V., England, G. W., & Lofquist, L. H. (1967). *Manual for the Minnesota Satisfaction Questionnaire* (Minnesota Studies in Vocational Rehabilitation: 22). Minneapolis: University of Minnesota.

West, M., Revell, W. G., & Wehman, P. (1992). Achievements and challenges: I. A five-year report on consumer and system outcomes from the Supported Employment Initiative. *Journal of the Association for Persons with Severe Handicaps, 17* (4), 227–235.

Westerheide, W. J., Lenhart, L., & Miller, M. C. (1975). Field test of a Service Outcome Measurement Form: Client change. *Monograph No. 3.* Oklahoma City, OK: Department of Rehabilitation Services.

Wilgosh, L., Mueller, H. H., & Rowat, W. (1994). Employer views on reasons for employment failure of employees with and without intellectual impairments. *Canadian Journal of Rehabilitation, 8* (2), 79–86.

Wood-Dauphinee, S. (1998). Competing conceptual frameworks for assessing rehabilitation outcomes. *Canadian Journal of Rehabilitation, 11* (4), 165–167.

Workforce Investment Act of 1998, 29 U.S.C. § 2801 *et seq.* (1998) (Session law # is P.L. 105-220).

Wright, G. N., & Remmers, H. H. (1960). *Manual for the Handicap Problems Inventory.* Lafayette, IN: Purdue Research Foundation.

Zivolich, S., Shueman, S. A., & Weiner, J. S. (1997). An exploratory cost-benefit analysis of natural support strategies in the employment of people with severe disabilities. *Journal of Vocational Rehabilitation, 8* (3), 211–221.

Zivolich, S., & Weiner-Zivolich, J. S. (1997). A national corporate employment initiative for persons with severe disabilities: A 10-year perspective. *Journal of Vocational Rehabilitation, 8* (1), 75–87.

Chapter 15

Assessment of Career Development and Maturity

Terry L. Blackwell, Stephen J. Leierer, and Douglas C. Strohmer

The need for career services across the life span has become more evident given the changing nature and availability of work and the corresponding demands on today's workers to engage in repeated occupational and learning transitions (McMahon, Patton, & Tatham, 2003). Paralleling the changing workforce demographics is the movement that views career development as a process that spans an individual's work life and affects occupational choice, efficacy, and behavior (Ginzberg, 1984; Gottfredson, 2002; Super, Savickas, & Super, 1996; Vondracek, Lerner, & Schulenberg, 1986). This process can have special significance for rehabilitation professionals providing services for people with disabilities who often have more limited career development opportunities than those who are not disabled (Shahnasarian, 2001; Szymanski & Vancollins, 2003).

Individuals entering the job market for the first time can expect to hold more than nine jobs by the time they are in their mid-30s, according to U.S. Department of Labor, Bureau of Labor Statistics (http://www.bls.gov). Many individuals within the labor force experience what has been termed "late, delayed, or impaired" career development (LoCascio, 1964, 1974). Manuele (1984) describes these as adults who frequently

> come from educationally disadvantaged backgrounds and have histories of unemployment or underemployment in low-level, poorly paying jobs . . . [whose] career development patterns often reveal limited aspiration and goal striving, previous histories of educational failure, limited use of resources, lack of involvement in career choice, planning and decision making. (p. 101)

Included within this group are people with disabilities, who comprise more than 19% of the population and rank as one of the fastest growing segments of the U.S. population and yet are often unemployed (U.S. Census Bureau). In issues affecting career development for people with disabilities, Szymanski and Vancollins (2003) identify five areas likely to further disadvantage individuals from the workforce.

1. Job insecurity in the changing labor market has increased because of company mergers and downsizing; increased use of temporary workers combine with disability compensation strategies, which may limit incentives for these workers.
2. Today's workforce is dependent on technology and, unfortunately, the accessibility and/or affordability of technology limits the ability of workers with disabilities to keep pace with other workers. In this way, workers with disabilities may become more isolated and fall behind their coworkers.
3. People with cognitive disabilities likely face unique challenges. While the workplace is fast-paced and knowledge dependent, the expectations and preparation may mandate people with cognitive disabilities

to a competitive disadvantage (Falvey, Bishop, & Gage, 1993). Train-ing programs for these clients will require supports and strategies that focus on the fluid and dynamic nature of many work environments.

4. Changing policies regarding people with disabilities are evolving because of increased competition for jobs between people with dis-abilities and other groups experiencing high unemployment. Like-wise, the independence and choice goals of clients with disabilities have been juxtaposed to the needs of the disability and caregiving industries (Szymanski, Johnston-Rodriquez, Millington, Rodriguez, & Lagergren, 1995).

5. Stress in the work environment has been recognized as an important influence on the effect of disability (Fougeyrollas & Beauregard, 2001; Hahn, 1989). Szymanski (1989) has noted that increased stress in the work environment may intensify disability-related stress.

This chapter will focus on a selected sampling of instruments that may be incorporated in the assessment process to assist individuals in their career development and decision making. Special emphasis will be given to working with people from diverse backgrounds and with disabilities. Although many of the instruments reviewed are developed for self-assessment, in general, ap-plication in the career decision-making process will be most effective when used in conjunction with professional support (Bobek & Gore, 2004). When using these instruments in counseling with clients, rehabilitation professionals are encouraged to keep in mind Patterson's notion of client-centered assess-ment (Patterson & Watkins, 1982). In a client-centered assessment the client is involved in question development, test selection, and interpretation of the results. By taking this "client involvement" approach to the assessment process, clients are more likely to be committed to the process and act on the results of assessment.

Career Maturity and Decision Making

In defining career development, Brown and Brooks (1996) describe it as a lifelong process of getting ready to choose, choosing, and typically continu-ing to make choices from among the many occupations available in our soci-ety. Central to this developmental approach is the concept of career maturity, which, broadly defined, refers to an individual's readiness to make informed, age-appropriate career decisions that are both realistic and consistent over time (Crites, 1976; Levinson, Ohler, Caswell, & Kiewra, 1998; Savickas, 1984; Super, Crites, Hummel, Moser, Overstreet, & Warnath, 1957). Assessment of an individual's career maturity is an important part of the developmental model. The assessment typically includes tests that measure abilities, interests, and values for exploring an individual's level of career maturity (Knapp-Lee, 1996; Sharf, 2006). Some authors have suggested that the assessment process also incorporate a measure of cultural identity (Blustein & Ellis, 2000; Hartung et al., 1998).

Assessment of an individual's level of career maturity requires the use of reliable and valid instruments in order to help the person make important career decisions (Bobek & Gore, 2004). The model of career maturity proposed by Crites (1971) "consists of affective and cognitive dimensions. The cognitive dimension is composed of decision-making skills; the affective dimension includes attitudes toward the career decision-making process" (Patton & Creed, 2001, p. 336). In addition, when working with individuals from diverse backgrounds, the rehabilitation professional needs to "consider the role of economic, educational, social and political opportunities that form socio-structural realities and perceptions—both of which can and often do influence the career decision-making processes of women and members of racial and ethnic minority groups" (Luzzo & MacGrogor, 2001) as well as individuals with disabilities who represent a diversity in gender, age, race, ethnicity, religion, sexual orientation, disability, language, and socioeconomic status.

Assessment Issues

Rehabilitation professionals will typically gather assessment data from a wide variety of sources when working with individuals on career development and decision-making activities. These data include both quantitative scores obtained from standardized tests and related instruments and qualitative data obtained through interviews and observations (Berven, 1984; Blackwell & Guglielmo, 2001; Reid, 1997; Sink, Gannaway, & Cottone, 1987).

Ethically, the responsible use of testing and other assessment information requires appropriate levels of competence and sound professional judgment. Competency requires that the test user keep current with developments in the areas of testing and assessment and adhere to his or her respective ethical standards and guidelines and relevant federal and state laws concerning assessment of individuals with disabilities. Users also need to be knowledgeable of existing research on the effects of a particular disability on specific test performance (Patterson & Blackwell, 2005).

When selecting an instrument for use in the assessment process, the rehabilitation professional needs to know the types of people the test was standardized for and if the instrument is appropriate for the individual being served. Caution must be exercised when interpreting scores for individuals not represented in the norming groups. Next, the test user needs be knowledgeable about the technical properties of the test and how reliable and valid the instrument is (Blackwell & Guglielmo, 2001). Test manuals and independent reviews of tests provide information on reliability and validity.

A reliable instrument is needed to produce dependable, repeatable, and consistent information about people taking the test. General guidelines for interpreting reliability coefficients of a test are as follows: .90 and up = *excellent*;

.80–.89 = *good*; .70–.79 = *adequate*; below .70 = *may have limited applicability* (U.S. Department of Labor, 2000a).

Validity is what gives meaning to the test scores and indicates how useful the test will be. Test validity is established in reference to specific groups, and it is the responsibility of the test user to determine if the instrument can be used appropriately with the particular type of individual who will be tested. Ethically, the ultimate responsibility for ensuring that validity evidence exists for the conclusions reached in using a test is with the test user (U.S. Department of Labor, 2000a).

Best practices would further suggest that rehabilitation professionals strive in their assessments to understand how the values, interests, thoughts, and perceptions of people with disabilities are influenced by the environmental and ecological factors related to the work world. They must understand the economic and employment context in which the individual lives, the impact of disability for that individual, and the prevailing cultural and social views regarding the individual's particular disability (Szymanski & Vancollins, 2003).

In the selection and use of tests, the rehabilitation professional may find the following checklist useful in facilitating ethical behavior in the assessment process:

- Have I used only those tests or assessment techniques for which I am qualified to administer, score, and interpret?
- Have I based my assessment activities on relevant research, proper techniques, and validity for the task at hand?
- Have I used the latest available edition of a given assessment instrument?
- Do I know the uses and applications, standardization, limitations, reliability, and validity of the tests or other assessment instruments I plan to use with the client?
- Do I know the limits of the tests or instruments I am using for assessing or making predictions from?
- Have I identified those factors (e.g., gender, age, race, ethnicity, religion, sexual orientation, disability, language, or socioeconomic status) that would require me to change how I would normally administer or interpret the assessment results? (Blackwell & Guglielmo, 2001)

Review of Selected Assessment Instruments

Osborn and Zunker (2006) asserted that

perhaps the greatest area of growth in the field of career assessment has been in the area of career development inventories. These inventories are designed to measure different aspects of career development that could interfere with an individual's progress toward career maturity. Other concepts measured by contemporary career development inventories include career maturity, levels of dysfunctional thinking, anxiety, self-esteem/efficacy, and cognitive clarity. In addition, the inventories may focus on career decision-making. (p. 190)

The following is a representative sampling of some selected instruments that may be useful in looking at the influence of specific characteristics on an individual's career preparation, career exploration, career selection, and career performance. However, it must be kept in mind that the use of assessment in career planning and development requires looking at a number of variables, including aptitudes, values, needs, interests, personality, and other characteristics relevant to an individual's career development.

Career Attitudes and Strategies Inventory (CASI)

John L. Holland and Gary D. Gottfredson

Purpose: Assess career attitudes and behaviors

Publication date: 1994

Population: Adults

Administration: Self-administered; individual and group

Time: 35 minutes

Reading level: Not specified

Languages: English

Norms: Employed adults

Subtests, scales, scores: Reports scores for CASI scales: Job Satisfaction, Work Involvement, Skill Development, Dominant Style, Career Worries, Interpersonal Abuse, Family Commitment, Risk-Taking Style, Geographic Barriers. Raw scores converted to *T*-scores

User qualifications: No special qualifications required

Available from: Psychological Assessment Resources, Inc. (800–331–8378) or www.parinc.com

Description: The *Career Attitudes and Strategies Inventory* (CASI) is a 130-item, self-scoring, self-interpreted inventory designed to measure "some common attitudes, feelings, experiences, and obstacles" that influence adult careers (Holland & Gottfredson, 1994, p. 1). Responses to the CASI provide interpretations on nine scales: Job Satisfaction, Work Involvement, Skill Development, Dominant Style, Career Worries, Interpersonal Abuse, Family Commitment, Risk-Taking Style, and Geographic Barriers. While the CASI was developed to be self-scoring and self-interpretive, Kinnier (1998) cautions that "although the interpretation of each scale seems fairly straightforward, the implications of the scores for a person's career development and choice are more complex and best addressed in counseling" (p. 184). The manual does provide a number of brief illustrative case profiles for professional reference and guidelines for becoming a "competent user" (p. 23).

Norms for this third version of the CASI consisted of 747 adults, age 17 to 77. Ethnic makeup was predominately European American (79%) and female (64%), with 97% of the sample having a grade 12 education or higher. The authors report occupational distribution was large, "ranging from laborers to executives" (p. 33).

The reliability coefficients (alpha) for the third version of the CASI ranged from .76 to .92. An average interval of 13-day test-retest reliabilities for a small sample of working adults ranged from .66 to .94. Evidence of validity was based primarily on correlational analysis. Overall, Kinnier (1998) finds that "tests of validity (mainly convergent and discriminant correlations) are generally encouraging" (p. 185).

Counseling considerations: The CASI can be a useful tool in the exploratory phase of career development for assessing an individual's career attitudes and behaviors. However, caution must be exercised when using this instrument with individuals with special needs who are not represented in the norms. Brown (1998) concludes that the CASI might best be used as "a pre-interview survey, a device to generate discussion, or to identify potentially problematic areas that would benefit from further exploration" (p. 183).

Career Beliefs Inventory (CBI)

John D. Krumboltz

Purpose: Identify beliefs that may be blocking career goals

Publication date: 1991

Population: Age 13 and up

Administration: Self-administered; individual or group

Time: 20–30 minutes

Reading level: 8th grade

Languages: English

Norms: Junior high, high school, and adult students; employed and unemployed adults

Subtests, scales, scores: 26 scales, divided into 5 categories: My Current Career Situation, What Seems Necessary for My Happiness, Factors that Influence my Decisions, Changes I am Willing to

Make, and Efforts I am Willing to Initiate. Scale scores are weighted and range from 10 to 50.

User qualifications: No restrictions, but best if given by a counselor, preferably one trained in career guidance and assessment

Available from: Consulting Psychologists Press (800-624-1765) or www.cpp.com

Description: The *Career Beliefs Inventory* (CBI) is designed as a counseling tool that can be used to identify beliefs as they relate to occupational choice and the pursuit of a career. The inventory can be administered to groups or individually from grade 8 to adult. The CBI is a 96-item paper-and-pencil, self-scorable inventory written at an 8th-grade reading level. Items are grouped into 26 scales organized under 5 headings (all items are rated using a 5-point Likert format). Scores are reported for the following scales: Administrative Index, Employment Status, Career Plans, Acceptance of Uncertainty, Openness, Achievement, College Education, Intrinsic Satisfaction, Peer Equality, Structured Work Environment, Control, Responsibility, Approval of Others, Self–Other Comparisons, Occupation/College Variation, Career Path Flexibility, Post-Training Transition, Job Experimentation, Relocation, Improving Self, Persisting While Uncertain, Taking Risks, Learning Job Skills, Negotiating/Searching, Overcoming Obstacles, and Working Hard. The 10-page CBI self-scorable booklet also includes 4 pages of interpretive information to help clients understand their scores for each of the 26 scales. In addition, there is an accompanying workbook, *Exploring Your Career Beliefs,* that can be used to provide activities to promote further exploration of career beliefs and integration of *Strong Interest Inventory* or *Myers-Briggs Type Indicator* results (Osborn & Zunker, 2006).

Norms for the CBI are based on a sample of more than 7,500 people in the United States and Australia. Data are provided for eight different groups broken down by sex, employment status, and maturity level (adult, college student, school student), with varying numbers for each group. No evidence is presented on the representation of people of minority backgrounds or disability status. Evidence for reliability and validity was found to be relatively weak (Bolton, 1995; Guion, 1995; Wall, 1994). However, the test user must keep in mind the "instrument was developed for providing information about career beliefs that can be used in career counseling but not as the basis for selection or classification" (Osborn & Zunker, 2006, p. 195).

Counseling considerations: The CBI was developed as a counseling tool designed to help people identify career beliefs that may be preventing them from achieving their career goals. As such, it will be most useful when administered at the beginning of the counseling process. The resulting scores can help the counselor more quickly target the beliefs and assumptions most likely in need of examination. In addition, the CBI allows counselors to open up important areas that are typically ignored in traditional forms of career counseling (e.g., ways of responding to the possibility of failure). The CBI makes career counseling more complete; it legitimizes the exploration of important attitudes and assumptions (Kumboltz, 1992). While all of the content areas covered would be applicable to individuals with disabilities, areas that specifically target disability are not. In this regard, the counselor will need to add issues unique to the individual's disability status.

Career Decision-Making System–Revised (CDM-R)

Thomas F. Harrington and Arthur J. O'Shea

Purpose: Assess abilities, interests, and work values

Publication date: 2000

Population: Middle school students to adults in transition

Administration: Self-administered; individual or group

Time: 20 minutes (Level 1), 30–40 minutes (Level 2)

Reading level: 4th grade (Level 1—middle school and individuals with limited reading ability). 7th grade (Level 2—high school and college students, adults)

Languages: English, Spanish

Norms: Junior high, high school, and special education students; college and university students; Spanish students; employed adults

Subtests, scales, scores: Reports scores for six interest areas: Crafts, Scientific, The Arts, Social, Business, and Office Operations. Interest scale raw scores range from 0 (low) to 40 (high).

User qualifications: No restrictions, but best if given by a counselor, preferably one trained in career guidance

Available from: Pearson Assessments (800-627-7271) or http://ags .personassessments.com

Description: *The Career Decision-Making System–Revised* (CDM-R) is an "assessment and information package designed to provide step-by-step guidance through the career decision process" (Kelly, 2005). The CDM-R is available in two forms. Level 1 is a 96-item interest survey, designed for "younger students and people of all ages with limited reading ability" (p. 7). Level 2 consists of 120-items and is designed for high school and college students and adults with "stronger reading skills" (p. 7). Levels 1 and 2 are available in English and Spanish. Both levels yields scores for six interest scales that parallel Holland's RAISEC model: Crafts (Realistic), Scientific (Investigative), The Arts (Artistic), Social (Social), Business (Enterprising), and Office Occupations (Conventional) (Kelly, 2005). Findings from the interest survey are combined with a listing of career choices, school subjects, work values, abilities, and future plans. This information is incorporated into a model for career decision making (Harrington & O'Shea, 2000). The manual is very informative, providing clear and practical guidelines for administration, scoring, and interpretation of the CDM-R. Additionally, a number of case studies are presented to illustrate the interpretive process.

The manual reports internal consistency reliabilities for the six interest scales ranging from .88 to .93 for Level 1 and .92 to .95 for Level 2. The median alpha coefficient for the Spanish version was .87. One-month median test-retest reliabilities for unemployed adults and high school and college students ranged from .79 to .91. The median 5-month retest reliabilities for high school and college students ranged from .75 (college females) to .82 (college males). No retest reliabilities were reported for the Spanish version. Parallel form reliability for a sample of 10th-grade students ranged from .81 to .94. Evidence of validity based on correlations with related measures, occupational and academic group comparisons, follow-up, and cross-cultural studies is also presented. Overall, Kelly (2005) found that the CDM-R "appears to have good predictive validity."

Counseling considerations: The CDM-R has been described as providing a "convenient link between interest testing and career exploration" (Kelly, 2005). It is designed for use to facilitate career planning, select college majors, choose training or retraining programs, and prepare for entering the job market (p. 7). Because the CDM-R is not interpreted in a normative manner, this can make the instrument an attractive addition for incorporation in the career assessment and exploration process for individuals from diverse backgrounds and with disabilities.

Career Decision Scale (CDS)

Samuel H. Osipow, Clarke G. Carney, Jane Winer, Barbara Yanico, and Maryanne Koschier

Purpose: Measure career indecision

Publication date: 1987

Population: High school and college students, adults

Administration: Self-administered; individual or group

Time: 10–15 minutes

Reading level: Not specified

Languages: English

Norms: Adolescent and adult

Subtests, scales, scores: Provides indecision score based on sum of self-ratings

User qualifications: Undergraduate degree in psychology, counseling, speech-language pathology, or closely related field plus satisfactory completion of coursework in test interpretation, psychometrics and measurement theory, educational statistics, or a closely related area or licensure or certification from an agency/organization that requires appropriate training and experience in the ethical and competent use of psychological tests

Available from: Psychological Assessment Resources, Inc. (800-331-8378) or www.parinc.com

Description: The *Career Decision Scale* (CDS) is used to measure career certainty and indecision. The scale contains 19 items and consists of the CDS-Indecision scale, which provides a measure of career indecision, and the CDS-Certainty scale, which indicates the respondent's degree of certainty about having made a career decision. The CDS-Indecision scale has 16 items and the CDS-Certainty scale has two items; there also is an open-ended question that allows respondents to present their concerns in their own words. Responses on the Indecision and the Certainty subscales are reported in this study. Participants responded to items by indicating on a 4-point Likert-type scale whether the item was *not at all like me* to *exactly like me*. Higher scores on the CDS-Indecision subscale indicate greater indecision; higher scores on CDS-Certainty indicate greater certainty. Internal consistency coefficients have been consistently reported in the .80 range (Hartman, Fuqua, & Hartman, 1983). Test-retest reliabilities have been reported in the range of .61 to .90 (Hartman, Utz, & Farnum, 1979). Internal reliability coefficients in our study were .89 for CDS-Indecision and .73 for CDS-Certainty. Concurrent validity (Hartman & Hartman, 1982), construct validity (Hartman et al., 1983), and predictive validity (Hartman, Fuqua, Blum, & Hartman, 1985) have all been adequately demonstrated (Patton & Creed, 2001).

Counseling considerations: Harmon (1994) points out that if the test user "is looking for an overall measure of career indecision for use in counseling [or] evaluation . . . there is probably no better measure" (p. 261). This information may be particularly useful when working with individuals with disabilities in the early career counseling and planning stages for developing specific interventions and evaluation strategies.

Career Thoughts Inventory (CTI)

James P. Sampson, Jr., Gary W. Peterson, Janet G. Lenz, Robert C. Reardon, and Denise E. Saunders

Purpose: Assist in career problem solving and decision making

Publication date: 1996

Population: High school and college students, adults

Administration: Self-administered; individual or group

Time: 7–15 minutes

Reading level: 6.4 grade for CTI, 7.7 grade for workbook

Languages: English

Norms: High school, college students, and adults

Subtests, scales, scores: Reports total score plus three construct scale scores for Decision Making Confusion, Commitment Anxiety, and External Conflict. Raw scores converted to *T*-scores and percentiles.

User qualifications: Undergraduate degree in psychology, counseling, speech-language pathology, or closely related field plus satisfactory completion of coursework in test interpretation, psychometrics and measurement theory, educational statistics, or a closely related area or licensure or certification from an agency/organization that requires appropriate training and experience in the ethical and competent use of psychological tests (PAR, 2006).

Available from: Psychological Assessment Resources, Inc. (800-331-8378) or www.parinc.com

Description: The *Career Thoughts Inventory* (CTI) is a 48-item, self-administered, career assessment instrument designed to help individuals identify an "individual who is likely to need counseling assistance; to identify the nature of an individual's career problems; and to help an individual identify, challenge, and alter negative career thoughts that interfere with effective career decision making" (PAR, 2006). An accompanying workbook for the CTI (Sampson, Peterson, Lenz, Reardon, & Saunders, 1996b) assists clients to understand the nature of their negative thoughts as well as how much help they are likely to need in order to make effective use of career services.

The CTI uses a 4-point rating scale (*Strongly Disagree* to *Strongly Agree)*, with the test booklet designed as a carbonless form that combines the answer, scoring, and profile sheets (Fontaine, 2001).

The CTI yields a CTI Total score (a single global indicator of negative thinking in career problem solving and decision making) as well as scores on three construct scales. The three construct scales are used to identify specific areas of thought dysfunction

(Fontaine, 2001): Decision Making Confusion (14 items reflecting an inability to initiate or sustain the decision-making process as a result of disabling emotions and/or a lack of understanding about the decision-making process itself), Commitment Anxiety (10 items measuring an inability to make a commitment to a specific career choice, accompanied by generalized anxiety about the outcome of the decision-making process that perpetuates the indecision), and External Conflict (5 items assessing an inability to balance the importance of one's own self-perceptions with the importance of input from significant others, resulting in a reluctance to assume responsibility for decision making) (Sampson, Peterson, Lenz, Reardon, & Saunders, 1996a).

Sampson et al. (1996a) reported internal consistency coefficient alphas for high school students, college students, adults, and clients seeking career services ranging from .93 to .97 for CTI total score, .90 to .94 for the DMC scale, .79 to .91 for the CA scale, and .74 to .81 for the EC scale. Four week test-retest reliability for all four scales ranged from .52 (EC) to .86 (CTI). The manual discusses construct, content, convergent, and criterion-related validity.

Counseling considerations: The CTI is a well-designed, theoretically based, reliable, and valid measure of dysfunctional career thoughts (Fontaine, 2001). The format of the CTI contributes to its ease of administration and interpretation, thereby facilitating the career counseling process by eliminating the need to interrupt the process for assessment. The counseling process is further enhanced by the addition of a workbook that allows the client and counselor to move from needs assessment to interventions. The CTI can be a particularly useful tool for rehabilitation professionals working with people with disabilities to assist them to identify, challenge, and alter maladaptive thinking that may impair their ability to solve career problems and make effective career decisions.

My Vocational Situation (MVS)

John L. Holland, Denise Daiger, and Paul G. Power

Purpose: Assess difficulties in vocational decision making

Publication date: 1980

Population: High school, college, and adults

Administration: Self-administered; individual or group

Time: 5–10 minutes

Reading level: 8th grade

Languages: English

Norms: High school and college students, adults

Subtests, scales, scores: Reports scores for three measures: Vocational Identity, Occupational Information, and Barriers. Scores expressed as raw scores in reference to means and standard deviations of norm groups.

User qualifications: No special qualifications are required.

Available from: Psychological Assessment Resources, Inc. (800-331-8378) or www.parinc.com

Description: *My Vocational Situation* (MVS) is "intended as a screening device for locating people in high schools, colleges, and adult programs who need intensive career counseling because of poor vocational identity" (Lunneborg, 1985, p. 1026). MVS provides measures of Vocational Identity, Occupational Information, and Barriers. Vocational Identity is defined as having "a clear and stable picture of one's goals, interests, personality, and talents" (Holland, Daiger, & Power, 1980, p. 1). The Vocational Identity scale consists of 18 true/false items; the score is the total number of false responses. The authors describe the Occupational Information and Barriers scales as "useful check lists" that may be "helpful for identifying specific needs or problems that are often neglected or that go unrecognized" (p. 7). The Occupational Information scale has four yes/no items that indicate the individual's need for career information. The Barriers scale consists of four yes/no items that identify four "perceived external obstacles to a chosen occupational goal" (p. 1). Scoring for the Occupational Information and the Barriers scales is the total number of no responses. High scores for all three scales are in the favorable direction.

Psychometric support for the MVS is sparse. The reliability estimates were reported to range from .86 to .89 for the Vocational Identity scale; .39 to .79 for the Occupational Information scale; and .23 to .66 for the Barriers scale for high school students, college students, and workers. Evidence of validity for the MVS "is not strong" (Lunneborg, 1985, p. 1027) based on construct correlations.

Counseling considerations: Although the MVS is designed as a self-exploration tool to help counselors in assessing client needs for vocational assistance, Westbrook (1985) asserts that "more research is needed before it can be used to make decisions about individuals" (p. 1029). The MVS can be useful for quickly differentiating clients according to the need levels (Osborn & Zunker, 2006). In using the MVS, counselors may start to look at some of the issues related to vocational identity, lack of information about occupations and training, and personal and environmental barriers that individuals with disabilities may experience to assist with development of subsequent plans for intervention.

O★NET® Work Importance Locator–Version 3.0 (WIL)

U.S. Department of Labor, Employment and Training Administration

Purpose: Assess work values

Publication date: 1998

Population: Adolescent and adult

Administration: Self-administered; individual or group

Time: 15–45 minutes

Reading level: 8th grade

Languages: English

Norms: Vocational and college students, displaced workers, employed and unemployed adults

Subtests, scales, scores: Reports scores for six work values: Achievement, Independence, Recognition, Relationships, Support, and Working Conditions. Score summaries with focus on two highest work values.

User qualifications: Not reported

Available from: Printed version and supporting documents are available for purchase from the U.S. Government Printing Office (GPO) (202-512-1800). No-cost electronic components are available at http://www.onetcenter.org/WIL.html.

Description: The *O★NET Work Importance Locator* (WIL) is one of three interactive instruments from the U.S. Department of Labor's set of *O★NET Career Exploration Tools.* Used singularly or in concert with the *O★NET Interest Profiler* and the *O★NET Ability Profiler,* the WIL is designed to assess those aspects or conditions of work that are important to people in a job or career. The WIL is used to help individuals gain an awareness of their work values and then be able to link these findings to the world of work via the occupations within the *O★NET OnLine* database as well as to occupational information in CareerOneStop.

The WIL is based on the earlier work of Rounds, Henly, Dawis, Lofquist, and Weiss (1981) and the *Minnesota Importance Questionnaire* (MIQ). Clients use a simple card-sorting format to rank the importance of 20 cards, each describing an aspect of work that satisfies one of six broad work values. The six work values are updated versions of the work values defined in Dawis and Lofquist's (1984) *Theory of Work Adjustment:* Achievement, Independence, Recognition, Relationships, Support, and Working Conditions. Scoring and interpretation are straightforward, using the *Work Value Card Sorting Sheet* and *O★NET Work Importance Locator Score Report* (*Work Importance Locator User's Guide,* 2000b).

The *O★NET Work Importance Locator: User's Guide* (2000b) provides discussion on how the WIL was developed with detailed instructions on administration and interpretation of results. Although some information is provided on reliability and validity of the WIL, the information presented is fairly sparse. Test–retest reliability ranged from .35 to .58 for a 2-month period, using a sample of vocational/technical and community college students. Using the same sample of students, an analysis of reliability estimates obtained from alternative forms of the WIL and the WIP (the computerized version) produced correlations ranging from .70 to .80 for the six work value scores. Internal reliability of the WIL revealed a median coefficient alpha of .20 for a sample of employment service clients and junior college students, indicating low internal consistency among items. Evidence of construct validity is reported from a single study that examined the scores between the scores on the WIL and those on the MIQ. Correlations between the work values scores on the two instruments were fairly low, ranging from .30 to .49. While the authors assert that "further evidence of validity should be forthcoming in the next few years" (p. 44), Kelley (2005) asserts that psychometric support for the MIL is marginal at this time.

Counseling considerations: The WIL can serve as a helpful starting point in beginning the career exploration process. However, there are several cautionary points to keep in mind when using the instrument. As Michael (2005) notes, while "the WIL has been built upon sound theoretical principles and its items parallel those from a measure that has been shown to be psychometrically sound, the reliability estimates of test scores are low to moderate depending upon the method employed." Also, Michael reports that the validity evidence provided is "marginal." Further, there is no indication to suggest the inclusion of individuals with disabilities in the norms and how this might affect the interpretation of scores. The WIL will likely best be utilized by "employing it in conjunction with information obtained from other O★NET career counseling tools," assessing abilities and interests, along with the individual's experience, education, and motivation. The authors emphasize that the results should not be used for employment or hiring decisions or applicant screening for jobs or training programs.

Super's Work Values Inventory–revised (SWVI-r)

Donald E. Super and Donald G. Zytowski

Purpose: Assess relative importance of selected attributes of occupations and jobs

Publication date: 2001

Population: Middle school, high school, and college students; adults

Administration: Self-administered; individual or group

Time: 15 minutes

Reading level: 6th grade

Languages: English

Norms: Adolescents and adults

Subtests, scales, scores: Reports scores for 12 work values: Income, Creativity, Mental Challenge, Prestige, Variety, Achievement, Independence, Co-Workers, Work Environment, Supervision, Security, and Lifestyle. Raw scores are converted to percentiles and given a rank order of importance.

User qualifications: Not reported

Available from: National Career Assessment Services (800-314-8972) or www.ncasi.com or www.kuder.com

Description: *Super's Work Values Inventory–revised* (SWVI-r) is a 72-item self-report inventory designed to measure the relative importance of 12 work values important in career choice and development (Zytowski, 2006). The SWVI-r is one of three assessment instruments in the Kuder Career Planning System (KCPS), "available exclusively online at http://www.kuder.com, with keyboard administration and instantaneous scoring and reporting" (p. 3). The SWVI-r can be combined with the *Kuder Career Search* (KCS) and *Kuder Skills Assessment* (KSA) from the Internet-based KCPS to produce interests, skills, and work values assessments with an electronic career portfolio and resume builder, resources for educational and occupational exploration, and administrative database management system.

 The SWVI-r uses a five-level response format (*1 = Not important at all* to *5 = Crucial*) with results provided in a 2-page, graphic on-screen report. Included in the report are links to "definitions of the values; educational and occupational information resources; the individual's Career Portfolio; and person-match job sketches that illustrate work values operating in various jobs" (pp. 3–4). The manual also provides links from the SWVI-r work values to the work needs of the "Occupational Units" in the O★NET database. Psychometric data for conducting an adequate evaluation of the SWVI-r is missing from the online manual.

Counseling considerations: The SWVI-r presents a useful career development assessment measure that can be used "to help individuals sharpen their sense of what is important to them in a job or occupation, to guide their educational and occupational exploration and planning" (p. 6). The instrument has some very practical application when working with people from diverse backgrounds and with disabilities. The SWVI-r can provide a nice starting point for subsequent career counseling and plan development activities when combined as an assessment in the KCPS.

Vocational Decision-Making Interview–Revised

Thomas Czerlinsky and Shirley K. Chandler

Purpose: Assess vocational decision-making skills and potential decision-making problem areas of people with disabilities

Publication date: 1993

Population: Middle school to adult

Administration: Structured interview, administered verbally

Time: 20–40 minutes

Reading level: 4th grade, nonreaders

Languages: English

Norms: Variety of individuals with disabilities

Subtests, scales, scores: Reports scores on three scales: Decision-Making Readiness, Employment Readiness, and Self-Appraisal. Raw scores converted to *T*-scores and percentiles

User qualifications: Professionals who have training or experience in interviewing techniques and knowledge of the "world of work, the career development process, and the vocational preparation and needs of individuals with various disabilities" (p. 18).

Available from: JIST Publishing (800-648-5478) or www.jist.com.

Description: The *Vocational Decision-Making Interview–Revised* (VDMI-R) is a 54-question, individually administered, structured interview, designed to be assess those "aspects of vocational decision making that are important to individuals with disabilities" (Czerlinsky & Chandler, 1999, p. 3). The VDMI-R is based on the *Decision-Making Interview* (DMI) developed by Strohmer (1979) and consists of three scales: Decision-Making Readiness, Employment Readiness, and Self-Appraisal. The 17-question Decision-Making Readiness scale relates to Opportunities and Requirements, Tasks and Duties, Rewards and Punishments, Acquisition of Information, and Skills in Choosing; the Employment Readiness scale contains 11 questions that refer to Coercion, Lack of Reinforcement, Economics, and Mobility; and the 23 question Self-Appraisal scale relates to Needs, Beliefs and Interests, Abilities, Personality, Prior Success, Responsibility/Control, and Anxiety/Fear.

Normative comparisons are obtained for each of the three scales as well as a VDMI-R total score, which are recorded on the "VDMI-R Scoring Profile." Raw scores are converted to *T*-scores and percentiles. The norms for the VDMI-R include 592–690 (depending on the scale) individuals with disabilities, including mental retardation, learning disabilities, physical or sensory disabilities, traumatic head injuries, and severe/chronic mental illness (Czerlinsky & Chandler, 1999). Reliability studies reported in the manual show "satisfactory internal consistency" for the three scales. Test-retest reliabilities for the VDMI-R after a 1-week period were reported to range from .62 to .80 for a sample of clients receiving vocational rehabilitation. Using a sample of students from several special education settings, the test-retest from 2 weeks to a full school year ranged from .55 to .87. Although several research studies are provided in the manual to document discriminant, content, and predictive validity, the evidence presented is of a general nature.

Counseling considerations: The VDMI-R provides a useful tool in addressing the needs of a population (individuals with disabilities) who may have difficulty responding to many of the more traditional career assessment instruments (Tiffany, 2001). It has applicability for both students and adults with a variety of disabilities, including low reading skills, learning disabilities, sight limitations or blindness, mental retardation, chronic mental illness, brain injuries, and sensory disabilities, in assisting with individual decision making as well as for program planning (Czerlinsky & Chandler, 1999). Although the VDMI-R is designed for use with individuals with a variety of disabilities, it would not be appropriate for use with individuals who lack the cognitive skills needed to effectively participate in the interview process.

Conclusion

Effective career decision making is a developmental process that requires a knowledge of self, interests, values, and preferences as these relate to the world of work. Central to this developmental process is the concept of career maturity, which, broadly defined, refers to an individual's readiness to make informed, age-appropriate career decisions that are both realistic and consistent over time (Crites, 1976; Levinson, Ohler, Caswell, & Kiewra, 1998; Savickas, 1984; Super, Crites, Hummel, Moser, Overstreet, & Warnath, 1957). Assessment of an individual's career maturity is an important part of this developmental model and may be particularly relevant for individuals with disabilities as their life and work experience, as well as their experience in making vocational and educational decisions, is frequently limited.

This chapter presented a selection of instruments that may be incorporated into assessment to assist individuals in the career development and decision-making process. Because many of the instruments presented are developed for self-assessment with professional support, consideration must be given for selection of instruments sufficiently sensitive to the special life events and characteristics when used with people from diverse backgrounds and with disabilities. Professional interpretation will also require an understanding of the environmental context and impediments that could affect the usefulness of these test results. As test users, rehabilitation professionals must be mindful of their ethical responsibilities for the selection and use of these instruments in order to stay abreast of the field and developments in this continually growing area of assessment.

References

Berven, N. L. (1984). Assessment practices in rehabilitation counseling. *Journal of Applied Rehabilitation Counseling, 15,* 9–14.

Bobek, B. L., & Gore, P. A. (2004, March). *Inventory of Work-Related Values: 2001 Revision.* (ACT Research Report Series 2004-3). Iowa City, IA: American College Testing.

Bolton, D. L. (1995). Review of the Career Beliefs Inventory. In J. C. Conoley & J. C. Impara (Eds.), *Twelfth mental measurements yearbook* [Electronic version]. Retrieved September 6, 2006, from http://www.unl.edu/buros.

Blackwell, T. L., & Guglielmo, D. E. (2001). Ethics and assessment. *Journal of Applied Rehabilitation Counseling, 32*(1), 10–14.

Blustein, D. L., & Ellis, M. V. (2000). The cultural context of career assessment. *Journal of Career Assessment*, 8, 379–390.

Brown, D., & Brooks, L. (Eds.). (1996). *Career choice and development* (3rd ed.). San Francisco: Jossey-Bass.

Brown, M. B. (1998). Review of the Career Attitudes and Strategies Inventory: An Inventory for Understanding Adult Careers. In J. C. Impara & B. S. Plake (Eds.), *The thirteenth mental measurements yearbook* (pp. 182–183). Lincoln, NE: Buros Institute of Mental Measurements.

Crites, J. (1971). *The maturity of vocational attitudes in adolescence.* Washington, DC: American Personnel and Guidance Association.

Crites, J. (1976). A comprehensive model of career development in early adulthood. *Journal of Vocational Behavior, 9,* 105–118.

Czerlinsky, T., & Chandler, S. K. (1999). *Vocational Decision-Making Interview administration manual.* Indianapolis, IN: JIST Works.

Falvey, M. A., Bishop, K. D., & Gage, S. T. 1993). Mental retardation. In M G. Browdin, F. Tellez, & S. K. Brodwin (Eds.), *Medical, psychosocial, and vocational aspects of disability* (pp. 165–177). Athens, GA: Elliot & Fitzpatrick.

Fontaine, J. H. (2001). Review of the Career Thoughts Inventory. In B.S. Plake & J.C. Impara (Eds.), *The fourteenth mental measurements yearbook* (pp. 228–230). Lincoln, NE: Buros Institute of Mental Measurements.

Fougeyrollas, P. & Beauregard, L. (2001). Disability: An interactive person-environment social creation. In G. L. Albrecht, K. D. Seelman, & M. Bury (Eds.), *Handbook of disability studies* (pp. 171–194). Thousands Oaks, CA: Sage.

Ginzberg, E. (1984). Career development. In D. Brown & L. Brooks (Eds.), *Career choice and development: Applying contemporary theories to practice* (pp. 169–191). San Francisco: Jossey-Bass.

Gottfredson, L.S. (2002). Gottfredson's theory of circumscription, compromise, and self-creation. In D. Brown & Associates (Eds.), *Career choice and development* (4th ed., pp. 85–148). San Francisco: Jossey-Bass.

Guion, R.M. (1995). Review of the Career Beliefs Inventory. From J. C. Conoley & J. C. Impara (Eds.), *Twelfth mental measurements yearbook* [Electronic version]. Retrieved September 6, 2006, from http://www.unl.edu/buros.

Hahn, H. (1989). The politics of special education. In D. K. Lipsky & A. Gartner (Eds.), *Beyond separate education: Quality education for all* (pp. 225–241). Baltimore: Paul H. Brookes.

Harmon, L. W. (1994). Review of the Career Decision Scale (CDS). In J. T. Kapes, M. M. Mastie, & E. A. Whitfield (Eds.), *A counselor's guide to career assessment instruments* (3rd ed., pp. 258–262). Alexandria, VA: National Career Development Association.

Harrington, T. F., & O'Shea, A. J. (2000). *The Harrington-O'Shea Career Decision-Making System Revised manual.* Circle Pines, MN: American Guidance Service.

Hartman, B., Fuqua, D., Blum, C., & Hartman, P. (1985). A study of the predictive validity of the Career Decision Scale in identifying longitudinal patterns of career indecision. *Journal of Vocational Behavior, 27,* 202–209.

Hartman, B., Fuqua, D., & Hartman, P. (1983). The construct validity of the Career Decision Scale administered to high school students. *Vocational Guidance Quarterly,* 31, 250–258.

Hartman, B., & Hartman, P. (1982). The concurrent and predictive validity of the Career Decision Scale adapted for high school students. *Journal of Vocational Behavior, 20,* 244–252.

Hartman, B., Utz, P., & Farnum, S. (1979). Examining the reliability and validity of an adapted scale of educational-vocational undecidedness in a sample of graduate students. *Journal of Vocational Behavior, 15,* 224–230.

Hartung, P. J., Vandiver, B. J., Leong, F. T., Pope, M., Niles, S. G., & Farrow, B. (1998). Appraising cultural identity in career-development assessment and counseling. *Career Development Quarterly,* 46, 276–293.

Holland, J. L., Daiger, D. C., & Power, P. G. (1980). *My Vocational Situation.* Palo Alto, CA: Consulting Psychologists Press.

Holland, J. L., & Gottfredson, G. D. (1994). *Career Attitudes and Strategies Inventory: An inventory for understanding adult careers.* Lutz, FL: Psychological Assessment Resources.

Kelley, K. N. (2005). Review of the O*NET Work Importance Locator. In R. A. Spies & B. S. Plake (Eds.), *Sixteenth mental measurements yearbook* [Electronic version]. Retrieved June 30, 2006, from http://www.unl.edu/buros.

Kelly, K. R. (2005). Review of The Harrington-O'Shea Career Decision-Making System-Revised, 2005 Update. From R. A. Spies & B. S. Plake (Eds.), *Sixteenth mental measurements yearbook* [Electronic version]. Retrieved June 30, 2006, from http://www.unl.edu/buros.

Kinnier, R. T. (1998). Review of the Career Attitudes and Strategies Inventory: An Inventory for Understanding Adult Careers. In J. C. Impara & B. S. Plake (Eds.), *The thirteenth mental measurements yearbook* (pp. 184–185). Lincoln, NE: Buros Institute of Mental Measures.

Knapp-Lee, L. J. (1996). Use of the COPES, a measure of work values, in career assessment. *Journal of Career Assessment,* 4, 429–443.

Krumboltz, J. D. (1992). Challenging troublesome career beliefs. Ann Arbor, MI: ERIC Clearinghouse on Counseling and Personnel Services No. ED347481.

Levinson, E. M., Ohler, D. L., Caswell, S., & Kiewra, K. (1998). Six approaches to the assessment of career maturity. *Journal of Counseling & Development,* 76, 475–482.

LoCascio, R. (1964). Delayed and impaired vocational development: A neglected aspect of vocational development theory. *Personnel and Guidance Journal,* 885–887.

LoCascio, R. (1974). The vocational maturity of diverse groups: Theory and measurement. In D.E. Super (Ed.). *Measuring vocational maturity for counseling and evaluation* (pp. 123–133). Washington, DC: National Vocational Guidance Association.

Lunneborg, P. W. (1985). Review of My Vocational Situation. In J. V. Mitchell, Jr. (Ed.), *The Ninth Mental Measurements Yearbook* (pp. 1026–1027). Lincoln, NE: Buros Institute of Mental Measures.

Lusso, D. A., & MacGregor, M. W. (December 2001). Practice and research in career counseling and development—2000—annual review. *Career Development Quarterly*. Retrieved June 20, 2006, from http://www.findarticles.com/p/articles/mi_m0JAX/is_2_50/ai_81762548.

Manuele, C. A. (1984). Modifying vocational maturity in adults with delayed career development. *Vocational Guidance Quarterly*, 33, 101–112.

McMahon, M., Patton, M., & Tatham, P. (2003). *Managing life, learning and work in the 21st century*. Retrieved June 20, 2006, from http://www.dest.gov.au/sectors/career_development/publications_resources/profiles/life_learning_and_work.htm..

Michael, W. B. (2005). Review of the O★NET Work Importance Locator. From R. A. Spies & B. S. Plake (Eds.), *Sixteenth mental measurements yearbook* [Electronic version]. Retrieved June 30, 2006, from http://www.unl.edu/buros.

Osborn, D. S., & Zunker, V. G. (2006). *Using assessment results for career development* (7th ed.). Belmont, CA: Thomson/Brooks/Cole.

Patterson, C. H., & Watkins, C. E., Jr. (1982). Some essentials of a client-centered approach to assessment. *Measurement and Evaluation in Guidance*, 15, 103–106.

Patterson, J. B., & Blackwell, T. L. (2005). Ethics and ethical decision making in rehabilitation counseling. In R. M. Parker, E. D. Szymanski, & J. B. Patterson (Eds.), *Rehabilitation counseling: Basics and beyond* (4th ed., pp. 89–116). Austin, TX: PRO-ED.

Patton, W., & Creed, P. A. (2001). Developmental issues in career maturity and career decision status. *Career Development Quarterly*, 49(4), 336–351.

Reid, C. (1997). Rehabilitation client assessment. *Rehabilitation Education*, 11, 211–219.

Sampson, J. P., Jr., Peterson G. W., Lenz, J. G., Reardon, R. C., & Saunders, D. E. (1996a). *Career Thoughts Inventory–Professional manual*. Odessa, FL: Psychological Assessment Resources.

Sampson, J. P., Jr., Peterson G. W., Lenz, J. G., Reardon, R. C., & Saunders, D. E. (1996b). *Improving your career thoughts: A workbook for the Career Thoughts Inventory*. Odessa, FL: Psychological Assessment Resources.

Savickas, M.L. (1984). Career maturity: The construct and its appraisal. *Vocational Guidance Quarterly*, 32, 222–231.

Schriner, K. (2001). A disability studies perspective on employment issues and polices for disabled people: An international view. In G. Albrecht, K. D. Seelman, & M. Bury (Eds.), *Handbook of disability studies* (pp. 642–662). Thousand Oaks, CA: Sage.

Shahnasarian, M. (2001). Career rehabilitation: Integration of vocational rehabilitation and career development in the twenty-first century. *Career Development Quarterly*. Retrieved June 20, 2006, from http://www.highbeam.com/library/docFree.asp?DOCID=1G1:72703670.

Sharf, R. S. (2006). *Applying career development theory to counseling* (4th ed.). Belmont, CA: Thomson/Brooks/Cole.

Sink, J. M., Gannaway, T. W., & Cottone, R. R. (1987). Psychological testing versus assessment in counseling and a critical response to canon 7–"assessment." *Journal of Applied Rehabilitation Counseling*, 18, 35–37.

Strohmer, D. C. (1979). *The Decision-Making Interview*. Menomonie, WI: Rehabilitation Research and Training Institute, University of Wisconsin–Stout.

Super, D. E., Crites, J. O., Hummel, R. C., Moser, H. P., Overstreet, P. L., & Warnath, C. F. (1957). *Vocational development: A framework for research*. New York: Teachers College Press, Columbia University.

Super, D. E., Savickas, M. L., & Super, C. M. (1996). The life-span, life-space approach to careers. In D. Brown, L. Brooks, & Associates (Eds.), *Career choice and development* (3rd ed., pp. 121–178). San Francisco: Jossey-Bass.

Szymanski, E. M. (1989). Disability, job stress, the changing nature of careers, and career resilience portfolio. *Rehabilitation Counseling Bulletin, 42,* 279–289.

Szymanski, E. M., Johnston-Rodriquez, S., Millington, M. J., Rodriguez, B. H., & Lagergren, J. (1995). The paradoxical nature of disability services. Illustrations from supported employment and implications for rehabilitation counseling. *Journal of Applied Rehabilitation Counseling, 26,* 17–22.

Szymanski, E. M., & Vancollins, J. (2003). Career development of people with disabilities: Some new and not so new challenges. *Australian Journal of Career Development,* 12(1), 9–16.

Tiffany, D. W. (2001). Review of the Vocational Decision-Making Interview–Revised. In B. S. Plake & J. C. Impara (Eds.), *The fourteenth mental measurements yearbook* (pp. 1313–1314). Lincoln, NE: Buros Institute of Mental Measures.

U.S. Census Bureau. (nd). *People with disabilities*. Retrieved June 19, 2006, from www.census .gov/hhes/www/disability.html.

U.S. Department of Labor. (2000a). *O*NET testing and assessment: An employer's guide to good practices*. Washington, DC: Author.

U.S. Department of Labor. (2000b). *O*NET Work Importance Locator user's guide*. Washington, DC: Author.

U.S. Department of Labor. (nd). *Average number of jobs started by individuals from age 18 to age 36 in 1978–2000 by age and sex*. Retrieved June 20, 2006, from http://www.bls.gov/nls/ nlsy79r19.supp.htm

Vondracek, F. W., Lerner, R. M., & Schulenberg, J .M. (1986). *Career development: A life span approach*. Hillsdale, NJ: Erlbaum.

Wall, J. E. (1994). Review of the Career Beliefs Inventory (CBI). In J. T. Kapes, M. M. Mastie, & E. A. Whitfield (Eds.), *A counselor's guide to career assessment instruments* (3rd ed., pp. 253–257). Alexandria, VA: National Career Development Association.

Westbrook, W. B. (1985). Review of My Vocational Situation. In J. V. Mitchell, Jr. (Ed.), *The Ninth Mental Measurements Yearbook* (pp. 1027–1029). Lincoln, NE: Buros Institute of Mental Measures.

Wise, R., Charner, I., & Randour, M. A. (1978). A conceptual framework for career awareness in career decision-making. In J. Whitely & A. Resnikoff (Eds.), *Career counseling* (pp. 216–231). Monterey, CA: Brooks/Cole.

Zytowski, D. G. (May, 2006). *Super's Work Values Inventory–revised: Technical manual version 1.0*. Retrieved September 14, 2006, from http//www.kuder.com/publicweb/swv_manual .aspx.

Chapter 16

Assessment of Individuals With Visual Impairments

John T. Gallagher and William R. Wiener

The number of individuals who are severely visually impaired in the United States has been estimated to be 4.3 million (Nelson & Dimitrova, 1993). Eighty-two percent of those individuals are older than age 55. The prevalence of severe visual impairment increases drastically as the population ages. At the ages of 0–17 years the prevalence of severe visual impairment is 1.5 per 1,000 in the general population. By the ages of 55–64, it has risen to 28.4 per 1,000, and by age 85+, it is found to be 210.6 per 1,000. The number of elderly people with visual impairments is expected to grow as the elderly population grows. However, medical and surgical advances in treating trauma, tumors, and premature birth are also expected to increase the population of individuals with visual impairment. This could possibly be offset with significant advances in other areas of medical treatment such as with diabetes, one of the leading causes of blindness. At this point it seems safe to predict that the psychological examiner and the rehabilitation counselor will face more and more situations where the person to be evaluated will have some degree of visual impairment.

Psychologists and rehabilitation counselors specializing in the assessment of individuals with visual impairments are few. Yet individuals with such disabilities present a number of assessment challenges that are unique and require innovative approaches. A referral to an assessment specialist is usually desirable; however, more often than not this will not be feasible. Therefore, this chapter introduces the general psychological examiner and rehabilitation counselor to the assessment of people with are blind or visually impaired and equips them with some knowledge and tools to meet the challenge. The focus will be on issues of assessment ordinarily confronting the psychological examiner and not assessment issues that are generally the province of other professionals dealing with people who are visually impaired. For example, assessment of visual acuity, visual fields, and other aspects of visual efficiency will not be addressed. Likewise, assessment of mobility skills, independent living skills, and other adaptive skills will not be specifically addressed; but, of course, the examination of various abilities, as typically done by the psychologist or rehabilitation counselor, will bear on these skills. It is also incumbent on any examiner to be alert to undiagnosed vision problems.

Use of Tests With People Who Are Visually Impaired

A standardized test is designed to measure specific aspects of human performance and will yield scores that can be compared with scores of a similar population. Caution is necessary when taking tests originally designed and normed for sighted people and trying to use the tests with people who are visually impaired. Differences in life experiences and in methods of test administration can make the comparisons less valid. Tests for people who are visually impaired are usually adapted by changing the medium of presentation and/or the method of response. For example, print items on a test may be enlarged, translated into Braille, or read to the examinee. In a similar way, a test that requires physical manipulation of objects may require a more complete orientation to the task, tactual modifications, or changes in administration. Such modifications may render the results less comparable to those of the population on which the test was normed. It is therefore best to use tests that are normed for the population being tested. However, such norms are not often available, and the examiner must utilize tests that are not normed on the population and that have been modified to suit that population. In this situation, the examiner must interpret the results with this distinction in mind. Typical adaptations may include the use of enlarged print, increased contrast, magnifying aids, closed-circuit television (CCTV) systems, writing guides, slates and styluses for Braille, Perkins Braillers, electronic Braille note takers, computers with voice synthesis, computers with screen magnification, tape recorders, and substitution of tactual or auditory stimuli for visual stimuli.

Since the earliest years of formal psychological testing, there have been efforts to develop psychological testing materials appropriate for individuals with little or no useful vision. Irwin and Goddard (1914, 1976) and Hayes (1929) are notable individuals who have launched early efforts to adapt existing tests for people who are blind. There have also been attempts to develop tests specifically for people who are blind. Likewise, there have been tests developed for the sighted population that have not been adapted but have been normed on subjects who are visually impaired. In addition, some tests that are neither adapted nor normed might be considered appropriate or marginally appropriate for people who are blind.

The Challenge of Developing Tests for People Who Are Blind or Visually Impaired

The development of formal psychological tests for use with the population of people with visual impairment is a daunting task. For years, potentially meaningful tests and test items have been developed for use with this population (Scholl & Schnur, 1976), but these are typically unavailable and slip quickly into obscurity (see, for example, Taylor & Ward, 1990). This is partly due to less demand for these tests than for tests with other populations, but it is also due to problems inherent within test development itself. The population of people with visual impairment is very diverse along many dimensions. This diversity is especially notable in the area of visual impairment itself. Some individuals may have normal visual acuity but limited fields of vision, while others may have their fields riddled with scotomas. Others may have better vision at some times and under some conditions than they have at others times and under other conditions. Still others, as in Balint's syndrome (Rafal, 1997), may see one object well but see no others. Even in conditions where individuals with partial vision have similar impairments with small differences in acuity, there may be large differences in visual function. Other impairments, such as auditory impairment, neurologic impairments, and mental retardation, are also found to a greater degree among people with visual impairment than among people who do not have visual impairments.

Considering this diversity, establishing normative data for a test for people who are visually impaired can be complex (Hull & Mason, 1993). Should there be separate norms for different levels of vision? How would these levels of vision be defined and divided? One solution has been to blindfold all individuals with partial vision on certain tests to make them equivalent to individuals with no useful vision. While this may be sensible in terms of making comparisons among the individuals, at the same time it may not show the individuals' true capabilities. Should a test be normed also for the sighted population for comparison to this group, blindfolded or not?

As a practical matter it is difficult to gather sufficient numbers of children or adults who are visually impaired to develop standardized normed tests. With adults one might attempt to gather normative data in adult rehabilitation centers for people who are blind and perhaps supplement this with using volunteers from local consumer groups. It can quickly be seen that selection bias will be strong using these methods. Furthermore, the variability of adults selected this way and the coexisting impairments of other types make comparisons among people with visual impairment difficult. It might be argued that adults who are visually impaired should be divided into groups not just by age but also by factors such as length of blindness and presence of neurologic problems. Individuals whose vision impairment is due to involvement of the cerebral cortex are a very different group than those whose visual impairment is from pathology of the eye; for examples see Farah (1990), Weiskrantz (1986), or Groenveld, Jan, and Leader (1990). There are also specific subgroups such as people with peripheral neuropathies that interfere with tactile functioning. Such people's needs are great yet will require a specialized approach to testing and cannot be easily compared along certain dimensions to other persons with visual impairment. See Wolf-Schein (1998) for considerations in assessing individuals who are deaf and blind.

A test devised and normed on people with visual impairment is often supported on a theoretical or logical basis rather than by hard validity studies. Often, if the test is an adaptation of a test for the sighted, the implication is that the validity studies on this test with the sighted population will also be applicable to the test for people who are blind. Of course, this is an empirical question that is rarely answered.

Because of these difficulties it would appear that fewer test instruments for people with visual impairment are being developed today than in the past. However, dedicated researchers still take up the gauntlet to develop and validate instruments for this population. This chapter will attempt to present a selection of instruments currently available for various assessment purposes faced by the practicing psychologist and rehabilitation counselor.

Considerations in the Assessment of Individuals Who Are Visually Impaired

It is important, first of all, for the examiner who is asked to assess the child or adult with visual impairment to understand, somewhat, the personal experience of being visually impaired and to understand something about the conditions causing visual impairments. Personal accounts and professional accounts of individuals dealing with vision loss or growing up without vision are readily available (Kuusisto, 1998; Ringgold, 1991; Sacks, 1997). It is also important for the examiner to understand the definitions of blindness and have a rudimentary understanding of the more common causes of impaired vision.

The legal definition of blindness was developed as part of the 1935 Social Security Act for the purpose of indicating that a person has a disability great enough to cause economic hardship. Visual impairment and blindness are defined as reduction in visual acuity and/or visual field. A visual acuity of 20/200 or less in the better eye with the best possible ordinary correction is labeled as legal blindness A visual field that subtends an angular distance of no more than 20 degrees also classifies an individual as being legally blind (Koestler, 1976). Individuals with such an acuity or field loss may often have much remaining usable vision but may have difficulty reading or performing other tasks. Individuals who have acuity or field sufficient to serve as a useful source of information are classified as having low vision. These individuals may be able to use special optical aids to assist with many functional tasks. For example, near vision magnifiers, spectacles, or CCTV systems may be used for reading the printed page. In order to read signs or addresses, a monocular distance aid may be helpful. For individuals who cannot benefit from such optical or electronic aids, Braille and talking books may be the methods of choice for reading. Independent travel for these individuals may require the use of a long cane or a guide dog to preview the area ahead for obstacles, changes in terrain, and possible drop-offs.

The visual pathologies of glaucoma, cataracts, diabetic retinopathy, and macular degeneration (Newell, 1996) most commonly contribute to legal blindness or low vision. Glaucoma reduces the individual's visual field. This condition occurs due to elevated pressure within the eye caused by improper drainage of a fluid called aqueous humor. The increased pressure pushes against the arteries supplying blood to the retina. The pressure, if unchecked, may damage the optic nerve (Vaughan, Asbury, & Riordan-Eva, 1995). Treatment includes reducing the pressure through the use of medications or through surgery to open up the drainage mechanism. The clouding of the lens of the eye is a condition known as a cataract. This process is usually slow and may take many years to develop. Changes in the proteins of the lens are responsible for creating this opacity. A surgical procedure that removes the lens can restore vision. The lens is then replaced with an intraocular implant or with an external lens (Vaughan et al., 1995). Another frequent cause of visual impairment is diabetic retinopathy. The person with diabetes often experiences leaking vessels in the retina that can distort vision and eventually lead to the development of new fragile vessels (neovascularization) that can pull the retina forward and further reduce vision (Vaughan et al., 1995). Photocoagulation and removal of the damaged vitreous can extend useful vision. Macular degeneration is a pathology that breaks down the cells in the macula, the part of the retina that contains the greatest concentration of cones and is responsible for the most acute vision (Vaughan et al., 1995). With this pathology there is a loss of central acuity but the individual is left with peripheral vision. Macular degeneration is the most common cause of visual impairment in those older than 40 years of age.

Other pathologies that affect vision are retinitis pigmentosa, optic atrophy, retinopathy of prematurity, and retinal detachment. Publications are available that can give a preliminary introduction to these pathologies (American Foundation for the Blind, 1975, 1987; Jose, 1993; National Federation of the Blind, 1989; Van Son, 1989). A more detailed description of these eye pathologies and the procedures available for remediation can be found in Vaughan and colleagues (1995).

It is particularly important for the examiner to pay attention to the effect that various pathologies might have on the individual's functioning and how this might affect the assessment procedures. For example, good central visual acuity but very limited visual fields might mislead someone to use tests involving visual scanning without consideration of how much the examinee might differ from the normative group in the ability to perceive the material. Similarly reduced visual acuity must be taken into consideration with any visual testing material.

Generally, the examiner testing the person who is visually impaired should pay special attention to the environmental needs of the individual. Many individuals with some vision are particularly sensitive to lights and glare. Examinees should not have to look toward a window or toward light fixtures. The lighting in the room should be able to be modified until it is most suitable to the individual taking the test. Likewise, glare and contrast should be considered with testing material that is of a visual nature (Collins-Moore & Osborn, 1984).

It is important to pay attention to the auditory environment. Background noise and other distractions should be minimized. For individuals with hearing impairments, extra consideration may need to be given to assure that the individual can understand the directions being given. This may include modifying voice tone and volume to meet the needs of the examinee. Having the examinee repeat the directions is often helpful. If the individual requires sign language and the examiner is not proficient in this language, an interpreter may need to be included in the testing process. The environment should be reviewed to be sure environmental hazards undetectable by a cane will not pose a danger. All individuals working with persons who are visually impaired should take the opportunity to learn methods of acting as a sighted guide from a certified orientation and mobility specialist. Typically, these methods include walking one half-step ahead of the person who is blind and having the individual hold on to the guide's arm just above the elbow. In this way the person who is blind will be able to feel body movements through the arm and respond accordingly. In the course of establishing rapport with the examinee, extra time should be taken to orient the individual to the room and, when appropriate, to the testing materials. Extra time should be taken to explain the procedures and what the examinee is to expect. The examinee should not be concerned about using sight oriented words, such as "see" and "look," as such terms are common in our culture and are typically used by and with persons who are visually impaired.

The evaluation of the client who is visually impaired very much requires the examiner to think in terms of psychological assessment rather than psychological testing (Matarazzo, 1990). That is, the examiner should not approach the evaluation through strict rote scoring and interpreting of a series of standardized tests, but rather as a flexible approach that considers the results in light of the particular individual undergoing the examination. This requires not only careful consideration of how to answer the referral questions but also a particular understanding of the individual being assessed, his or her impairments, and how those impairments interact with the results and interpretation. For example, knowing whether an individual's visual impairment is progressive or stable is important because it influences how much the results will predict future behavior. Consider the situation of a person with deteriorating low vision but sufficient vision for a visual test of spatial ability; a blindfolded test of tactile spatial ability may be more predictive of future spatial adjustment than a visual–spatial test. Psychological test reports to rehabilitation or school personnel are often more helpful with the inclusion of concrete examples of the examinee's functioning rather than just normative comparisons (Groenveld, 1990).

It is important to understand each examinee's needs, not only with regard to environmental considerations, but also with regard to the materials to be used. For example, the individual may need large-print material. An examiner who is seeing many individuals with visual impairment will find it convenient to have materials in various sizes of large print and to have the examinee indicate what size print is most comfortable. The examiner might do well to have several kinds of magnifiers on hand for use by the examinee as experience shows that individuals very often do not have magnifiers with them. Some types of testing involve depriving an individual who is partially sighted of vision for a particular task. It is usually preferable to use a blindfold for this unless the individual is uncomfortable being blindfolded. The examiner should have disposable blindfolds or blindfolds that can be sterilized between use. Eye diseases can be passed from one individual to another via unclean blindfolds, and the examiner should ensure that disease transmission does not occur. Some subjects may prefer to use some type of a screen preventing them from seeing the test materials rather than being blindfolded. Some test manufacturers provide these screens with their instruments (e.g., the *Comprehensive Vocational Evaluation System for the Blind* [Dial et al., 1991b]), but most do not. The screen can be a dark cloth draped over a frame to form a curtain that the individual can pass his hand under. The examiner should also have something that can darken the windows. Papers and materials of different shades and felt-tipped pens (to make heavy marks) should also be on hand. The examiner might also find useful a guide translating Braille letters into script letters so that he or she can get a minimal orientation to the Braille material that he or she is using and help the Braille reader find the desired starting place. In settings where many individuals with visual impairment are tested, it may be practical to have a CCTV available for magnification of materials and a computer with a voice synthesis program such as JAWS (http://www.freedomscientific.com) or Freedom Box (http://www.freedombox.info).

Adapting Tests for People Who Are Visually Impaired

Tests given to sighted people in written format are usually adapted in several ways for use with people who are visually impaired. Without formally modifying the material, the examiner might read the items to the individual taking the test. This might seem straightforward, but it is not always so. For example, individuals can become confused by items presented in a negative way that do not seem to be as confusing when given in a written format. For example, when the item "I have not had headaches during the last 6 months" is answered "false," "no," or "disagree," it means that the individual has had headaches during the past 6 months. Individuals can become easily confused by such items. It is, therefore, incumbent on the examiner reading such an item to either change the item to read in a more positive way or to elaborate on the response possibilities. That is, the examiner should either say, "I have had headaches during the past 6 months" or "I have not had any headaches in the past six months; answering true means you have had no headaches and answering false means that you have had headaches." The examiner will have to use clinical judgment as to how much this rewording has changed the nature of the test. The same considerations might be made for any tests that are given in a format of audio recording or voice computer reading.

Giving tests in a large-print version would seem to be the most straightforward way of adapting test materials. An individual needing large-print test materials may very well need a large-print answer sheet as well. Answers on an answer sheet that is an enlargement of one scored by a computer or scoring keys would have to be transferred to the original answer sheet before scoring. Many people who are visually impaired and able to read large print are unable to sustain reading for long periods of time. Therefore, individuals who can read large print should always be asked about their testing preferences.

Braille versions of tests are typically available in a Grade II Braille format. If an individual is a Braille reader, it should be ascertained if he or she can read the more advanced Grade II format as opposed to Grade I Braille. Likewise, not all Braille readers will be familiar with the Nemeth code needed for Braille mathematics materials. The examiner might also note that publishers who provide Braille versions of their tests may not provide for a way for the Braille reader to record responses. We have most often met this problem by having the examinee record responses either on a cassette tape recorder or by making responses in Braille on blank pieces of Braille paper, being sure to number each response.

When administering a test originally intended for sighted people to people who are visually impaired, it is important to remember that some items may have content that implies the use of sight. For example, several comprehension questions from the *Wechsler Intelligence Scales* imply the use of vision. It is appropriate for the sighted examiner to substitute the word "I" for "you" when administering these items. "What should you do if you see an unconscious person on the street?" could be changed to "What should I do if I see an unconscious person on the street?" Rewording these types of items presumably makes the testing more fair. Other changes might also be appropriate, and an examiner should consider his or her materials and what will be fair for the person with visual impairment. For example, if giving a vocabulary test where the sighted subject is asked to define words spoken by the examiner but also has the advantage of seeing these words printed, the examiner can provide large print or Braille versions of these word lists, as appropriate, or can spell the words verbally after saying them.

A final note on test adaptations should be made. In situations where a test publisher indicates the availability of versions of a test developed and normed for sighted people but adapted for use on people who are blind, this typically means that there are large-print, audio-recorded, or Braille versions available. It does not usually mean that item content has been modified to meet the needs of people with visual impairment or that norms are available for people who are visually impaired. When obtaining such tests from a publisher, examiners should ask questions to clarify exactly what is available.

Tests for Use With Individuals Who Are Visually Impaired

The remainder of this chapter is devoted to describing tests currently available for the examinee who is visually impaired. Of course, it is understood that test results will be integrated with interview and background information. In certain settings, observational data might also be useful, whether informal or formalized through rating scales. It is particularly important to pay attention to medical reports, rehabilitation reports, educational reports, and examinations of visual functioning. In clinical settings, the use of formalized interview formats designed for psychiatric diagnosis, such as the *Structured Clinical Interview* for *DSM-IV Axis I Disorders–Clinical Version* (First, Gibbon, Spitzer, & Williams, 1997), may be preferable to the use of testing instruments for psychopathology. This is true since some experiences of clients who are visually impaired differ so significantly from those of the sighted groups used to norm tests for psychopathology. In general, it will take the skill and judgment of the examiner to integrate testing results with the interview and background information, taking into account the characteristics of the individual being assessed, the deviations from the standardized procedures used, and the ways that the individual differs from the normative groups. Assessing people who are visually impaired very much entails considered judgment as opposed to straightforward, rote interpretation of test results.

Comprehensive Vocational Evaluation System

It would be ideal to have a battery of tests that comprehensively evaluates various dimensions of importance for adolescents or adults who are visually impaired. Such a battery of tests would be normed on a large representative group of people who are visually impaired with information available relating to degrees of visual impairment, age of onset of visual impairment, and any other coexisting disabilities. The data from such a comprehensive battery would be useful in educational, vocational, rehabilitation, mental health, and neuropsychological settings. Furthermore, the ideal battery, while comprehensive, would not be so time-consuming and complex that it would be rarely used. There is currently one test battery that comes closest to the ideal: the *Comprehensive Vocational Evaluation System* (CVES) developed by Jack Dial and his colleagues (Chan et al., 1993; Dial et al., 1991a, 1991b). This battery of tests is being increasingly used by agencies serving people who are visually impaired.

The CVES is organized around five factors: verbal–cognitive, sensory, motor, emotional functioning, and adaptive behavior. Components of the test battery include the *Cognitive Test for the Blind,* the *Haptic Sensory Discrimination Test,* the *McCarron Assessment of Neuromuscular Development* (MAND-VI Edition), the *Observational-Emotional Inventory–Revised,* the *Emotional Behavior Checklist,* and the *Survey of Functional Adaptive Behaviors.* Supplemental to this battery of tests developed by McCarron and Dial are specialized administration procedures and norms for people with visual impairment using the *Wide Range Achievement Test–Revised* or *Wide Range Achievement Test–Third Edition.* The normative group for the CVES included 421 subjects, 55 percent of whom were men. The mean age was 26 years. These subjects were selected out of 1,100 who were assessed as not having a coexisting disability. Almost all of the subjects were clients of the Texas Division for Blind Services.

The *Cognitive Test for the Blind* is an intelligence test that forms the heart of the CVES. From this test can be derived verbal, performance, and full-scale measures of intellectual ability. There are five verbal subtests:

1. Auditory Analysis requires the individual to reproduce nonsense words of increasing length, thus getting at phonemic analysis.
2. The Immediate Digit Recall subtest requires the subject to repeat a series of digits forward and backward, as in the usual digit-span task, except the digits are presented at a slightly slower rate.
3. Language Comprehension and Memory requires receptive language abilities and verbal memory.
4. Verbal memory is also involved in Letter–Number Learning, but this subtest stresses sequential abilities and learning over trials.
5. The Vocabulary subtest requires the individual to define words given by the examiner; as such, it is a measure of word knowledge and verbal expression.

The five performance subtests of the *Cognitive Test for the Blind* require that the subject be able to manipulate objects and perceive objects tactually.

1. The Haptic Category Learning Test is a tactile adaptation of *Halstead's Category Test* (Reitan & Wolfson, 1985), an established test of concept formation.
2. The Haptic Category Memory Test assesses incidental memory from the Haptic Category Learning Test in a recognition format.
3. Haptic Memory Recognition also requires memory for tactilely appreciated items in a recognition format.
4. Spatial Pattern Recall also requires memory but puts a heavy emphasis on the comprehension of spatial patterns such as is seen in visual tests with block design types of items.
5. The Spatial Analysis subtest requires spatial analysis and construction with no memory component.

As is clear from the paragraphs above, memory plays a major role in the assessment of verbal and performance abilities in the *Cognitive Test for the Blind*. Another component of the CVES, the *Haptic Sensory Discrimination Test,* requires only a working memory of a few seconds. This test calls for the assessment of haptic discrimination of shape, size, texture, and configuration. Each hand is tested separately using a counterbalanced format.

The *McCarron Assessment of Neuromuscular Development* (MAND-VI) is an assessment of fine and gross motor abilities. Included are measures of grip strength, finger-tapping speed, turning, slow and steady movement, and fine-motor tasks such as putting beads on a rod. Balance measures and finger-to-nose movements are also included. Norms are available not only for adults who are visually impaired but for sighted children and adults as well. This gives this test broad applicability.

The *Observational-Emotional Inventory–Revised* and the *Emotional Behavior Checklist* are rating scales of observed behavior and/or historical information. These are designed to measure such emotional factors as self-concept, socialization, depression, anxiety, and impulsivity. The *Survey of Functional Adaptive Behaviors* deals with various aspects of basic adaptive skills such as use of money and transportation so that independent functioning may be assessed.

It is clear that the CVES attempts to measure a number of areas crucial to the functioning of adults who are visually impaired. A number of agencies dealing with clientele who are visually impaired use the test. But with the total package costing more than $4,500 in the year 2007, the test likely will be too expensive for the individual practitioner not specializing in this type of assessment. Components of the system are available separately. But when separate tests and individual subtests are used, the overall factor breakdown advocated by the authors is not possible.

Although the CVES is the most promising instrument available for assessment of adults who are blind or visually impaired, it does have shortcomings. A major shortcoming is that the normative group is not stratified as to age. With the average age of the normative group being 26, we recommend caution in using this battery of tests with individuals who are older than 50 years of age. With the normative group being limited to one area of the country, individuals using this test battery frequently may want to develop local norms. The battery is also time-consuming; the authors indicate that testing time for the full battery will be approximately 6 hours. On the positive side, the CVES is at the center of an ongoing body of research that is examining different subgroups as well as predictive validity (Dial et al., 1991a; Joyce et al., 2000; Joyce et al., 2004; McGee Hall, 1994; Nelson et al., 2001; Nelson et al., 2002a, 2002b; O'Brien, 1992; Rabeck, 1994;). Miller and Skillman (2003) surveyed assessment professionals working with the visually impaired and found individuals using the *Cognitive Test for the Blind* to be highly satisfied with the instrument.

Wechsler Adult Intelligence Scale–Third Edition

Most examiners will use the verbal portion of the *Wechsler Adult Intelligence Scale–Third Edition* (WAIS-III; Wechsler, 1998) to assess verbal intelligence. This, of course, is the latest edition of the well-established intelligence test for adults. The advantage over some other tests that have verbal intelligence scales is that the WAIS-III uses no pictorial stimuli for the verbal portion of the test. The CVES makes allowances for the individual who wishes to use the WAIS-III verbal portion along with the performance section of the *Cognitive Test for the Blind*. The verbal subtests of the WAIS-III include Vocabulary (which measures word knowledge and expression); Similarities (which measures verbal abstract classification); Arithmetic (which measures mathematical reasoning and mental calculation); Digit Span (which measures attention and working memory);

Information (which measures general cultural knowledge), Comprehension (which measures social understanding and reasoning); and a supplemental subtest, Letter Number Sequencing (which measures working memory). The test is appropriate for individuals aged 16–89 years and is normed on a national sample. We have found the Comprehension subtest to be particularly useful in assessing the social judgment of clients who are visually impaired (social judgment is often a problem for the young adult who is congenitally blind). Performance subtests from the WAIS-III are not appropriate for individuals without useful vision. They are also typically not appropriate for examinees who are legally blind with low vision, but they could be used cautiously in certain cases. Results in such cases cannot really be used to determine performance IQ scores but rather to give a rough idea of functioning in certain visual task situations.

Haptic Intelligence Scale for Adult Blind

The *Haptic Intelligence Scale for Adult Blind* (Shurrager & Shurrager, 1964) was designed as a performance scale for people who are blind to go with the *Wechsler Adult Intelligence Scale* (WAIS; Wechsler, 1955) verbal scale. The Haptic performance scale uses subtests that are clever adaptations of Wechsler performance subtests. These subtests are Digit Symbol (which measures processing speed and new learning), Block Design (which measures spatial analysis and construction), Object Assembly (which measures part-to-whole construction), and Object Completion (which requires tactile identification and detection of missing parts of objects). Additionally, there are two subtests having no parallel in the WAIS: Pattern Board and Bead Arithmetic. Pattern Board involves reproduction from memory of patterns of pegs in a pegboard, while Bead Arithmetic involves use of an adapted abacus. This final subtest is inappropriate for use with individuals who have had experience with an abacus, as the subtest is designed to assess how well the individual can learn to use this instrument.

The *Haptic Intelligence Scale for Adult Blind* (Shurrager & Shurrager, 1964) can be administered to most subjects in approximately 1 hour and is well-tolerated and easily understood by most examinees. Individuals with some useful vision are generally blindfolded during administration. Norms are broken out for six age groups ranging from 16 to 64 years of age. Normative tables are based on 700 cases with representatives from each region of the country. Clearly, this is one of the most carefully normed tests for people who are visually impaired. Unfortunately, this test has never been updated, so the normative group is four decades old and the resulting score no longer corresponds to the latest edition of the WAIS. That is, with the normative group tending to do better on the WAIS with each revision, the Haptic norms today tend to overestimate the equivalent Wechsler performance IQ (Flynn, 1984).

The performance subtests of the Haptic are somewhat easier to administer than the performance subtests of the *Cognitive Test for the Blind,* but the difference is not great. Examiners might find the Haptic preferable for older adults and the more updated *Cognitive Test for the Blind* preferable for younger adults.

Of course, when the *Cognitive Test for the Blind* comes out with new norms stratified by age, this recommendation could change.

Brief Intelligence Tests

There is often a need for a brief measure of verbal intelligence. Several well-established instruments are available; we have used the *Wide Range Intelligence Test* (WRIT) on occasion (Glutting et al., 2000). More often, we will use the *Wechsler Abbreviated Scale of Intelligence* (WASI; The Psychological Corporation, 1999). This test has two verbal subtests—Vocabulary and Similarities—and provides a good prediction of WAIS-III Verbal IQ results. Both the WRIT and WASI correlate highly with WAIS-III Verbal IQ. The *Slosson Intelligence Test–Revised* (SIT-R3; Slosson, 2002) has a modification available for blind subjects with a supplemental manual for people who are visually impaired/blind (Larson, 2002). While these brief tests are useful, they should not be substituted for the more complete intelligence tests (*Wechsler Adult Intelligence Scale–Third Edition, Cognitive Test for the Blind*) if intellectual functioning requires close examination.

Wide Range Achievement Test–Revised and Wechsler Individual Achievement Test

Achievement tests of reading, spelling, writing, and mathematics would generally not need to be normed on populations of people who are visually impaired, as grade-equivalent scores are often the results desired. The problem lies mainly in getting them into a Braille or large-print format that is useable by the examinee.

The only individual achievement test we know of that has been normed on adults who are visually impaired is the *Wide Range Achievement Test–Revised* (WRAT-R; Jastak & Wilkinson, 1984). The normative group is that used in the CVES. Administration procedures cited in the CVES publication (Dial et al., 1991b) involve use of Braille, large-print, or verbal administration as appropriate to the person taking the test. Braille or large-print versions of this test are not generally available and would have to be made by the examiner. A subsequent edition of this test, WRAT-3 (Wilkinson, 1993), has not been normed on people who are visually impaired, but the test materials are already in relatively large print. The WRAT-R has three subtests: Reading, Spelling, and Arithmetic. The Reading subtest is simply individual word recognition and does not include reading in context or reading comprehension. Spelling requires the individual to spell individual words that are dictated. Arithmetic involves solving written calculation problems and does not include story problems.

The advantage of the WRAT-R, in addition to being normed on adults who are visually impaired, is it samples a wide range of abilities up to a 12th grade level. The disadvantage is the lack of available adapted materials and the limited achievement skills that are assessed. We have found that using the Listening Comprehension and Written Expression sections of the *Wechsler Individual Achievement Test* (WIAT) and WIAT-II (Psychological Corporation, 1992, 2002) can provide useful achievement information even for those recently blinded with no ability to read or write.

Wechsler Memory Scale–Third Edition

The *Wechsler Memory Scale–Third Edition* (WMS-III) has been standardized on the same normative group that is used for the WAIS-III (Wechsler, 1997). The WMS-III has verbal memory items that can easily be given to subjects who are visually impaired and have adequate hearing. Given the high rate of coexisting neurologic difficulties in adults who are blind, it is, at times, important to evaluate aspects of memory functioning. The subtests of the WMS-III can be analyzed individually or through a complex of index and composite scores. For example, there are scores involving immediate memory, working memory, learning slope, and retention over time. Verbal memory subtests include subtests that sample memory for paragraphs, paired association, and word list learning. Additionally, there are mental control and information orientation measures.

The advantages of the WMS-III are that it is recently developed, normed on a wide range of ages, and directly comparable to the WAIS-III. There are no norms on people who are visually impaired, but theoretically those who are visually impaired would not be particularly disadvantaged on verbal memory tests. The disadvantage is that there is no way to give the nonverbal memory items to those individuals.

Paced Auditory Serial Addition Test and Oral Trailmaking

The ability to process information quickly and engage in some mental processing while holding something else in mind is important in a number of settings. The *Paced Auditory Serial Addition Test* was developed for neuropsychological applications (Gromwall & Sampson, 1974; Spreen & Strauss, 1998). This test is administered using an audiotape, with the examiner recording the subject's verbal responses. Concentration, mathematical calculation, working memory, and simultaneous processing are required for success in this endeavor. It is a demanding speed test that many subjects find frustrating (Tombaugh, 2006). As such, the examiner can judge not only the individual's processing ability but also the individual's ability to respond to a frustrating task.

Should the examiner desire a briefer assessment of speed and simultaneous processing, *Oral Trailmaking* (Abraham, Axelrod, & Ricker, 1996; Ricker & Axelrod, 1994) is an oral version of the *Trailmaking Test* (Reitan & Wolfson, 1985), which has been shown to have high ecological validity as a test of executive functioning (Chaytor et al., 2006). The use of this test with people who are visually impaired has not been studied. A consistent ratio has been found between *Oral Trailmaking* and the *Trailmaking Part B* performance across age levels. *Oral Trailmaking* was found to be faster by a ratio of 2.44 to 1. Presumably, then, comparisons can be made to norms for the *Trailmaking Test* (Spreen & Strauss, 1998; Strauss, Sherman, & Spreen, 2006). However, Braille readers may have an advantage at this task because of the correspondence of numbers and letters. An alternate test of simultaneous processing might be used, such as the *Category Switching Test* from the Delis-Kaplan Executive Function System (Delis, Kaplan, & Kramer, 2001).

Benton Sound Recognition

The accurate perception and discrimination of different environmental sounds can be measured by the *Benton Auditory Discrimination Test* (Spreen & Strauss, 1998). The identification of sounds on this test is rather simple for most individuals but may show deficits in individuals who are significantly impaired. This test does not evaluate assessment of the source of the sound but only the discrimination of the nature of the sound. The direction of the source of the sound can be assessed informally or by using the CUBE from Valpar (discussed later).

Visual Object and Space Perception Battery and Developmental Test of Visual Perception

Adults who have some vision but appear to have a visual perception problem can be assessed using the *Visual Object and Space Perception Battery* (Warrington & James, 1991). This battery is particularly useful for individuals with cortical blindness, where visual perception and integration could be a problem. This test was normed in Great Britain but is available in the United States through Northern Speech Services. More familiar in format to American users but requiring greater visual acuity is the *Developmental Test of Visual Perception, Adolescent and Adult* (DTVP-A; Reynolds et al., 2002). The six subtests are useful if the examinee has sufficient acuity for them.

Valpar Component Work Sample and Conceptual Understanding through Blind Evaluation

Available through Valpar is a battery of tests called the *Valpar Component Work Sample* (Valpar, 1980b). This battery evaluates sighted individuals' ability to perform various mental and physical tasks. Measurements of intelligence are not included. The publisher offers tactile and verbal modifications of some of the work samples with "B-kits" to allow testing of individuals who are visually impaired. Components include small tools, size discrimination, upper-extremity range of motion, simulated assembly, whole-body range of motion, and measurement. The *Conceptual Understanding through Blind Evaluation* (CUBE; Valpar, 1980a) is a multipurpose test battery to evaluate various skills and abilities related to loss of vision. The CUBE battery includes five parts: Tactual Percepts, Mobility/Discrimination Skill, Spatial Organization and Memory, Assembly and Packaging, and Audile Perception.

The advantage of these Valpar batteries is that they are fairly comprehensive in terms of the physical aspects of work behavior. They are expensive and require lengthy testing time, however (the CUBE alone costs more than $4,000). These are more likely to be used in rehabilitation or work training settings, not in independent examiners' offices.

Purdue Pegboard Test and Minnesota Rate of Manipulation

The *Purdue Pegboard Test* (Tiffin, 1968) was developed for the sighted and involves motor speed and coordination along with eye–hand coordination. The results can be examined for the speed of each hand individually, the speed of the hands together, and the speed of an assembly task. Norms for individuals who are visually impaired (Vander Kolk, 1980) are available. These norms include adults with low vision as well as those with no useful vision. Vander Kolk also presents detailed guidelines for use and interpretation. Thus, an individual taking this test could be compared to norms for people who are visually impaired as well as to norms available for the sighted.

The *Minnesota Rate of Manipulation Test* was studied by Roberts and Bauman (1944). They used the Displacing and Turning subtests with special administrative and training procedures for blind subjects and found that the results corresponded so closely to that of sighted subjects that separate norms were not needed. A more recent study by Needham and Eldridge (1990) calls such an approach into question as they found performance of blind subjects to be markedly different. Until this difference can be resolved, we are not recommending using this test with reference to norms. Rather, we recommend the use of the *Purdue Pegboard Test*.

Right–Left Orientation Test

It can be easily appreciated that spatial orientation is important to individuals who are blind. The *Right–Left Orientation Test* (Benton et al., 1994) is a straightforward test of an individual's ability to respond to commands related to right and left from his own perspective and from another's perspective. The examiner may wish to informally add items related to compass directions to this test.

Items such as "If you are facing south, what direction is on your right?" can be helpful in ascertaining a person's understanding in this area.

Self-Directed Search

We know of no vocational interest tests with norms for people who are visually impaired. The *Self-Directed Search–Form E* is available in audiotape format, and *Form R* is available on the Internet (Holland, 1994). This test does not have an answer format or norms for people who are visually impaired, but the examiner interested in vocational interest assessment using Holland's typology may wish to use this instrument. Holland's interest and occupational types are Realistic, Investigative, Artistic, Social, Enterprising, and Conventional (Holland, 1992).

Scales of Independent Behavior–Revised

Riverside Press publishes a 40-item short form of the *Scales of Independent Behavior–Revised* specifically designed for the visually impaired (Knowlton et al., 1996). This scale yields a Broad Independence Score and a General Maladaptive Score. Specific areas of functioning assessed include motor skills, social interaction, communicating, personal living skills, and community living skills.

Sixteen Personality Factor Questionnaire

Matching individuals to jobs can also be accomplished by the use of personality tests. Personality patterns can be compared to those of individuals in different work settings. For example, social extroverts are more likely than social introverts to be found in sales positions. We have used the *Sixteen Personality Factor Questionnaire* (16PF) for this purpose (Cattell, 1968; Cattell, Cattell, & Cattell, 1993). A version of the 16PF found in the *Clinical Analysis Questionnaire* (Cattell & Krug, 1975) has few enough items to be read to the client, yet it can maintain the integrity of the longer version of the test. The 16PF is a factor analytically derived test that produces scores on 16 primary personality factors and 5 secondary personality factors. Special scores can also be calculated on areas such as leadership, creativity, and freedom from accidents. This instrument has been revised (Cattell et al., 1993) and is available for computer administration. We prefer to use the older version (Cattell, 1968) of this test because of the availability of the shorter form (as mentioned above). Interpretation with a vocational emphasis requires the use of manuals (Cattell, Eber, & Tatsuoka, 1970; Krug, 1981). The interpretation of personality patterns, however, is fairly straightforward, and even the inexperienced examiner can understand the results. It can easily be seen how understanding the individual in terms of concepts such as independence, expediency, conscientiousness, self-assuredness, adventuresomeness, and anxiety could be useful in working with individuals who are visually impaired.

Millon Clinical Multiaxial Inventory–III

Clinicians desiring tests of psychopathology can find computer-administered and audio versions of the *Minnesota Multiphasic Personality Inventory–2* (MMPI-2; Hathaway & McKinley, 1989) as well as shortened versions of the MMPI (Vincent et al., 1984) or the *Personality Assessment Inventory* (Morey, 1989) that could be read to the client. We recommend the use of the *Millon Clinical Multiaxial Inventory–III* (MCMI-III; Millon, 1994) because the full form of the test is already brief and is available on recording or computer. The MCMI-III is a 175-item true/false test that is computer scored to yield scores on various scales of psychopathology and personality disorder. There are some safeguards for response bias. Each scale compares the individual with various groups of individuals with psychopathology. Again, norms are not available on the population of people who are visually impaired. Caution should be used in accepting and using the interpretations made by the computer due to population differences.

Zung Depression Scale and Geriatric Depression Scale

Examiners often want a quick assessment of depressive symptomatology when working with consumers who are visually impaired. The *Beck Depression Scale* (Corcoran & Fischer, 1987) presents problems when given in a verbal format. We prefer using the *Zung Depression Scale* (Corcoran & Fischer, 1987) because it is easier to give verbally. A resulting score simply compares the individual to patients who are and are not depressed in inpatient and outpatient settings. There is no comparison to people with visual impairments. The resulting score may tend to make individuals who have recently lost their vision look more depressed than they are, however, especially if they are in poor health. Therefore, particular attention to the content of items is important. When health problems are a significant issue or when the individual is elderly, we recommend use of the *Geriatric Depression Scale* (Corcoran & Fischer, 1987; Strauss, Sherman, & Spreen, 2006). This scale requires a simple "yes" or "no" response and does not have many of the items related to physical dysfunction. The *Geriatric Depression Scale* is a simple type of symptom checklist that lends itself well to verbal administration.

Loevinger Sentence Completion Test

Sentence completion measures have occasionally been used with people who are blind. These tests can be given verbally or in large-print format quite easily.

We recommend the use of the *Loevinger Sentence Completion Test* (Loevinger, 1970) because it assesses the important dimension of ego maturity. Maturity of an individual's thinking is often key to adjustment and participation in rehabilitation. This test was not developed for people who are visually impaired, but it does adapt very easily. The greatest difficulty with this instrument is that it requires considerable skill and time to score the person's ego development level. There may also be some projective value of the responses that the clinician may wish to consider in interpreting results. As with any sentence completion test, item stems can be added to bring out unique responses pertaining to the individual's functioning. Items such as "losing my vision has been" and "my hope for the future is" might be useful additions.

Conclusion

Only readily available tests have been reviewed and recommended in this chapter. Although the selection is sparse, we have some hope for the future. We hope to soon see stratified age norms for the CVES. We also hope to see the updating of certain tests such as the *Haptic Intelligence Scale for Adult Blind*. The future may hold publication of newer tests through the work of Mangiamelli and Peters (1999) or others of whom we are yet unaware.

Given the diversity and uniqueness of the population of people who are visually impaired, anyone performing psychological assessments with individuals from this group will have to use considerable caution and judgment. This advice applies not only in selecting instruments but also in interpreting their results. It is our hope that this chapter will help the examiner faced with this challenge and thus benefit people with visual impairments.

References

Abraham, E., Axelrod, B. N., & Ricker, J. H. (1996). Application of the Oral Trail Making Test to a mixed clinical sample. *Archives of Clinical Neuropsychology, 11*(8), 697–701.

American Foundation for the Blind. (1975). *Not without sight* (Video). New York: Author.

American Foundation for the Blind. (1987). *Low vision, questions and answers: Definitions, devices, services.* New York: Author.

Benton, A. L., Sivan, A. B., Hamsher, K., Varney, N. R., & Spreen, O. (1994). *Contributions to neuropsychological assessment* (2nd ed.). Orlando, FL: Psychological Assessment Resources.

Cattell, R. B. (1968). *Sixteen personality factor questionnaire, Edition R.* Champaign, IL: Institute for Personality and Ability Testing.

Cattell, R. B., Cattell, A. K., & Cattell, H. B. (1993). *Sixteen Personality Factor Questionnaire, Fifth Edition,* Champaign, IL: Institute for Personality and Ability Testing.

Cattell, R. B., Eber, H. W., & Tatsuoka, M. M. (1970). *Handbook for the 16PF.* Champaign, IL: Institute for Personality and Ability Testing.

Cattell, R. B., & Krug, S. (1975). *Clinical Analysis Questionnaire*. Champaign, IL: Institute for Personality and Ability Testing.

Chan, F., Lynch, R. T., Dial, J. G., Wong, D. W., & Kates, D. (1993). Applications of the McCarron-Dial System in vocational evaluation: An overview of its operational framework and empirical findings. *Vocational Evaluation and Work Adjustment Bulletin*, Summer, 57–65.

Chaytor, N., Schmitter-Edgecombe, M., & Burr, R. (2006). Improving the ecological validity of executive functioning assessment. *Archives of Clinical Neuropsychology, 21 (3)*, 217–227.

Collins-Moore, M. S., & Osborn, K. N. (1984). Assessing the visually handicapped child. In S. J. Weaver (Ed.), *Testing children: A reference guide for effective clinical and psychoeducational assessment*. Kansas City, MO: Test Corporation of America.

Corcoran, K., & Fischer, J. (1987). *Measures for clinical practice: A source book*. New York: The Free Press.

Delis, D. C., Kaplan, E., & Kramer, J. H. (2001). *Delis-Kaplan Executive Function System*. San Antonio, TX: The Psychological Corporation.

Dial, J. G., Chan, F., Mezger, C., Parker, H. J., Zangler, K., Wong, D. W., et al. (1991a). Comprehensive vocational evaluation system (CVES) for visually impaired/blind individuals: A validation study. *Journal of Visual Impairment and Blindness, 85*, 153–157.

Dial, J. G., Mezger, C., Gray, S., Massey, T., Chan, F., & Hull, J. A. (1991b). *Comprehensive vocational evaluation systems: A systematic approach to vocational, educational and neuropsychological assessment of the visually impaired and blind*. Dallas, TX: McCarron-Dial Systems.

Farah, M. J. (1990). *Visual agnosia: Disorders of object recognition and what they tell us about normal vision*. Cambridge, MA: Massachusetts Institute of Technology Press.

First, M. B., Gibbon, M., Spitzer, R. L., & Williams, J. B. W. (1997). *Structured Clinical Interview for DSM-IV Axis I Disorders: Clinical Version*. North Tonawanda, NY: Multi-Health Systems.

Flynn, J. R. (1984). The mean IQ of Americans: Massive gains 1932 to 1978. *Psychological Bulletin, 95*, 29–51.

Glutting, J., Adams, W., & Sheslow, D. (2004). *Wide Range Intelligence Test*. Wilmington, DE. Wide Range.

Groenveld, M. (1990). The dilemma of assessing the visually impaired child. *Developmental Medicine and Child Neurology, 32*, 1105–1113.

Groenveld, M., Jan, J. E., & Leader, P. (1990). Observations on the habilitation of children with cortical visual impairment. *Journal of Visual Impairment and Blindness*, January, 11–17.

Gromwall, D., & Sampson, H. (1974). *The psychological effects of concussion*. New Zealand: Auckland University Press.

Hathaway, S. R., & McKinley, J. C. (1989). *Minnesota Multiphasic Personality Inventory–2*. Minneapolis, MN: National Computer Systems.

Hayes, S. F. (1929). The new revision of the Binet intelligence tests for the Blind. *Teachers Forum, 2*, 2–4.

Holland, J. L. (1992). *Making vocational choices: A theory of vocational personalities and work environments*. Odessa, FL: Psychological Assessment Resources.

Holland, J. L. (1994). *Self-Directed Search Form E–4th Edition*. Odessa, FL: Psychological Assessment Resources.

Hull, T., & Mason, H. (1993). Issues in standardizing psychometric tests for children who are blind. *Journal of Visual Impairment and Blindness*, May, 149–150.

Irwin, R. B., & Goddard, H. H. (1976). Adaptation of the Binet-Simon Tests (original work published in 1914). In G. Scholl and R. Schneer (Eds.), *Measures of psychological, vocational, and educational functioning in the blind and visually handicapped* (pp. 17–20). New York: American Foundation for the Blind.

Jastak, S., & Wilkinson, G. S. (1984). *Wide Range Achievement Test–Revised*. Wilmington, DE: Jastak Assessment Systems.

Jose, R. T (Ed.). (1993). *Understanding low vision*. New York: American Foundation for the Blind.

Joyce, A., Dial, J., Nelson, P., & Hupp, G. (2000). Neuropsychological predictors of adaptive living and work behaviors [Abstract]. *Archives of Clinical Neuropsychology, 15,* 665.

Joyce, A., Isom, R., Dial, J., & Sandel, M. (2004). Implications of perceptual–motor differences with blind populations. *Journal of Applied Rehabilitation Counseling, 35*(3), 3–7.

Kirchner, C., Schmeidler, E., & Todorov, A. (1999). *Looking at employment through a lifespan telescope: Age, health and employment status of people with serious visual impairment*. Mississippi State, MS: Rehabilitation Research and Training Center on Blindness and Low Vision.

Knowlton, M., Lee, I., Buininks, R. H., Woodcock, R. W., Weatherman, R. F., & Hill, B. K. (1996). *Scales of Independent Behavior–Revised: Short Form for the Visually Impaired*. Itasca, IL: Riverside.

Koestler, F. (1976). *The unseen minority: A social history of blindness in the United States*. New York: David McKay.

Krug, S. E. (1981). *Interpreting 16PF profile patterns*. Champaign, IL: Institute for Personality and Ability Testing.

Kuusisto, S. (1998). *Planet of the blind*. New York: Bantam Doubleday Dell.

Larson, S. (2002). *Slosson Intelligence Test–Revised: Supplemental Manual for Visually Impaired/Blind*. East Aurora, NY: Slosson Educational Publications.

Loevinger, J. (1970). *Measuring ego development* (Vols. 1 and 2). San Francisco: Jossey-Bass.

Mangiamelli, L. J., & Peters, L. (1999). A non-visual battery for assessment of spatial abilities *Archives of Clinical Neuropsychology, 14*(1), 86.

Matarazzo, J. D. (1990). Psychological assessment versus psychological testing. *American Psychologist, 45*(9), 999–1017.

McGee Hall, J. M. (1994). *Neuropsychological functioning of adult subjects with diabetic retinopathy compared to a normal blind population*. Unpublished doctoral dissertation, University of North Texas, Denton, TX.

Miller, J., & Skillman, G. (2003). Assessors' satisfaction with measures of cognitive ability applied to persons with visual impairment. *Journal of Visual Impairment and Blindness*, December, 769–774.

Millon, T. M. (1994). *Millon Clinical Multiaxial Inventory–III*. Minneapolis, MN: National Computer Systems.

Morey, L. C. (1989). *Personality Assessment Inventory*. Odessa, FL: Psychological Assessment Resources.

National Federation of the Blind. (1989). *Blindness and disorders of the eye*. Baltimore: Author.

Needham, W. E., & Eldridge, L. S. (1990). Performance of Blind Vocational Rehabilitation Clients on the Minnesota Rate of Manipulation Test. *Journal of Visual Impairment and Blindness, 84*(4), 182–185.

Nelson, K. A., & Dimitrova, G. (1993). Severe visual impairment in the United States and in each state, 1990. *Journal of Visual Impairment and Blindness, 87,* 80.

Nelson, P., Dial, J., & Joyce, A. (2002a). Validation of the Cognitive Test for the Blind as an assessment of intellectual functioning. *Rehabilitation Psychology, 47,* 184–193.

Nelson, P., Dial, J., & Joyce, A. (2002b). Detecting brain injury in adults with visual impairment or blindness [Abstract]. *Archives of Clinical Neuropsychology, 17,* 715–867.

Nelson, P., O'Brien, E., Dial, J., & Joyce, A. (2001). Neuropsychological correlates of retinopathy of prematurity (ROP) compared to other causes of blindness [Abstract]. *Archives of Clinical Neuropsychology, 16,* 766–767.

Newell, F. W. (1996). *Ophthalmology: Principles and practices* (8th ed.). St Louis, MO: Mosby.

O'Brien, E. P. (1992). *Neuropsychological sequelae of adult subjects with retinopathy of prematurity compared to other blind populations.* Unpublished doctoral dissertation, University of North Texas, Denton, TX.

Psychological Corporation. (2002). *Wechsler Individual Achievement Test–Second Edition.* San Antonio, TX: Author.

Psychological Corporation. (1992). *Wechsler Individual Achievement Test (WIAT).* San Antonio, TX: Psychological Corporation.

Rabeck, D. D. (1994). *Neuropsychological functioning of blind subjects with learning disabilities compared to those with blindness alone.* Unpublished doctoral dissertation, University of North Texas, Denton, TX.

Rafal, R. D. (1997). Balint syndrome. In T. E. Feinbert and M. J. Farrah (Eds.), *Behavioral neurology and neuropsychology* (pp. 337–356). New York: McGraw-Hill.

Reitan, R. M., & Wolfson, D. (1985). *The Halstead-Reitan Neuropsychological Test Battery: Theory and clinical interpretation.* Tucson, AZ: Neuropsychology Press.

Reynolds, C. R., Pearson, N. A., & Voress, J. K. (2002). *Developmental Test of Visual Perception–Adolescent and Adult.* Austin, TX: PRO-ED.

Ricker, J. H., & Axelrod, B. N. (1994). Analysis of an oral paradigm for the trail making test. *Assessment, 1,* 47–51.

Ringgold, N. P. (1991). *Out of the cornea of my eyes: Living with vision loss in later life.* New York: American Foundation for the Blind.

Roberts, J. R., & Bauman, M. K. (1944). *Motor skills tests adapted to the blind.* Minneapolis, MN: Minnesota Educational Test Bureau.

Sacks, O. (1997). *The island of the colorblind.* New York: Knopf.

Scholl, G., & Schnur, R. (1976). *Measures of psychological, vocational, and educational functioning in the blind and visually handicapped.* New York: American Foundation for the Blind.

Shurrager, H. C., & Shurrager, P. S. (1964). *Haptic Intelligence Scale for Adult Blind.* Chicago: Stoetling.

Slosson, R. L. (2002). *Slosson Intelligence Test–Revised.* East Aurora, NY: Slosson Educational Publications.

Spreen, O., & Strauss, E. (1998). *A compendium of neuropsychological tests* (2nd ed.). New York: Oxford.

Strauss, E., Sherman, E., & Spreen, O. (2006). *A Compendium of Neuropsychological Tests: Administration, Norms and Commentary, Third Edition.* New York: Oxford.

Taylor, R. E., & Ward, K. M. (1990). The tale of our search for the tactile Progressive Matrices. *American Psychologist, 45*(1), 69.

Tiffin, J. (1968). *Purdue Pegboard Test.* Lafayette, IN: Lafayette Instrument.

Tombaugh, T. (2006). A comprehensive review of the Paced Auditory Serial Addition Test (PASAT). *Archives of Clinical Neuropsychology, 21,* 53–76.

Valpar International. (1980a). *Conceptual understanding through blind evaluation.* Tucson, AZ: Author.

Valpar International. (1980b). *Valpar Component Work Sample.* Tucson, AZ: Author.

Van Son, A. R. (1989). *Diabetes vision impairment and blindness.* New York: American Foundation for the Blind.

Vander Kolk, C. J. (1980). *Assessment and planning with the visually impaired.* Baltimore: University Park Press.

Vaughan, D. G., Asbury, T., & Riordan-Eva, P. (1995). *General ophthalmology* (14th ed.). Norwalk, CT: Appleton and Lange.

Vincent, K. R., Castillo, I. M., Hauser, R. I., Zapata, J. A., Stuart, H. J., Cohn, C. K., et al. (1984). *MMPI-168 codebook.* Norwood, NJ: Ablex.

Warrington, E. K., & James, M. (1991). *The Visual Object and Space Perception Battery.* Bury St. Edmunds, UK: Thames Valley Test Co.

Wechsler, D. (1955). *Wechsler Adult Intelligence Scale.* New York: Psychological Corporation.

Wechsler, D. (1997). *Wechsler Memory Scale–Third Edition.* San Antonio, TX: Psychological Corporation.

Wechsler, D. (1998). *Wechsler Adult Intelligence Scale–Third Edition.* San Antonio, TX: Psychological Corporation.

Weiskrantz, L. (1986). *Blindsight: A case study and implications.* Oxford, England: Clarendon Press.

Wilkinson, G. S. (1993). *Wide Range Achievement Test–Third Edition.* Wilmington, DE: Jastak Associates.

Wolf-Schein, E. G. (1998). Considerations in assessment of children with severe disabilities including deaf-blindness and autism. *International Journal of Disability, Development and Education. 45*(1), 35–55.

Chapter 17

Assessment of Individuals Who Are Deaf or Hard of Hearing

Shawn P. Saladin

Estimates of the number of people in the United States who have hearing loss vary widely due to differences in data collection procedures, but one trend is clear—the number of people with hearing loss is growing (Kochkin, 2005; Lucas, Schiller, & Benson, 2004; Pleis & Coles, 2002). The 1994 *National Health Interview Survey* reported that nearly 22 million people had hearing difficulties, ranging from mild hearing loss to total absence of hearing (National Center for Health Statistics, 1996). In 2001, estimates suggested that more than 28.4 million people had some level of hearing loss, with approximately 3.4% of the U.S. population reporting significant or complete hearing loss (Lucas et al., 2004). Kochkin (2005) predicts an even sharper increase to 52 million people with hearing loss by the year 2050. However, many rehabilitation professionals are unfamiliar with the communication-related, educational, vocational, and behavioral ramifications of hearing loss and the related impact on assessment.

Assessments can be an important part of the rehabilitation process and rehabilitation service provision. Assessments when properly conducted, and assessment results when properly applied, can help guide career and personal counseling, vocational training, provision of assistive technology, job placement, and medical and psychological treatments (Parker & Bolton, 2005). Whether providing or purchasing intellectual, psychological, vocational, and other assessment of clients who have hearing loss, rehabilitation professionals need information about instruments and techniques that can be used effectively with the population (Braden, 1994; Vernon & Andrews, 1990). Lack of information may result in the selection and use of inappropriate instruments and procedures, which in turn may negatively affect service provision and vocational accommodations. The purpose of this chapter is threefold: to familiarize the reader with the definitions and terminology related to the assessments of people with hearing loss; to discuss several key issues that affect most standardized assessments of people with hearing loss; and to review a selection of assessment instruments and related accommodations, including a brief section on the assessment and accommodation of individuals who are both Deaf and blind.

Definitions of Hearing Loss

Developing stable definitions of deafness and hearing loss presents a range of challenges because the population is very diverse, not only in terms of age and ethnicity, but also in etiology, age of onset, educational background, and personal identity. While some definitions of hearing loss rely on audiometric test results expressed numerically, other definitions rely on functional reports. Still other definitions are cultural and are grounded in personal choices about self-identification. As a result, variability among definitions of hearing loss exists and many definitions have significant subjectivity.

The author wishes to acknowledge the contribution of McCay Vernon to the field of assessment of the deaf.

Medical and Functional Definitions

Pure-tone audiometry is a well-established standardized method of quantifying hearing loss (American National Standards Institute, 1996, 1997, 2003). The technique measures the softest sound a person can hear measured in decibels (dB) for each ear at various frequencies, which are measured in hertz (Hz), to establish an auditory sensitivity threshold (Wilber, 1999). Generally, an individual's results at three specific frequencies are averaged, providing an indicator of how much hearing a person has in each ear without amplification. With a threshold of 0 to 25 dB, a person will be identified as having no loss of hearing ability. A person with mild hearing loss usually has a threshold of 26 to 40 dB, while a person with a mild-to-moderate hearing loss generally has a 41 to 55 dB threshold. An individual will have a moderate hearing loss with a 56 to 70 dB threshold and a severe hearing loss if his or her threshold ranges from 71 to 90 dB. Persons with a 90-decibel threshold or greater are identified as having a profound hearing loss (Tye-Murry, 2004).

Functionally, a person with a mild hearing loss may experience a slight decrease in speech recognition if background noise is present. With a mild to moderate loss, a person will likely need face-to-face communication to comprehend at least half of a conversation and may have some problems understanding conversation in group settings. Having a moderate loss usually results in significant difficulty in group settings and significant difficulty in face-to-face verbal conversations. An individual with a severe hearing loss is not likely to recognize voices or environmental noises, while a person who has a profound hearing loss usually relies on visual methods of communication and may only detect sounds through vibrations. From this perspective, people whose threshold is in the mild, mild-to-moderate, and moderate categories are usually considered *hard of hearing,* while people with results in the severe and profound categories would be labeled *deaf* (Flexor, 1999; Moores, 1996; Tye-Murry, 2004).

Cultural Definitions and Appropriate Terminology

Capitalizing the terms *Deaf* or *Deafness* is appropriate when the terms are used to refer to people with hearing loss who identify as part of the Deaf sociolinguistic and cultural group. When these terms are not capitalized, no reference to membership in the cultural community is implied (Lane, Hoffmeister, & Bahan, 1996; Padden & Humphries, 2005). Thus, the blended phrase *Deaf or hard of hearing* is used here to be maximally inclusive and culturally sensitive. It is interesting to note that Deaf culture typically makes no distinction between person-first language and phrases such as *Deaf person,* finding either option equally acceptable (Baker-Shenk & Cokely, 1980).

Both audiometric and functional definitions focus on the level and severity of loss of hearing. However, a cultural definition also exists that is not focused on hearing status. Over the last two decades, a definition of Deafness that represents a particular view of life manifested by the mores, beliefs, and language that are particular to Deaf people has emerged. Identifying oneself as culturally Deaf does not reflect or imply any specific medical status of hearing. In fact, hearing status is one of the least important criteria used to delineate group membership; acceptance of Deaf values, rejection of Deafness as impairment, and the use of American Sign Language (ASL) are more highly valued (Padden & Humphries, 2005). Within Deaf culture, the term *hearing impaired* denotes a negative medical paradigm that pathologizes differences in hearing status and negates the cultural component of Deafness (Baker-Shenk & Cokely, 1980). As such, the Deaf cultural community has rejected it.

General Issues in Assessment

Increasingly, educational settings and rehabilitation settings at all levels require participation in standardized assessment for screening, eligibility, and placement services. In addition, many employment settings now require standardized assessments in the form of certification or licensure examinations or for promotions after hire (Johnson, 2005). However, people who are Deaf or hard of hearing often do not perform well on the types of standardized assessment instruments used in these settings (Loew, Cahalan-Laitusis, Cook, & Harris, 2005; Martin & McCrone, 1990); even exceptionally bright and well-educated Deaf people may experience significant difficulties (Mounty & Martin, 2005). Often, assessment challenges arise due to deficits in English language literacy and limited real-world and social knowledge resulting from experiences of linguistic and social isolation, which can begin at a very early age (Holt, Traxler, & Allen, 1997; Lane, 1992; Lane et al., 1996; Schein, 1989; Smart, 2001). Additionally, the inappropriate use of sign language as an accommodation may negatively affect assessment of people who are Deaf or hard of hearing (Allen, 1994a; Ladd, 2003; Rogers, 2005).

Literacy and Related Academic Skills

Reduced literacy and language access are at the root of many of the problems encountered in standardized testing of Deaf and hard-of-hearing individuals (Loew et al., 2005). Many Deaf and some hard-of-hearing people find English difficult to learn. While people who hear well learn language primarily through hearing and speech interactions, the ability to hear speech is not available or is seriously restricted for Deaf or hard-of-hearing learners. For individuals whose hearing loss occurred before the acquisition of speech, English is effectively a foreign language. Often, when teaching reading in a mainstream school, a phonological approach is used, creating significant difficulties for students with hearing loss. Other typical methods of developing English literacy have also been found to be inappropriate for students with hearing loss (Lipton & Gold-stein, 1997). As a result, many Deaf or hard-of-hearing people have English reading skills at the 3rd grade level or less (Elliot, 1987; Holt et al., 1997). Developing some understanding of the linguistic and educational isolation that results in limitations in English language literacy and other academic skill deficits is important to understanding the challenges faced in assessing Deaf or hard-of-hearing individuals (Gallaudet Research Institute [GRI], 2003a; Holt et al., 1997). All of these problems are interrelated, creating a cascade of concerns.

Linguistic Isolation

Linguistically, Deaf and hard-of-hearing people may be divided into those who speak and read English and, hence, are amenable to standard written questionnaires and those who do not or who do so poorly. For Deaf and hard-of-hearing individuals, when the hearing loss is congenital or prelingual, the impact on language development is most severe and linguistic isolation often occurs (Allen, 1994b; Hindley, 2000; Lipton & Goldstein, 1997). In addition, Vess and Douglas (1995) note that the learning styles of people who have prelingual or early hearing loss may be largely situated in experiential contexts. As a result, limitations in conceptual knowledge and abstract thinking occur. However, linguistic isolation is just one way people who are Deaf or hard of hearing become separated from larger society.

Social Isolation

Social isolation is a serious concern for Deaf and hard-of-hearing individuals, and it can begin at a very early age (Smart, 2001). It is estimated that about 90% of parents and 79% of siblings of Deaf or hard-of-hearing children are hearing, but most do not master ASL or other modes of manual communication and so may be unable to fully connect with the Deaf or hard-of-hearing child (GRI, 2003a). While residential schools for the Deaf have existed for more than a century, recent research indicates that approximately 75% of Deaf and hard-of-hearing students spend all or part of their school day in a public school resource or self-contained classroom, where they are often the only individual with a hearing loss (GRI, 2003a; Osgood, 2005). Because of such placements, Deaf or hard-of-hearing youth miss opportunities to fully participate in school and community environments and miss many rich opportunities for social learning. Efforts have been made to integrate Deaf and hard-of-hearing students with hearing peers, but while sign language interpreters are often available in the classroom, interpreters are rarely available on playgrounds, in school cafeterias, and in other social settings (Osgood, 2005). Difficulties with social learning, interactions, and behaviors can result in an inability to recognize and respond to environmental stimuli and marked difficulties in comprehension (Holt et al., 1997; Smart, 2001).

Test Construction

The difficulties experienced due to English language literacy problems and a lack of real-world and social knowledge are compounded by the typical construction and language used in standardized tests—probably the most basic challenge in assessment of Deaf and hard-of-hearing individuals (Mounty & Martin, 2005; Weinstock & Mounty, 2005). For instance, many types of assessments include questions that consist of an incomplete sentence, also called an incomplete stem, followed by multiple-choice options that complete the sentence stem. However, incomplete stems can be very difficult for Deaf or hard-of-hearing individuals. People whose native language is not English or who have limited access to English acquisition understand a complete question better than questions comprised of an incomplete statement that is completed by one of the multiple-choice options (Massad, 2005). Questions or items stated in the negative; questions made up of multiple subordinate clauses; questions with qualifiers; and test items that are excessively complex, ambiguous, or idiomatic may also be difficult for Deaf or hard-of-hearing test takers, yet these question formats are commonly found in various standardized assessments (Mounty & Martin, 2005; Weinstock & Mounty, 2005).

In addition to difficulties associated with various formats used for test construction, items may also be more subtly biased due to constructs of language. Native language fluency is complex and involves much more than mastery of grammatical rules; voice register, nuances of inflection and tone, and formal and informal usages are all part of native fluency. It is due to these aspects of language that one is able to conclude that although a sentence is technically constructed correctly, it just doesn't "sound" right. These types of questions are generally labeled *sound-based* and are especially challenging for prelingually Deaf or hard-of-hearing consumers (Weinstock & Mounty, 2005, p. 29). If possible, the rehabilitation professional should thoroughly review tests for formats, grammatical constructs, and sound-based vocabulary known to pose difficulties for Deaf test takers (Ragosta, 2005). It may also be helpful to prepare consumers for the types of constructions and language used in standardized assessments by providing opportunities for practice and study (Weinstock & Mounty, 2005). If using an assessment tool that contains problematic construction is not avoidable, language-related and other accommodations may be needed.

Sign Language as an Accommodation

Translating a written test into manual communication is known as *sight translation* (Rogers, 2005, p. 111) and initially seems to be a reasonable accommodation for individuals whose literacy difficulties pose challenges in assessment situations. However, assessment accommodations through sign language interpretation are much more complex than simply arranging for an interpreter's attendance (Johnson, Kimball, & Brown, 2001; Rogers, 2005). Foremost, it is critical to recognize that not all individuals who are Deaf or hard of hearing are fluent in the use of sign language. Second, the significant variability within and among signed languages may affect both the expressive accuracy and the receptive understanding of content. Additionally, live translations can vary from interpreter to interpreter due to differences in language skills, competencies, and familiarity with the testing procedures, content of the test, and preferred communication style of the client (Blennerhassett, 2000; Rogers, 2005).

Sign Language Fluency

Many types of manual communication are used in the United States, but the most common are ASL and Signed English. However, many Deaf people are not fluent enough in either ASL or Signed English to use these languages in formal assessment situations (Rogers, 2005). It is estimated that nearly 10% of severely and profoundly Deaf students attend oral schools and do not learn to communicate or comprehend in any oral or manual mode (Allen, 1994b; Ladd, 2003). Thus, the test taker may not receive all of the instructions or information necessary to perform at his or her full ability (Blennerhassett, 2000; Schick, Williams, & Kupermintz, 2006).

Translation Issues

Signed languages, like most spoken languages, are changeable and subject to the regional and ethnic dialects and personal preferences. The regional variations in syntax and vocabulary of ASL, along with wide use of self-, family-, and school-created signs, can all affect meaningful transliteration (Braden, 1994; Lipton & Goldstein, 1997), and, although Signed English includes standardized combinations of specific ASL word signs with spoken English syntax, it is prone to nonstandard alterations due to regional differences and the omission of signs by hearing users (Braden, 1994; Lipton & Goldstein, 1997). Any translation can change the construct being measured, whether the translation is oral to oral or oral to manual (Gierl, 2000; Loew et al., 2005). The process of translation may result in shortened interactions between the person administering an evaluation and the person being evaluated, and the seating arrangements necessary for translation and interpretation may interfere with the testing materials, alter the standardized delivery of the instrument, or otherwise interfere with the testing situation (Blennerhassett, 2000).

Interpreter Skills and Bias

The knowledge, skills, and abilities of the sign language interpreter are of critical importance to the use of sign language as a meaningful accommodation in standardized assessment situations (Gierl, 2000; Loew et al., 2005). However, even the use of a very well-qualified interpreter may not result in full access to and comprehension of content (Schick et al., 2006). Proper interpretation focuses on meaning rather than words alone. If it is necessary to use an interpreter because the professional administering an assessment cannot sign, the interpreter should ideally be fluent not only in manual communication but also in psychology and testing; otherwise, results are not likely to meet high standards of validity (Raifman & Vernon, 1996).

The use of an interpreter also has the potential for introducing bias into the testing situation or for invalidating test results because they were obtained under nonstandard procedures (Johnson et al., 2001; Loew et al., 2005). For instance, if language is the construct being assessed, either directly or indirectly, translation would not be appropriate. And, just as the process of translation may inadvertently omit information needed to answer a test item correctly (Johnson et al., 2001), the hand shapes or directionality of a sign shape used by an interpreter may provide information that reveals an answer to a test question (Blennerhassett, 2000). In fact, Rogers (2005) notes that it is not unusual for test administrators to become suspicious of interpreters and to interrupt or even withdraw interpreting services during assessment.

Assessments in Rehabilitation Settings

Despite broad concerns about and challenges to the use of standardized testing for persons who are Deaf or hard of hearing, there will be instances in rehabilitation settings when such testing is necessary and desirable. Test selection may depend on two broad factors: the nature of the consumer and the nature of the test. Etiological factors, age of onset, the presence of other disabilities, preferred mode of communication, and other social and educational experiences may further affect formal assessments (Zieziula, 1986). Depending on the reason for referral and the age of the client, a complete psychological assessment battery may include intelligence testing, psychiatric testing and screening for brain injury, educational achievement testing, and aptitude and interest testing, which the rehabilitation professional may compile along with case history data.

Assessment of Intellectual Functioning

Braden (2001) notes that the key difficulty in assessing the cognitive abilities of people who are Deaf or hard of hearing is differentiating between language deficits, cognitive deficits, and language deficits resulting from cognitive deficits. Ideally, diagnosticians address the difficulty through the use of multiple forms of assessment (Braden, 2001). When a person who is Deaf or hard of hearing possesses exceptional language abilities, it may be proper to use a verbal test. However, if this is not the case, an inaccurate psychological evaluation may result (Vernon, 1996). For an intelligence test to be valid with most clients who are prelingually Deaf or hard of hearing, a nonverbal performance-type instrument is recommended (Braden, 1994).

A number of intelligence tests specifically developed for individuals who are Deaf or hard of hearing are no longer in print and not available to clinicians through the publishers. Although some of these out-of-print instruments may remain in circulation through photocopies and other reproductions, with no recent norms, no psychometric updates or improvements, and no revisions to bring them conceptually and contextually up to date, the use of such instruments is not recommended. Examples of tests in this category include the *General Aptitude Test Battery for the Deaf* (U.S. Department of Labor, 1982), the *Hearing Measurement Scale* (Noble & Atherley, 1970), and the *Hiskey-Nebraska Test of Learning Aptitude* (Hiskey, 1966). Spragins (1997) notes that PRO-ED, Inc., continues to stock the Hiskey-Nebraska record forms, although the author cautions that the test norms developed in 1966 have never been revised and have little relevance today. Despite the unavailability of these tests, other instruments are available and useful in rehabilitation-related assessment. Brief reviews of several instruments follow.

Wechsler Adult Intelligence Scale–Third Edition

The *Wechsler Adult Intelligence Scale–Third Edition* (WAIS-III; Wechsler, 1997) is the most commonly used test of intelligence for adults, and portions of the instrument have been used with Deaf or hard-of-hearing consumers (Collins & Hunter, 2001; Flanagan, McGrew, & Ortiz, 2000; Gregory, 1999; Kaufman & Lichtenberger, 1999). Most often, the Performance Scale of the WAIS-III is selected for use in assessing Deaf or hard-of-hearing individuals. The Performance Scales are appropriate for people aged 16 to 89 years. Although there are no norms or specific instructions for use with Deaf or hard-of-hearing people, it is possible to use demonstrations or manual communication to accommodate the needs of Deaf or hard-of-hearing test takers. However, individuals with receptive language limitations may still have difficulty understanding the tasks (Blennerhassett, 2000). The WAIS-III Performance Scale is best used as one part of a multifactor evaluation to ensure a "best" measure of the student's performance. It may be necessary to administer at least two Performance Scales for results to approach the reliability and validity of a full IQ test (Braden, 1994).

Leiter-R

The *Leiter-R* (Roid & Miller, 1997) is a test that has been widely administered to individuals in special populations. Because the format requires no verbal instructions or responses, the *Leiter-R* has been used successfully with individuals who have hearing loss, including individuals outside of the typical age range of 2 to 20 years old (Tsatsanis, Dartnall, Cicchetti, Sparrow, Klin, & Volkmar, 2003). The test manual does not suggest any special accommodations or instructions for use with Deaf individuals; however, most of the required tasks are self-evident and others may be demonstrated (Roid & Miller, 1997). Although the nonverbal format of the instrument makes it an appealing choice for assessing people who are Deaf or hard of hearing, there are some concerns. Particularly, no norms for people who are Deaf or hard of hearing are available, administration time can be lengthy when used with Deaf people, and costs are high per individual administration (Spragins, 1997).

Test of Nonverbal Intelligence–Third Edition

The *Test of Nonverbal Intelligence–Third Edition* (TONI-3; Brown, Sherbenou, & Johnsen, 1997) is a brief, language-free measure appropriate for people aged 6 through 89. Using the TONI-3, the test administrator may use gestures or manual communication to convey instructions to the participant, who then points to response choices (Spragins, Blennerhassett, & Mullen, 1993). There are no norms available for Deaf or hard-of-hearing populations. Interestingly, the developers suggest development of local or specialized norms, so it is possible that some organizations have done so. A valuable feature of the TONI-3 is the use of geometric patterns rather than activity scenarios or storyboards, so it may be less affected by deficits in real-world and social knowledge that may exist for individuals who are Deaf or hard of hearing than other measures. This instrument is best used in combination with other formal and informal evaluative measures (Spragins, 1997).

Raven's Progressive Matrices

Raven's Progressive Matrices (Raven, 1948; Raven, Court, & Raven, 1977) is a series of three nonverbal tests of reasoning ability based on completion of a matrix design. The Standard Progressive Matrices, which are suitable for people ranging in age from 6 to 80 years, and the Advanced Progressive Matrices, which are suitable for high-functioning older children and adults, are most relevant to rehabilitation settings and have been successfully used with individuals who are Deaf or hard of hearing (Blennerhassett, Strohmeier, & Hibbett, 1994; Naglieri & Welch, 1991). As with many instruments, normative data and standardized instructions for Deaf individuals have not been developed. Task requirements can be conveyed nonverbally by demonstration, gesturing, and pointing, although it has been reported that task requirements are usually evident. In studies completed in Deaf residential settings, the Matrices have been shown to correlate significantly with other measures of intellectual abilities (Blennerhassett et al., 1994). The Matrices are recommended as a supplemental measure within a more comprehensive test of intellectual abilities. The test is not recommended for use with individuals who are impulsive (Spragins, 1997).

Comprehensive Test of Nonverbal Intelligence

The *Comprehensive Test of Nonverbal Intelligence* (CTONI; Hammill, Pearson, & Wiederholt, 1997) is a nonverbal measure of reasoning that may be administered using pantomime or other manual communication (Drossman, Maller, & McDermott, 2001). Because the CTONI includes sequential reasoning tasks, it could be biased for Deaf or hard-of-hearing individuals, who are known to have difficulty in sequences or seriating (Spragins, 1997). The authors note that the instrument is appropriate when assessing individuals with speech or language differences. The test manual reports successful use with students who are Deaf or hard of hearing and moderate to high subtest correlations with other intelligence measures (Hammill et al., 1997). According to Spragins (1997), the CTONI appears to be an appropriate instrument for assessing Deaf or hard-of-hearing individuals, although results should be interpreted with some caution.

Although the IQ scores of older youth and adults are more reliable than those of children who are Deaf or hard of hearing, low scores in particular should be considered questionable in the absence of other supporting evidence. Because there are many reasons why an individual may perform below capacity, there is a greater possibility that a low IQ score is incorrect. However, there are almost no conditions that can lead to performance that is above capacity, so high IQ scores are likely to be correct (Vernon & Hammer, 1996). Braden (2001) cautions against the presumption that any test that yields a low score for an individual who is Deaf or hard of hearing has inherent bias; indeed, sometimes people simply do not perform well or have actual deficits in the areas under investigation. Since the use of manual communication alters standardization and can affect results, the administrator should note what type of communication was used and what modifications were made (Spragins, 1997).

To conclude, a valid appraisal of intelligence may be a critical piece of a holistic assessment for rehabilitation purposes and is most important for individuals who are Deaf or hard of hearing. Unfortunately, there have been cases where Deaf or hard-of-hearing individuals have been misidentified as having intellectual disabilities. In other cases, Deaf or hard-of-hearing individuals have been refused proper vocational rehabilitation because inappropriate tests were used (Vernon & Andrews, 1990). Selecting the performance-based or nonverbal sections of an instrument can be a useful adaptive strategy for reducing or eliminating verbal bias; however, it should be done cautiously. Most importantly, it should not be assumed that a performance-based scale equates to using a nonverbal measure since many performance scales actually require lengthy English instructions (Gibbins, 1989).

Psychiatric Assessment and Brain Injury Screening

Serious mental illnesses can and do occur in people who are Deaf and hard of hearing. In fact, as many as half of all Deaf or hard-of-hearing people may have experienced some mental health condition (Allen, 1994a; Hindley, Kitson, & Leach, 2000). The manifestations of mental illnesses, especially psychotic disorders, in people who are Deaf or hard of hearing can be very different from those experienced by hearing people. In particular, disruptions in sensory and linguistic functioning are often primary symptoms of mental illness. It is generally valid in the hearing population to assume that individuals are fluent in their native language and that disruptions in fluency are evidence of neurological or psychiatric problems; unfortunately, the same is not true for individuals who are deaf or hard of hearing. Deaf or hard-of-hearing people may have sensory and language experiences that are very different from those experienced by hearing people, making it difficult to determine typicality (Elliott, 1987; Evans & Elliott, 1981).

Misdiagnoses of mental illness are common among Deaf and hard-of-hearing people, due to a variety of test administration challenges and the social and behavioral differences and perceptual differences associated with severe hearing loss (Blennerhassett, 2000; Brauer, 1993; Briccetti, 1994; Kitson & Thacker, 2000; Moores, 1978; Rosen, 1967; Vernon & Andrews, 1990). Dickert (1988) found that service providers consistently rated Deaf clients as needing more supervision and medication in spite of rating them as less mentally ill than hearing clients, suggesting that the service providers did not fully grasp the needs of the population.

As previously discussed, it is not uncommon for Deaf or hard-of-hearing people to have minimal language skills, whether oral or manual. Yet many instruments for assessing psychiatric functioning depend on extensive verbal or written interchanges and on the rapport built between the participant and administrator. As a result, few psychiatric tests have had wide application with adults or children who are Deaf or hard of hearing. However, several have shown utility and are commonly used. Some instruments may also be used in conjunction with neurological and audiological diagnostic techniques to screen for possible brain injury, which appears more frequently among individuals who are Deaf, especially those who are likely to be referred for psychological evaluation (Braden, 1994; Morgan & Vernon, 1994).

Rorschach Ink Blot

The *Rorschach Ink Blot* test (Rorschach, 1942) is a well-known instrument that requires the participant to respond to a set of 10 cards, each containing an abstract inkblot. While comprehensive overviews of the administration, scoring, and interpretation procedures are available, the effectiveness of the instrument is highly dependent on the administrator's skills (Exner, 2001; Spragins, 1997). Use of the Rorschach system with Deaf or hard-of-hearing individuals may be limited to persons who have good English skills or who are late deafened; individuals who do not have good communication skills may be limited in their ability to give adequate responses or have difficulty expanding on their responses. Schwartz, Mebane, and Malony (1990) found that the Rorschach could be used appropriately with Deaf participants who had some postsecondary education, some fluency in English, and interactions with the hearing community if administered by a psychologist who is knowledgeable about Deaf culture and Deaf test takers.

Minnesota Multiphasic Personality Inventory

The *Minnesota Multiphasic Personality Inventory* (MMPI; Butcher, Dahlstrom, Graham, & Tellegen, 1989) is a popular and well-established personality assessment for which an ASL version has been developed, titled the *Brauer Gallaudet MMPI-168* (Brauer, 1992). The ASL version of the MMPI has been found to reliably capture the same constructs as the English version. However, the two versions share some limitations, including the overidentification of participants as "disturbed" (Riley-Glassman, 1989). Research also indicates that the ASL version is very lengthy (LaVigne & Vernon, 2003) and in need of more conceptually and culturally meaningful translation (Brauer, 1992). Additionally, the ASL MMPI may be vulnerable to differences in perceptions of the personality and signing style of the sign language interpreter on items sensitive to the participant, a phenomenon known as *signer effect* (Brauer, 1992, p. 380).

Bender Visual Motor Gestalt Test

The *Bender Visual Motor Gestalt Test* (Bender-Gestalt) was developed by Lauretta Bender in 1938, and original normative data included individuals with various disabilities including brain injury. While multiple versions of the Bender-Gestalt test exist, the most relevant to rehabilitation settings is the *Bender Visual Motor Gestalt Test, Second Edition* (Bender Gestalt–II; Brannigan & Decker, 2003). Although early research suggested the instrument was not useful for individuals who are Deaf (Bolton, 1972; Bolton, Donoghue, & Langbauer, 1973), the instrument is frequently used for screening and identifying neurological difficulties among people who are Deaf or hard of hearing (Spragins, 1997; Vernon & Andrews, 1990). An advantage of the Bender Gestalt–II is that an objective scoring system is available. As with the instruments previously discussed, the lack of norms for Deaf or hard-of-hearing individuals is a disadvantage. Even though it is widely used, little research exists indicating that participants who are Deaf or hard of hearing fully understand the test instructions (Spragins, 1997). The instrument can be a valuable tool when used in conjunction with other tests and background information rather than as a stand-alone assessment (Bender, 1938; Koppitz, 1963).

Memory-for-Designs Test

The *Memory-for-Designs Test* (MFD; Graham & Kendall, 1960) may be a good tool for assessing people who are Deaf or hard of hearing. The instrument consists of 15 designs on stimulus cards that are shown to the participant for 5 seconds. Then, the designs are reproduced by the test taker, with high error scores indicating lower performance. This test has a precise scoring technique that controls for variation in age, intelligence, and vocabulary level; however, the instrument has a mixed research record and no specific norms for persons with hearing loss (Mandes & Gessner, 1989). On the positive side, the MFD has been found to be sensitive to subtle age-related changes in the brain, as well as demonstrated discrimination between cognitive deficits related to brain injury and cognitive deficits unrelated to an acquired injury. However, some studies have shown that the MFD reports a high number of false-negative results, so it is best used in conjunction with other data (Mandes & Gessner, 1989).

Projective Drawing Techniques

Little research supports the use of the projective techniques with Deaf or hard-of-hearing participants, and the expectations for such participants are not well-established. People who are Deaf or hard of hearing may differ from hearing people in visual–motor functioning, which may affect projective drawings and interpreted results (Schwartz et al., 1990). In fact, drawings completed by youth who are Deaf or hard of hearing are known to differ from those of hearing youth (Briccetti, 1994; Spragins, 1997). Some projective methods, including the *Draw-A-Person: Screening Procedure for Emotional Disturbance* (DAP: SPED; Machover, 1949), have been shown to misclassify the emotional functioning of Deaf and hard-of-hearing individuals and should be used cautiously if at all (Briccetti, 1994). Despite these limitations, projective techniques are used with Deaf and hard-of-hearing individuals (Schwartz et al., 1990). Spragins (1997) suggests that drawing can provide a nonthreatening way to begin an assessment battery and may help build rapport by fostering communication between the participant and the administrator through discussion of drawings. The *House-Tree-Person* (HTP; Buck, 1948) is an evaluating technique appropriate for individuals older than 3 years old that is frequently used with Deaf or hard-of-hearing individuals (Spragins, 1997). The HTP uses an approach in which the participant creates three drawings and then interprets them to the test administrator. Normative data are provided through a series of books containing qualitative analyses of a wide variety of drawings, and there are no objective scoring criteria (Buck, 1992; Burns, 1987).

In summary, psychiatric evaluation of individuals who are Deaf or hard of hearing may be much more complex than intelligence testing. It is necessary to interpret test results in light of an in-depth understanding of the impact of hearing loss, personal experiences with the individual, and case history data. Some research suggests that in order to effectively assess the emotional functioning of a person who is Deaf or hard of hearing, the examiner must be fluent in manual communication (Brauer, 1993). At a minimum, Levine (1981) and Blennerhassett (2000) suggest that mental health professionals working with people who are Deaf or hard of hearing need a good understanding of Deaf culture and the developmental implications of Deafness in order to better understand typicality as it applies to the group (*Gallaudet University School Psychology Handbook,* 1994, p. 46; Kitson & Thacker, 2000). Generally, it may be of value for rehabilitation professionals to view with skepticism results reported by examiners who are unfamiliar with Deaf and hard-of-hearing people.

In connection with personality evaluation, it is important to note that the confusion and apparent disassociation reflected in the writing of Deaf and hard-of-hearing people with poor verbal skills is usually only the result of the language deficiency and rarely indicate an equally altered thought process (Brauer, 1993). Paper-and-pencil personality measures may be appropriate for individuals who are hard of hearing with well-developed expressive and receptive language ability; however, the problems of test administration and interpretation may make the results questionable (Heller, 1987; Vernon & Andrews, 1990). Last, there is some question as to whether the norms for the personality structure of people without hearing loss are appropriate for clients who are Deaf or hard or hearing (Heller, 1987). It is possible that Deafness alters the perceived environment sufficiently to bring about an essentially different organization of personality and make normality for a person who is Deaf or hard of hearing different from normality for a person with no difficulty hearing. This issue is heavily debated by scholars in the field of Deafness (Vernon & Andrews, 1990) and should be considered when discussing the personality assessment of those with severe hearing loss. Nonetheless, a complete neuropsychological evaluation should be done if screening tools yield positive results.

Achievement Testing

At times it may be necessary for professionals working with consumers who are Deaf or hard of hearing to obtain a measure of the individual's level of educational achievement. In rehabilitation or closely related settings, quantifying an individual's academic knowledge, skills, and abilities may aid in the development of an appropriate rehabilitation plan, needed training or education, and meaningful job placement (Spragins, 1997). However, there are several challenges to using standardized achievement tests with deaf or hard-of-hearing individuals, especially in selecting and sequencing an appropriate instrument, in conveying the test instructions and content, and in adapting the measures to the population (Allen, White, & Karchmer, 1983). Efforts to improve achievement test reliability and validity for people who are Deaf or hard of hearing have resulted in recommendations for use of the *Peabody Individual Achievement Test–Revised/Normative Update* (Spragins, 1997) and extensive normative and administrative research on several editions of the *Stanford Achievement Test* (GRI, 2003b).

Peabody Individual Achievement Test–Revised/Normative Update

The *Peabody Individual Achievement Test–Revised/Normative Update* (PIAT-R/NU; Markwardt, 1997) is a commonly used achievement screening instrument. It is a multiple-choice tool that has no time limits. The format allows for pointed responses and may be appropriate for individuals with hearing loss or other communication disorders (Markwardt, 1997; Spragins, 1997). The Normative Update (Markwardt, 1997) was standardized for a population aged 5 through 22 years, so it has value to rehabilitation professionals working with young adults in transition. Deaf or hard-of-hearing individuals were not included in the normative sample (Markwardt, 1997). Nonetheless, the test items appear to be reflective of the curricular content typical in most U.S. public schools, so the content is likely relevant to Deaf or hard-of-hearing individuals who participated in mainstream or inclusive school settings. The content may have limited relevance to individuals who were educated in residential schools or other special educational settings, although increasingly these programs are in line with public school guidelines (Spragins, 1997).

Stanford Achievement Tests

The *Stanford Achievement Test for the Hearing Impaired* (SAT-HI; Harcourt, Brace, & Jovanovich, 1973) was developed from the sixth edition of the *Stanford Achievement Test* (SAT-6; Harcourt, Brace, & Jovanovich, 1972) for the purpose of measuring the academic achievement of individuals who are either Deaf or hard of hearing (French, 1987; Kelly & Braden, 1990; Trybus & Jensema, 1976). The instrument included the most extensive standardization for Deaf or hard-of-hearing individuals of any available instrument (Blennerhassett, 2000; Harcourt, Brace, & Jovanovich, 1973; Spragins et al., 1993). The SAT-HI included the same items as the SAT-6 but combined subtests in higher-level mathematics with subtests in lower-level reading into a single test booklet (Trybus & Jensema, 1976; Trybus & Karchmer, 1977; Wolk & Zieziula, 1985). Since the development of the instrument, the GRI has continued to address the need for norms for Deaf and hard-of-hearing individuals by developing norms for subsequent editions of the Stanford, although use of the label "for the Hearing Impaired" has been eliminated. These newer editions are popular assessment measures for use with Deaf or hard-of-hearing individuals (Allen, 1984; Kelly & Braden, 1990; Spragins, 1997).

Stanford Achievement Test–Eighth Edition

The *Stanford Achievement Test–Eighth Edition* (SAT-8; The Psychological Corporation, 1992) was normed with deaf and hard-of-hearing students about a year after its initial release (Spragins, 1996). Research indicates that individuals who attended nonintegrated school settings had lower SAT-8 scores than did individuals who attended special day or residential programs. Interestingly, individuals who attended integrated local educational programs performed best. However, the researchers caution that it is not clear if students performed better due to the integrated setting or if individuals were placed in integrated settings due to higher functioning initially (Holt, 1993; Spragins, 1996).

Stanford Achievement Test–Ninth Edition

The *Stanford Achievement Test–Ninth Edition* (SAT-9; Harcourt Assessment, 1996a) used with Deaf or hard-of-hearing participants is identical to that used in assessing hearing individuals (GRI, 1996a). The SAT-9 is available in eight difficulty levels (Harcourt Assessment, 1996b). Because it is essential to select a battery that is at a level appropriate to the person being tested, various technical manuals to assist in selection of subtest levels appropriate for Deaf and hard-of-hearing participants are available, as are guides for result interpretation (Allen, 1996; GRI, 1996b, 1996d, 1996e; Holt, 1994; Holt et al., 1997; Traxler, 1996). Additionally, special norms for Deaf students are available, making this instrument an appealing choice (Center for Assessment and Demographic Studies, 1989, 1991; GRI, 1996c). While the SAT-9 has a number of advantages, some limitations exist. The SAT-9 subtests in mathematics are more dependent on verbal information than in previous editions and may be more difficult for individuals with more severe hearing loss. Additionally, the instrument has been more useful with average rather then well-advanced test takers, making it difficult to determine an actual achievement level for high-performing participants (Spragins, 1997).

Stanford Achievement Test–Tenth Edition

Unlike previous editions, the *Stanford Achievement Test–Tenth Edition* (SAT-10; Harcourt Assessment, 2002) is not timed, removing the need for extended time as an accommodation. The publisher reports that (a) the wide use of untimed high-stakes assessments in schools nationwide, (b) a growing body of research indicating that ability is more critical in assessment than rate of answering and student performance has little relationship to the time used to complete the test, and (c) an interest in accommodating individuals with disabilities influenced the change (Case, 2004). The GRI provides screening tests in reading and mathematics for use with the SAT-10, and it is possible for results to indicate the need to administer more than one level of SAT-10 subtests to an individual (GRI, 2003b).

In sum, when interpreting results of achievement tests with Deaf persons, it is important to be aware that only about 2% of graduates from day and residential schools for the Deaf attain a 10th-grade level in educational achievement, 41% reach 7th- or 8th-grade levels, 27% reach 5th- or 6th-grade levels, and approximately 30% are at or below a 3rd-grade level or have no functional literacy (GRI, 2003a). Research demonstrates that individuals with mild to moderate hearing losses score significantly higher on standardized achievement measures than individuals who have severe or profound hearing loss. The presence or absence of additional conditions further influences performance; individuals who have an additional disability or multiple disabilities along with hearing loss perform much less well than individuals who have a hearing loss only (Holt, 1993; Spragins, 1996).

Aptitude and Interest Testing

In public rehabilitation, more Deaf and hard-of-hearing consumers are placed in noncompensated jobs than any other disability group (Capella, 2003). Since a goal of many rehabilitation services is competitive, gainful, full-time employment, meaningful work-related assessments of consumers who are Deaf or hard of hearing are an appropriate professional tool. Aptitude and interest testing is often a basic part of a thorough psychological assessment, particularly with teenagers and adults in the process of vocational exploration and choice. Although hundreds of aptitude and interest tests are available to assist in discovering the particular abilities that a client may have, many are verbal and few may be readily accessible to individuals who are Deaf or hard of hearing. In many instances, general aptitude may be more appropriately and thoroughly assessed with intelligence or achievement measures (Spragins, 1996; Spragins et al., 1993). Interest tests, too, are often highly verbal and may have limited utility for people who are congenitally or profoundly Deaf. A key to choosing from among the myriad options involves selecting an instrument for consumers who are Deaf or hard of hearing that is not primarily dependent on language or literacy, such as the *Reading Free Vocational Interest Inventory: 2* (Becker, 2000) and the *Geist Picture Interest Inventory–Revised* (Geist, 1988).

Reading Free Vocational Interest Inventory: 2

Reading-Free Vocational Interest Inventory: 2 (RFVII: 2; Becker, 2000) is a picture-format, reading- and writing-free interest inventory appropriate for ages 13 and older. The RFVII has been used successfully with Deaf or hard-of-hearing individuals, and the pictorial items may be described by the examiner or an interpreter using manual communication as needed (Spragins et al., 1993). Using the RFVII, an individual is exposed to a wide range of occupations, indicating preferences by selecting one of three drawings depicting job tasks from the unskilled, semiskilled, and skilled levels. Because it was designed for people with learning or intellectual disabilities, it focuses more on work preferences at the unskilled and semiskilled levels than on skilled employment options, limiting its utility for many Deaf or hard-of-hearing individuals. While learning skilled trades offers economic benefit and possible economic security, vocational education comprised of training programs geared toward manual labor or trade-specific work may be viewed as limiting (Leakey, 1993).

Geist Picture Interest Inventory–Revised

The *Geist Picture Interest Inventory–Revised* (GPII-R; Geist, 1988) is a widely used measure of vocational and leisure interests. It is suitable for age groups spanning late junior high to adulthood so it may be useful in transition planning. It is also helpful that it requires little reading and can be self-administered. The GPII-R includes separate male and female general interest areas (Geist, 1988). The *Geist Picture Interest Inventory: Deaf: Male* (GPII: D: M; Geist, 1962) was developed from the first edition of the instrument for use with Deaf or hard-of-hearing males only. A large normative sample was selected from students at Gallaudet University, 20 residential schools, and a group of employed Deaf men, among others. Although the instrument is one of the very few to provide norms for Deaf consumers, the usability of the GPII: D: M is limited by its gender specificity (Zieziula, 1986).

Historically, the school experiences of people who are deaf or hard of hearing have centered on vocational training programs rather than academic or college-bound tracks (Leakey, 1993), and their rehabilitation experiences have focused more on basic restoration and interpreting services and less on postsecondary education (Capella, 2003). Some individuals who are Deaf or hard of hearing may prematurely reject or forgo certain career choices due to perceived barriers and limited awareness of available options and accommodations (Punch, Creed, & Hyde, 2006). Often, the occupational interests and employment trends of individuals who are Deaf or hard of hearing reflect typical school and service provisions experiences. Research indicates that people who are Deaf or hard of hearing are less likely than hearing peers to be employed in white-collar jobs and tend to have significantly lower levels of family income than hearing adults (Allen, 1994a; Brodwin, Parker, & DeLaGarza, 1996; Lucas et al., 2004). However, individuals who participate in work- and career-related experiences as young adults are more aware of their own vocational aptitudes and interests and are more likely to consider a wider variety of career options than those who do not participate in such programs. Additionally, early participation in career exploration and development activities, including aptitude and interest assessments, has been shown to positively affect career decision-making skills (Schroedel, 1991).

Communication Skills Appraisal

Because a major challenge associated with hearing loss is in the area of communication, it is important to include an evaluation of communication skills in a comprehensive assessment. A thorough appraisal may include audiological testing for an evaluation of current hearing function; changes in hearing status may determine the selection of evaluative instruments. Importantly, assessments should be responsive to the anticipated purposes and contexts of a person's communication skills since individuals tend to communicate differently in different situations due to cultural factors, gender, age, the relative formality or informality of the settings, educational background, and social status (Hoemann, 1986). An individual's abilities in written, spoken, and signed language may all potentially be assessed.

Assessment of Written and Spoken Language

Competence in written and spoken language may have a role in the types and levels of occupations that are available to the individual, so assessment of literacy skills may be important. Along with other achievement or academic ability measures, the Spelling, Language, Reading Comprehension, and Word Reading subtests of the SAT-10 may all provide good information regarding a person's language-related abilities and achievement (Mounty et al., 2005). In addition, speech and speech reading should be quantified. Speech and speech reading are best evaluated by well-trained speech and language professionals who will evaluate speech sound production; fluency; and other aspects of speech, language, and hearing. Although an evaluation of an individual's speech-reading skills can be valuable, the rehabilitation professional is cautioned that many adults and children who are Deaf do not speak or speech read well, and while the ability to speech-read is an asset, even the most skilled speech readers may find this an inadequate way to obtain important information (Vernon, 1996).

Sign Language Skill Assessment

Sign language skills should be evaluated because they may be highly useful across a variety of settings and create the option of using a sign language interpreter when appropriate. In general, there are both direct and indirect methods with which to evaluate sign language abilities (Mounty et al., 2005). Direct methods involve the use of more formal and specific language activities or tasks in order to measure specific responses. The *Signed Language Development Checklist* (SLDC; Mounty, 1994), the *Gallaudet University American Sign Language Proficiency Interview* (GU-ASLPI; Center for American Sign Language Literacy, 2000), along with more general language proficiency interviews are all examples of direct measures. These tools all utilize a question-and-answer format in order to assess how well the participant uses a target language. Although checklists and proficiency interviews are widely used, the methodology is not without criticism (Mounty et al., 2005). Johnson (2001) suggests that a person may not have the opportunity to fully demonstrate his or her language skills since questions-and-answer formats do not recreate real-life conversational situations and do not include a realistic conversational exchange.

Indirect communication appraisals include the collection of language samples in natural situations or settings. Using indirect naturalistic methods involves observing and recording language in settings typical to the individual, such as the home, classroom, or workplace, and then rating or coding the results to develop a profile of proficiency (Mounty et al., 2005; Reeves & Newell, 2000). Although naturalistic assessments may result in more breadth and depth than more formalized approaches, they are also vulnerable to variations in data collection and analysis related to the philosophy and expertise of the evaluator. However, by combining direct and indirect communication assessment methods and then considering results within the context of other information, a more holistic view of individual ability may be gained (Mounty et al., 2005).

To summarize, in any communication skills assessment, it is crucial that rehabilitation professionals not confuse difficulty in communication with lack of intelligence. A person who is congenitally Deaf can have a very high IQ, yet have written language that is not grammatically correct or, in some cases, not understandable. Those who work with adults or children who are Deaf need to be aware of these factors in order to better facilitate fair and meaningful evaluations for individuals who are Deaf or hard of hearing, and it is important for evaluators to be professionally prepared in language testing.

Case History Data

The best psychiatric and psychological evaluations are often based largely upon background information (Vernon & Andrews, 1990). In addition to the various formal and informal assessments used in comprehensive rehabilitation service planning and provision, a review of case history data including educational, medical, and social services records is a valuable source of information. Case history data can be especially important when serving consumers who are Deaf or hard of hearing since they may not be accurately evaluated by regular psychological procedures. Often, past case history data provide a good prediction of future needs. It is usually possible to obtain a great deal of information on young adults by contacting their schools, especially residential or large day programs. Integrated educational programs (i.e., facilities with both students who are deaf and those who are hearing) may also provide valuable data if they have teachers or consultants who are qualified to work with youth with hearing loss. An adult's case history may include information on past job performance, any particular concerns or assets, the circumstances that have led to the individual's success, and the specific educational and vocational skills that have been mastered.

Assessments of Persons Who Are Deaf-Blind

The majority of individuals who are Deaf-Blind have acquired one or both disabilities, but there are also distinct genetically based syndromes that cause Deaf-Blindness, including Usher syndrome (Kimberling & Möller, 1995), which causes congenital hearing loss or deafness and progressive blindness due to retinitis pigmentosa (Rönnberg, Samuelson, & Borg, 2002). Deaf-Blindness may also be acquired through the aging processes, brain injury, or infectious diseases affecting a person who already has a hearing loss or low or no vision. The legal definition of Deaf-Blindness adheres to the definitions for deafness and blindness, respectively. Individuals who are both Deaf and blind represent a very small fraction of the population. Accordingly, research related to the assessment needs of people who are Deaf-Blind may be hampered by the small sample size available for investigation (Loew et al., 2005). Additionally, the deaf-blind population is as heterogeneous and varied in etiology as the Deaf and hard-of-hearing population. Deaf-Blind consumers may present significant challenges relative to evaluation and diagnosis. While few instruments exist for assessment of individuals who are Deaf-Blind, the *Callier-Azusa Scale* (Stillman, 1978) and the *Functional Skills Screening Inventory* (Becker, Schur, Paoletti-Schelp, & Hammer, 1984) are noteworthy.

The *Callier-Azusa Scale*

The *Callier-Azusa Scale* (Stillman, 1978a) has been designed specifically for individuals who have both hearing and vision loss. The instrument is primarily for people who are older than 9 years of age and are low functioning (Vernon, Blair, & Lotz, 1979). The publisher indicates the instrument has been thoroughly field tested. Using direct observation to evaluate visual, auditory, and tactile development, the G edition assesses motor development, perceptual abilities, daily living skills, language development, and social skills (Stillman, 1978b). An H edition assesses communication abilities including symbolic skills, receptive and expressive abilities, and communication reciprocity (Stillman & Battle, 1985).

The *Functional Skills Screening Inventory*

The *Functional Skills Screening Inventory* (FSSI; Becker et al., 1984) was developed for use with individuals with moderate to severe disabilities, although not specifically for individuals who are Deaf, blind, or both. However, it has been used successfully with people who are Deaf-Blind (Hammer & Carlson, 1996). The FSSI evaluates basic functional skills and concepts, communication, personal care, domestic skills, work skills and concepts, community living skills, social awareness, and challenging behaviors and allows for the individual's functioning to be tracked over time. The scale emphasizes the individual's assets, rather than focusing on deficits (Becker et al., 1984; Hammer & Carlson, 1996).

Both the *Callier-Azusa Scale* and the FSSI rely on observer ratings and informant data, so both may have a high degree of subjectivity. For adults who are Deaf-Blind, an extensive case history is an excellent option for alternative assessment, although the danger of misdiagnosis may still exist. If possible, the client should have an extended evaluation at a facility like the Helen Keller National Center for Deaf-Blind Youths and Adults in Sands Point, New York (Vernon & Green, 1980). When such intensive evaluations are not practical, however, every effort should be made to provide meaningful assessment accommodations.

Accommodations for Individuals Who Are Deaf-Blind

Accommodations appropriate to consumers who are Deaf-Blind may be widely varied and are often provided in combination, making it difficult to determine which strategies or modifications were most useful (Loew et al., 2005). While facilitating the use of the sense of touch would appear to be the most obvious accommodation, research has indicated that many individuals who are Deaf-Blind prefer to use any residual vision as their preferred strategy. Preferences for residual vision are closely followed by residual hearing, perception of airflow, and sense of smell (Rönnberg et al., 2002). Above all, individual preferences should guide the choice of accommodations used by people who are Deaf-Blind. Thorough preparation and the opportunity to practice implementing and using accommodations in advance are critical aspects of accommodation success (Weinstock & Mounty, 2005; Zieziula, 1986). Braden (2001) further notes that appropriate accommodations for assessments may be guided by both clinical experience and intuition. Most importantly, accommodations should result from collaboration among the person being evaluated; the examiner; and other relevant service providers such as audiologists, interpreters, and caregivers.

Conclusion

A complete assessment battery for rehabilitation purposes may include intelligence testing, personality testing and screening for brain injury, educational achievement testing, aptitude and interest testing, communication skills evaluation, and a review of case history data. In some cases not all of this information will be needed, or, if needed, data may be obtained in part from records or other sources. Test selection may be influenced by the needs and preferences of the consumer and the nature of the assessment instrument. Etiological factors, age of onset, the presence of other disabilities, preferred mode of communication, and other social and educational experiences may further affect formal assessments (Zieziula, 1986). Throughout this chapter, four general principles have overarched all forms of assessments of individuals who are Deaf or hard of hearing. Several key themes related to the future directions of assessment of individuals who are Deaf or hard of hearing are also noteworthy.

General Assessment Principles

Four basic concepts are involved in effective assessment of individuals who are Deaf or hard of hearing, superseding specific considerations related to particular instruments. These broad recommendations are applicable to both selecting and administering tests.

1. Information obtained from assessment instruments that depend on verbal language for either administration or evaluation of performance is generally not appropriate for individuals who are Deaf or hard of hearing because such instruments measure primarily the individual's language limitations due to Deafness, not the intelligence, personality, abilities, achievement, or other characteristics of the individuals (Mounty & Martin, 2005; Weinstock & Mounty, 2005).

2. Consumers who are congenitally hard of hearing may be more diagnostically similar to a person who is congenitally Deaf than their functional speech and response to sound might indicate. Thus, it may be appropriate to assess hard-of-hearing individuals using measures found to work well for individuals with profound hearing loss in addition to tests for individuals without hearing loss in order to obtain the most valid results. Careful attention should be paid to the use of instruments that are primarily screening techniques, not in-depth procedures, and results should be interpreted and applied accordingly.

3. The use of standardized assessment instruments should be one part of a more comprehensive approach to assessing individuals who are Deaf or hard of hearing that includes case history data and a thorough records review. It is of critical importance to obtain complete background information on clients who are Deaf since they may not be

accurately evaluated by regular psychological procedures. The best psychiatric and psychological evaluations are often based 75% on background information (Vernon & Andrews, 1990).

4. Tests administered by professionals who are not experienced with clients who are Deaf or hard of hearing are prone to more error than those given by professionals who are very familiar with the special needs of individuals who are Deaf or hard of hearing. Because of the dearth of research demonstrating the type of responses that could be anticipated from Deaf or hard-of-hearing individuals, examiners need considerable familiarity with and understanding of Deaf culture and other educational and social issues related to Deafness. With any instrument, it is important for the examiner to note the accommodations provided and the degree to which the participant appears to have understood the evaluation (Spragins, 1997; Spragins et al., 1993).

Future Directions

The future directions of assessment of individuals who are Deaf or hard of hearing seem to be most likely influenced by trends in increasing diversity, trends toward the medical treatment and management of hearing loss, and trends related to the issue of high stakes testing. Allen (1994a) notes that the increase in diversity within the Deaf and hard-of-hearing population will need a commensurate diversification of service plans and options from rehabilitation and related professionals. Additionally, cochlear implants and other augmentative sensory aids and prostheses have become more sophisticated and gained greater acceptance, including within the Deaf community, providing some Deaf and hard-of-hearing people more access to sound than ever before (Christiansen & Leigh, 2002; National Center for Health Statistics, 2002). Rehabilitation professionals will need greater familiarity with the technologies available and the costs, benefits, and limitations of the latest options. Last, it is likely that the use of high stakes testing will increase in secondary, postsecondary, and employment settings (Johnson, 2005). Professional guidance in preparation and study materials and in developing appropriate accommodations is linked to success on high stakes measures for individuals who are Deaf and hard of hearing (Johnson, 2005; Weinstock & Mounty, 2005; Zieziula, 1986). Communication, experience, and knowledge facilitate optimal outcomes for both rehabilitation professionals and consumers who are Deaf or hard of hearing.

References

Allen, T. E. (1984, April). *Out-of-level testing with the Stanford Achievement Test (Seventh Edition): A procedure for assigning students to the correct battery level.* Paper presented at the annual meeting of the American Educational Research Association, New Orleans, LA.

Allen, T. E. (1994a). *Who are the deaf and hard-of-hearing students leaving high school and entering postsecondary education?* Retrieved May 19, 2006, from http://gri.gallaudet.edu/Annual Survey/whodeaf.html.

Allen, T. E. (1994b). *How many people in the USA and Canada use ASL as a primary language and how many use it as their second or other language?* Washington, DC: Gallaudet Research Institute, Gallaudet University.

Allen, T. E. (1996). *Stanford Achievement Test, 9th Edition, and WISC-III and their use with deaf and hard-of-hearing students: Progress report.* Retrieved June 25, 2006, from http://www.gallaudet.edu/~cadsweb/satprogr.html.

Allen, T. E., White, C. S., & Karchmer, M. A. (1983). Issues in the development of a special edition for hearing-impaired students of the seventh edition of the Stanford Achievement Test. *American Annals of the Deaf, 128*(1), 34–39.

American National Standards Institute. (1996). *Specification for audiometers (ANSI S3.6-1996).* New York: Author.

American National Standards Institute. (1997). *Method for manual pure-tone threshold audiometry (ANSI S3.21-1978).* New York: Author.

American National Standards Institute. (2003). *Maximum permissible ambient noise levels for audiometric test rooms* (ANSI S3.1-1999). New York: Author.

Baker-Shenk, C., & Cokely, D. (1980). *American Sign Language: A teacher's resource text on grammar and culture.* Silver Spring, MD: TJ Publishers.

Becker, H., Schur, S., Paoletti-Schelp, M., & Hammer, E. (1984). *The Functional Skills Screening Inventory.* Amarillo, TX: Functional Resources Enterprises.

Becker, R. L. (2000). *Reading Free Vocational Interest Inventory: 2 (RFVII:2).* Columbus, OH: Elbern.

Bender, L. (1938). *A visual motor gestalt test and its clinical use.* New York: American Orthopsychiatric Association.

Blennerhassett, L. (2000). Psychological Assessments. In N. Kitson & P. Hindley (Eds.), *Mental health and deafness* (pp. 185–205). London: Whurr Publishers LTD.

Blennerhassett, L., Strohmeier, S. J., & Hibbett, C. (1994). Criterion-related validity of Raven's Progressive Matrices with deaf residential school students. *American Annals of the Deaf, 139*(2), 104–110.

Bolton, B. (1972). Quantification of two projective tests for deaf clients. *Journal of Clinical Psychology, 28*(4), 554–556.

Bolton, B., Donoghue, R., & Langbauer, W. (1973). Quantification of two projective tests for deaf clients: A large sample validation study. *Journal of Clinical Psychology, 29*(2), 249–250.

Braden, J. (1994). *Deafness deprivation and IQ.* New York: Plenum Press.

Braden, J. P. (2001). The clinical assessment of deaf people's cognitive abilities. In M. D. Clark, M. Marschark, & M. Karchmer (Eds.), *Context, cognition, and deafness* (pp. 14–37). Washington, DC: Gallaudet University Press.

Brannigan, G. G., & Decker, S. L. (2003). *Bender Visual Motor Gestalt Test, Second Edition: Bender-Gestalt II.* Itasca, IL: Riverside Publishing.

Brauer, B. A. (1992). The signer effect on MMPI performance of deaf respondents. *Journal of Personality Assessment, 58*(2), 380–388.

Brauer, B. A. (1993). Adequacy of a translation of the MMPI into American Sign Language for use with deaf individuals: Linguistic equivalency issues. *Rehabilitation Psychology, 38*(4), 247–260.

Briccetti, K. A. (1994). Emotional indicators of deaf children on the Draw-A-Person test. *American Annals of the Deaf, 139*(5), 500–505.

Brodwin, M. G., Parker, R. M., & DeLaGarza, D. (1996), Disability and accommodation. In E. M. Szymanski & R. M. Parker (Eds.), *Work and disability: Issues and strategies in career development and job placement* (pp. 165–207). Austin, TX: PRO-ED.

Brown, L., Sherbenou, R. J., & Johnsen, S. K. (1997). *Test of Nonverbal Intelligence-Third Edition (TONI-3).* Austin, TX: PRO-ED.

Buck, J. (1948). The H.T.P. technique: A qualitative and quantitative scoring manual. *Journal of Clinical Psychology, 4,* 151–159.

Buck, J. (1992). *The House-Tree-Person projective drawing technique: Manual and interpretive guide (revised).* Los Angeles, CA: Western Psychological Services.

Burns, R. C. (1987). *Kinetic-House-Tree-Person Drawings: An interpretative manual.* Los Angeles: Western Psychological Services.

Butcher, J., Dahlstrom, W., Graham, J., & Tellegen, A. (1989). *Minnesota Multiphasic Personality-Inventory II.* Minneapolis, MN: Regents of the University of Minnesota.

Capella, M. E. (2003). Evaluating differences in demographics, services, and outcomes for vocational rehabilitation consumers with hearing loss versus consumers with other disabilities. *Journal of Rehabilitation, 69*(3), 39–46.

Case, B. J. (2004). *It's about time: Stanford Achievement Test Series, tenth edition (Stanford 10).* San Antonio, TX: Harcourt Assessment.

Center for American Sign Language Literacy. (2000). *American Sign Language Assessment.* Washington, DC: Gallaudet University.

Center for Assessment and Demographic Studies. (1989). *Administering the 8th edition Stanford Achievement Test to hearing impaired students.* Washington, DC: Gallaudet Research Institute.

Center for Assessment and Demographic Studies. (1991). *Stanford Achievement Test 8th edition form J: Hearing impaired norms booklet.* Washington, DC: Gallaudet Research Institute.

Checklist (Revised). Washington, DC: Gallaudet University.

Collins, J. M., & Hunter, J. E. (2001, April). *Problems with the WAIS Intelligence Test 1938–1997.* Symposium Presentation at the Annual Conference of the Society for Industrial and Organizational Psychologists, San Diego.

Dickert, J. (1988). Examination of Bias in Mental Health Evaluation of Deaf Patients. *Social Work, 33*(3), 273–274.

Drossman, E. R., Maller, S. J., & McDermott, P. A. (2001). Core profiles of school-aged examinees from the national standardization sample of the Comprehensive Test of Nonverbal Intelligence. *School Psychology Review, 30*(4), 586–598.

Elliot, H. (1987). Educational history. In H. Elliot, L. Glass, & J. Evans (Eds.), *Mental health assessment of deaf clients: A practical manual* (pp. 71–75). London: Taylor & Francis.

Evans, J. W., & Elliott, H. (1981). Screening criteria for the diagnosis of schizophrenia in deaf patients. *Archives of General Psychiatry, 38*(7), 787–790.

Exner, J. E., Jr. (2001). *A Rorschach Workbook for the Comprehensive System* (5th ed.). Asheville, NC: Rorschach Workshops.

Flanagan, D. P., McGrew, K. S., & Ortiz, S. O. (2000). *The Wechsler Intelligence Scales and Gf-Gc theory: A contemporary approach to interpretation.* Boston: Allyn & Bacon.

Flexor, C. (1999). *Facilitating hearing and listening in young children.* Clifton Park, NY: Delmar Learning.

French, D. B. (1987). Validity, test bias, and the use of the Special Edition of the Stanford Achievement Test for the Hearing Impaired (SAT-HI) with Canadian students. *ACEHI Journal, 13*(3), 104–116.

Gallaudet Research Institute. (1996a). *Achievement Testing of Deaf and Hard-of-hearing Students: The 9th Edition Stanford Achievement Test.* Washington, DC: Gallaudet University.

Gallaudet Research Institute. (1996b). *Stanford Achievement Test. Conversion Tables: Stanford 9 Scaled Scores to SAT-8 Scaled Scores*. Washington, DC: Gallaudet University.

Gallaudet Research Institute. (1996c). *Stanford Achievement Test, 9th Edition, Form S: Norms booklet for Deaf and hard-of-hearing students*. Washington, DC: Gallaudet University.

Gallaudet Research Institute. (1996d). *Stanford Achievement Test, 9th Edition. Administration procedures for deaf and hard-of-hearing students*. Washington, DC: Gallaudet University.

Gallaudet Research Institute. (1996e). *Stanford Achievement Test, 9th Edition. Screening procedures for deaf and hard-of-hearing students*. Washington, DC: Gallaudet University.

Gallaudet Research Institute. (2003a). *Regional and national summary report of data from the 2002–2003 annual survey of deaf and hard-of-hearing children and youth*. Washington, DC: Author.

Gallaudet Research Institute. (2003b). *Frequently asked questions about the Stanford Achievement Test 10th edition with deaf and hard-of-hearing students*. Washington, DC: Gallaudet University.

Gallaudet University School Psychology Handbook. (1994). *Communication Policy*. Washington, DC: Gallaudet University.

Geist, H. (1962). *The Geist Picture Interest Inventory: Deaf form: Male*. Los Angeles: Western Psychological Services.

Geist, H. (1988). *Geist picture interest inventory-Revised (GPII-R)*. Beverly Hills, CA: Western Psychological Services.

Gibbins, S. (1989). The provision of school psychological assessment services for the hearing impaired. *Volta Review, 91*(2), 95–103.

Gierl, M. J. (2000). Construct equivalence on translated achievement test. *Canadian Journal of Education, 25*(4), 280–296.

Graham, F., & Kendall, B. (1960). *Memory-for-Designs Test: Revised General Manual*. Missoula, MT: Psychological Test Specialists.

Gregory, R. J. (1999). *Foundations of intellectual assessment: The WAIS-III and other tests in clinical practice*. Needham Heights, MA: Allyn & Bacon.

Hammer, E., & Carlson, R. (1996). Using the Intervener Model with adults who are Deaf-Blind. *Journal of Vocational Rehabilitation, 7*(1), 125–128.

Hammill, D. D., Pearson, N. A., & Wiederholt, J. L. (1997). *Comprehensive Test of Nonverbal Intelligence (CTONI)*. Austin, TX: PRO-ED.

Harcourt Assessment, The Psychological Corporation. (1996a). *The Stanford achievement test* (9th ed.). San Antonio, TX: Author.

Harcourt Assessment, The Psychological Corporation. (1996b). *Stanford Achievement Test Series: Technical data report* (9th ed.). San Antonio, TX: Author.

Harcourt Assessment, The Psychological Corporation. (2002). *The Stanford achievement test* (10th ed.). San Antonio, TX: Author.

Harcourt, Brace, & Jovanovich. (1972). *The Stanford Achievement Test* (6th ed.). San Antonio, TX: Harcourt Assessments.

Harcourt, Brace, & Jovanovich. (1973). *The Stanford Achievement Test for the Hearing Impaired*. San Antonio, TX: Harcourt Assessments.

Heller, B. (1987). Mental health assessment of deaf persons: A brief history. In H. Elliot, L. Glass, & J. W. Evans (Eds.), *Mental health assessment of deaf clients* (pp. 9–20). Boston: Little, Brown & Co.

Hindley, P. (2000) Child and adolescent psychiatry. In P. Hindley & N. Kitson (Eds.), *Mental Health and Deafness* (pp. 43–74). London: Whurr Publishers.

Hindley, P., Kitson, N., & Leach, V. (2000). Forensic psychiatry and deaf people. In P. Hindley & N. Kitson (Eds.), *Mental health and deafness* (pp. 206–231). London: Whurr Publishers.

Hiskey, M. S. (1966). *Hiskey-Nebraska Test of Learning Aptitude*. Lincoln, NE: Union College Press.

Hoemann, H. W. (1986). *Introduction to American Sign Language.* Bowling Green, OH: Bowling Green Press.

Holt, J. A. (1993). Stanford Achievement Test–8th Edition for deaf and hard-of-hearing students: Reading Comprehension subgroup results. *American Annals of the Deaf,* Online edition. Retrieved April 23, 2007, from http://gri.gallaudet.edu/Assessment/sat-read.html.

Holt, J. A. (1994). Classroom attributes and achievement test scores for deaf and hard-of-hearing students. *American Annals of the Deaf, 139*(4), 430–437.

Holt, J. A., Traxler, C. B., & Allen, T. E. (1997). Interpreting the scores: A user's guide to the 9th edition Stanford Achievement Test for students who are deaf or hard-of-hearing. *Gallaudet Research Institute Technical Report, 97,* 1.

Johnson, E., Kimball, K., & Brown, S. O. (2001). American sign language as an accommodation during standards-based assessments. *Assessment for Effective Intervention, 26*(2), 39–47.

Johnson, M. (2001). *The art of nonconversation: A reexamination of the validity of the oral proficiency interview.* New Haven: Yale University Press.

Johnson, R. C. (2005). Epilogue: Fort Monroe revisited. In J. L. Mounty & D. S. Martin (Eds.), *Assessing deaf adults: Critical issues in testing and education* (pp. 174–179). Washington, DC: Gallaudet University Press.

Kaufman, A. S., & Lichtenberger, E. O. (1999). *Essentials of WAIS-HI Assessment.* New York: Wiley.

Kelly, M., & Braden, J. (1990). Criterion-related validity of the WISC-R Performance Scale with the Stanford Achievement Test-Hearing-Impaired Edition. *Journal of Special Education, 26*(3), 235–252.

Kimberling, W. J., & Möller, C. (1995). Clinical and molecular genetics of Usher syndrome. *Journal of the American Academy of Audiology, 6*(1), 63–72.

Kitson, N., & Thacker, A. (2000). Adult psychiatry. In P. Hindley & N. Kitson (Eds.). *Mental health and deafness* (pp. 75–98). London: Whurr Publishers.

Kochkin, S. (2005). MarkeTrak VII: Hearing loss population tops 31 million people. *The Hearing Review, 12*(7), 16–29.

Koppitz, E. (1963). *The Bender-Gestalt Test for Young Children: Koppitz scoring system.* New York: Grune & Stratton.

Ladd, P. (2003). *Understanding deaf culture: In search of deafhood.* Buffalo, NY: Multilingual Matters.

Lane, H. (1992). *The mask of benevolence: Disabling the deaf community.* New York: Alfred A. Knopf.

Lane, H., Hoffmeister, R., & Bahan, B. (1996). *A journey into the deaf world.* San Diego, CA: Dawn Sign Press.

LaVigne, M., & Vernon, M. (2003). An interpreter isn't enough: Deafness, language, and due process. *Wisconsin Law Review, 5,* 844–935.

Leakey, T. A. (1993). Vocational education in deaf American and African-American communities. In J. V. Van Cleve (Ed.), *Deaf history unveiled: Interpretations from the new scholarship* (pp. 74–91). Washington, DC: Gallaudet University Press.

Levine, E. S. (1981). *The psychology of early deafness.* New York: Columbia University Press.

Lipton, D. S., & Goldstein, M. F. (1997). Measuring substance abuse among the deaf. *Journal of Drug Issues, 27*(4), 733–754.

Loew, R., Cahalan-Laitusis, C., Cook, L., & Harris, R. (2005). Access considerations and the provision of appropriate accommodations: A research perspective from a testing organization. In J. L. Mounty & D. S. Martin (Eds.), *Assessing deaf adults: Critical issues in testing and evaluation* (pp. 37–53). Washington, DC: Gallaudet University Press.

Lucas, J. W., Schiller, J. S., & Benson, V. (2004). *Summary health statistics for U.S. adults: National health interview survey, 2001: Vital & health statistics, 10(218). (DHHS Publication No. PHS 2004-1546).* Hyattsville, MD: U.S. Department of Health and Human Services.

Machover, K. (1949). *Personality projection in the drawing of the human figure.* Springfield, IL: Charles C. Thomas.

Mandes, E., & Gessner, T. (1989). The principle of additivity and its relation to clinical decision making. *Journal of Psychology: Interdisciplinary and Applied, 123*(5), 485–490.

Markwardt, F. C. Jr. (1997). *Peabody Individual Achievement Test Normative Update (PIAT-R NU).* Circle Pines, MN: American Guidance Service.

Martin, D. S., & McCrone, W. (1990). Testing the hearing-impaired teacher: Is fairness possible? *Journal of Personnel Evaluation in Education, 3*(2), 169–178.

Massad, C. E. (2005). Considerations in developing licensing tests that are accessible for all candidates. In J. L. Mounty & D. S. Martin (Eds.), *Assessing deaf adults: Critical issues in testing and evaluation* (pp. 65–74). Washington, DC: Gallaudet University Press.

Moores, D. (1978). *Educating the Deaf: Psychology, principles, and practices.* Boston: Houghton Mifflin.

Moores, D. F. (1996). Educational options for the deaf and hard-of-hearing. In R. L. Schow & M. A. Nerbonne (Eds.), *Introduction to audiologic rehabilitation* (3rd ed., pp. 264–286). Boston: Allyn & Bacon.

Morgan, A., & Vernon, M. (1994). A guide to the diagnosis of learning disability in deaf and hard-of-hearing individuals. *American Annals of the Deaf, 139*(3), 358–370.

Mounty, J. (1994). *Signed language development checklist.* Princeton, NJ: Educational Testing Service.

Mounty, J. L., Gordon, J. M., Mitchiner, B. S., & Arellano, L. (2005). *Faculty assessment project.* Washington, DC: Gallaudet University.

Mounty, J. L., & Martin, D. S. (2005). *Assessing deaf adults: Critical issues in testing and evaluation.* Washington, DC: Gallaudet University Press.

Naglieri, J., & Welch, J. (1991). Use of Raven's and Naglieri's nonverbal matrix tests. *Journal of the American Deafness and Rehabilitation Association, 24*(3), 98–103.

National Center for Health Statistics. (1996). *Vital and health statistics series 10,(200).* Washington, DC: Author.

National Center for Health Statistics. (2002). *Trends and differential use of assistive technology devices: United States, 1994.* Washington, DC: Author.

Noble, W., & Atherley, G. (1970). The Hearing Measurement Scale: A questionnaire for the assessment of auditory disability. *Journal of Auditory Research, 10,* 229.

Osgood, R. (2005). *The history of inclusion in the United States.* Washington, DC: Gallaudet University Press.

Padden, C., & Humphries, T. (2005). *Inside deaf culture.* Cambridge, MA: Harvard University Press.

Parker, R. M., & Bolton, B. (2005). Psychological assessment in rehabilitation. In R. M. Parker, E. M. Szymanski, & J. B. Patterson (Eds.), *Rehabilitation counseling: Basics and beyond* (4th ed., pp. 307–334). Austin, TX: PRO-ED.

Pleis, J. R., & Coles, R. (2002). *Summary health statistics for U. S. adults: National health interview survey, 1998. Vital & Health Statistics 10(209).* Washington, DC: National Center for Health Statistics.

Psychological Corporation. (1992). *The Stanford Achievement Test* (8th ed.). San Antonio, TX: Author.

Punch, R., Creed, P. A., & Hyde, M. B. (2006). Career barriers perceived by hard-of-hearing adolescents: Implications for practice from a mixed-methods study. *Journal of Deaf Studies and Deaf Education, 11*(2), 224–237.

Ragosta, M. (2005). Historical reflections on testing individuals who are deaf and hard-of-hearing. In J. L. Mounty & D. S. Martin (Eds.), *Assessing deaf adults: Critical issues in testing and evaluation* (pp. 11–23). Washington, DC: Gallaudet University Press.

Raifman, L. J., & Vernon, M. (1996). Important implications for psychologists of the American with Disabilities Act: Case in point, the patient who is deaf. *Professional Psychology: Research and Practice, 27*(4), 372–377.

Raven, J. C. (1948). *Progressive Matrices.* New York: Psychological Corporation.

Raven, J. C., Court, J. H., & Raven, J. (1977). *Raven's Progressive Matrices and Vocabulary Scales.* New York: Psychological Corporation.

Reeves, J. B., & Newell, W. (2000). The sign language skills classroom observation: A process for describing sign language proficiency in classroom settings. *American Annals of the Deaf, 145*(4), 315–341.

Riley-Glassman, N. D. (1989). Discriminating clinic from control groups of deaf adults using a short form of the Brauer-Gallaudet American Sign Language translation of the Minnesota Multiphasic Personality Inventory. *Dissertation Abstracts International, 50*(5-B). (AAT No. 8919056)

Rogers, P. (2005). Sign language interpretation in testing environments. In J. L. Mounty & D. S. Martin (Eds.), *Assessing deaf adults: Critical issues in testing and evaluation* (pp. 109–122). Washington, DC: Gallaudet University Press.

Roid, G. H., & Miller, L. (1997). *The Leiter International Performance Scale—Revised.* Chicago: Stoelting Company.

Rönnberg, J., Samuelsson, E., & Borg, E. (2002). Exploring the perceived world of the deaf-blind: On the development of an instrument. *International Journal of Audiology, 41*(2), 136–142.

Rorschach, H. (1942). *Psychodiagnostics.* Berne, Switzerland: Hans Huber.

Rosen, A. (1967). Limitations of personality inventories for assessment of deaf individuals as illustrated by research with the MMPI. *Journal of Rehabilitation of the Deaf, 1*(2), 47–52.

Schein, J. D. (1989). *At home among strangers.* Washington, DC: Gallaudet University Press.

Schick, B., Williams, K., & Kupermintz, H. (2006). Look who's being left behind: Educational interpreters and access to education for deaf and hard-of-hearing students. *Journal of Deaf Studies and Deaf Education, 11*(1), 3–20.

Schroedel, J. G. (1991) Improving the career decisions of deaf seniors in residential and day high schools. *American Annals of the Deaf, 136*(4), 330–338.

Schwartz, N. S., Mebane, D. L., & Malony, H. N. (1990). Effects of alternate modes of administration on Rorschach performance on deaf adults. *Journal of Personality Assessment, 54*(3), 671–683.

Smart, J. (2001). *Disability, society, and the individual.* Austin, TX: PRO-ED.

Spragins, A. B. (1996). *Reviews of four types of assessment instruments used with deaf and hard-of-hearing students: Tests of academic skills.* Gallaudet Research Institute. Retrieved April 23, 2007, from http://gri.gallaudet.edu/~catraxle/ACADEMIC.html.

Spragins, A. B. (1997). *Reviews of four types of assessment instruments used with deaf and hard-of-hearing students: 1997–1998 update.* Gallaudet Research Institute. Retrieved April 23, 2007, from http://gri.gallaudet.edu/~catraxle/reviews.html.

Spragins, A. B., Blennerhassett, L., & Mullen, Y. (1993). *Review of five types of assessment instruments used with deaf and hard-of-hearing students.* Washington, DC: Gallaudet University Press.

Stillman, R. (1978a). *Callier-Azusa Scale.* Dallas, TX: University of Texas at Dallas.

Stillman, R. (1978b). *Callier-Azusa Scale (G), cognitive development subscale.* Dallas, TX: University of Texas at Dallas.

Stillman, R., & Battle, C. (1985). *Callier-Azusa Scale (H), scales for the assessment of communicative abilities.* Dallas, TX: University of Texas at Dallas.

Traxler, C. B. (1996). *Frequently Asked Questions about the Stanford Achievement Test. Gallaudet Research Institute.* Retrieved April 23, 2007, from http://gri.gallaudet.edu/~catraxle/sat-faq.html.

Trybus, R. J., & Jensema, C. (1976). *The development, use, and interpretation of the 1973 Stanford Achievement Test, Special Edition for Hearing Impaired Students.* Washington, DC: Gallaudet University.

Trybus, R. J., & Karchmer, M. A. (1977). School achievement scores of hearing-impaired children: National data on achievement and growth patterns. *American Annals of the Deaf, 122*(2), 62-69.

Tsatsanis, K. D., Dartnall, N., Cicchetti, D., Sparrow, S. S., Klin, A., & Volkmar, F. R. (2003). Concurrent validity and classification accuracy of the Leiter and Leiter-R in low-functioning children with autism. *Journal of Autism and Developmental Disorders, 33*(1), 23–30.

Tye-Murry, N. (2004). *Foundations of aural rehabilitation: Children, adults, and their family members* (2nd ed.). Clifton Park, NY: Thomson Learning.

U.S. Department of Labor. (1982). *USES General Aptitude Test Battery for the Deaf: GATB for the Deaf.* Washington, DC: Author.

Vernon, M. (1996). Psychosocial aspects of hearing impairment. In R. L. Show & M. A. Nerbonne (Eds.), *Audiologic rehabilitation* (pp. 229–263). Needham, MA: Simon & Schuster.

Vernon, M., & Andrews, J. F. (1990). *The psychology of deafness: Understanding deaf and hard-of-hearing people.* White Plains, NY: Longman Press.

Vernon, M., & Green, D. (1980). A guide to the psychological assessment of deaf-blind adults. *Visual Impairment and Blindness, 74*(6), 229–230.

Vernon, M., & Hammer, E. (1996). The state of evaluation and diagnosis of deaf-blind people: Psychological and functional approaches. *Journal of Vocational Rehabilitation, 6*(2), 133–141.

Vernon, M., Blair, R., & Lotz, S. (1979). Psychological evaluation and testing of children who are deaf-blind. *School Psychology Digest, 8,* 291–295.

Vess, S. M., & Douglas, L. S. (1995). Program planning for children who are deaf or severely hard-of-hearing. In A. Thomas & J. Grimes (Eds.), *Best practices in school psychology–III* (pp. 1123–1133). Washington, DC: National Association of School Psychologists.

Wechsler, D. (1997). *WAIS-III Administration and Scoring Manual.* San Antonio, TX: Psychological Corporation.

Weinstock, R. B., & Mounty, J. L. (2005). Test-taking for deaf and hard-of-hearing individuals: Meeting the challenges. In J. L. Mounty & D. S. Martin, (Eds.), *Assessing deaf adults: Critical issues in testing and evaluation* (pp. 27–36). Washington, DC: Gallaudet University Press.

Wilber, L. A. (1999). Pure-tone audiometry: Air and bone conduction. In F. E. Musiek & W. F. Rintelmann (Eds.), *Contemporary perspectives in hearing assessment* (pp. 1–20). Boston, MA: Allyn & Bacon.

Wilkinson, G. S., & Robertson, G. J. (2006). *The Wide Range Achievement Test* (4th ed.). Wilmington, DE: Wide Range.

Wolk, S., & Zieziula, F. R. (1985). Reliability of the 1973 edition of the SAT-HI over time: Implications for assessing minority students. *American Annals of the Deaf, 130*(4), 285–290.

Zieziula, F. R. (Ed.). (1986). *Assessment of hearing-impaired people: A guide for selecting psychological, educational, and vocational tests.* Washington, DC: Gallaudet College Press.

Chapter 18

Assessment of Adults With Intellectual Disabilities

Sandra E. Hansmann and Irla Lee Zimmermann

Th his chapter provides a brief history of the concept of intellectual disability, also termed mental retardation, followed by discussion of current terminology trends and accepted definitions, focusing on definitions by the World Health Organization (WHO), the American Psychiatric Association (APA), and the American Association on Mental Retardation (AAMR). The chapter then critically reviews a variety of available instruments for evaluating individuals with intellectual disabilities in rehabilitation settings and concludes with a summary and suggested future directions for this unique area of assessment.

The Concept of Intellectual Disabilities

Hippocrates, often labeled the father of medicine, mentioned the condition of intellectual disabilities as early as 400 BCE, associating it with skull deformities. In the second century CE, the Greek physician Galen discussed different levels of mental skills (Miller, O'Callaghan, Keogh, & Whitman, 1994). Over the centuries, treatment of individuals with intellectual disabilities has varied widely and has been closely related to the beliefs and customs of a given era, culture, and location (Biasini, Grupe, Huffman, & Bray, 1999). For instance, during the Middle Ages, some individuals were persecuted, some were used as royal court fools, and still others were favored as holy innocents (Biasini, Grupe, Huffman, & Bray, 1999; Miller, O'Callaghan, Keogh, & Whitman, 1994). Circumstances changed little until the 19th century, when associations and schools were formed to serve the needs of individuals with cognitive differences and efforts were made to distinguish between people with intellectual disabilities and people with psychiatric disabilities (Scheerenberger, 1987).

Early in the 20th century, intelligence tests were introduced, resulting in the first modern definitions and diagnostic labels of intellectual disability. Increasing attempts were made to differentiate between the impact of genetics and that of environment on intellectual development, resulting in new diagnostic categories. Unfortunately, the diagnoses were often then used to consign individuals to institutions (Stevens & Martin, 1999).

In more recent years, a radical change has taken place in attitudes toward people with intellectual disabilities (McDermott, Martin, & Butkus, 1999). Increasing focus is placed on the strengths rather than the weaknesses of the individual (Polloway, 1997), and these changes are reflected in the terminology used in relation to people with intellectual disabilities, the definitions of intellectual disability, and assessment instruments for the group. Most changes reflect a desire to avoid some of the stigma associated with labeling (Baroff, 1999; Sandieson, 1998). Significantly, new trends involve defining and discussing intellectual disabilities in a way that promotes greater sensitivity to needs and characteristics of an individual (Smith, 1997).

Terminology

When considering the concept across history, the evolution of the language and terminology used to characterize intellectual disability is notable. While terms such as *idiot* and *moron* once had specific functional meanings and were considered acceptable medical terms, these words have become completely un-acceptable. New, less stigmatizing terms are now preferable. Depending on the source, terms such as *developmental disability, cognitive disability,* and *mentally challenged* have all been widely used (Biasini et al., 1999). Depersonalizing phrases such as *the mentally retarded* have been replaced by person-first language, as in the phrase *individual with mental retardation.* Many advocates, families, and organizations now support replacement of all forms of reference to *retardation,* deeming the term and all its variants hurtful and stigmatizing (Bellini, 2003; Iacono, 2002; Leicester & Cooke, 2002). For example, the former Association for Retarded Citizens has become The Arc and has adopted the term *cognitive disability* in place of any references to mental retardation. Similarly, the American Association on Mental Retardation is considering a name change to the American Association on Intellectual Disabilities in an effort to recognize consumer and family preferences and to reflect current practices within both American and international communities. Although some critics have expressed concern over a lack of precision (Greenspan, 1997; MacMillan, Gresham, & Siperstein, 1993), supporters of the new name view it as representative of a paradigm shift recognizing human needs over those of institutions (AAMR, 2002). Accordingly, this chapter uses the term *intellectual disability.*

Definitions of Intellectual Disability

The primary components of modern definitions of intellectual disability—childhood origination, significant limitation in cognition or intellect, and difficulties in adaptive behaviors—have been stable since the early 20th century (Bellini, 2003; Scheerenberger, 1987). Current conceptualizations of intellectual disabilities reflect positive changes in public attitudes and a desire for a function-based definition, although most definitions remain grounded at least in part in quantifiable intelligence quotient (IQ) scores on comprehensive, standardized measures of intelligence. Although there is no single universal definition, definitions developed by the WHO *International Classification of Diseases Guide for Mental Retardation* (WHO, 1996), the *Diagnostic and Statistical Manual of Mental Disorders–Fourth Edition–Text Revision* (DSM–IV–TR; American Psychiatric Association [APA], 2000), and the AAMR (2002) are widely used.

World Health Organization Definition

The WHO publishes the *International Classification of Diseases* (ICD; WHO, 1996) as a tool for standardizing diagnostic classifications of health conditions around the world. The ICD, now in its 10th edition (ICD 10), includes the *Guide for Mental Retardation* (WHO, 1996). The guide retains the term *mental retardation* as used in prior editions but includes new alpha–numeric codes. Mental disorders are identified with the letter "F"; specific subcategories are further identified with numbers 00 through 99. Mental retardation has a categorical designation of F70 through F79 (WHO, 1996). The ICD 10 *Guide for Mental Retardation* states:

> Mental retardation is a condition of arrested or incomplete development of the mind, which is characterized by impairment of skills manifested during the developmental period, which contribute to the overall level of intelligence, i.e. cognitive, language, motor and social abilities . . .

> Adaptive behavior is always impaired, but in protective social environments when support is available this impairment need not be at all obvious in individuals with mild intellectual disabilities. (p. 1)

The diagnostic guidelines also make specific recommendations with regard to the assessment of intellectual functioning, indicating that culturally appropriate standardized tests administered individually should be used for diagnostic purposes. The WHO notes assessments should also consider the presence of other conditions, such as language problems and physical or sensory disabilities (WHO, 1996). The codes F70 through F73 cover a range of severity that includes mild, moderate, severe, and profound intellectual disability, respectively. In addition to the severity codes, the classification system includes "other mental retardation" (F78), used when additional limitations are present that make determination of function difficult, and "unspecified mental retardation" (F79), used when evidence of an intellectual disability exists but cannot be quantified (Biasini et al., 1999; WHO, 1996).

American Psychiatric Association Definition

Like the ICD 10 (WHO, 1999) definition, the definition of intellectual disability provided by the APA in the DSM-IV-TR (APA, 2000) requires consideration of both general intellectual functioning and adaptive skill limitations. According to the DMS-IV-TR:

> The essential feature of mental retardation is significantly subaverage general intellectual function (Criterion A) that is accompanied by significant limitations in adaptive functioning in at least two of the following skills areas: communication, self-care, home living, social/interpersonal skills, use of community resources, self-direction, functional academic skills, work, leisure, health, and safety (Criterion B). The onset must occur before age 18 (Criterion C). (p. 41)

The definition also specifies four degrees of impairment: mild, moderate, severe, and profound. Delays in at least 2 of 10 areas of adaptive skills are also necessary for a diagnosis, and delays should be quantified by assessments other than office screenings (APA, 2000; Biasini et al., 1999).

American Association on Mental Retardation Definition

As previously noted, the AAMR has been instrumental in developing conceptual frameworks and terminology relevant to intellectual disabilities. However, the most recent definition from the AAMR has retained the term *mental retardation* (MR) because it is used in so many government regulations and laws, although other AAMR publications have eliminated it (Bellini, 2003). The definition states:

> Mental retardation is a disability characterized by significant limitations both in intellectual functioning and in adaptive behavior as expressed in conceptual, social, and practical adaptive skills. This disability originates before the age of 18. (p. 8)

Five assumptions are critical to application of this definition of MR. First, functional limitations in learning and in performance of activities of daily living should be considered contextually in relation to age, environment, peers, and culture. Second, the definition assumes that considerations of cultural and linguistic diversity and communication differences along with sensory, motor, and behavioral factors have been part of a valid assessment process. Further, definitions of mental retardation must recognize that strengths often coexist with limitations, and the purpose of describing limitations is to develop a big picture of needed supports, rather than to list deficits. Finally, the definition assumes that with meaningful, individualized support over the lifespan, individual functioning will usually improve (AAMR, 2002; Bellini, 2003).

While the various definitions have unique components, the common thread across the DSM-IV-TR, AAMR, and ICD-10 is cognitive impairment—subaverage or below typical intellectual functioning. The definitions also agree that onset must occur before adulthood, defined as age 18 for both DSM-IV TR and AAMR, and specified as during the developmental period by the ICD-10. The current definitions also specify an accompanying deficit in adaptive behavior; to be diagnosed with mental retardation, an individual must manifest not only low cognitive skills but also limited ability to adapt to the demands of society, with allowances being made for age, sociocultural background, and community settings (AAMR, 2002; APA, 2000; WHO, 1996).

Assessing Intellectual Disabilities

Implicit in the preceding definitions and specifically stated in the AAMR essential assumptions is the assumption that whatever instrument is used, it must be appropriate and must accommodate individual needs (AAMR, 2002; WHO,

1996). A routine and stereotyped use of assessment measures throws little light on the prognosis of persons with intellectual disabilities, either vocationally or in terms of adjustment to the community (Anastasi & Urbina, 1997; Nezu, Nezu, & Gill-Weiss, 1992). Correctly used, however, assessment measures can be invaluable in assessing the individual's skills and pinpointing the intellectual and personality strengths and weaknesses for eventual vocational programming (Brolin, 1976; Decola, 1997).

Many service and support eligibility decisions are based on various standardized assessment scores, so it is critical for evaluations to be sensitive enough to establish whether a diagnosis of intellectual or other developmental disability is warranted (Biasini et al., 1999). Following are discussions and brief summaries of some commonly used screening tools and comprehensive assessments related to cognitive functioning. Then, reviews and discussions of several assessments of adaptive behavior, personality, and achievement are included. Last, a selection of interest inventories and instruments for social and vocational assessments are discussed.

Measures of Cognitive Functioning

The following section describes the contribution of several frequently used and accepted measures for assessment of the cognitive functioning of adults with intellectual disabilities. It is beyond the scope of this chapter to provide detailed psychometric reviews and evaluations; however, brief descriptions of the selected instruments are provided, along with discussions of basic features, assets, and known and potential limitations that are of particular relevance to individuals with intellectual disabilities.

Screening instruments for general cognitive functioning are useful for a variety of reasons. Often, the focus or purpose of an evaluation requires only a global estimate of intellectual function, such as during a primarily vocational assessment (Kaufman, 1990). Additionally, an individual previously diagnosed may benefit from an expeditious check of current intellectual status (Anastasi & Urbina, 1997; Zimmerman, Covin, & Woo-Sam, 1986). The continuing focus on managed care has also affected the use of screening instruments—time restrictions and cost containment has led to an increasing interest in short measures (Piotrowski, 1999), and objective screening instruments can often provide clearer evidence of the need for in-depth evaluation. With any brief screening instrument, care should be used in interpretation and application of the results (Frauenhoffer, Ross, Searight, & Piotrowski, 1998; Parker, 1993).

The *Wechsler Abbreviated Scale of Intelligence*

Variations of Wechsler scales for measuring intellectual functioning have been in use for many years. Across various fields, evaluators have used pieces of more comprehensive Wechsler instruments to make their own versions of brief functional assessments, although such practices are psychometrically questionable

(Stano, 2004). The *Wechsler Abbreviated Scale of Intelligence* (WASI; Psychological Corporation, 1999a) offers an alternative to do-it-yourself adaptations and builds on the reputation of the popular Wechsler measures.

The WASI was normed with a national sample of 2,245 children and adults ranging from 6 to 89 years of age, although the sample did not include individuals with intellectual disabilities (Psychological Corporation, 1999a). The WASI includes four subtests in Vocabulary, Similarities, Block Design, and Matrix Reasoning. Together, the subtests make up the instrument's Verbal and Performance scales, yielding the Verbal and Performance IQ scores (Psychological Corporation, 1999a). When all four subtests are included, administration time is about 30 minutes, although an estimated IQ can be obtained from administration of the two-subtest form, which can be completed in about 15 minutes (Stano, 2004).

Some WASI subtests include very basic picture items for the purpose of extending the floor of the scale, enhancing its use with people with intellectual disabilities (Psychological Corporation, 1999b). According to Stano (2004), the WASI has been administered to several small clinical groups including individuals with intellectual disabilities, and useful information relevant to rehabilitation services was obtainable, especially when the four-subtest form was used rather than the two-subtest form.

Peabody Picture Vocabulary Test–Third Edition

The *Peabody Picture Vocabulary Test–Third Edition* (PPVT-III; Dunn & Dunn, 1997) has replaced the *Peabody Picture Vocabulary Test–Revised* (Dunn & Dunn, 1981), which was a commonly used measure of language for individuals with intellectual disabilities (Pickett & Flynn, 1983). The PPVT-III is a nonverbal multiple-choice test designed to evaluate the receptive English language comprehension of children and adults, standardized with 2,725 people aged 2 to 90+ years. People with intellectual disabilities were not included in the development of norms (Dunn & Dunn, 1997).

The PPVT-III is very brief; administration time is only 11 to 12 minutes, which may be especially advantageous in some settings and with individuals with decreased attention span. However, the instrument is not free of limitations for people with intellectual disabilities. A major criticism of the instrument is the sole reliance on receptive language as a measure of comprehension. Additionally, the format, which consists of pointing to one picture out of four, may favor the possibility of guessing. Guessing can be of particular concern in evaluating participants with intellectual disabilities who may be prone to guessing as a form of acquiescence (Kilsby, Bennert, & Beyer, 2002).

Kaufman Brief Intelligence Test–Second Edition

The *Kaufman Brief Intelligence Test–Second Edition* (KBIT-2; Kaufman & Kaufman, 2004) is useful for screening of verbal and nonverbal intelligence, standardized for ages 4 through 90. Administration of the KBIT-2 requires about 20 minutes. The instrument consists of a vocabulary section, assessing knowledge of words and their meanings, along with a matrices section, using pictures and abstract designs without words. The KBIT-2 may be a valuable tool for determining the need for a comprehensive assessment for individuals who appear to have cognitive deficits, although it was not normed with individuals with intellectual disabilities. Standardization was otherwise intensive; using a sample matching recent U.S. census data, the measure was conormed with other measures of cognitive functioning (Kaufman & Kaufman, 2004).

The prior version, the KBIT (Kaufman & Kaufman, 1990), demonstrated adequate reliability and validity (Parker, 1993) and served well as a screening test of ability and as an indicator of the need for more comprehensive testing (Walters & Weaver, 2003). The KBIT-2 offers some improvements over the older version that may be important in assessing people with intellectual disabilities, including receptive and expressive vocabulary items that do not require literacy. Additionally, new packaging includes brightly colored items designed to appeal to less mature or reluctant participants and may have appeal for individuals with intellectual disabilities (Kaufman & Kaufman, 2004). The format of the KBIT-2 allows for the assessment of verbal versus nonverbal intelligence independently, allowing a clinician to make some differentiation between language deficits and cognitive deficits.

Slosson Intelligence Test–Revised 2002 Edition

The *Slosson Intelligence Test–Revised 2002 Edition* (SIT-R3; Slosson, Nicholson, & Hibpshman, 2002) was designed to provide a quick estimate of general verbal cognitive ability. The authors caution that the SIT-R3 is not meant to be used alone in making placement decisions; rather, it should serve as an indication of the need for further, more in-depth assessment (Slosson, Nicholson, & Hibpshman, 2002). It may also be used to confirm other findings as part of a comprehensive battery.

The SIT-R3 was standardized with 1,854 people ranging in age from 4 to 65 years old (Slosson, Nicholson, & Hibpshman, 2002). Items are derived from the following cognitive domains: general information, similarities and differences, vocabulary, comprehension, digit span, arithmetic, visual–motor, and auditory memory for sentences. The SIT-R3 is an individually administered untimed test—a benefit for people with intellectual disabilities. Although it was designed primarily for students, the authors note particular utility for adults with intellectual or psychiatric disabilities. The instrument allows for IQ scores as low as 36, so it is suitable for persons with mild to moderate intellectual disabilities. In addition to psychologists and diagnosticians, counselors, special educators, and social workers are noted as appropriate test administrators, so it would be appropriate for use in rehabilitation-related setting by rehabilitation professionals.

Test of Nonverbal Intelligence–Third Edition

The *Test of Nonverbal Intelligence–Third Edition* (TONI-3; Brown, Sherbenou, & Johnsen, 1997) is a brief language-free measure of intelligence, aptitude, problem solving, and abstract reasoning (Brown, Sherbenou, & Johnsen, 1997). It is comprised of 50 items containing problem-solving tasks that progressively increase in complexity and difficulty. The TONI-3 was standardized with a national sample of 3,000 people aged 6 through 89 years (Plake & Impara, 2001). The instrument has been used with populations dually diagnosed with autism and intellectual disability and has been normed with various special populations. The TONI-3 has also correlated well with other similar measures (Brown, Sherbenou, & Johnsen, 1997; Edelson, 2005).

The TONI-3 is considered especially suitable for adults with intellectual disabilities in that is not timed, and does not require reading, writing, speaking, or listening. As a completely nonverbal and largely motor-free measure, the TONI-3 is appropriate for non-English speakers and for persons who do not speak or read English well. In addition, The TONI-3 uses geometric pattern matching and pattern deletions, and thus is not limited due to lack of real-world and social knowledge, making it useful for assessing individuals who have both intellectual disabilities and autism (Edelson, 2005).

Comprehensive Measures of Intelligence

While brief measures and screening tools are very useful in many settings, they are not the recommended instruments for establishing a diagnosis or for developing an educational or rehabilitation plan. Most definitions of intellectual disability retain a strong focus on IQ scores quantifiable by comprehensive measures of intelligence. Comprehensive measures of intelligence have a lengthy history, with the first conceptualization of intelligence testing emerging in the mid-19th century. Modern intelligence tests followed shortly after the turn of the century and have been subject to revisions and improvements ever since (Wasserman & Tulsky, 2005).

But despite years of refinements, comprehensive measures of IQ are not without limitations, some of which are related to individual instruments, as discussed below. Some, however, are broader. In particular, Mather and Wendling (2005) note that an exclusionary focus on global IQ scores can be detrimental to planning and service provision because such scores are a limited view of an individual's actual abilities and skills. Even the most comprehensive test battery provides only an impression of an individual's performance at a given point in time and relative only to a select normative group (Mather & Wendling, 2005). Rehabilitation professionals are urged to cautiously apply professional judgment in developing and interpreting assessment data even from seemingly thorough comprehensive batteries and to sensitively convey assessment results to consumers and their families (Parker & Bolton, 2005).

Stanford-Binet Intelligence Scales–Fifth Edition
Since the Stanford-Binet was first developed, it has been revised several times to give us the current *Stanford-Binet 5* (SB-5; Roid, 2003). A wide-ranging,

individually administered test battery, the updated Stanford-Binet remains one of the most popular intelligence assessment instruments currently in use (Roid & Barram, 2004). The SB-5 is expected to be a meaningful measure for individuals with disabilities, including people with intellectual disabilities, due to improvements in design, procedure, and norms.

The SB-5 yields Verbal, Performance, and Full-Scale IQ scores through coverage of five cognitive factors, which are assessed both verbally and nonverbally to better evaluate individuals with communication difficulties: Fluid Reasoning, Knowledge, Quantitative Reasoning, Visual–Spatial Processing, and Working Memory. According to the test manual, improvements in the measurement of these cognitive factors make the test a better indicator for clients with special needs, including individuals with intellectual disabilities (Roid, 2003). Procedures of the SB-5 also allow for adaptation of the test to the functional level of the participant. With such tailoring, the SB-5 could be useful for assessing persons with low-end functioning, especially since the scale range has been extended to measure lower areas of functioning (Roid & Barram, 2004).

The SB-5 normative sample was closely matched to the 2000 United States Census and included 4,800 people ranging in age from 2 to 85+ years; however, people with intellectual disabilities were not included. While several studies have demonstrated reliability and validity of earlier editions for people with intellectual disabilities (Bower & Hayes, 1995; Dacy, Nelson, & Stoeckel, 1999), and Stanford-Binet instruments generally have performed well in assessing mild to moderate intellectual disabilities (Biasini et al., 1999), no literature yet exists for the SB-5. Nonetheless, previous concerns regarding the adequacy of the standardization for adults who have intellectual disabilities (Kaufman, 1990) appear to have been addressed (Spies & Plake, 2005). It is most critical to note that Stanford-Binet instruments overall have not been designed to test individuals with severe or profound levels of deficit (Biasini et al., 1999).

Wechsler Adult Intelligence Scale–Third Edition

The *Wechsler Adult Intelligence Scale–Third Edition* (WAIS-III; Wechsler, 1997) has replaced its predecessor, the *Wechsler Adult Intelligence Test–Revised* (WAIS-R; Wechsler, 1981) and will probably take over its position as the most commonly used test of intelligence for adults with mild to moderate intellectual disability (Kaufman & Lichtenberger, 1999). Generally, Wechsler scales have been recommended for use with people with intellectual disabilities because they capitalize on the extensive research and normative efforts of previous editions of the Wechsler (DeVinney, Kamneatz, Chan, & Hattori, 1998). The combination of verbal and performance scales making up the WAIS-III is particularly useful for assessing persons with intellectual disabilities, whose often minimal formal education may limit their verbal abilities. Changes in WAIS-III construction have added items at the lower levels of the various subtests, and these appear to correct WAIS-R limitations that had overestimated low IQ scores (Kaufman & Lichtenberger, 1999; Zimmerman, Covin, & Woo-Sam, 1986).

Despite improvements, some limitations are noteworthy. Although lower floors were developed to enhance utility for people with more significant intellectual disabilities, the test is still primarily constructed to assess intellectual functioning for persons with IQ scores greater than 50. Individuals who are unable to complete the initial subtest items are assigned an automatic standard score of at least 1 and a full IQ of 47 to 50 depending on age. Thus, for individuals who are lower functioning, scores may be highly inaccurate and not reveal a consistent verbal-performance profile (Kaufman & Lichtenberger, 1999). It has been recommended that participants have raw score credit in a total of six subtests—three verbal subtests and three performance subtests—before making an assumption of applicable results (Biasini et al., 1999).

Kaufman Adolescent and Adult Intelligence Test

The *Kaufman Adolescent and Adult Intelligence Test* (KAIT; Kaufman & Kaufman, 1993) was developed in part as a response to criticisms of other measures as defining intelligence too narrowly (Flanagan, Alfonso, & Flanagan, 1994). The KAIT is an individually administered measure of general intelligence, standardized for individuals aged 11 through 85 and older. No special populations were included in the standardization sample (Conoley & Impara, 1995).

The KAIT includes both a standard and expanded test battery, the latter of which Kaufman and Kaufman (1993) recommend for clinical, neuropsychological, and psychoeducational application. A unique feature of the KAIT is that it includes allowable teaching procedures, so that test takers are able to comprehend each task to the greatest extent possible. Furthermore, the KAIT provides a supplementary measure of mental status for individuals with severe impairments consisting of 10 simple questions involving general and personal information, arithmetic, and reading, enabling assessment of both orientation and attention (Kaufman & Kaufman, 1993).

Flanagan, Genshaft, and Boyce (1999) praise the instrument, noting that "overall the KAIT is a well-organized and well-constructed battery of innovative and stimulating tests" (p. 62). The de-emphasis of the KAIT on speed and motor proficiency can be valuable in assessing individuals with intellectual disabilities, and the authors suggest accommodating people with disabilities further through elimination of speed and motor factors altogether (Kaufman & Kaufman, 1993). However, KAIT subtests do require vocal responses (Flanagan, Alfonso, & Flanagan, 1994), so the instrument may not be appropriate for individuals who have communication disorders or difficulty in oral communication, including some individuals with intellectual disabilities.

Comprehensive Test of Nonverbal Intelligence

The *Comprehensive Test of Nonverbal Intelligence* (CTONI; Hammill, Pearson, & Wiederholt, 1997) is individually administered orally or in pantomime to measure nonverbal reasoning. The test was standardized using a sample of 2,500 individuals in the United States, Canada, and Panama with people ages 6 through 90. Administration time is 60 minutes. The Nonverbal Intelligence

Quotient (NIQ) composite score is a "general measure of nonverbal ability for spatial reasoning and nonverbal symbolic reasoning" (Drossman, Maller, & McDermott, 2001, p. 588).

Responding to pictures of common objects such as toys, animals, and people, along with geometric designs, participants indicate their answers by pointing to alternative choices. Oral and written responses are not required at all. Additionally, no object manipulation is required. The CTONI is considered appropriate for several special populations, including people with intellectual disabilities, individuals with speech or language differences, or people with physical disabilities for whom other measures might be considered inappropriate or biased (Hammill, Pearson, & Wiederholt, 1997).

A computerized version, the *Comprehensive Test of Nonverbal Intelligence–Computer Administered* (CTONI-CA), is also available and can be administered entirely on a desktop computer. However, the primary advantages of the CTONI-CA are to the person administering the test since scoring errors are eliminated and the system allows for immediate viewing and printing of results (Hammill, Pearson, & Wiederholt, 1997). The lack of human interaction and problems understanding and using the technology could pose significant barriers for persons with intellectual and other disabilities.

Woodcock-Johnson III Tests of Cognitive Ability

The *Woodcock-Johnson III* (WJ III; Woodcock, McGrew, & Mather, 2001a) is a test of general intellectual abilities that includes 31 subtests of broad and narrow cognitive abilities to provide an assessment of multiple types of intelligence across tests of cognitive abilities and achievement (Schrank, 2005; Woodcock, McGrew, & Mather, 2001a). The *Woodcock-Johnson III Tests of Cognitive Ability* (WJ III COG; Woodcock, McGrew, & Mather, 2001c) is a part of the larger WJ III and thus shares the same norm group, which included 8,818 participants ranging in age from 2 to 90 years old.

Because the test administrator actually establishes the floor and ceiling for each subtest (Schrank, 2005), the design of this instrument may allow for better adaptation of the material to the needs of a participant with an intellectual disability than other tests. The instrument has been used successfully to assess adults with learning and intellectual disabilities (Hawkins, Eckland, James, & Foose, 2003; Mather & Woodcock, 2001). However, the WJ III COG norm sample consisted of English-only speakers; thus, it may not be appropriate for persons from culturally or linguistically diverse backgrounds. It is also important to recognize that many WJ III COG subtests require a great deal of preparation and training on the part of the test administrator, and results may be dependent on the examiner's skill levels and experience (Ortiz & Dynda, 2005).

Leiter International Performance Scale–Revised

The *Leiter International Performance Scale–Revised* (Leiter-R; Roid & Miller, 1997) is the most recent revision of the *Leiter International Performance Scale*

(Leiter, 1948), a venerable nonverbal intelligence test that has been widely administered to individuals in special populations, particularly individuals who cannot be productively assessed with measures such as Wechsler scales. Because the format requires no verbal instructions or responses and minimized physical output, the older edition of the Leiter has been used with individuals who have autism, intellectual disability, or hearing loss or who are non–English-speaking (Tsatanis, Dartnall, Cicchetti, Sparrow, Klin, & Volkmar, 2003), despite having norms that were widely considered inadequate (Kampaus, 1993).

The most recent revision of the instrument, however, includes changes to the content and the format and is grounded in current theoretical models of intelligence (Tsatanis et al., 2003). The authors note the revised instrument includes batteries for Visualization and Reasoning and Attention and Memory, with 10 subtests each, and the standard scores now use a mean of 100 and a standard deviation of 15, consistent with other comprehensive measures (Roid & Miller, 1997). For the revisions, the authors also used a stratified random normative sample of persons 2 to 20 years of age and included special groups including persons with learning disabilities and intellectual disability. The latest version consists of 20 subtests and requires 60 minutes to administer, resulting in three composite scores in Fluid Reasoning (suitable for all ages), Fundamental Visualization (suitable for children 2 to 5 years of age), and Spatial Visualization, for the 11- to 20-year-old age range (Roid & Miller, 1997).

Adaptive Behavior Instruments

As previously noted, current definitions of intellectual disabilities include benchmarks for cognitive functioning along with statements of differences in adaptive behavior. Indeed, regardless of IQ score, a diagnosis of intellectual disabilities cannot be made unless the individual is also unable to successfully adapt to his or her current environment (AAMR, 2002; APA, 2000; WHO, 1996). Therefore, it is necessary to include a measure of adaptive functioning in assessments of intellectual disability (Biasini et al., 1999). However, adaptive ability remains a difficult concept to define and measure, influenced by the reality that different skills and abilities are required in different environments (Sparrow, Balla, & Cicchetti, 1984). Furthermore, the adequacy of adaptive behavior depends greatly on the acceptance and tolerance of the social or work setting involved (Polloway, 1997).

Adaptive behavior instruments have been proliferating over the years. In fact, there are more than 200 adaptive measures available (Biasini et al., 1999). Increasingly, these instruments meet standards of psychometric quality and combine both criterion and normative referencing. Many measures involve the cooperation of a knowledgeable informant, typically a parent or teacher, with additional information as needed gathered from direct observation. The test taker may be encouraged to serve as his or her own informant, although not all individuals with intellectual disabilities will be able to do so (Bruininks,

Woodcock, Weatherman, & Hill, 1996). While a variety of instruments are available, the DSM-IV (APA, 1994) specifically notes the *Vineland Adaptive Behavior Scale* (VABS; Sparrow et al., 1984) and the *Adaptive Behavior Scale* (Nihira, Leland, & Lambert, 1993) as appropriate tools for adaptive assessment of people with intellectual disabilities.

Vineland Adaptive Behavior Scales

The *Vineland Adaptive Behavior Scales* (Sparrow et al., 1984) has been one of the most widely used adaptive scales for adults with intellectual disabilities, although the primary normative sample was comprised of children ranging in age from infancy to age 18. However, VABS supplemental standardization samples included individuals with cognitive disabilities, including adults who are low functioning (Anastasi & Urbina, 1997; Biasini et al., 1999). Providing a norm-referenced assessment of adaptive behavior, it provides useful criteria for identifying deficits in the domains of communication, daily living skills, socialization, and motor skills.

Consisting of a semistructured interview and questionnaire, the VABS uses items that measure personal and social skills used in daily situations. The VABS results in scores across four domains and an Adaptive Behavior Composite score that can be expressed in standard scores, percentile ranks, and age equivalents. An optional Maladaptive Behavior domain can be included to measure challenging behaviors. Although the VABS does not specifically cover the 10 DSM-IV adaptive skills areas, it has generally proved to be particularly suitable for individuals with intellectual disabilities in community settings (Sparrow et al., 1984). The DSM-IV-TR and AAMR guidelines recommend that this tool be used in conjunction with developmental, medical, and educational histories and teacher evaluation (AAMR, 2002; APA, 2000).

Vineland Adaptive Behavior Scales–Second Edition

The *Vineland Adaptive Behavior Scales–Second Edition* (Vineland II; Sparrow, Cicchetti, & Balla, 2005) is the most recent revision of the *Vineland Adaptive Behavior Scales*. The test was designed to provide the adaptive information needed for diagnoses of intellectual disabilities, autism, and other developmental delays. The Vineland II differs in some important ways from the VABS and offers several appealing features for rehabilitation professionals. Primarily, it has expanded standardization norms and an expanded age range, increasing its utility for adults. Three forms—the Survey Interview, Expanded Interview, and Parent/Caregiver Rating Form—are appropriate for evaluation of persons from birth to age 90; the Expanded Form will be released in 2007. The Teacher Rating Form is appropriate in school settings for children and young adults ages 3 to 21 (Sparrow et al., 2005).

The Vineland II has a three-domain structure related to the broad areas of adaptive functioning described by the AAMR. Included are Communication,

Daily Living, and Socialization domains, which correspond to Conceptual, Practical, and Social domains under the AAMR (2002) guidelines. The authors have incorporated content changes, creating items that are more relevant to current daily tasks and skills and improving classification of moderate to profound intellectual disabilities (Sparrow et al., 2005). In addition, the expanded age range allows for greater use of the instrument in the identification of changes over time, especially for older adults.

Adaptive Behavior Scale, Second Edition
Part One–Residential and Community Version

The *Adaptive Behavior Scale, Second Edition* (ABS: 2, Lambert, Nihira, & Leland, 1993), is a broad adaptive behavior scale that is available in two versions: School (ABS-S: 2; Lambert et al., 1993) and Residential and Community (ABS-RC: 2; Nihira, Leland, & Lambert, 1993). The ABS-RC: 2 is a brief instrument requiring an administration time of 15 to 30 minutes. It was designed especially for use with individuals with intellectual disabilities, ages 18 to 80, and is relevant to rehabilitation counseling and other adult rehabilitation–related settings. Items are presented in a questionnaire that can be completed by the individual or by an individual familiar with the client. The ABSRC: 2 was standardized with more than 4,000 individuals with developmental disabilities in 43 states who lived in either residential or community settings (Nihira et al., 1993).

Although it is widely used, the instrument has some drawbacks. Items on maladaptive behaviors are rated only by how often they occur, rather than by occurrence and severity. Thus, a minor behavioral concern occurring frequently could be rated as more maladaptive than an endangering behavior that occurs occasionally. Additionally, the instrument includes a number of negatively worded items that could be quite challenging (Hill, 2001). Although ABSRC: 2 results are considered of value for clinical or criterion-referenced assessment of deficits, results may be less pertinent for diagnostic decisions (Anastasi & Urbina, 1997).

Achievement Tests

Comprehensive intelligence tests are generally good predictors of educational achievement for individuals with intellectual disabilities (Biasini et al., 1999). Although intelligence tests are more comprehensive than achievement tests, measures of achievement can be beneficial in the assessment of clients with intellectual disabilities. Comparing IQ results and achievement results may be a useful way to determine if an individual is functioning at full potential and may help target areas needing support or remediation. Achievement testing usually measures an individual's grasp of factual information and depends largely upon formal educational experience. However, quantifying the extent of academic progress can be important to vocational and independent living plans for a person with an intellectual disability (Biasini et al., 1999).

Wide Range Achievement Test, Fourth Edition

The *Wide Range Achievement Test,* now in its fourth edition (WRAT 4; Wilkinson & Robertson, 2006), has been one of the most widely used adult achievement measures (Kaufman, 1990; Wilkinson, 1993). The WRAT 4 is a rapid measure of reading recognition, spelling, and arithmetic and includes Sentence Comprehension as a new reading achievement measure. It was standardized with a national stratified sample of 3,000 individuals ranging in age from 5 to 94 years. The instrument was normed by both age and grade, making it particularly suitable for persons with intellectual disabilities.

The WRAT 4 was designed to collect initial information for educational or vocational assessment processes and to determine minimum levels of skills needed in some educational or vocational setting, rather than to serve as a formal diagnostic of intellectual functioning (Wilkinson & Robertson, 2006). The instrument includes four subtests labeled Word Reading, Sentence Comprehension, Spelling, and Math Computation, noted here in the order of recommended administration.

Administration time is linked to age, skill, and behavior and so may vary when used with individuals with intellectual disabilities. The test kit includes Blue and Green Forms that can be used interchangeably and are useful when rapid retesting is needed without practice effects. The two forms can also be administered together in a Combined Form. Interestingly, the Combined Form includes a performance observation for qualitative assessment, useful in developing a more holistic understanding of the consumer.

Peabody Individual Achievement Test–Revised/Normative Update

The *Peabody Individual Achievement Test–Revised/Normative Update* (PIAT-R/NU; Markwardt, 1997) supersedes the *Peabody Individual Achievement Test–Revised* (PIAT-R; Markwardt, 1987), a commonly used achievement measure for clients with intellectual disabilities. The Normative Update was standardized for a population aged 5 through 22, so it may be most valuable to rehabilitation professionals who work with children or young adults in transition. According to the author, students who receive special education services were included in the age and grade normative samples in representative proportions (Markwardt, 1997).

Unlike some other measures of achievement, no writing is involved, which may be advantageous in assessing people with intellectual disabilities. The PIAT-R/NU offers another advantage as well—in the reading comprehension measure and reading recognition section. Scores can be expressed as age equivalents or grade equivalents, and the score system allows for standard scores (mean = 100, standard deviation = 15) as low as 65. The format allows respondents to point to response items and is appropriate for many students with physical, communication, or intellectual disabilities. The manual provides instructions for additional accommodations for student with disabilities (Markwardt, 1997).

Kaufman Functional Academic Skills Test

The *Kaufman Functional Academic Skills Test* (K-FAST; Kaufman & Kaufman, 1994) differs from the previously covered achievement tests in that it was designed especially for transition-aged youth and adults. The measure was standardized for ages 15 to 85+ with a sample of 1,424 people and requires only 15 to 25 minutes administration time. The K-FAST allows for either verbal or motor responses and provides age-based standard scores of arithmetic and reading, as well as a composite score.

According to the manual, the K-FAST is best used as a supplement to other cognitive or adaptive assessments, and while it can be administered and scored by a range of professionals and paraprofessionals, interpretation should be done only by qualified administrators (Kaufman & Kaufman, 1994). Because the instrument focuses on content appropriate for adult independent living, such as budgeting and understanding labels when shopping, it is particularly useful for vocational assessment of people with intellectual disabilities.

Woodcock-Johnson III Tests of Achievement

As previously discussed, the *Woodcock-Johnson III* (WJ III; Woodcock, McGrew, & Mather, 2001a) is a battery of individually administered tests of general intellectual abilities (Schrank, 2005; Woodcock, McGrew, & Mather, 2001c). The *Woodcock-Johnson III Tests of Achievement* are a part of the larger WJ III (WJ III ACH; Woodcock, McGrew, & Mather, 2001b) and share the same norm group.

The WJ III ACH has two parallel forms, A and B, to allow for more frequent use with less practice effect concerns. Overall, 22 tests are grouped into curriculum-related groups: Reading, Mathematics, Written Language, Oral Language, and Academic Knowledge. The standard battery includes 12 tests including measures of word identification, spelling, writing fluency, math fluency, and applied problems, to name several. The extended battery includes an additional 10 tests covering oral comprehension, academic knowledge, spelling of sounds, and sound awareness. With a mixture of timed and untimed items, the standard battery takes 60 to 70 minutes to administer.

The WJ III ACH has a matching cognitive measure in the previously discussed *Woodcock-Johnson III Tests of Cognitive Ability* (WJ III COG), so fully conormed measures of intelligence and achievement are available when the batteries are used in combination (Blackwell, 2002; McGrew & Woodcock, 2001). Since the instrument was designed to allow the test administrator to tailor testing to an individual's ability level and to administer only subtests and items that are necessary, utility for individuals with cognitive disabilities has increased and testing time has been decreased (Blackwell, 2001; Woodcock, McGrew, & Mather, 2001c). Also, the WJ III ACH manual describes appropriate administrative accommodations for persons with special needs (Blackwell, 2002).

Mini-Battery of Achievement

The *Mini-Battery of Achievement* (MBA; Woodcock, McGrew, & Werder, 1994) is a brief test of basic skills and knowledge that has relevance to a variety of rehabilitation-related settings. It is suitable for individuals aged 4 to 90 years, and administration requires only 25 to 30 minutes. The MBA manual refers to the *Woodcock-Johnson Psycho-Educational Battery–Revised* (WJ-R; Woodcock & Johnson, 1989) technical manual for normative information since these instruments share a common sample. In fact, the MBA is a composite of WJ-R items; 101 items (38%) taken from the WJ-R, Form A, and 119 items (44%) taken from Form B (Woodcock, McGrew, & Werder, 1994).

The MBA manual provides suggested starting points for different school-based achievement levels. The battery is essentially untimed, although test administrators are directed to advance testing after spending a reasonable, not undue, amount of time per item (Woodcock, McGrew, & Werder, 1994). Most MBA items are open-ended questions or open-response statements, which can reduce concerns of guessing or acquiescence. With its broad range of coverage and rapid administration time, this battery could be a practical measure for adults with intellectual disabilities. However, the format may prove frustrating or difficult for individuals with significant intellectual disabilities. Although the MBA can be given by a wide variety of professionals and paraprofessionals, some of the instructions may be confusing to individuals with little or no background in assessment. Because of this concern, it has been recommended that only experienced examiners should administer the test (Michael, 1998).

Assessment of Psychiatric Disorders

Intellectual disabilities can exist concurrently with other conditions, including psychiatric disorders (Miller et al., 1994; WHO, 1996). In fact, individuals with intellectual disabilities are disproportionately diagnosed with personality, psychiatric, and other mental disorders, with rates approximately three to four times greater than the general population (Masi, 1998). There is growing interest in assessments for people with dual diagnoses of psychological disorders and intellectual disabilities, presenting a variety of challenges and a variety of approaches to evaluate psychopathology (Reiss, 1993; Wagner, 1991).

Unfortunately, traditional psychiatric assessment instruments often require reading and comprehension levels beyond what would be appropriate for persons with intellectual disabilities, however mild (Butcher, 1999). Nevertheless, some researchers have obtained useful information from instruments not designed for persons with intellectual disabilities through modifications, such as reading test items aloud and providing simplified explanations of items when needed (McDaniel & Harris, 1999). Doing so is problematic, however, since individuals with intellectual disabilities tend to respond to open-ended or less structured questions in unreliable or invalid ways (Kilsby, Bennert, & Beyer, 2002; Ollendick, Oswald, & Ollendick, 1993). A more productive approach appears to be the use of rating scales, which may overcome differences stemming from the verbal limitations of the participant (McLean, 1993), and several specific measures have been developed for use with adults with intellectual disabilities.

Psychopathological Instrument for Mentally Retarded Adults

According to the authors, the *Psychopathological Instrument for Mentally Retarded Adults* (PIMRA; Matson, Kazdin, & Senatore, 1984) was the first dual-diagnosis assessment instrument intended for persons with mild to moderate intellectual disabilities. It has not been retitled in person-first terminology. The PIMRA is a brief assessment device based on the DSM-IV (APA, 1994). It is useful for persons age 16 and older and covers eight categories of mental disorders: schizophrenia, affective, psychosexual, adjustment, anxiety, somatoform, personality, and inappropriate mental adjustment.

Despite being developed more than 20 years ago, the instrument remains available and in use in the United States, the United Kingdom, and several other countries (Balboni, Battagliese, & Pedrabissi, 2000). The psychometric properties are good, and recent research suggests good reliability and validity (Balboni, Battagliese, & Pedrabissi, 2000; Gustafsson & Sonnander, 2005). Norms were based on a total sample of 600 individuals with intellectual disabilities from Texas, Pennsylvania, and Illinois. The instrument consists of two structured interviews organized around two checklists, one for ratings by others and one for self-report. Each category is assessed by seven or eight items that can be rated by the client or by an informant, such as a parent or other family member, a teacher, or a counselor who knows the person well. It is important to note that the informant version may be more useful than the self-report if respondents are lower functioning (Sovner & Pary, 1993; Swiezy, Matson, Kirkpatrick-Sanchez, & Williams, 1995). In fact, the self-report interview and checklist are not to be used if the individual is not verbal or otherwise unable to respond or understand the questions (Matson, 1988).

Reiss Screen for Maladaptive Behavior

The *Reiss Screen for Maladaptive Behavior* (Reiss, 1988) is a well-known and widely utilized tool that serves as a broad screening assessment for the presence or absence of psychopathology (Walsh & Shenouda, 1999). The instrument consists of 36 items using a combination of three different but related screening methods. First, the instrument uses a rating scale linked to the severity of challenging behaviors. The second method links ratings to specific diagnoses, and the third method screens for less common but critical symptoms such as suicidal behaviors. The total score provides a measure of severity. National norms were delineated into categories of mild and severe intellectual disability so validity for either group could be established, offering greater confidence in the Reiss Screen for the population.

Each item on the instrument refers to a psychiatric symptom or behavioral category rather than to a specific observable behavior, including Aggressive Behavior, Psychosis, Paranoia, Depression (behavioral signs), Depression (physical signs), Dependent Personality Disorder, and Avoidant Disorder (Reiss, 1988; 1997). Although the *Reiss Screen for Maladaptive Behavior* has not been revised, the instrument has been well-researched and is regarded as appropriate for persons with intellectual disabilities (Reiss, 1997; Sturmey, Burcham, & Shaw, 1996; Walsh & Shenouda, 1999).

Vocational Assessment

A prominent rehabilitation goal is placement in the work setting (Muklewicz & Bender, 1988), and a growing number of individuals with disabilities have become likely candidates for vocational rehabilitation (Muklewicz & Bender, 1988). Vocational assessments can have an important role in broader career development activities undertaken by special education and rehabilitation professionals with young adults and adults with intellectual disabilities. These assessments can aid in the identification of employment interests, career goals, and occupational skills and ultimately foster vocational satisfaction for adults with intellectual disabilities (Wadsworth, Milsom, & Cocco, 2004).

The assessment of adults with intellectual disabilities in a vocational setting typically seeks to answer a series of questions, determined by the referring source, using information based primarily on tests, observations, and interviews (Decola, 1997). Considerations of vocational potential, interests, and social and prevocational functioning as proposed by Amble and Peterson (1979) have also stood the test of time and remain relevant today. Rumrill and Roessler (1999) note that assessments tend to focus on occupational choice. However, for most people, occupational choices are not fixed and may change as the individual has more life experiences (Szymanski & Hanley-Maxwell, 1996; Wadsworth, Milsom, & Cocco, 2004). As part of an ongoing evaluative process for occupational choice, measures of interest are often sought, and interest inventories are popular measures. Two vocational interest inventories noted to be especially appropriate for persons with intellectual disabilities are reviewed, followed by discussion of several appropriate social, prevocational, and vocational skills assessments.

Reading Free Vocational Interest Inventory: 2

The *Reading Free Vocational Interest Inventory: 2* (RFVII: 2; Becker, 2000) is a picture-format, nonreading interest inventory designed specifically for individuals with intellectual disabilities or learning disabilities in vocational or technical schools, job training programs, or sheltered workshop settings (Becker, 2000). The measure focuses on work preferences primarily at the unskilled and semi-skilled levels. Using picture cards depicting unskilled, semiskilled, and skilled job tasks, the instrument allows consideration of a wide range of jobs. No reading or writing is required, and the pictorial items may be described by the examiner for individuals needing further assistance.

This measure has separate norms for people who have intellectual disabilities or learning disabilities or who are employed in sheltered workshop or similar settings. The manual provides T scores, percentiles, and ratings for various areas of interest including automotive trades, building trades, clerical jobs, work in animal care, jobs in the food service industry, and work related to medical care. Job categories also include employment in horticulture, house-keeping, personal service, laundry service, and materials handling.

The inventory has been shown to have reliability for use with persons with intellectual disabilities and is appropriate for ages 13 and older. It can be used individually or in groups and is brief, with an administration time of about 20 minutes. Prior editions of the RFVII: 2 appeared to predict job retention (Becker, Schull, & Cambell, 1981), but thus far no predictive studies have been published using the current instrument. Nonetheless, the format and norma-tive sample support this measure as useful in vocational interest assessment for people with intellectual disabilities.

GEIST Picture Interest Inventory–Revised

Geist Picture Interest Inventory–Revised (GPII-R; Geist, 1988) is a widely used, simplified measure of vocational and leisure interests suitable for consumers with intellectual disabilities. To identify vocational and personal leisure inter-ests, the participant circles one picture in a series of three depicting the voca-tional or hobby-related scene he or she prefers. A motivation questionnaire, to explore motivation behind occupational choices, can be administered sepa-rately. However, the GPII-R is gendered in construction, using separate male and female general interest areas. The author defends the separation, noting that gender stereotypes do influence vocational choice (Geist, 1988).

This inventory may be administered individually or with groups, and it can be scored in only a few minutes, so it may be both time- and cost-effective in rehabilitation settings. It is suitable for age groups spanning late junior high to adulthood so it may be useful in transition planning. Rehabilitation profes-sionals are encouraged to be aware of possible gender stereotyping and to allow vocational exploration outside of traditional roles (Danker-Brown, Sigelman, & Flexer, 1978).

Scales of Independent Behavior–Revised

While not a completely work-related assessment, the *Scales of Independent Be-havior–Revised* (SIB-R; Bruininks, Woodcock, Weatherman, & Hill, 1996) may prove to be particularly suitable for vocational assessment of people with intellectual disabilities. The SIB-R is based on a standardization sample of 2,182 individuals ranging in age from infancy to 80 years old. The SIB-R assesses four adaptive behavior clusters: motor skills, social interaction and communication skills, personal living skills, and community living skills. The latter cluster consists of items measuring behavior related to successful employment. The SIB-R also contains a detailed scale of problem behavior, measuring internalized, externalized, and asocial maladaptive aspects. Scores can be expressed as standard scores, percentiles, ranks, and age scores. Both frequency of occurrence and severity of the problem are assessed (Bruininks, Woodcock, Weatherman, & Hill, 1996).

A particular contribution of the SIB-R is the Support Score, which is a weighted measure of maladaptive and adaptive behavior used to determine the support, supervision, and resources an individual needs. Six broad levels of support (pervasive, extensive, frequent, limited, intermittent, and infrequent or no support) can be determined. The SIB-R, unlike the previously discussed measures, covers the levels of support required and offers normative data for adults who are not disabled, enhancing its value for determining vocational adjustment. This scale may provide some objectivity in assessing the "levels of support" concept described in the AAMR definition of intellectual disability (Bruininks, Woodcock, Weatherman, & Hill, 1996).

Work Samples

Although the inclusion of work samples in vocational assessment has been a popular strategy (Menchetti, Rusch, & Owens, 1983), there are several drawbacks to their use (Singer, 1977). Foremost, work samples often are not readily available in rehabilitation counseling settings. The materials required are often expensive and cumbersome and are more likely to be found in a training program setting. Additionally, time constraints may affect work sample use since the time needed for a thorough and realistic sample could require days or weeks (Jewish Employment and Vocational Services, 1976; Singer, 1977).

Critically, work samples often have limited validity or predictive value for a population of persons with intellectual disabilities, even for those with mild disabilities (Irvin, Gersten, Taylor, Close, & Bellamy, 1981). Work samples have been faulted as measuring products of prior learning and neglecting progress made on the job itself. They often do not duplicate well the exact characteristics of specific job clusters and bypass the social aspects that are most often associated with job retention (Black & Rojewski, 1998). In the field of personnel selection, work samples have been used to predict job performance, to evaluate training or job readiness, to identify specific and broad abilities and skills, as a criterion for hiring, and as a criterion for validating other types of more formalized test batteries (Jackson, Harris, Ashton, McCarthy, & Tremblay, 2000). However, the use of sheltered workshops and supported employment programs allows for an opportunity for individuals to be evaluated on the job and receive training at the same time (West, Johnson, Cone, Hernandez, & Revell, 1998).

Conclusion

The concept of intellectual disabilities dates to antiquity. However, through the centuries, definitions have evolved and societal attitudes toward persons with intellectual disabilities have changed (Biasini et al., 1999; Miller et al., 1994). No longer are individuals castigated or permanently institutionalized. Despite difficulties, people with intellectual disabilities are seen as persons who possess skills of potential benefit to society. Although modern definitions of intellectual disability have changed little, the terminology used to classify functioning and to characterize individuals has undergone dramatic revisions (Bellini, 2003; Iacono, 2002; Leicester & Cooke, 2002; McDermott, Martin, & Butkus, 1999).

Assessment of individuals with intellectual disabilities is the process wherein current deficits can be identified and talents recognized in order to better view the individual as a total entity possessing unique cognitive and social adaptation skills. By combining assessments such as norm-referenced tests, observations, and more informal measures, the rehabilitation professional can lay a firm foundation for making decisions (Biasini et al., 1999; Sattler, 1992). Fortunately, there are both new and well-established measures available for assessing individuals with intellectual disabilities. However, none can be accepted without question or caveat (Kamphaus, Petoskey, & Morgan, 1997; American Psychiatric Association, 2000). When integrating findings from standardized measures with background data and clinical impressions, the limitations of standardized instruments must be recognized.

The future of assessment of adults with intellectual disabilities is likely to embrace three major trends. First, the trend toward the use of person-first language paired with less stigmatizing terms is likely to continue, fueled by a philosophical shift toward human needs over institutional conveniences and strongly supported by consumers and their advocates (AAMR, 2002; Biasini et al., 1999). A second important trend includes addressing the rehabilitation needs of individuals whose intellectual deficits are mild yet who are unable to adjust or adapt to an increasingly complex society. It is this population that the new AAMR (2002) definition of intellectual disabilities seeks to address. A third trend involves the increasing belief that work has therapeutic and self-validating qualities to it and that adults with intellectual disabilities, even those who appear to have profound disabilities, must be allowed an opportunity to join the workforce and become productive citizens. Such an approach has been increasingly expressed in mandated programs laid out by legislation and supported employment program development (Wehman, West, & Kregel, 1999). Across all of these trends, the role of rehabilitation will be paramount.

Authors' Note

We wish to acknowledge the contributions of James M. Woo-Sam, PhD, co-author of previous editions of this chapter.

References

Amble, B. R., & Peterson, G. (1979). Rehabilitation counselors: The use of psychological reports. *Rehabilitation Counseling Bulletin, 22,* 127–130.

American Association on Mental Retardation. (2002). *Mental retardation: Definition, classification, and systems of support* (10th ed.). Washington, DC: Author.

American Psychiatric Association. (1994). *Diagnostic and statistic manual of mental disorders: DSM-IV* (4th ed.). Washington, DC: Author.

American Psychiatric Association. (2000). *Diagnostic and statistic manual of mental disorders: DSM-IV-TR.* Washington, DC: Author.

Anastasi, A., & Urbina, S. (1997). *Psychological testing.* Upper Saddle River, NJ: Prentice Hall.

Balboni, H., Battagliese, G., & Pedrabissi, L. (2000). The psychopathology inventory for mentally retarded adults: Factor structure and comparisons between subjects with or without dual diagnosis. *Research in Developmental Disabilities, 21*(4), 311–321.

Baroff, G. S. (1999). General learning disorder: A new designation for intellectual disabilities. *Intellectual Disabilities, 37,* 68–70.

Becker, R. L. (2000). *Reading Free Vocational Interest Inventory: 2 (RFVII: 2).* Columbus, OH: Elbern Publications.

Becker, R. L., Schull, C., & Cambell, K. (1981). Vocational interest evaluation of trainable mentally retarded adults. *American Journal of Mental Deficiency, 85,* 350–356.

Bellini, J. (2003). Mental retardation: Definition, classification, and systems of supports. *Mental Retardation, 41*(2), 135–140.

Biasini, F. J., Grupe, L., Huffman, L., & Bray, N. W. (1999). Mental retardation: A symptom and a syndrome. In S. Netherton, D. Holmes, & C. E. Walker (Eds.), *Comprehensive Textbook of Child and Adolescent Disorders* (pp. 6–23). New York: Oxford University Press.

Black, R. S., & Rojewski, J. W. (1998). The role of social awareness in the employment success of adolescents with mild intellectual disabilities. *Education and Training in Intellectual Disabilities and Developmental Disabilities, 33,* 144–161.

Blackwell, T. L. (2002). Test Review: Woodcock, R.W., McGrew, K.S., & Werder, J.E. (1994). Woodcock-McGrew-Werder Mini-Battery of Achievement. *Rehabilitation Counseling Bulletin, 45*(2), 121–122.

Bower, A., & Hayes, A. (1995). Relations of scores on the Stanford Binet fourth edition and form L-M: Concurrent validation study with children who have intellectual disabilities. *American Journal on Intellectual Disabilities, 99,* 555–558.

Brolin, D. E. (1976). *Vocational preparation of retarded citizens.* Columbus, OH: Charles E. Merrill.

Brown, L., Sherbenou, R. J., & Johnsen, S. K. (1997). *Test of Nonverbal Intelligence–Third Edition (TONI-3).* Austin, TX: PRO-ED.

Bruininks, R. H., Woodcock, R. W., Weatherman, R. F., & Hill, B. K. (1996). *Scales of Independent Behavior–Revised (SIB-R).* Chicago: Riverside.

Butcher, J. N. (1999). *A beginner's guide to the MMPI-2.* Washington, DC: American Psychological Association.

Conoley, J. C., & Impara, J. C. (Eds.). (1995). *The Twelfth Mental Measurements Yearbook.* Lincoln, NE: Buros Institute of Mental Measurements.

Dacy, C. M., Nelson, W. M., & Stoeckel, J. (1999). Reliability, criterion-related validity, and qualitative comments of the fourth edition of the Stanford Binet Intelligence Scale with a young adult population with intellectual disability. *Journal of Intellectual Disability Research, 43,* 179–184.

Danker-Brown, P., Sigelman, C. K., & Flexer, R. W. (1978). Sex bias in vocational programming for handicapped students. *The Journal of Special Education, 12*(4), 451–458.

Decola, K. L. (1997). Increasing self-determination through vocational assessment for persons with intellectual disabilities. *Vocational Evaluation & Work Adjustment Bulletin, 30,* 51–55.

DeVinney, D. J., Kamnetz, B., Chan, F., & Hattori, K. (1998). Wechsler scale short forms in vocational assessment and evaluation settings. *Vocational Evaluation & Work Adjustment Bulletin, 31,* 4–10.

Drossman, E. R., Maller, S. J., & McDermott, P. A. (2001). Core profiles of school-aged examinees from the national standardization sample of the Comprehensive Test of Nonverbal Intelligence. *School Psychology Review, 30*(4), 586–598.

Dunn, L. M., & Dunn, L. M. (1981). *Peabody Picture Vocabulary Test–Revised.* Circle Pines, MN: American Guidance Services.

Dunn, L. M., & Dunn, L. M. (1997). *Peabody Picture Vocabulary Test–Third Edition.* Circle Pines, MN: American Guidance Services.

Edelson, M. G. (2005). A car goes in the garage like a can of peas goes in the refrigerator: Do deficits in real-world knowledge affect the assessment of intelligence in individuals with autism? *Focus on Autism and Other Developmental Disabilities, 20,* 2–9.

Flanagan, D. P., Alfonso, V. C., & Flanagan, R. (1994). A review of the Kaufman Adolescent and Adult Intelligence Test: An advancement in cognitive assessment? *School Psychology Review, 23,* 512–525.

Flanagan, D. P., Genshaft, J. L., & Boyce, D. M. (1999). Review of Kaufman, A.S., & Kaufman, N. L. (1993) Kaufman Adolescent and Adult Intelligence Test (KAIT). *Journal of Psychoeducational Assessment, 17,* 62–89.

Frauenhoffer, D., Ross, M. J., Searight, H. R., & Piotrowski, C. (1998). Psychological test usage among licensed mental health practitioners: A multidisciplinary survey. *Journal of Psychological Practice, 4,* 28–33.

Geist, H. (1988). *Geist picture interest inventory–Revised (GPII-R).* Beverly Hills, CA: Western Psychological Services.

Greenspan, S. (1997). Dead manual walking? Why the 1992 AAMR Definition needs redoing. *Education and Training in Intellectual Disabilities and Developmental Disabilities, 32,* 180–190.

Gustafsson, C., & Sonnander, K. (2005). A psychometric evaluation of a Swedish version of the psychopathology inventory for mentally retarded adults (PIMRA). *Research in Developmental Disabilities, 26,* 183–201.

Hammill, D. D., Pearson, N. A., & Wiederholt, J. L. (1997). *Comprehensive Test of Nonverbal Intelligence (CTONI).* Austin, TX: PRO-ED.

Hawkins, B. A., Eklund, S. J., James, D. R., & Foose, A. K. (2003). Adaptive behavior and cognitive function of adults with Down Syndrome: Modeling change with age. *Mental Retardation, 41*(1), 7–28.

Hill, B. (2001). *Adaptive and maladaptive behavior scales.* Retrieved June 2, 2006, from http://www.assessmentpsychology.com/adaptivebehavior.htm.

Horn, J. L., & Cattell, R. B. (1967). Age differences in fluid and crystallized intelligence. *Acta Psychologica, 26,* 107–129.

Iacono, T. (2002). Words. *AAC Augmentative and Alternative Communication, 18,* 215–216.

Irvin, L. K., Gersten, R., Taylor, V. E., Close, D. W., & Bellamy, G. T. (1981). Vocational skill assessment of severely mentally retarded adults. *American Journal of Mental Deficiency, 85,* 635–638.

Jackson, D. N., Harris, W. G., Ashton, M. C., McCarthy, J. M., & Tremblay, P. F. (2000). How useful are work samples in vocational studies? *International Journal of Selection and Assessment, 8*(1), 29–33.

Jewish Employment and Vocational Services. (1976). *Work sample evaluation system.* Philadelphia: Author.

Kamphaus, R. W. (1993). *Clinical assessment of children's intelligence.* Boston: Allyn & Bacon.

Kamphaus, R. W., Petoskey, M. D., & Morgan, A. W. (1997). *A history of intelligence test interpretation.* In D. P. Flanagan, J. L. Genshaft, & P. L. Harrison (Eds.), *Contemporary Intellectual Assessment* (pp. 32–47). New York: The Guilford Press.

Kaufman, A. S. (1990). *Assessing adolescent and adult intelligence.* Boston: Allyn & Bacon.

Kaufman, A. S., & Kaufman, N. L. (1990). *Administration and Scoring Manual for Kaufman Brief Intelligence Test (K-BIT).* Circle Pines, MN: American Guidance Service.

Kaufman, A. S., & Kaufman, N. L. (1993). *Manual for Kaufman Adolescent and Adult Intelligence Test (KAIT).* Circle Pines, MN: American Guidance Service.

Kaufman, A. S., & Kaufman, N. L. (1994). *Kaufman Functional Academic Skills Test (KFAST).* Circle Pines, MN: American Guidance Service.

Kaufman, A. S., & Kaufman, N. L. (2004). *Kaufman Test of Educational Achievement–Second Edition.* Circle Pines, MN: American Guidance Service.

Kaufman, A. S., & Lichtenberger, E. O. (1999). *Essentials of WAIS-HI Assessment.* New York: Wiley.

Kilsby, M., Bennert, K., & Beyer, S. (2002). Measuring and reducing acquiescence in vocational profiling procedures for first time job-seekers with mental retardation. *Journal of Vocational Rehabilitation, 17,* 287–299.

Lambert, N., Nihira, K., & Leland, H. (1993). *AAMR Adaptive Behavior Scale–School* (2nd Ed.). Austin, TX: PRO-ED.

Leicester, M., & Cooke, P. (2002). Rights not restrictions for learning disabled adults: A response to Spiecker and Steutel. *Journal of Moral Education, 31*(2), 181–187.

Leiter, R. G. (1948). *Leiter International Performance Scale.* Chicago: Stoelting.

MacMillan, D. L., Gresham, F. M., & Siperstein, G. N. (1993). Conceptual and psychometric concerns about the 1992 AAMR definition of intellectual disabilities. *American Journal of Intellectual Disabilities, 98,* 325–335.

Markwardt, F. C., Jr. (1987). *Peabody Individual Achievement Test (PIAT-R NU).* Circle Pines, MN: American Guidance Service.

Markwardt, F. C., Jr. (1997). *Peabody Individual Achievement Test Normative Update (PIAT-R NU).* Circle Pines, MN: American Guidance Service.

Masi, G. (1998). Psychiatric illness in mentally retarded adolescents: Clinical features. *Adolescence, 33,* 425–434.

Mather, N., & Wendling, B. J. (2005). Linking cognitive assessment results to academic interventions for students with learning disabilities. In D. P. Flanagan & P. L. Harrison (Eds.), *Contemporary intellectual assessment: Theories, tests and issues* (pp. 269–294). New York: The Guilford Press.

Mather, N., & Woodcock, R. W. (2001). Application of the Woodcock-Johnson Tests of Cognitive Ability–Revised to the diagnosis of learning disabilities. In A. S. Kaufman & N. L. Kaufman (Eds.), *Specific learning disabilities and difficulties in children and adolescents: Psychological assessment and evaluation* (pp. 55–96). New York: Cambridge University Press.

Matson, J. L. (1988) *The PIMRA Manual.* Orlando Park, IL: International Diagnostic Systems.

Matson, J. L., Kazdin, A. E., & Senatore, V. (1984). Psychometric properties of the Psychopathology Inventory for Mentally Retarded Adults. *Applied Research in Mental Retardation, 5,* 881–889.

McDaniel, W. F., & Harris, D. W. (1999). Mental health outcomes in dually diagnosed individuals with intellectual disabilities assessed with the MMPI-168 (L)s: Case studies. *Journal of Clinical Psychology, 55,* 487–496.

McDermott, S., Martin, M., & Butkus, S. (1999). What individual, provider, and community characteristics predict employment of individuals with intellectual disabilities? *American Journal of Intellectual Disabilities, 104,* 346–355.

McGrew, K. S., & Woodcock, R. W. (2001). *Woodcock-Johnson III technical manual.* Itasca, IL: Riverside Publishing.

McLean, W. E. (1993). Overview. In J. L. Matson & R. P. Barrett (Eds.), *Psychopathology in the mentally retarded* (pp. 1–16). Boston: Allyn & Bacon.

Menchetti, B., Rusch, F. R., & Owens, P. (1983). Vocational training. In J. L. Mason & S. E. Breuning (Eds.), *Assessing the mentally retarded* (pp. 247–284). New York: Grune & Stratton.

Michael, W. B. (1998). Review of the Woodcock-McGrew-Werder Mini-Battery of Achievement. In J. C. Impara & B. S. Plake (Eds.), *The Thirteenth Mental Measurements Yearbook* (pp. 1140–1141). Lincoln, NE: Buros Institute of Mental Measurements.

Miller, C. L., O'Callaghan, M. F., Keogh, D. A., & Whitman, T. L. (1994). Intellectual disabilities. In V. B. Van Hasselt & M. Hersen (Eds.), *Advanced abnormal psychology.* New York: Plenum Press.

Miller, P. S. (1999). The Equal Employment Opportunity Commission and people with intellectual disabilities. *Intellectual Disabilities, 37,* 162–167.

Muklewicz, C., & Bender, M. (1988). *Competitive job finding guide for persons with handicaps.* Austin, TX: PRO-ED.

Nezu, C. M., Nezu, A. M., & Gill-Weiss, M. J. (1992). *Psychopathology in persons with intellectual disabilities.* Champaign, IL: Research Press.

Nihira, K., Leland, H., & Lambert, N. (1993). *AAMR Adaptive Behavior Scale–Residential and Community* (2nd ed.). Austin, TX: PRO-ED.

Ollendick, T. H., Oswald, D. P., & Ollendick, D.G. (1993). Anxiety disorders in mentally retarded persons. In J. L. Matson & R. P. Barrett (Eds.), *Psychopathology in the mentally retarded* (pp. 41–85). Boston: Allyn & Bacon.

Ortiz, S. O. & Dynda, A. M. (2005). Use of intelligence test with culturally and linguistically diverse populations. In D. P. Flanagan & P. L. Harrison (Eds.), *Contemporary intellectual assessment: Theories, tests and issues* (pp. 545–556). New York: The Guilford Press.

Parker, L. D. (1993). The Kaufman Brief Intelligence Test: An introduction and review. *Measurement & Evaluation in Counseling & Development, 26,* 152–156.

Parker, R. M., & Bolton, B. (2005). Psychological Assessment in Rehabilitation. In R. M. Parker, E. M. Szymanski, & J. B. Patterson (Eds.), *Rehabilitation counseling: Basics and beyond* (4th ed., pp. 307–334). Austin, TX: PRO-ED.

Pickett, J. M., & Flynn, P. T. (1983). Language assessment tools for mentally retarded adults: Survey and recommendations. *Intellectual Disabilities, 21,* 244–247.

Piotrowski, C. (1999). Assessment practices in the era of managed care: Current status and future directions. *Journal of Clinical Psychology, 55,* 787–796.

Plake, B. S., & Impara, J. C. (Eds.). (2001). *The fourteenth mental measurements yearbook.* Lincoln, NE: Buros Institute of Mental Measurements.

Polloway, E. A. (1997). Developmental principles of the Luckasson et al., (1992). AAMR definition of intellectual disabilities: A retrospective. *Education and Training in Intellectual Disabilities and Developmental Disabilities, 32,* 174–178.

Psychological Corporation. (1999a). *Wechsler Abbreviated Scale of Intelligence.* San Antonio, TX: Author.

Psychological Corporation. (1999b). *Wechsler Abbreviated Scale of Intelligence Manual.* San Antonio, TX: Author.

Reiss, S. (1988). *The Reiss Screen for Maladaptive Behavior test manual.* Orland Park, IL: International Diagnostic Systems.

Reiss, S. (1993). Assessment of psychopathy in persons with intellectual disabilities. In J. L. Matson & R. P. Barrett (Eds.), *Psychopathology in the Mentally Retarded.* Boston: Allyn & Bacon.

Reiss, S. (1997). Comments on the Reiss Screen for Maladaptive Behavior and its factor structure. *Journal of Intellectual Disability Research, 41,* 346–354.

Roid, G. H. (2003). *The Stanford-Binet Intelligence Scales–Fifth Edition.* Itasca, IL: Riverside Publishing.

Roid, G. H. & Barram, R. A. (2004). *Essentials of Stanford-Binet intelligence scales (SB5) assessment.* Hoboken, NJ: John Wiley & Sons.

Roid, G. H., & Miller, L. (1997). *The Leiter International Performance Scale–Revised.* Chicago: Stoelting Company.

Rumrill, P. D., Jr., & Roessler, R. T. (1999). New directions in vocational rehabilitation: A "career development" perspective on "closure." *Journal of Rehabilitation, 65* (Jan–March), 26–33.

Sandieson, R. (1998). A survey on terminology that refers to people with intellectual disabilities/developmental disabilities. *Education and Training in Intellectual Disabilities and Developmental Disabilities, 33,* 290–295.

Sattler, J. M. (1992). *Assessment of children* (3rd ed.). San Diego: Jerome M. Sattler, Publisher, Inc.

Scheerenberger, R. C. (1987). *A history of intellectual disabilities: A quarter century of promise.* Baltimore: Paul H. Brookes.

Schrank, F. A. (2005). Woodcock-Johnson III Test of Cognitive Abilities. In D. P. Flanagan & P. L. Harrison (Eds.), *Contemporary intellectual assessment: Theories, tests and issues* (pp. 371–401). New York: The Guilford Press.

Serr, R., Lavay, B., Young, D., & Greene, G. (1994). Dexterity and bench assembly work productivity in adults with mild intellectual disabilities. *Education and Training in Intellectual Disabilities and Developmental Disabilities, 29,* 165–171.

Singer, T. (1977). *Vocational evaluation system.* Rochester, NY: The Singer Educational Division.

Slosson, R. L., Nicholson, C., & Hibpshman, T. L. (2002). *Slosson Intelligence Test–Revised 2002 Edition.* East Aurora, NY: Slosson Educational Publications Inc.

Smith, J. D. (1997). Intellectual disabilities as an educational construct: Time for a new shared view? *Education and Training in Intellectual Disabilities and Developmental Disabilities, 32,* 168–173.

Sovner, R. & Pary, R. J. (1993). Affective disorders in developmentally disabled persons. In J. L. Matson & R. P. Barrett (Eds.), *Psychopathology in the Mentally Retarded* (2nd ed., pp. 87–147). Boston: Allyn & Bacon.

Sparrow, S. S., Balla, D. A., & Cicchetti, D. V. (1984). *Vineland Adaptive Behavior Scales.* Circle Pines, MN: American Guidance Service.

Sparrow, S. S., Cicchetti, D. V., & Balla, D. A. (2005). *Vineland Adaptive Behavior Scales, Second Edition.* Circle Pines, MN: American Guidance Service.

Spies, R. A., & Plake, B. S. (Eds.). (2005). *The sixteenth mental measurements yearbook.* Lincoln, NE: Buros Institute of Mental Measurements.

Stano, J. (2004). Test Review of the Wechsler Abbreviated Scale of Intelligence. *Rehabilitation Counseling Bulletin, 48*(1), 56–57.

Stevens, P., & Martin, N. (1999). Supporting individuals with intellectual disability and challenging behavior in integrated work settings: An overview and a model for service provision. *Journal of Intellectual Disabilities Research, 43,* 19–29

Sturmey, P., Burcham, J. A., & Shaw, B. (1996). The frequency of REISS screen diagnoses in a community sample of adults with mental retardation. *Behavioral Interventions, 11*(2), 87–94.

Swiezy, N. B., Matson, J. L., Kirkpatrick-Sanchez, S., & Williams, D. E. (1995). A criterion validity study of the schizophrenia subscale of the Psychopathology Instrument for Mentally Retarded Adults (PIMA). *Research in Developmental Disabilities, 16,* 75–80.

Szymanski, E. M., & Hanley-Maxwell, C. (1996). Career development of people with developmental disabilities: An ecological model. *Journal of Rehabilitation, 62,* 48–55.

Tsatsanis, K. D., Dartnall, N., Cicchetti, D., Sparrow, S. S., Kiln, A., & Volkmar, F. R. (2003). Concurrent validity and classification accuracy of the Leiter and Leiter-R in low-functioning children with autism. *Journal of Autism and Developmental Disorders, 33*(1), 23–30.

Wadsworth, J., Milsom, A., & Cocco, K. (2004). Career development for adolescents and young adults with mental retardation. *Professional School Counseling, 8*(2), 141–147.

Wagner, P. A. (1991). Developmentally based personality assessment of adults with intellectual disabilities. *Intellectual Disabilities, 29,* 87–92.

Walsh, K. K., & Shenouda, N. (1999). Correlations among Reiss Screen, the Adaptive Behavior Scale II, and Aberrant Behavior Checklist. *American Journal of Mental Retardation, 104*(3), 236–248.

Walters, S. O., & Weaver, K. A. (2003). Relationships between the Kaufman Brief Intelligence Test and the Wechsler Adult Intelligence Scale–third edition. *Psychological Reports, 92*(3), 1111–1115.

Wasserman, J. D., & Tulsky, D. S. (2005). A history of intelligence assessment. In D. P. Flanagan & P. L. Harrison (Eds.), *Contemporary intellectual assessment: Theories, tests and issues* (pp. 2–22). New York: The Guilford Press.

Wechsler, D. (1981). *Manual for the Wechsler Adult Intelligence Test–Revised.* San Antonio, TX: The Psychological Corporation.

Wechsler, D. (1997). *Wechsler Adult Intelligence Test—III administration and scoring manual.* San Antonio, TX: The Psychological Corporation.

Wehman, P., West, M., & Kregel, J. (1999). Supported employment program development and research needs: Looking ahead to the year 2000. *Education and Training in Intellectual Disabilities and Developmental Disabilities, 34,* 3–19.

West, M., Johnson, A., Cone, A., Hernandez, A., & Revell, G. (1998). Extended employment support: Analysis of implementation and funding issues. *Education and Training in Intellectual Disabilities and Developmental Disabilities, 33,* 357–366.

Wilkinson, G. S. (1993). *Wide Range Achievement Test–3.* Wilmington, DE: Wide Range.

Wilkinson, G. S. & Robertson, G. J. (2006). *The Wide Range Achievement Test* (4th ed.). Wilmington, DE: Wide Range.

Woodcock, R. W., & Johnson, M. B. (1989). *Woodcock-Johnson Psycho-Educational Battery–Revised.* Allen, TX: DLM Teaching Resources.

Woodcock, R. W., McGrew, K. S., & Mather, N. (2001a). *Woodcock-Johnson III.* Itasca, IL: Riverside.

Woodcock, R. W., McGrew, K. S., & Mather, N. (2001b). *Woodcock-Johnson III Tests of Achievement.* Itasca, IL: Riverside.

Woodcock, R. W., McGrew, K. S., & Mather, N. (2001c). *Woodcock-Johnson III Tests of Cognitive Ability.* Itasca, IL: Riverside.

Woodcock, R. W., McGrew, K. S., & Werder, J. E. (1994). *Woodcock-McGrew-Werder Mini-Battery of Achievement.* Chicago: Riverside Publishing Company.

World Health Organization. (1996). *International Classification of Diseases, Tenth Edition: Guide for Mental Retardation.* Geneva: Author.

Zimmerman, I. L., Covin, J., & Woo-Sam, J. M. (1986). A longitudinal comparison of the WISC-R and WAIS-R. *Psychology in the Schools, 23,* 148–151.

Chapter 19

Assessment in Psychiatric Rehabilitation

Kim L. MacDonald-Wilson and Patricia B. Nemec

Psychiatric rehabilitation assessment is not to be confused with traditional psychiatric diagnosis. A rehabilitation assessment and a traditional psychiatric diagnosis are very different. The goal is different; the process is different; the tools are different. Yet, each provides useful and meaningful information, each requires training to implement, and each has a role in a comprehensive treatment and rehabilitation intervention. Traditional psychiatric diagnosis focuses on the medical impairment—that is, the pathological condition and symptom development over time—while rehabilitation assessment focuses on the skills and the resources the person needs to achieve his or her overall rehabilitation goal, which names the particular role and environment in which the person wishes to live, learn, or work. Rather than assigning particular diagnostic categories, the rehabilitation assessment lists and describes the critical skills and resources needed for success and satisfaction in the goal environment. The purpose of the traditional psychiatric diagnostic procedure is to assign a diagnostic label to describe the person's pathological condition, and it is selected based on descriptions and observations of the person's history, signs, and symptoms. In contrast, the rehabilitation assessment identifies both existing and needed skills and resources, which are selected based on their likely impact on goal achievement, on the perspectives of the person setting the goal (along with the views of his or her significant others, if relevant), and on objective evaluation of skill performance and resource accessibility.

Because the goals of the two approaches are so different, it would be expected that the diagnostic procedures would be different. Just as psychiatric knowledge and specific diagnostic techniques are needed by a practitioner to conduct a psychiatric diagnosis, unique knowledge and techniques are needed by a practitioner to conduct a psychiatric rehabilitation assessment.

The Empirical Foundation for a Psychiatric Rehabilitation Assessment

Developments in psychiatric rehabilitation assessment reported in this chapter are anchored in empirical studies conducted during the last several decades by many researchers from a variety of disciplines. In a series of reviews of this research literature, William Anthony and his colleagues at the Boston University Center for Psychiatric Rehabilitation have concluded that the rehabilitation outcome of persons with psychiatric disabilities is a function of their skills and supportive resources in the community.

In the initial review of this body of research, Anthony and Margules (1974) concluded that persons with long-term psychiatric disabilities can learn a variety of skills regardless of their symptoms and that these skills, when properly integrated into a comprehensive rehabilitation program that provides support for the use of these skills in the community, can have a significant impact on rehabilitation outcome. Since that 1974 literature review, several other reviews and studies also have concluded that rehabilitation outcome is a function of skills and the supportive resources in a person's community (Anthony, 1979, 1994; Anthony & Jansen, 1984; Anthony & Liberman, 1986; Arns & Linney, 1995; Cohen & Anthony, 1984; Cook & Razzano, 2000; Dion & Anthony, 1987; Tsang, Lam, Ng, & Leung, 2000).

Given that rehabilitation outcome is a function of skills and resources, it makes sense that the improvement of skills and resources be the focus of psychiatric rehabilitation interventions. *It follows logically that if rehabilitation interventions are designed to improve an individual's skills and supports, then rehabilitation assessments should evaluate his or her present and needed skills and supports.*

Traditional psychiatric diagnostic procedures do *not* provide much information relevant to prescribing a rehabilitation intervention. A number of studies and reviews of the research literature report that only a modest or no significant relationship exists among rehabilitation outcome, psychiatric diagnostic labels, and/or descriptions of the person's symptom patterns (Anthony, 1994; Anthony, Rogers, Cohen, & Davies, 1995; Arns & Linney, 1995; Ikebuchi, Iwasaki, Sugimoto, Miyauchi, & Liberman, 1999). More recent studies have found modest relationships between negative symptoms and vocational outcomes, particularly when concurrent vocational outcomes and not future vocational outcomes are considered (Bell & Lysaker, 1995; Hoffman, Kupper, Zbinden, & Hirsbrunner, 2003; Rogers, Anthony, Cohen, & Davies, 1997). A 2004 meta-analysis of diagnostic and demographic variables supports the conclusion that a diagnosis of schizophrenia is related to vocational outcomes, although effect sizes and the number of studies included were small (Wewiorski & Fabian, 2004). However, recent reviews of the literature conclude that, although there are modest relationships between negative symptoms, or diagnosis and vocational outcomes, the strongest predictors are social skills, work history, and premorbid functioning (Cook & Razzano, 2000; Tsang et al., 2000), suggesting that a rehabilitation assessment of skills and functioning provides more relevant information for rehabilitation outcomes than traditional measures of symptoms or diagnosis.

In summary, the empirical literature suggests two conclusions. First, the present psychiatric diagnostic system collects and organizes diagnostic information that is not descriptive, prescriptive, or predictive with respect to rehabilitation outcome. Thus, a unique assessment procedure is needed for psychiatric rehabilitation. Second, a psychiatric rehabilitation assessment needs to focus on describing a person's skills and environmental supports in relation to his or her overall rehabilitation goals.

Components of Psychiatric Rehabilitation Assessment

The psychiatric rehabilitation assessment evaluates a person's skills and supports in the context of the environments in which he or she chooses to live, learn, work, and socialize. The assessment contains three components: an overall rehabilitation goal, a functional assessment, and a resource assessment. The overall rehabilitation goal identifies the particular environments in which the person chooses to live, learn, work, or socialize during the next 6–18 months. A goal environment may be one where the person currently is and where he or she wants to stay; or the environment may be one to which the person desires to move within the next year or two. After the goal environment has been determined, assessment instruments may then be used to complement the interview process to help the individual figure out what skills and supports need to be developed to maximize his or her success and satisfaction in each chosen goal environment.

The overall rehabilitation goal typically is established during a series of interviews in which the person's satisfaction and dissatisfaction with his or her current environments and his or her choice of future environments are explored. The overall rehabilitation goal is critical to the assessment because the hope of its achievement motivates the person to engage in the assessment. In addition, the overall rehabilitation goal focuses both the practitioner and the individual setting the goal on those skills and supports that are relevant to success in that particular environment. In addition, the overall rehabilitation goal focuses subsequent assessments by limiting the skills and supports assessed to those that are relevant to satisfaction and success in that goal environment. The following are examples of overall rehabilitation goals:

- To live at Mulberry House with my girlfriend until November 2008
- To work in transitional employment by June 2008
- To study at a supported learning program at Worcester State College by fall 2009

Establishing a person's overall rehabilitation goal at the beginning of the psychiatric rehabilitation process is consistent with the philosophy and principles of psychiatric rehabilitation (Anthony, Cohen, Farkas, & Gagne, 2000; Hughes & Weinstein, 2000; Pratt, Gill, Barrett, & Roberts, 2006), of good mental health practice (New Freedom Commission, 2003; Rapp & Goscha, 2005), and of high-quality health-care service delivery (Institute of Medicine, 2001). Self-determination, which includes setting personally meaningful goals, is a cornerstone for the new driving vision of the U.S. Substance Abuse and Mental Health Services Administration (SAMHSA, 2006).

Setting goals affects performance whether a person has a disability or not. A number of early experimental studies have shown the positive effects of setting goals (Locke, Shaw, Saari, & Latham, 1981). Personalized goals affect performance by targeting a specific outcome, mobilizing efforts and strategies to achieve that outcome, and increasing persistence (Locke et al., 1981). A specific goal and detailed planning for how to achieve that goal increase the likelihood that the goal will be reached (Gollwitzer, 1996).

Taking the time to work with an individual to set his or her overall rehabilitation goals is also important because, if this process is neglected, the practitioner and the individual very likely may be pursuing different goals without knowing it. Research evidence suggests that assessments of individuals by practitioners and assessments by individuals themselves often have little or no agreement on items as diverse as potential for recovery (Blackman, 1982), desired outcomes (Berzinz, Bednar, & Severy, 1975), rehabilitation issues (Leviton, 1973), perceptions of needs (Phelan et al., 1995; Slade, Phelan, & Thornicroft, 1998), and the existence of functional skills (Dellario, Anthony, & Rogers, 1983). For example, Dimsdale, Klerman, and Shershow (1979) studied a group of people in a psychiatric inpatient facility where the staff viewed insight as the primary goal. The individuals themselves, however, placed insight at the bottom of their list of goals. Other research indicates that when clients' and practitioners' goals are incongruent, clients do not appear to profit from therapy, are disappointed with their care, and often fail to comply with their treatment activities (Lazare, Eisenthal, & Wasserman, 1975; Noble, Douglas, & Newman, 2001; Tryon & Winograd, 2002). This finding is not exclusive to mental health and psychiatric rehabilitation services (Cruz & Pincus, 2002; Vermeire, Hearnshaw, Van Royen, & Denekens, 2001).

Sometimes the reasons for not involving people with psychiatric disabilities in goal-setting stem from the mistaken belief that they are unable to make decisions or choices. Some authors have suggested that the decision-making difficulties experienced by individuals with psychiatric disorders may be more related to treatment environments and interaction than to symptoms or impairments (Estroff, Patrick, Zimmer, & Lachiotte, 1997; Goffman, 1961; Ryan, 1976; Schmieding, 1968). Other researchers hold the view that impaired decision-making ability or poor goal-setting is an inherent component of mental illness, especially psychosis. For example, negative symptoms, one of the major problems associated with schizophrenia, include withdrawal, lack of goal-directed behavior, and low motivation. While some people with schizophrenia may struggle with some decisions and some decision-making processes (Ernst & Paulus, 2005; Shumway, Sentell, Chouljian, Tellier, Rozewicz, & Okun, 2003), they still wish to be involved in making treatment decisions (Hamann, Cohen, Leucht, Busch, & Kissling, 2005) and often have the capacity to make decisions when adequately informed (Grisso & Appelbaum, 1995; Stiles, Poythress, Hall, Falkenbach, & Williams, 2001). Psychiatric rehabilitation interventions also can be used to increase the knowledge needed to make an informed decision and to improve decision-making skills (Rapp & Goscha, 2005).

Apart from the question of whether persons with psychiatric disabilities can make their own choices or state their own needs, most mental health and rehabilitation practitioners agree that setting goals in treatment is important. Unfortunately, for many years mental health professionals resisted adopting goal-setting as a regular part of their practice (Holroyd & Goldenberg, 1978) and, in particular, goal-setting that reflected the consumer's perspective about desired rehabilitation outcomes (Farkas, Cohen, & Nemec, 1988).

Several studies examining vocational programs and program participant preference have reported on the relationship between participant choice and rehabilitation outcome (Becker, Drake, Farabaugh, & Bond, 1996; Bell & Lysaker, 1996). Becker et al. (1996) found that participants in a supported employment program who obtained employment in their *chosen* employment areas were more satisfied with their jobs and remained in their jobs twice as long as those who worked in nonpreferred job areas. Bell and Lysaker (1996) randomly assigned three groups of veterans in a vocational program to three different conditions: (1) those required to work at least 20 hours a week; (2) those required to work at least 10 hours a week but who could, if they wished, work up to 20 hours; and (3) those who *chose* to work as few or as many hours as they wanted up to a maximum of 20 hours a week. Participants who were permitted to choose the number of hours worked actually worked more hours per week than people in the other conditions and reported a greater reduction in symptoms than participants required to work at least 10 hours per week. In summary, the research clearly supports the importance of helping individuals choose their overall rehabilitation goals during the first stages of the assessment process.

In psychiatric rehabilitation assessment, it is only after a person sets an overall rehabilitation goal that more formal assessment instruments are used to assess the person's skills and supports in relation to the demands of the chosen goal environment(s).

Psychiatric Rehabilitation Assessment Interview

The psychiatric rehabilitation assessment typically involves a practitioner conducting a series of interviews with a client. Two principles guide the assessment interview. First, the practitioner attempts to maximize the involvement of the client in the interview process. Second, the information collected during the interview is recorded in a way that maximizes the client's understanding and ownership of the assessment results.

Involving the client in the interview means facilitating the client's active participation in completing each of the tasks that are part of doing a rehabilitation assessment. An important ingredient of the assessment process is the interpersonal skill of the person conducting the assessment (Anthony, Pierce, & Cohen, 1980). Several practitioner skills serve to involve the client in the assessment. These skills include orienting, giving instructions, requesting information, and demonstrating understanding throughout the interview.

Orienting means that the practitioner describes the task, the purpose of the task, and the roles of both the practitioner and client. The orientation gives a clear picture of what will happen and how the client is expected to participate. This sort of preparation or "role induction" contributes to positive outcomes in counseling relationships (Orlinsky, Grawe, & Parks, 1994) and can be especially valuable for individuals who lack experience or knowledge of expectations from a counseling-type interaction (Noble et al., 2001; Sue, Zane, &

Young, 1994; Walitzer, Dermen, & Connors, 1999). The way the practitioner orients the client is important. The practitioner should use language that the client is likely to understand, pace the orientation to maintain the client's attention and interest, and frequently check on the client's understanding of what the practitioner has previously said. An orientation at the beginning of a functional assessment might sound like this (the practitioner is speaking):

> "The first task in functional assessment is listing critical behaviors. The goal of listing is to write a list of all the skills that you need to successfully achieve your goal of living at home with your family. First, you and I will name the behaviors your family expects you to do, and second, you will tell me about the things that you want to be able to do. I will be asking you questions and summarizing what you say to make sure that I understand what you are saying. I want you to honestly share your thoughts and feelings. Also, please ask questions when you are unclear about something. Just to make sure that I'm being clear now, please tell me, in your own words, what will happen next."

Giving instructions is similar to orienting in that both provide direction. Giving instructions, however, specifically directs a person to perform a particular action or set of actions. The instructions tell a person what exact steps to follow. For example, the practitioner might give instructions during the functional assessment like this:

> "Read over this list of types of mental health services, and circle the ones that you have used in the past month."

Giving instructions can be combined with reorienting as needed to provide structure to the interview. For example, a practitioner might remind someone of the focus of the assessment by saying, "Remember that we're here to figure out what work skills you have. Right now I would like you to answer my questions with your feelings and experiences from your last job, rather than talking about your roommate."

Requesting information encourages participation rather than directly telling the client how to be active. Requesting information is asking for facts, opinions, and feelings. Requesting information encourages someone to talk about a particular topic. Open-ended questions are especially valuable for encouraging dialogue. For example, the relatively narrow open-ended question, "What did you like best about living in the rooming house?" is likely to encourage participation more than the direct and closed-ended question, "Did you live on the ground floor?" or the very broad, "How are things at home now?" Indirect leads (Gerber, 1986) provide another way of inviting discussion, such as, "Tell me about a time when you asked a teacher for help," or "Give me an example of something your sister does that bugs you."

Demonstrating understanding is capturing in words what the client is feeling or thinking. Demonstrating understanding—also known as active listening (see, for example, Egan, 2007) and paraphrasing or reflecting feelings (see, for example, Carkhuff, 2000)—tells the individual that the practitioner is listening and helps clarify the individual's perspective. In the following sample dialogue that might occur in response to the indirect lead about the irritating sister, the practitioner demonstrates understanding of the client's feelings and view of the situation:

> Client: "What bugs me? She treats me bad. She never listens."

> Practitioner: "You're angry with her because she hurts you."

> Client: "Yeah, I keep trying to tell her that she's cruel to me, but she just doesn't listen. Maybe she doesn't care."

> Practitioner: "You think it doesn't matter to her that you are upset about how she treats you."

The practitioner's interpersonal skills facilitate client involvement and are key to developing an active partnership (Danley, MacDonald-Wilson, & Hutchinson, 1998; Mosher & Burti, 1992; Rapp & Goscha, 2005) during the assessment. However, many people with severe psychiatric disabilities have difficulties participating in an interview where active participation is expected. They may be accustomed to psychiatric interviews that focus on their symptoms, maladaptive behaviors, and probable causes of impairment (Kramer & Gagne, 1997). People who have spent years receiving mental health services may be "trained" to wait for direct questions and then to provide only the information requested. Negative experiences, lack of trust, and difficulty concentrating can interfere with someone's ability to connect. When a person does not participate in an interview without assistance, the practitioner needs to work at connecting and can benefit from using the practitioner skills described. Facilitating participation is important and may take time. No one should be prematurely dismissed as "unready" or "unable" to participate. Rather, practitioners should assume that lack of client participation is an indication that the practitioner needs to change his or her approach.

A structured assessment instrument can be used to supplement the rehabilitation assessment interview. Ideally, an instrument is used to save time, money, and/or effort while providing the same information that would otherwise be obtained through the interview or direct observation. Another benefit of using a test in psychiatric rehabilitation assessment is that a "good" test—one that is valid and reliable—provides some standardization. This may be important if the goal of assessment is comparison of program participants to one another, to certain norms, or to themselves at different points in time. In this way, tests can provide assessment information that could only be estimated from an interview (e.g., IQ aptitude scores, interest profiles).

Most structured instruments are beneficial if incorporated at the initial stages of exploration, providing some structure and a "shortcut" for gathering information. In addition, the use of instruments may be especially beneficial with individuals who need structure and/or who are limited in their verbal expression. Novice interviewers also may benefit from having a structured format, as might any interviewer who, without a structured or standardized procedure, may omit assessment of some important area.

In clinical assessment situations, the assessment process itself must begin and end with the individual. Before any instruments are used, the practitioner attempts to obtain the person's own perspective on his or her skill and resource needs, strengths, and deficits. The assessment can then proceed to acquiring information from significant others, testing, and/or observations in simulated environments. The practitioner must use the information collected by such standardized instruments in a conservative way. The information is just one source of data. Indeed, it is the focus and conduct of the assessment process, rather than the assessment instruments, that are the foundation for a valid assessment. Frey (1984) noted the limitations of assessment instruments: "Any attempt to capture, through single measures, an individual's status in a way that reflects all that is important to the rehabilitation process is ostentatious, to say the least" (p. 35).

One response to this predicament is to teach practitioners general assessment skills and how to use a specific instrument or assessment battery. Psychiatric rehabilitation assessment skills permit the practitioner to conduct a truly personalized and comprehensive assessment. Without a skilled practitioner, assessment can revert to a simple checklist of functioning, seemingly independent of the client's high-priority goals and the specific requirements of his or her preferred environment.

From the many instruments available, the practitioner must select the instrument most relevant to the specific assessment situation. However, there are certain critical characteristics of assessment instruments that can facilitate selection of a relevant and useful instrument. These critical characteristics are similar to the characteristics that are important in recording assessment information: A useful instrument will be clear, brief, environmentally specific, and skills- and/or resources-oriented.

Clear: As discussed earlier, the practitioner involves the client throughout the assessment interviews. The individual also should be involved in the administration of any assessment instruments. The instrument itself, the process of administration, and the results all need to be comprehensible to the client. The language of the instrument must be fairly simple and concrete. Language such as "gets lost" or "runs into walls" is preferable to "gross spatial and perceptual disorientation." Similarly, "arrives on time" may be preferable to "punctual." The use of the instrument must be clearly relevant to the client's situation. The practitioner using a particular instrument is aware of the reasons for the choice and needs to communicate these reasons to the individual. An orientation to the process and purpose of using an instrument is given, along with good instructions.

Brief: Brevity and simplicity in administering an instrument will facilitate its use within the assessment interview. A brief instrument will be easier to integrate into the assessment and less likely to change the interview from individualized exploration to rote and mechanical measurement. In addition, a brief instrument is more likely to be completed consistently than a lengthy instrument that taxes the patience of both client and practitioner.

Environmentally specific: Identification of the environment in which the person is expected to function is required for a meaningful assessment of his or her level of functioning. Ideally, then, an assessment instrument would determine performance within a particular environment. A standardized instrument, by definition, cannot provide adequate specificity if designed for broad use. It may be developed for use in a particular type of environment, such as a rooming house or a transitional employment program, but would still miss some of the environmental requirements of a particular rooming house or a specific transitional employment placement. An instrument could be developed for an environment by tailoring it to the requirements of that setting. For a treatment program, such an assessment instrument could be based on the entrance and exit criteria for the program. A skills–oriented assessment might list the skills a person must demonstrate to be admitted to the program and the skills required before the person could leave as a "successful graduate." With some attention, such an instrument could be reliable and valid, offering the opportunity for program evaluation data collection and clinical assessment.

Skill/resource focused: For use in the functional assessment part of the psychiatric rehabilitation assessment, an instrument needs to be skills oriented and, ideally, will assess both skill strengths and skill deficits. Skill-focused instruments need to contain items that are behavioral, observable, and measurable. Items that are skill focused identify behaviors or actions that could be observed or demonstrated. In addition, such instruments need to specify actual skills (e.g., "introducing yourself" or "shampooing hair") rather than activities that require mastery of multiple skills (e.g., "verbal communication," "dependability," or "maintaining personal hygiene"). Separate instruments may be needed that focus on resources and supports, indicating resources (e.g., low-cost transportation) that are needed, available, and accessible to the client.

Documenting assessment results is another potential area for developing a partnership between the individual and the practitioner. Once all the data are gathered, the assessment information should be recorded and organized in such a way that the individual understands the completed assessment because developing a partnership requires an opportunity for the individual to access and review the assessment results. Of course, the information gathered from a psychiatric rehabilitation assessment also must be recorded in a way that is consistent with the record-keeping requirements of the agency and/or funding source.

Psychiatric Rehabilitation Assessment Instruments

The focus on outcome assessment in psychiatric rehabilitation services has increased with the relatively new emphasis on evidence-based practice (Drake,

Merrens, & Lynde, 2005). Outcome assessment can occur at the level of the individual, the program, and/or the system (Blankertz & Cook, 1998), or as the new International Classification of Functioning, Disability and Health describes, it can occur at the level of the body, the individual, and society (World Health Organization, 2001). At the individual level, one can examine clinical outcomes, satisfaction, and service utilization (Sederer, Dickey, & Hermann, 1996). In the clinical outcome area, literally hundreds of assessment instruments, varying greatly in their focus, exist for use with persons with psychiatric disabilities. Some measures focus on psychiatric diagnosis and symptoms, some on cognition and neuropsychological functions, some on behavior and skills, some on functioning and status, and some on resources or needs (both those needed by and/or available to the person with a psychiatric disability). The preponderance of the assessment literature for people with psychiatric disabilities is in the area of psychiatric symptoms and diagnosis and on neuropsychological or cognitive functions. Readers are referred to Glynn (1998) and the chapters on assessment of psychopathology and neuropsychological assessment in this volume for additional detail.

Many instruments, particularly those that claim to measure functioning, contain items from a variety of domains (Derogatis, 1994; Eisen, Dill, & Grob, 1994; Ware, Snow, Kosinski, & Gandek, 1993). A number of literature reviews have surveyed a variety of existing instruments potentially useful to psychiatric rehabilitation assessment and outcomes assessment. Sederer and Dickey (1996) review a number of instruments useful in outcome assessment in clinical practice, including those that focus on global well-being, functioning, symptoms, satisfaction, and service use. Dickerson (1997), Scott and Lehman (1998), and Wykes (1998) reviewed instruments that assess the social adjustment and social functioning of people with psychiatric disorders. A recent focus on social cognition has prompted a review of instruments that examine the cognitive component of social functioning (Corrigan & Penn, 2001). Phelan, Wykes, and Goldman (1994) and Goldman, Skodol, and Lave (1992) offered a review of global scales, discussing their strengths and problems. Wallace (1986) and Vaccaro, Pitts, and Wallace (1992) have reviewed functional assessment instruments for people with severe psychiatric disabilities.

Assessment of Functioning

Functioning refers to activities or performance, "a natural or proper action for which a person, office, thing or organization is fitted or employed" (Webster's, 1990, p. 677). An assessment of functioning may focus on global functioning or specific evaluation of skills and behaviors. Global measures might emphasize performance in particular roles (e.g., spouse, worker), performance in particular domains (social, emotional, psychological), or status (employment, educational, residential) to indicate functioning. At times, global functioning instruments also include measures of symptoms. Global measures focus on the outcome of functioning (e.g., has been employed full time, is married, has friends), whereas skill assessments focus on specific sets of behaviors (e.g., initiating conversations, expressing feelings, budgeting money). Functional assessment in psychiatric rehabilitation involves the latter. However, measures of global functioning are often used in outcome assessment approaches and are mistaken at times for assessments of skills. Some measures of functioning often used with people with psychiatric disabilities include the *Behavior and Symptom Identification Scale-32* (BASIS-32; Eisen et al., 1994), the *Global Assessment of Functioning* (GAF; APA, 2000; Goldman, Skodol, & Lave, 1992), the *Role Functioning Scale* (RFS; Goodman, Sewall, Cooley, & Leavitt, 1993), the *Multnomah Community Ability Scale* (Barker, Barron, McFarland, & Bigelow, 1994), and the *Life Skills Profile* (Rosen, Hadzi-Pavlovic, & Parker, 1989). While these measures are useful in determining improvements in various types of functioning, few of them contain items that measure specific skills. Most contain items that measure larger activities (i.e., activities of daily living, social competence, symptom management) that require mastery of a variety of skills.

Measures that are reliable and valid are needed both to assess the outcome and effectiveness of service programs and to provide clinically relevant data on the skills and resources, strengths, and needs of the individual to plan interventions to address those needs. Typically, skill and resource assessments are process types of measures, not outcome measures. Ultimately, the effectiveness of psychiatric rehabilitation interventions lies in demonstrating changes in roles or status, the outcome of improvements in skills and resources. However, this chapter focuses on reviewing assessment instruments that can be used in the psychiatric rehabilitation process with individuals, in conducting functional and resource assessments.

Skills-Oriented Instruments

A number of instruments that measure skills have been developed for use with persons with psychiatric disabilities. Table 19.1 summarizes the instruments for assessing skills, and Table 19.2 summarizes instruments for assessing resources. The next section is a description of instruments assessing skills related to particular environments—the living, learning, working, or social environments.

Living Environments
The *St. Louis Inventory of Community Living Skills* (SLICLS) is a brief instrument and was designed to focus on discrete community living skills to be used to evaluate rehabilitation programs, to specify a residential placement, or to measure the impact of skills training interventions (Evenson & Boyd, 1993). It is a 15-item instrument rated on a 7-point scale indicating skill level and help needed, from 1 = *few or no skills,* 2 = *needs substantial help or improvement,* 3 = *needs moderate help or improvement,* 4 = *skill level not clear or not observed,* 5 = *has moderate skills,* 6 = *has substantial skills,* to 7 = *self-sufficient, very adequate skills.* Each item is given descriptors, or examples of skills reflected in the item

(text continues on p. 548)

TABLE 19.1.
Instruments for Assessing Skills

Skills: Living-Community Environments

Instrument	Assessment Method	# Items	Rating Scale	Scales/Sample Items	Clear ?	Brief ?	Skills Incl.?	Skills +	Skills −	Env. Spec.
Atascadero Skills Profile (Vess, 2001)	Consensus of team rating	34	5-pt scale: 0 = skills consistently absent or completely inadequate to 4 = skills consistently present and adequate	10 Domains: Behavior, Medication, Substance abuse, Assault, Suicide, Self-care, Independent living, Sexual deviance, Interpersonal, Leisure	M	Y 10 min	M	Y	Y	Y
Brief Instrumental Functioning Scale (Sullivan, Dumenci, Burnam, & Koegel, 2001)	Self-report	6	3-pt scale: can do alone, needs help, don't know if can do alone	Take medications, Fill out benefits application, Budget money, Use city buses, Set up job interview by phone, Find an attorney	Y	Y	M	Y	Y	N
Client Assessment of Strengths, Interests and Goals (CASIG) and Staff Observations and Client Information (SOCI [aka CASIG-I; Wallace, Lecomte, Wilde, & Liberman, 2001)	Structured interview with consumer and informants	~100 with follow-up prompts	Varies by section: Skills rated by yes-no-not apply	8 Domains: Goals, Social and independent living skills, Medication practices, Quality of life, Quality of treatment, Symptoms, Unacceptable community behaviors, Specific goals	Y	N 45–90 min	Y	Y	Y	Y

Note. Y = yes; N = no; M = moderately; Incl. = included; Env. Spec. = environmentally specific.

(continues)

TABLE 19.1. Continued.

Skills: Living-Community Environments (Continued)

Instrument	Assessment Method	# Items	Rating Scale	Scales/Sample Items	Clear?	Brief?	Skills			Env. Spec.
							Incl.?	+	–	
Independent Living Skills Survey (ILSS-I, ILSS-SR; Wallace, Liberman, Tauber, & Wallace, 2000)	Informant-report and / Self-report interview	ILSS-I, 103 / ILSS-SR, 61 + 9 for interviewer	ILSS-I: 5-pt scale (always to never, and no opportunity to do) / ILSS-SR: 3-pt scale (yes, no, not apply)	ILSS-I 12 Domains: Appearance & clothing, Personal hygiene, Care of personal possessions, Food preparation & storage, Health maintenance, Money management, Transportation, Leisure & community, Job seeking, Job maintenance, Eating,[a] Social relations[a]	Y	M / 20–30 min	Y	Y	Y	Y
St. Louis Inventory of Community Living Skills (Evenson & Boyd, 1993)	Clinician rating of observed behavior	15	7-pt scale: 1 = few to no skills to 7 = very adequate skills, self-sufficient	Sample items: Personal hygiene, Communication, Handling money, Sexuality, Problem solving, Health practices	M	Y / 3 min	M	M	M	Y
UCSD Performance-Based Skills Assessment (UPSA; Patterson et al., 2001)	Performance rating of 5 task areas	5	Points awarded in each area for performance of subtasks	5 Task areas: Household chores, Communication, Finance, Transportation, Planning recreational activities	Y	M / 30 min	M	N	N	Y

Note. Y = yes; N = no; M = moderately; Incl. = included; Env. Spec. = environmentally specific.

(continues)

TABLE 19.1. *Continued.*

Skills: Learning–Educational Environments

Instrument	Assessment Method	# Items	Rating Scale	Scales/Sample Items	Clear ?	Brief ?	Skills Incl.?	Skills +	Skills –	Env. Spec.
Views About College Questionnaire (Stein, 2005)	Self-report	20	5-pt scale, extent of agreement with statements	Suggested Domains: Aspirations and plans; Perceived social support and acceptance; Perceived intellectual and emotional capacity for college	M	Y	N	N	N	M

Skills: Working Environments

Instrument	Assessment Method	# Items	Rating Scale	Scales/Sample Items	Clear ?	Brief ?	Skills Incl.?	Skills +	Skills –	Env. Spec.
Situational Assessment Scales to Assess Work Adjustment (WA) and Interpersonal Skills (IS) (Rogers, Hursh, Kielhofner, & Spaniol, 1990)	Rating of observed behavior in work setting	WA, 21 IS, 14	4-pt scale: 1 = cause to be fired to 4 = above acceptable performance; Behavioral anchors on each rating for each item	2 Scales: Work Adjustment (WA) Interpersonal Skills (IS)	Y	M	Y	Y	Y	Y
Standardized Assessment of Work Behaviour (Griffiths, 1973)	Rating of observed behavior in work setting	25	Each item is a 5-point continuum from strength (i.e., does complicated jobs) to deficit (i.e., can only do simple jobs)	5 Scales: Task Competence Response to supervision Relationship with others Work motivation Confidence-initiative	M	Y	M	Y	Y	Y

Note. Y = yes; N = no; M = moderately; Incl. = included; Env. Spec. = environmentally specific.

(continues)

TABLE 19.1. *Continued.*

Skills: Working Environments (Continued)

Instrument	Assessment Method	# Items	Rating Scale	Scales/Sample Items	Clear ?	Brief ?	Skills			Env. Spec.
							Incl.?	+	–	
Vocational Cognitive Rating Scale (VCRS; Greig, Hursh, Kielhofner, & Spaniol,, 2004)	Rating of observed behavior and brief interview with supervisor	16	5-pt scale: consistently inferior performance to consistently superior performance	Sample Items: Can remember instructions or begin tasks without a reminder; Starts tasks without prompting	Y	Y	Y	Y	Y	Y
Work Behavior Inventory (WBI; Lysaker, Bell, Bryson, & Zito, 1993)	Rating of observed behavior and brief interview with supervisor	36	5-pt scale: 1 = consistently inferior performance to 5 = consistently superior performance	5 Scales: Work Habits Work Quality Personal Presentation Cooperativeness Social Skills	M	Y	M	Y	Y	Y
Work-Related Self-Efficacy Scale (WRSES; Waghorn, Chant, & King, 2005)	Self-rating	37	11-pt scale: 0–100 in intervals of 10	4 Scales: Career Planning Skills Job Securing Skills Work-Related Social Skills General Work Skills	Y	Y	Y	N	N	M
Work-Related Social Skills Measure (Tsang & Pearson, 2000)	Self-report (SR) and observation of role-play (RP) performance	SR, 10 RP, 2	SR 6-pt scale: 1 = always difficult to 6 = not difficult at all; RP 5-pt scale: 0 = poor performance to 4 = normal performance	SR Sample Items: Make appointment for job interview, Resolve conflict with coworker RP Situations: Participating in job interview, requesting urgent leave	Y	Y	M	N	Y	Y

Note. Y = yes; N = no; M = moderately; Incl. = included; Env. Spec. = environmentally specific.

(continues)

TABLE 19.1. *Continued.*

Skills: Social

Instrument	Assessment Method	# Items	Rating Scale	Scales/Sample Items	Clear?	Brief?	Skills			Env. Spec.
							Incl.?	+	–	
Assessment of Interpersonal Problem Solving Skills (AIPSS; Donahoe et al., 1990)	Interviewer rating of response to video vignettes and role play	13 vignettes	Accuracy for vignettes; Quality of role-played performance	Identify the problem Generate alternatives Select alternative Perform role-play solution	M	N	Y	Y	Y	N
Communication Skills Questionnaire (Takahashi, Tanaka, & Miyaoka, 2006)	Self-report, family rating, or clinician rating	29	5-pt scale: 1 = poor to 5 = always good 3-pt scale: 0 = poor to 2 = almost always good	General communication skills Interpersonal communication skills—cooperative and assertive communication skills	Y	Y	M	Y	Y	N
Simulated Social Interaction Test (SSIT; Curran, 1982)	Rating role-play performance	8 role plays	11-pt scale of social skill	Global social skill	M	N	N	N	N	N
Social Problem Solving Assessment Battery (SPSAB; Sayers, Bellack, Wade, Bennett, & Fong, 1995)	Role-play Test (RPT) Rating Role play performance	6 role plays	5-pt scales with behavioral anchors for each behavior	Overall quality of problem solving; Clarity; Negotiation; Persistence; Interest; Fluency; Affect	M	M	M	M	M	N

Note. Y = yes; N = no; M = moderately; Incl. = included; Env. Spec. = environmentally specific.

(continues)

TABLE 19.1. *Continued.*

Skills: Social (Continued)

Instrument	Assessment Method	# Items	Rating Scale	Scales/Sample Items	Clear ?	Brief ?	Skills			Env. Spec.
							Incl.?	+	–	
Social Problem Solving Assessment Battery (SPSAB; Sayers, Bellack, Wade, Bennett, & Fong, 1995) *(continued)*	Response Generation Test (RGT) Rating of responses to vignettes generated	6 video situations	3-pt scales of accuracy of problem and goals: 3 = most accurate 5-pt scales rating solutions (5 = better response)	Describe the problem Identify target person's goals Generate solutions	N	N	M	M	M	N
	Response Evaluation Test (RET) Subject rating of scenarios	12 audio-taped interactions	5-pt scale: 1 = ineffective to 5 = effective	Person rates scenarios in which target displays effective response and ineffective response	N	M	N	N	N	N

Note. Y = yes; N = no; M = moderately; Incl. = included; Env. Spec. = environmentally specific.

[a]Not contained in ILSS–SR.

TABLE 19.2.
Instruments for Assessing Resources

Instrument	Assessment Method	# Items	Rating Scale	Scales/Items	Clear ?	Brief ?	Env. Spec.	Resources		
								Needed	Avail	Access
Camberwell Assessment of Need (CAN; Phelan et al., 1995)	Interviewer rating of clinicians and individuals	22	Each item rated on the following: Need (3 pt: no need, met need, unmet need); Amount of Help received family (4 pt: none, low, moderate, high); Amount of help received/ provided staff (4 pt: none, low, moderate, high); Short version rates Need only	Sample items: Accommodation, Food, Selfcare, Physical health, Psychological distress, Drugs, Intimate relationships, Money	M	Y 25 min	M	Y	Y	Y
Camberwell Assessment of Need Short Appraisal Schedule (CANSAS; Andreasen, Caputi, & Oades, 2001)		12-item short form								
Instrumental Evaluation Support List (ISEL; Cohen, Mermelstein, Kamarck, & Hoberman, 1985)	Self-report	30	4-pt scale: definitely true, probably true, probably false, definitely false	Scales: Perceived availability of: tangible support, self-esteem support, appraisal help, belonging	Y	Y	M	N	M	N
Multidimensional Scale of Perceived Social Support (MSPSS; Cecil, Stanley, Carrion, & Swann, 1995; Zimet, Dahlem, Simet, & Farley, 1988)	Self-report	12	7-pt scale for degree of perceived social support: 1 = very strongly agree to 7 = very strongly disagree	3 Scales: Support from: family, friends, significant others	Y	Y	M	N	Y	N

(continues)

TABLE 19.2. *Continued.*

Instrument	Assessment Method	# Items	Rating Scale	Scales/Items	Clear?	Brief?	Env. Spec.	Resources Needed	Avail	Access
Needs and Resources Assessment (NARA; Corrigan, Buican, & McCracken, 1995, 1996)	Interview and self-report	13	# Needs and resources listed; Satisfaction rated 7-pt scale: 7 = delighted; Importance of Need rated 7-pt scale: 7 = most important	Sample Domains: Housing; Physical health; Mental health; Income & finances; Education; Family; Job status; Legal problems	M	M	N	Y	N	N
Personal Network Interview Schedule (PNI; Stein, Rappaport, & Seidman, 1995)/ *Social Network Scale* (SNS; Corrigan & Phelan, 2004)	Self-report in semi-structured interview	12 stage I/V	Varies by stage Numbers counted for network size; Density calculated as ratio of dyads of people in network who know each other to total dyads; Satisfaction, Obligation, and Mutuality rated on 5-pt scale by individual	Network size: overall, family, friends, professionals; Network density; Perception of satisfaction; Perception of mutuality; Perception of obligation	M	N	M	N	Y	Y
Workplace Climate Questionnaire (WCQ; Kirsh, 1999)	Self-report	25	5-pt scale of agreement	Sample items: I am able to adjust my working hours; My health-care benefits meet my needs; My supervisor is approachable	Y	Y	Y	M	Y	N

Note. Y = yes; N = no; M = moderately; Incl. = included; Env. Spec. = environmentally specific; Avail = available; Access = accessible.

(e.g., personal hygiene, such as bathing or showering, dental care, and general cleanliness; handling time, such as ability to keep appointments, return when due, participate in activities when scheduled, get to work on time). These items represent activity areas, with specific skills or behaviors listed under each activity area. Raters, who are someone who knows the person well, are instructed to rate behaviors that they observed in the last week, not their estimate of potential ability. Items cover skills in personal care/physical skills (personal hygiene, grooming, dress skills, self-care, health practices, meal preparation, clothing maintenance), social skills (communication, sexuality, leisure activities, use of resources), and intellectual skills (handling money, handling time, safety, problem solving). The instrument demonstrates good internal consistency and excellent inter-rater reliability, as well as construct and concurrent validity (Fitz & Evenson, 1995). It seems effective in differentiating between people in three levels of residential care compared with other measures of global functioning (Fitz, 1999) and has been validated with a Chinese sample in Hong Kong (Au, Tam, Tam, & Ungvari, 2005). Overall, the SLICLS is a moderately clear, very brief instrument that gathers information on activity areas, with skill descriptors representing those areas, although those specific skills are not separately rated. It may be a useful instrument to use clinically in identifying areas of skills needing further exploration.

The *Independent Living Skills Survey* (ILSS) is a performance-based measure of basic functional living skills of individuals with psychiatric disabilities (Wallace, Liberman, Tauber, & Wallace, 2000). There are two versions of the form—the informant version (ILSS-I) and the self-report version (ILSS-SR). The informant version is administered in person, by telephone, or by mail to providers in community facilities who have had the opportunity to observe the individual in the past 30 days. The self-report format can be administered on paper or in an interview. These measures are an update of an instrument first presented by Wallace (1986) in his review of functional assessment instruments. For the ILSS-I, items are rated on a 5-point scale from 0 = *never* to 4 = *always*. There is also a sixth response option, "no opportunity," for items in which the person has limited or no opportunity to perform or demonstrate a skill (e.g., preparing a meal in residences where meals are prepared by staff). For the ILSS-SR, items are answered Yes (1) or No (0), with the option of "not apply" if opportunities to perform the skill are not available. In both versions, scores are summed in each area and averaged. An area is not scored if three or fewer items are answered with "no opportunity" or "not apply." The original version of this scale did not include interpersonal skills and was added to the informant version. In addition, the self-report version does not contain items related to the functional area of eating. Internal consistency and stability for the ILSS-I were good to excellent, while the ILSS-SR was marginal to good across all functional areas within the instrument. Inter-rater agreement between self-reporting individuals and informants was moderate, attributed in part to the different formats of rating between versions. Validity testing indicated that the ILSS-SR total score could predict employment, could discriminate between individuals who participated in skills training interventions and those who did not, and could show improvements in skills after skill training. Overall, this instrument is clear, skill-focused, and moderately brief, due in part to its comprehensiveness. Its major advantage is that it provides detailed information on skills in a range of areas related to living in the community, making it extremely relevant for clinical use in functional assessment. Information can also be gathered from multiple perspectives, with two versions available.

The *Client Assessment of Skills, Interests, and Goals* (CASIG), and its informant version, the *Staff Observation and Client Information* (SOCI; also known as the CASIG-I), is a new measure that assesses treatment outcomes and embeds the assessment in the clinical process of planning and evaluating treatment (Wallace, Lecomte, Wilde, & Liberman, 2001). It includes sections on goals, social and independent living skills, medication practices and side effects, quality of life, quality of treatment, symptoms, unacceptable community behaviors, and specific goals related to previous sections of the interview.

What is novel about this instrument is that it incorporates assessing the person's goals for improved community functioning, his or her current functional and cognitive skills, medication practices, quality of life and treatment, symptoms, and unacceptable community behaviors. This intentional embedding strategy was used in order to improve incorporation of outcome measures and assessments in clinical practice. From a psychiatric rehabilitation perspective, it is useful because it incorporates the person's goals in five broad areas—residential, vocational/educational, social/family relationships, religion/spiritual, and physical/mental health—and then follows up with identifying specific goals related to other sections of the interview. The social/independent living skills section is a subset of items from the ILSS (Wallace et al., 2000) that focus on assessing performance in the past 90 days. Although only the social/independent living skills section directly assesses skills, individuals are asked about specific goals related to symptoms, medications and side effects, and unacceptable behaviors, which may generate additional specific skill or resource needs. The SOCI (or CASIG-I) is completed by an informant and administered as a questionnaire. Items about goals, quality of life, and quality of treatment are not included. Interviews were designed to be conducted by peer-interviewers (consumers). Internal consistency of the social and independent living skills scales ranged from marginal to excellent, and stability was good to excellent. Interrater reliability for the skills section was also adequate. A later study also provided evidence of construct, convergent, and discriminant validity with individuals in Canada (Lecomte, Wallace, Caron, Perreault, & Lecomte, 2004). Although clear, with multiple components (i.e., goals, satisfaction, symptoms, medications, skills), the CASIG is not brief. However, it is an excellent tool to integrate into a psychiatric rehabilitation assessment.

The *UCSD Performance-Based Skills Assessment* (UPBSA) is an instrument that rates performance of specific tasks in five areas—household chores, communication, finance, transportation, and planning recreational activities (Patterson, Goldman, McKibbin, Hughs, & Jeste, 2001). Individuals are given instructions to carry out tasks and points are awarded for performance of tasks in each area. Tasks are clear and easy to understand, although assessment requires at least 30 minutes to complete. Some adaptation of tasks for the local area may be required (i.e., using public transportation). Tasks are generally described in behavioral language, but the scoring system does not immediately yield a profile of specific skill strengths and deficits. This measure was validated with middle-aged and older adults with schizophrenia and successfully discriminated these participants from people without psychiatric disabilities.

The *Brief Instrumental Functioning Scale* (BIFS) is a six-item self-report measure that assesses ability to effectively negotiate daily activities, recently validated with people who are homeless (Sullivan, Dumenci, Burnam, & Koegel, 2001). Individuals are asked to rate themselves in six areas— take medications, fill out benefits application, budget money, use city buses, set up job interviews by telephone, and find an attorney. Ratings are done on a 3-point scale: 1 = *can do alone*, 2 = *need help*, and 3 = *don't know if I can do alone*. This measure is particularly useful in nonclinical settings where a quick assessment of functioning is needed. While this measure demonstrated high stability and successfully discriminated people with serious mental illness from those without, it is not comprehensive and may not be sensitive to change. Some of the areas of functioning assessed are larger activity areas that may require a number of skills to perform (e.g., filling out a benefits application, finding a lawyer) and would be useful as an initial exploration of skill strengths and deficits with individuals who may not be likely to engage in longer assessments, such as those who experience homelessness.

The *Atascadero Skills Profile* (ASP) is a 34-item instrument rated by consensus of treatment team members in contact with individuals with psychiatric disorders residing in forensic hospitals (Vess, 2001). Ten domains of behavior are rated—self-management of psychiatric symptoms (behavior), self-management of psychiatric symptoms (medication), substance abuse prevention skills, self-management of assaultive behavior, control of self-injurious or suicidal behavior, self-care, independent living skills, control of deviant sexual impulses and behaviors, interpersonal skills, and leisure and recreation skills. A team of professionals rate the individual by consensus using a 5-point scale from 0 = *skills consistently absent or completely inadequate* to 4 = *skills consistently present and adequate*. A number of items are moderately clear and reflect larger activity areas or require interpretation to rate (e.g., accepts need for medication; demonstrates adequate work skills; demonstrates social interactions that respect the privacy, property, and feelings of others), while others are written in clear skill language (e.g., recognizes internal precursors that escalate into violent behavior). The measure is relatively brief; yields a profile of strengths and deficits; and demonstrates good internal consistency, stability, construct validity, and sensitivity to change.

In summary, the ILSS is recommended when a comprehensive measure of independent living skills is needed, especially if both practitioner and self-report versions are desired. To more easily integrate an assessment of skills into a comprehensive clinical interview process that evaluates many areas related to psychiatric rehabilitation outcome, especially goal setting, use the CASIG. For a simpler and briefer review of living skills, the SLICLS is recommended.

A measure that focuses on performance of tasks, such as the UPBSA, may be useful with people who are more action oriented and enjoy doing activities. For special populations, the BIFS is useful with people who experience homelessness, and the ASP is useful with people residing in forensic hospitals. However, in using all of these instruments to assess skill functioning, in particular in living environments, it will be necessary to supplement these standardized measures to identify the unique skill demands of the desired goal environment.

Learning Environment

A review of the literature in supported education revealed few instruments that are available to assess the skills of students with disabilities, and those that are available have been used primarily with students with learning disabilities. Although academic assessment may include standardized achievement and literacy tests, there is little emphasis on the general student skills needed to succeed in educational settings, such as skills in note taking, test taking, using campus resources, and connecting with other students. One instrument in particular, the *Learning and Study Strategies Inventory* (LASSI), is reported to be widely used in college and university disability services offices for students with learning disabilities (Proctor, Prevatt, Adams, Hurst, & Petscher, 2006) but has not been validated with students with psychiatric disabilities. The instrument also appears to evaluate constructs other than learning strategies, such as attitudes, motivation, and anxiety about performance (Weinstein & Palmer, 2002). An extensive review of the literature on supported education programs developed specifically for people with psychiatric disabilities yielded no specific measures of student skills or behaviors used in evaluation of those services (Collins, Bybee, & Mowbray, 1998; Cook & Solomon, 1993; Mowbray, Collins, & Bybee, 1999; Unger, Anthony, Sciarappa, & Rogers, 1991).

Only one measure was identified that was developed for use with people with psychiatric disabilities that contained items assessing capacity and supports related to attending college—the *Views about College Questionnaire* (VCQ; Stein, 2005). This instrument was developed for a larger study about aspirations for college, perceptions of social support, and personal loss due to mental illness. The VCQ is a 20-item, self-report measure to assess an individual's views about starting or returning to college. Items are grouped into three areas or domains: aspirations and plans, perceived social support and acceptance, and perceived intellectual and emotional capacity for college. While the instrument appears brief and moderately clear, it is focused not on a specific college but on college in general, and the capacity items do not identify skills or even behaviors related to college. The instrument does a better job of capturing the intentions and perceived support needs for going to college at some time in the future and may best be used individually with an individual exploring further education, not as an assessment of skills or supports needed for success in a particular college. No reliability or validity data are available for this instrument.

Clearly, people with psychiatric disabilities considering educational or learning environments need information about the skills needed for success and satisfaction in particular settings. Given that there are no satisfactory instruments available specific to people with psychiatric disabilities, practitioners will need to conduct functional assessments individually, emphasizing the skills required for the particular settings in which the person wants to function. Professionals should consider developing and testing reliable and valid instruments that assess student skills.

Working Environment

One of the first documented situational assessment tools, the *Standardized Assessment of Work Behaviour* (a.k.a., the Griffiths; Griffiths, 1973, 1977) is a 25-item scale that assesses a broad range of skills (e.g., uses tools/equipment, communicates spontaneously, grasps instructions quickly) that make up five clusters: Task Competence, Response to Supervision, Relationship with Others, Work Motivation, and Confidence-Initiative. Designed to measure vocational skills of individuals with psychiatric disabilities, items are rated by clinicians or work supervisors based on observed behavior in a work setting on a continuum from skill strength (e.g., looks for more work) to skill deficit (e.g., waits to be given work). The Griffiths has also been used as a self-rating; there were significant differences between supervisor and self-ratings (Griffiths, 1975). Adequate reliability and validity data are available for this scale (Griffiths, 1973), including discriminating between employed and unemployed individuals after leaving the hospital work unit (Griffiths, 1977). Although developed initially for use in a hospital work unit, it has been used to rate work behavior in the community. In addition, it has been used as a standard for the development of more recent situational assessment tools, but it is not widely used today. The instrument is brief, and most of the items are written in behavioral or skill language. However, some of the items require some judgment to assess (e.g., doesn't fit in easily, has sensible attitude to authority) and may not be clear to the person being evaluated. In spite of the short amount of time needed to complete the instrument, however, significant time may be required to arrange a work setting in which to conduct the evaluation if one is not immediately available.

Another situational assessment instrument is the *Situational Assessment: Scales to Assess Work Adjustment and Interpersonal Skills* (Rogers, Hursh, Kielhofner, & Spaniol, 1990; Rogers, Sciarappa, & Anthony, 1991). Rogers et al. (1991) described the process of conducting a situational assessment, as well as the development of the situational assessment instrument. The instrument contains two separate scales consisting of 21 work adjustment skills and 14 interpersonal skills. Each item is rated by a clinician or supervisor on a 4-point rating scale (from 1 = *cause to be fired* to 4 = *above acceptable performance*), based on observation of the person in a preferred work environment. Extensive descriptors and behavioral anchors are provided for each rating on each item as a guide. Although internal consistency, inter-rater, and test-retest reliabilities were excellent, the sample was too homogeneous (few people obtained employment) to determine predictive validity. All items are clear and well-written using skill language and represent the general work and interpersonal skills required in most jobs (e.g., adjusts effort to work demand, initiates new work independently, converses with coworkers in a way that job gets done, asks for help when having difficulty with tasks). Both skill strengths and skill deficits can be identified. However, it does not appear to be a brief instrument; the procedure described for assessment included daily observation of 2-hour work periods over a period of 10 days in order to rate the individual's performance on these skills. While long, the detail and behavioral specificity provided make it particularly useful clinically in rehabilitation planning and skill development interventions.

The *Work Behavior Inventory* (WBI) is a 36-item work performance assessment instrument specifically designed for people with severe mental illness (Lysaker, Bell, Bryson, & Zito, 1993). This measure is intended for use in observing the person in a real work situation and consists of five subscales: work habits, work quality, personal presentation, cooperativeness, and social skills. Items are rated on a 5-point scale from *consistently inferior* to *consistently superior.* Examples of some of the items include the following: expresses positive feelings appropriately, accepts constructive criticism without becoming upset, and begins work tasks promptly. However, some items require judgment (i.e., appears interested in others; does not seem to tire easily) or describe the absence of a negative behavior (i.e., refrains from inappropriate joking).

This brief instrument has acceptable reliability and validity data. Interrater reliabilities on the subscales were excellent, and internal consistency was high. Concurrent validity between subscales on the *Work Personality Profile* was moderate to strong, and the WBI discriminated differences between samples of people with schizophrenia and people with substance abuse diagnoses (Bryson, Bell, Lysaker, & Zito, 1997). The WBI also predicted hours worked and money earned, but not future competitive employment, although it could identify those who did not work at all (Bryson, Bell, Greig, & Kaplan, 1999).

Because some items require judgment or describe the absence of a negative behavior, the instrument is only moderately clear and moderately uses skill or behavioral language in items. However, it is brief (with the caveat about arranging a work setting) and easy to use. It indicates both strengths and deficits and is specific to observation of behavior in a work environment. Its greatest strength is that it is in active use in a number of studies evaluating work performance, cognitive functioning, and symptoms of people with psychiatric disabilities (Bell & Bryson, 2001; Evans et al., 2004).

The *Vocational Cognitive Rating Scale* (VCRS) is a 16-item instrument designed to measure cognitive skills in the workplace, specifically developed for people with serious psychiatric disabilities (Greig, Nicholls, Bryson, & Bell, 2004). Each item is rated on a 5-point scale, from 1 = *consistently inferior performance* to 5 = *consistently superior performance,* yielding one total score for the scale. Behavioral anchors are provided for each rating on each item. Examples of items include the following: stays focused when performing a simple task, continues to work without slowing down when he or she sees or hears something interesting or different, and transitions smoothly from one task to another.

Ratings are accomplished by a clinician who has observed the individual for 15 minutes in the work setting and has interviewed the onsite supervisor.

Reliability and validity for the scale are good to excellent. Inter-rater reliability was excellent, and internal consistency was high. The VCRS successfully discriminated between people who had worked full time from those who had limited work experience. The scale also successfully predicted work performance scores and hours worked. Overall, the VCRS is a new, clear, brief, and skills-oriented instrument that describes skill strengths and deficits and is used specifically in the workplace with people with psychiatric disabilities. Its focus is on primarily cognitive behaviors and does not address social or physical skills needed in the workplace. The scale taps behaviors that research indicates are essential for success in the workplace, particularly for people who have schizophrenia or schizoaffective disorders.

The *Work-Related Self-Efficacy* (WSES) scale is a promising, recent self-report instrument intended to assess confidence in performance of core work-related activities and was specifically developed for people with psychiatric disabilities (Waghorn, Chant, & King, 2005). These core activities include career planning skills, job securing skills, work-related social skills, and general work skills. The authors propose that it may be used as a vocational counseling tool to facilitate communication about specific tasks, supports, and assistance needed to achieve positive work performance. The instrument consists of 37 items, and the individual rates his or her level of confidence in performing a specific activity on an 11-point rating scale (0–100) in intervals of 10. Examples of items include how confident the individual feels in his or her ability to do the following: identify personal work values, use a social network to identify job opportunities, cooperate with other workers to perform a task, and start work soon after arriving.

Internal consistency was fairly high. Test-retest reliabilities were also very strong and stable over time. Concurrent validity demonstrated moderate significant correlations of the composite WSES score with years since last employment, years of continuous employment, weeks worked in the previous year, and current employment.

Most items are clearly written, and the instrument is brief, uses skill or behavioral language, and is specific to work activities. One issue is that, although the items are worded in skill-oriented language, the individual is asked to rate confidence in performing the activities, not actual strength or deficit in performing the activity in a real work environment. The authors recommend using other measures of skill performance to supplement the self-efficacy rating. A major advantage is that this measure is one of the few to involve the individual in rating him- or herself, and items are clear and specific enough for opening discussion with the individual about actual skill levels. Additional testing of this measure as well as future alterations of the scale are needed to assess its promise.

A new brief instrument that is a combined performance and self-report measure is the untitled *work-related social skills* measure developed by Tsang and Pearson (2000). A brief self-administered checklist containing 10 items is rated by individuals on social skills that are used in securing and sustaining a job. Individuals rate themselves on a 6-point scale based on level of difficulty in performing the task, from 1 representing *Always difficult* to 6 representing *Not difficult at all*. Sample items are presented in mostly behavioral, observable language (i.e., request urgent leave from supervisor, help to instruct or demonstrate a task to a new colleague), although several items represent a component consisting of many skills or are otherwise general (e.g., participate appropriately in a job interview, avoid involvement in destructive gossip). A second component of the measure consists of two role-play situations with a confederate that are rated independently on three aspects reflecting the model of social skills proposed by Tsang and Pearson (1996): basic social survival skills (grooming, personal hygiene, politeness), basic social skills (voice quality, nonverbal components, and verbal components), and situation-specific ratings. The rater uses a 5-point scale with behavioral anchors reflecting each aspect rated, with 0 representing poor performance and 4 representing "normal" performance. Internal consistency and inter-rater reliabilities were adequate, although test-retest reliabilities for the self-administered checklist demonstrated some variability. The measure was able to discriminate between people with schizophrenia participating in rehabilitation programs in Korea and employed members from the trade unions without mental health diagnoses, but the applicability of this measure in the United States and additional validity studies must be conducted. It is a brief measure (approximately 30 minutes for both components) that is moderately clear and focused on the work environment, although it is not specific to the requirements of any one work environment. The measure is mentioned here because it is one of the only exclusive social skills measures related to work environments available that uses self-report and role-play performance methods.

The majority of instruments in the work skills area are situational assessment types of instruments—the Griffiths, the WBI, the *Situational Assessment Scales to Assess Work Adjustment and Interpersonal Skills,* and the VCRS. Situational assessments require time and cost to arrange a work site in which to observe the individual's work behaviors. However, they are ideal for conducting a psychiatric rehabilitation assessment because they assess skills in a real work setting. At times, the assessment site may be a work detail in a clubhouse or other rehabilitation program, which may require different skills than real jobs in the community. Practitioners must take care to tailor the assessment to those skills critical for success and satisfaction in the desired work setting. Their major advantage is that they are environmentally specific—that is, they are conducted in the environment of need. However, standardized instruments may not always capture skills essential to a particular environment that may not be necessary elsewhere. While the instrument itself may not take long to fill out, the set-up and observation periods may take some time. The WBI is the most frequently reported and validated instrument used of the three, but the *Situational Assessment Scales* are the most detailed and skill-oriented and may be easiest to use in conducting a functional assessment. Several other recent measures also focus on particular types of skills and may be useful in conducting a functional assessment—cognitive (the VCRS), social (the work-related social skills measure), and self-efficacy (the WRSES). Additional study must be done to validate these instruments and identify other measures using alternate methods of data collection to improve the choices of assessment tools available.

Social Environment

Although many of the instruments listed in living, learning, and working environment sections include social skills, behaviors, activities, or functioning items, there are several measures that specifically emphasize social or interpersonal skills. Many of these measures were developed to examine the effects of behavior therapy or skills training interventions used to increase the social skills of people with severe psychiatric disabilities. None of these measures are specific to a social role or environment but are assumed to be used in general social situations. For a more in-depth review of measures of social skills and social skills training, refer to Bellack (2004) and Wallace et al. (1980).

Several role-play tests assess social skills. The *Simulated Social Interaction Test* (SSIT) is a role-play test of social skills in dealing with eight simulated anxiety-provoking situations (Curran, 1982). Although this was a popular assessment tool to evaluate the outcomes of social skills training, this assessment measures global social skill in response to situations, does not provide information about specific social skills or components of social skill, and is not useful clinically in assessing specific social skills during a functional assessment.

More recent measures of social skills have incorporated recent research into the cognitive component of social skills. The *Assessment of Interpersonal Problem Solving Skills* (AIPSS) is a videotaped role-play test of social skills in which an individual is shown a series of interpersonal problem vignettes and is asked to identify the problem, describe a solution, and role play that solution. A trained rater then rates the various components or subscales of the receiving, processing, and sending skills model of social skills developed by Wallace (Donahoe, Carter, Bloem, Hirsch, Laasi, & Wallace, 1990).

The *Social Problem Solving Assessment Battery* (SPSAB) is a battery of three tests that incorporates a role-play test to measure social skills and problem-solving ability (Sayers, Bellack, Wade, Bennett, & Fong, 1995). The intent of the measure is to evaluate the skills that enable individuals to identify social problems, generate response alternatives, evaluate the effectiveness of responses, and carry out effective social solutions. One major feature of this tool was the involvement of family members, providers, and people with schizophrenia in identifying the problem situations. The battery contains three assessments: a Role-Play Test (RPT), a Response Generation Test (RGT), and a Response Evaluation Test (RET). The RPT contains six 3-minute role plays that involve a confederate. The role plays involve three types of social skill situations: initiating conversation, compromising and negotiating, and being assertive. The role plays are videotaped and rated independently by a trained rater on overall quality of problem solving, clarity, negotiation, persistence, interest, fluency, and affect. The information gathered may not be clear to the individual, and it takes some time to administer the instrument and to train raters. Some feedback about specific skills may be provided on three types of social situations, but the instrument was developed primarily as a research tool evaluating the effectiveness of social skills training and may have limited usefulness clinically. The RGT involves six videotaped interactions between two individuals who have a conflict or problem, and the individual being assessed attempts to describe the problem, identify the target person's goals, and propose solutions. Trained raters rate the accuracy of the problems and goals on 3-point scales and rate the solutions generated on 5-point scales on a number of characteristics. The instrument can provide feedback to individuals about their skills in identifying problems and goals and generating solutions, but the ratings need interpretation to provide that feedback and are not immediately clear. The RET consists of 12 audiotaped interactions, in which dyads demonstrate both effective and ineffective solutions to a social situation, and the individual rates each interaction on a 5-point scale of *effective* to *ineffective*. While useful in research, this tool may not be useful clinically in assessing interpersonal skills.

An instrument has been developed in Japan using a self-report, family-report, or clinician-report format, called the *Communication Skills Questionnaire* (CSQ; Takahashi, Tanaka, & Miyaoka, 2006). It was developed for clinical use in evaluating social skill training without using the cumbersome role-play measures listed previously. The CSQ is a 29-item questionnaire containing general communication skills (primarily nonverbal skills) and interpersonal communication skills, which in factor analysis yielded cooperative communication skills and assertive communication skills. Individuals themselves, family members, or clinicians rate the skills with respect to interpersonal relationships with family, friends, superiors, neighbors, and strangers. General communication skills are rated on a 5-point scale (1 = *Poor,* 2 = *Fairly,* 3 = *Sometimes good,* 4 = *Almost always good,* 5 = *Always good*), and Interpersonal communication skills are rated on a 3-point scale (0 = *Poor,* 1 = *Sometimes good,* 2 = *Almost always good*). Total scores are summed. Most interpersonal skills items are written in clear, behavioral language (e.g., asking a question, starting a conversation, expressing the need for help), while some of the general communication skills are less clear or behavioral (e.g., good appearance, eye contact, showing enthusiasm). The measure was tested on people in psychiatric hospitals and on people involved in psychiatric rehabilitation programs in the community, their family members, and medical personnel; a group of medical students without psychiatric diagnoses was the control group. Initial psychometric testing demonstrates good internal consistency, good test-retest reliability, and moderate inter-rater reliability among medical personnel. The instrument had adequate convergent validity and was able to discriminate between people with psychiatric diagnoses and those without diagnoses. The CSQ is a clear, brief measure using skill language for most of the items and appears easy to use clinically in assessing social skills and planning rehabilitation interventions. However, it is a new measure that has not yet been tested in the United States with people with psychiatric disabilities and does not currently predict functioning in particular living, learning, or working environments. It is a promising tool worthy of further investigation.

What appears to be missing from the social environment are tools that assess skills of people with psychiatric disabilities in performing valued social roles other than those in living, learning, and working environments. These might include measures of skill functioning in parenting roles, partner or intimate relationship roles, leadership roles, spiritual roles, and citizenship roles. In order to facilitate individual success and satisfaction in chosen roles and environments, the field must assess the skills and supports necessary for achieving those roles. Development of valid and reliable instruments in these domains is clearly a growth area for assessment in psychiatric rehabilitation.

Resource-Oriented Instruments

Few scales are currently in use that focus on supports or resources and that can be helpful clinically during a resource assessment. Most common are social support measures (see Cohen, Underwood, & Gottlieb, 2000, for a review). Assessments of other types of supports (e.g., income, mental health services) often focus on needs assessment and exist as a part of some checklists in use by state mental health systems or agencies but are not widely used (State of Alabama Department of Mental Health Services, 1984; Weiner, 1993). Needs assessment instruments often assess areas of function and, for poor areas of function, suggest a need for service to address it. The specific services and supports may not be listed or assessed. This lack of instruments poses challenges in identifying tools that can be used in conducting an individualized resource assessment with a person with a psychiatric disability, especially one that focuses on resources and supports needed for success and satisfaction in particular living, learning, working, or social environments.

A recent instrument is the *Needs and Resources Assessment Interview* (NARA; Corrigan, Buican, & McCracken, 1995). This interview or self-report instrument combines identification of needs in specific domains of functioning with a review of the resources required to meet the identified needs. Individuals are also asked to rate their satisfaction with functioning in each of the domains, as well as to rate the importance of the need. The domains reviewed include housing, physical health, dental health, mental health, income and finances, education, job status, friends, family, leisure time, spiritual life, legal problems, and drug-related problems.

The NARA has adequate internal consistency and test-retest reliability, particularly when structured as an interview versus a paper-and-pencil self-report instrument (Corrigan, Buican, & McCracken, 1996). Since this is a semi-structured interview to identify needs and resources to address those needs, some items may not be clear to all individuals. Ratings of satisfaction and importance may be useful in identifying needed resources and supports, but a limitation of this measure is that it only indirectly identifies a support or service need and does not assess availability or accessibility of needed resources.

A similar type of instrument is the *Camberwell Assessment of Needs* (CAN), a structured interview that focuses on 22 areas of functioning (Phelan et al., 1995). Needs are identified by asking about difficulties in each area. The individual is also asked about how much help is received from friends and relatives, as well as from service providers. The last section outlines the type of assistance needed as identified from the individual's perspective, and a care plan is developed.

A short version, the *Camberwell Assessment of Need Short Appraisal Schedule* (CANSAS), is also available (Andreasen, Caputi, & Oades, 2001). The CAN is widely used in Europe and is often used in instrument validation studies in the United States. In a comparison of mental health outcome assessment measures, only the CANSAS was found to provide information about both met needs and unmet needs and is useful both as a research tool and as a clinical tool (Salvi, Leese, & Slade, 2005). Overall, the CAN is clear; is relatively brief (25 minutes); and evaluates need, availability, and accessibility of supports. The CANSAS, while briefer, evaluates need only. Both assess resources in the broader social environment and in primarily living or community environments in general, but they do not specifically focus on supports for a particular environment. In addition, the CANSAS and the CAN are two of the few needs assessment instruments that actively incorporate the perspective of the individual, not relying solely on the rating of staff, which is essential particularly because there are differences in ratings between staff and individuals with psychiatric disabilities, especially in their ratings of unmet needs (Slade et al., 1998). Involvement of people with psychiatric disabilities is an essential component of assessment in psychiatric rehabilitation.

One measure of social support is the *Multidimensional Scale of Perceived Social Support* (MSPSS; Zimet, Dahlem, Zimet, & Farley, 1988). Although originally developed for nonpsychiatric populations, recent psychometric testing has been conducted with people diagnosed with schizophrenia, bipolar disorder, or major depression (Cecil, Stanley, Carrion, & Swann, 1995). The MSPSS is a 12-item self-report scale that assesses a person's perception of the adequacy of social support received from family, friends, and significant others. Individuals rate the degree of agreement with statements about perceived social support on a scale of 1–7, from *very strongly agree* to *very strongly disagree*. Subscales are available representing perceived social support from family, friends, and significant others. This scale is a clear, brief measure of the global "social" environment that evaluates the availability of support from the perspective of the individual. It does not evaluate other types of resources, nor does it assess the needed level of support or the accessibility of support. It is not focused on a particular social environment or role. The instrument demonstrated high reliability in internal consistency and adequate validity compared to the nonpsychiatric samples, although additional testing was recommended (Cecil et al., 1995).

There are several other types of social support measures. One is the *Personal Network Interview Schedule* (PNI; Stein, Rappaport, & Seidman, 1995), also known as the *Social Network Scale* (Corrigan & Phelan, 2004), which is a semi-structured, 12-stage interview that evaluates network size of family, friends, and professionals; network density; and perceptions of satisfaction, mutuality, and obligation. Total numbers of individuals in the support network are counted after an in-depth interview, and density is calculated by a ratio of dyads of people in the network who know one another to the total number of dyads available. Perceptions of satisfaction, mutuality, and obligation are rated by the individual on 5-point Likert scales. The scale is moderately clear, and not brief, but it is moderately specific to social environments. It indicates the availability and extent of supports but not necessarily the need or accessibility of identified supports. Higher levels of social support, using this instrument, have been associated with better recovery process (Corrigan & Phelan, 2004).

Another instrument that evaluates the availability of social support is the *Interpersonal Support Evaluation List* (ISEL; Cohen, Mermelstein, Kamarck, & Hoberman, 1985). Originally developed for use in the general population, it has been validated recently with people with psychiatric disabilities (Rogers, Anthony, & Lyass, 2004). The ISEL is a 30-item, self-report instrument focused on the perceived availability of support in four areas: tangible support (perceived availability of material aid), self-esteem support (perceived availability of a positive comparison when comparing oneself to others), belonging (perceived availability of someone to do things with), and appraisal help (perceived availability of someone to talk to about problems). Items are rated by the individual on how true he or she believes the statement to be about himself or herself. The instrument is brief and clear and pertains to the general social environment but not to supports needed in specific environments. In addition, the ISEL measures the perception of availability of support, but not actual availability of support, and does not evaluate need or accessibility of support.

A newer instrument that appears to measure supports in the workplace is the *Workplace Climate Questionnaire* (WCQ; Kirsh, 2000a, 2000b). Although designed to measure aspects of the social and structural environment of the workplace, a number of items in this brief self-report instrument reflect interpersonal supports (i.e., with supervisor, coworkers), benefits (health care, holidays, transportation), and accommodations (adjustments to work hours, help with solving problems). The WCQ is a 25-item, self-report measure of employees in the workplace. Participants rate each statement on a 5-point scale of agreement with the statement. The instrument is clear, brief, and specific to the employee's current work environment. It indirectly indicates the availability of supports identified but does not assess needed supports or accessibility of those supports. While the measure has reported adequate reliability and validity, additional testing is needed.

No one measure of social supports and other resources appears to capture the various types of supports and resources needed for people with psychiatric disabilities to achieve their goals, especially in particular living, learning, working, or social environments. Some combination of these various instruments integrated into an assessment process tailored to an individual would help identify the resource needs of the given individual.

Conclusion

Assessment in psychiatric rehabilitation is not instrument dominated. It requires a practitioner who is able to develop a trust-based relationship with the person. Practitioners who conduct such assessments must have good interpersonal skills (e.g., the ability to demonstrate understanding). The practitioner must be skilled in involving individuals in a psychiatric rehabilitation assessment process that the individuals themselves understand.

Most existing instruments lack many of the characteristics that would make an instrument useful for psychiatric rehabilitation assessment. Although increasing numbers of psychiatric assessment instruments are focusing on skill and resource assessments instead of a symptom and impairment focus, these instruments are still limited in their clinical application. The most obvious limitation is their lack of environmental specificity, with the possible exception of situational assessments in working environments. Existing instruments, because of their need to be standardized, provide information relevant to general environments rather than specific environments (e.g., a general work setting rather than a specific job site). To be used effectively, any assessment instrument must be integrated into the broader context of psychiatric rehabilitation, a process and partnership that is driven by the person's goal.

Authors' Note

We would like to acknowledge the contributions of William A. Anthony and the late Mikal R. Cohen, original authors of previous editions of this chapter.

References

American Psychiatric Association (APA). (2000). *Diagnostic and statistical manual of mental disorders* (4th ed., Text Revision). Washington, DC: Author.

Andreasen, R., Caputi, P., & Oades, L. G. (2001). Inter-rater reliability of the Camberwell Assessment of Need Short Appraisal Schedule. *Australian and New Zealand Journal of Psychiatry, 35,* 856–861.

Anthony, W. A. (1979). *Principles of psychiatric rehabilitation.* Austin, TX: PRO-ED.

Anthony, W. A. (1994). Characteristics of people with psychiatric disabilities that are predictive of entry into the rehabilitation process and successful employment outcomes. *Psychosocial Rehabilitation Journal, 17*(3), 3–13.

Anthony, W. A., Cohen, M. R., Farkas, M., & Gagne, C. (2000). *Psychiatric rehabilitation* (2nd ed.). Boston: Center for Psychiatric Rehabilitation, Boston University.

Anthony, W. A., & Jansen, M. (1984). Predicting the vocational capacity of the chronically mentally ill: Research and policy implications. *American Psychologist, 39,* 537–544.

Anthony, W. A., & Liberman, R. P. (1986). The practice of psychiatric rehabilitation: Historical, conceptual, and research base. *Schizophrenia Bulletin, 12,* 542–559.

Anthony, W. A., & Margules, A. (1974). Toward improving the efficacy of psychiatric rehabilitation: A skills training approach. *Rehabilitation Psychology, 21,* 101–105.

Anthony, W. A., Pierce, R., & Cohen, M. (1980). *The skills of diagnostic planning.* Baltimore: University Park Press.

Anthony, W. A., Rogers, E. S., Cohen, M., & Davies, R. R. (1995). Relationships between psychiatric symptomatology, work skills, and future vocational performance. *Psychiatric Services, 46*(4), 353–358.

Arns, P. G., & Linney, J. A. (1995). Relating functional skills of severely mentally ill clients to subjective and societal benefits. *Psychiatric Services, 46*(3), 260–265.

Au, R. W. C., Tam, P. W. C., Tam, G. W. C., & Ungvari, G. S. (2005). Cross-cultural validation of the St. Louis Inventory of Community Living Skills for Chinese patients with schizophrenia in Hong Kong. *Psychiatric Rehabilitation Journal, 29*(1), 34–39.

Barker, S., Barron, N., McFarland, B. H., & Bigelow, D. A. (1994). A community ability scale for chronically mentally ill consumers: Part I. Reliability and validity. *Community Mental Health Journal, 30*(4), 363–383.

Becker, D. R., Drake, R. E., Farabaugh, A., & Bond, G. R. (1996). Job preferences of clients with severe psychiatric disorders participating in supported employment programs. *Psychiatric Services, 47*(11), 1223–1226.

Bell, M. D., & Bryson, G. (2001). Work rehabilitation in schizophrenia: Does cognitive impairment limit improvement? *Schizophrenia Bulletin, 27*(2), 269–279.

Bell, M. D., & Lysaker, P. (1995). Psychiatric symptoms and work performance among persons with severe mental illness. *Psychiatric Services, 46*(5), 508–510.

Bell, M., & Lysaker, P. (1996). Levels of expectation for work activity in schizophrenia: Clinical and rehabilitation outcomes. *Psychiatric Rehabilitation Journal, 19*(3), 71–76.

Bellack, A. S. (2004). Skills training for people with severe mental illness. *Psychiatric Rehabilitation Journal, 27*(4), 375–391.

Berzinz, J. I., Bednar, R. L., & Severy, L. J. (1975). The problem of intersource consensus in measuring therapeutic outcomes: New data and multivariate perspectives. *Journal of Clinical Psychology, 84*(1), 10–19.

Blackman, S. (1982). Paraprofessional and patient assessment criteria of patient's recovery: Why the discrepancy? *Journal of Clinical Psychology, 37*(4), 903–907.

Blankertz, L., & Cook, J. A. (1998). Choosing and using outcome measures. *Psychosocial Rehabilitation Journal, 22*(2), 167–174.

Bryson, G., Bell, M. D., Greig, T., & Kaplan, E. (1999). The Work Behavior Inventory: Prediction of future work success of people with schizophrenia. *Psychiatric Rehabilitation Journal, 23*(2), 113–117.

Bryson, G., Bell, M. D., Lysaker, P., & Zito, W. (1997). The Work Behavior Inventory: A scale for the assessment of work behavior for people with severe mental illness. *Psychiatric Rehabilitation Journal, 20*(4), 47–55.

Carkhuff, R. R. (2000). *The art of helping* (8th ed.). Amherst, MA: HRD Press, Inc.

Cecil, H., Stanley, M. A., Carrion, P. G., & Swann, A. (1995). Psychometric properties of the MSPSS and NOS in psychiatric outpatients. *Journal of Clinical Psychology, 51*(5), 593–602.

Cohen, B., & Anthony, W. A. (1984). Functional assessment in psychiatric rehabilitation. In A. Halpern & M. Fuhrer (Eds.), *Functional assessment in rehabilitation* (pp. 79–100). Baltimore: Paul H. Brookes.

Cohen, S., Mermelstein, R., Kamarck, T., & Hoberman, H. M. (1985). Measuring the functional components of social support. In I. Sarason & B. Sarason (Eds.), *Social support: Theory, research, and applications* (pp. 73–94). Dordrecht, the Netherlands: Martinus Nijhoff.

Cohen, S., Underwood, L. G., & Gottlieb, B. H. (2000). *Social support measurement and intervention: A guide for health and social scientists.* New York: Oxford Press.

Collins, M. E., Bybee, D., & Mowbray, C. T. (1998). Effectiveness of supported education for individuals with psychiatric disabilities: Results from an experimental study. *Community Mental Health Journal, 34,* 595–613.

Cook, J. A., & Razzano, L. (2000). Vocational rehabilitation for persons with schizophrenia: Recent research and implications for practice. *Schizophrenia Bulletin, 26*(1), 87–103.

Cook, J. A., & Solomon, M. L. (1993). The Community Scholars Program: An outcome study of supported education for students with severe mental illness. *Psychosocial Rehabilitation Journal, 16,* 83–97.

Corrigan, P. W., Buican, B., & McCracken, S. (1995). The Needs and Resources Assessment Interview for severely mentally ill adults. *Psychiatric Services, 46*(5), 504–505.

Corrigan, P. W., Buican, B., & McCracken, S. (1996). Can severely mentally ill adults reliably report their needs? *Journal of Nervous and Mental Disease, 184*(9), 523–529.

Corrigan, P. W., & Penn, D. L. (2001). Introduction: Framing models of social cognition and schizophrenia. In P. W. Corrigan & D. L. Penn (Eds.), *Social cognition and schizophrenia* (pp. 3–37). Washington, DC: American Psychological Association.

Corrigan, P. W., & Phelan, S. M. (2004). Social support and recovery in people with serious mental illnesses. *Community Mental Health Journal, 40*(6), 513–523.

Cruz, M. & Pincus, H. A. (2002). Research on the influence that communication in psychiatric encounters has on treatment. *Psychiatric Services, 53*(10), 1253–1265.

Curran, J. P. (1982). A procedure for assessment of social skills: The simulated social interaction test. In J. P. Curran & P. M. Monti (Eds.), *Social skills training: A practical handbook for assessment and treatment* (pp. 348–373). New York: The Guilford Press.

Danley, K., MacDonald-Wilson, K., & Hutchinson, D. (1998). *The Choose-Get-Keep Approach to employment support: Operational Guidelines.* Boston: Center for Psychiatric Rehabilitation at Boston University.

Dellario, D. J., Anthony, W. A., & Rogers, E. S. (1983). Client-practitioner agreement in the assessment of severely psychiatrically disabled persons' functional skills. *Rehabilitation Psychology, 28,* 243–248.

Derogatis, L. R. (1994). *Symptom checklist-90-R (SCL-90-R) administration, scoring, & procedures manual* (3rd ed.). Minneapolis, MN: National Computer Systems.

Dickerson, F. B. (1997). Assessing clinical outcomes: The community functioning of persons with serious mental illness. *Psychiatric Services, 48*(7), 897–902.

Dimsdale, J., Klerman, G., & Shershow, J. (1979). Conflict in treatment goals between patients and staff. *Social Psychiatry, 14,* 1–4.

Dion, G. L., & Anthony, W. A. (1987). Research in psychiatric rehabilitation: A review of experimental and quasi-experimental studies. *Rehabilitation Counseling Bulletin, 30,* 177–203.

Donahoe, C. P., Carter, M. J., Bloem, W. D., Hirsch, G. L., Laasi, N., & Wallace, C. J. (1990). Assessment of interpersonal problem-solving skills. *Psychiatry, 53,* 329–339.

Drake, R. E., Merrens, M. R., & Lynde, D. W. (2005). *Evidenced-based mental health practice: A textbook.* New York: W. W. Norton.

Egan, G. (2007). *The skilled helper: A problem-management and opportunity-development approach to helping* (8th ed.). Pacific Grove, CA: Brooks/Cole Publishing Company.

Eisen, S. V., Dill, D. L., & Grob, M. C. (1994). Reliability and validity of a brief patient-report instrument for psychiatric outcome evaluation. *Hospital and Community Psychiatry, 45,* 242–247.

Ernst, M., & Paulus, M. P. (2005). Neurobiology of decision-making: A selective review from a neurocognitive and clinical perspective. *Biological Psychiatry, 58,* 597–604.

Estroff, S. E., Patrick, D. L., Zimmer, C. R., & Lachiotte, W. S. (1997). Pathways to disability income among people with severe, persistent psychiatric disorders. *Milbank Quarterly, 75*(4), 495–532.

Evans, J. D., Bond, G. R., Meyer, P. S., Kim, H. W., Lysaker, P. H., Gibson, P. J., et al. (2004). Cognitive and clinical predictors of success in vocational rehabilitation in schizophrenia. *Schizophrenia Research, 70*(2/3), 331.

Evenson, R. C., & Boyd, M. A. (1993). The St. Louis Inventory of Community Living Skills. *Psychosocial Rehabilitation Journal, 17*(2), 93–99.

Farkas, M. D., Cohen, M. R., & Nemec, P. B. (1988). Psychiatric rehabilitation programs: Putting concepts into practice. *Community Mental Health Journal, 24,* 7–21.

Fitz, D. (1999). Recommending client residence: A comparison of the St. Louis Inventory of Community Living Skills and global assessment. *Psychiatric Rehabilitation Journal, 23*(2), 107–112.

Fitz, D., & Evenson, R. C. (1995). A validity study of the St. Louis Inventory of Community Living Skills. *Community Mental Health Journal, 31*(4), 369–377.

Frey, W. D. (1984). Functional assessment in the '80s: A conceptual enigma, a technical challenge. In A. S. Halpern & M. J. Fuhrer (Eds.), *Functional assessment in rehabilitation* (pp. 11–43). Baltimore: Brookes.

Gerber, S. K. (1986). *Responsive therapy: A systematic approach to counseling skills.* New York: Human Sciences Press, Inc.

Glynn, S. M. (1998). Psychopathology and social functioning in schizophrenia. In K. T. Mueser & N. Tarrier (Eds.), *Handbook of social functioning in schizophrenia* (pp. 66–78). Needham Heights, MA: Allyn & Bacon.

Goffman, E. (1961). *Asylums: Essays on the social situation of mental patients and other inmates.* Garden City, NJ: Doubleday-Anchor.

Goldman, H. H., Skodol, A. E., & Lave, T. R. (1992). Revising Axis V for DSM-IV: A review of measures of social functioning. *American Journal of Psychiatry, 149*(9), 1148–1156.

Gollwitzer, P.M. (1996). The volitional benefits of planning. In P. M. Gollwitzer & J. A. Bargh (Eds.), *The psychology of action: Linking cognition and motivation to behavior* (pp. 287–312). New York: The Guilford Press.

Goodman, S. H., Sewell, D. R., Cooley, E. L., & Leavitt, N. (1993). Assessing levels of adaptive functioning: The Role Functioning Scale. *Community Mental Health Journal, 29*(2), 119–131.

Greig, T. C., Nicholls, S. S., Bryson, G. J., & Bell, M. D. (2004). The Vocational Cognitive Rating Scale: A scale for the assessment of cognitive functioning at work for clients with severe mental illness. *Journal of Vocational Rehabilitation, 21,* 71–81.

Griffiths, R. D. P. (1973). A standardized assessment of the work behavior of psychiatric patients. *British Journal of Psychiatry, 123,* 403–408.

Griffiths, R. D. P. (1975). The accuracy and correlates of psychiatric patients' self-assessment of their work behavior. *British Journal of Social and Clinical Psychology, 14,* 181–189.

Griffiths, R. D. P. (1977). The prediction of psychiatric patient's work adjustment in the community. *British Journal of Social and Clinical Psychology, 16,* 165–173.

Grisso, T., & Appelbaum, P. S. (1995). The MacArthur treatment competence study: III. Abilities of patients to consent to psychiatric and medical treatments. *Law and Human Behavior, 19,* 149–174.

Hamann, J., Cohen, R., Leucht, S., Busch, R., & Kissling, W. (2005). Do patients with schizophrenia wish to be involved in decisions about their medical treatment? *American Journal of Psychiatry, 162*(12), 2382–2384.

Hoffman, H., Kupper, Z., Zbinden, M., & Hirsbrunner, H. (2003). Predicting vocational functioning and outcome in schizophrenia outpatients attending a vocational rehabilitation program. *Social Psychiatry and Psychiatric Epidemiology, 38,* 76–82.

Holroyd, J., & Goldenberg, I. (1978). The use of goal attainment scaling to evaluate a ward-treatment program for disturbed children. *Journal of Clinical Psychology, 34,* 732–739.

Hughes, R. A., & Weinstein, D. (2000). *Best practices in psychosocial rehabilitation.* Columbia, MD: International Association of Psychosocial Rehabilitation Services.

Ikebuchi, E., Iwasaki, S., Sugimoto, T., Miyauchi, M., & Liberman, R. (1999). The factor structure of disability in schizophrenia. *Psychiatric Rehabilitation Skills, 3*(2), 220–230.

Institute of Medicine Committee on Quality of Health Care in America. (2001). *Crossing the quality chasm: A new health system for the 21st century.* Washington, DC: National Academies Press.

Kirsh, B. (2000a). Factors associated with employment for mental health consumers. *Psychiatric Rehabilitation Journal, 24*(1), 13–21.

Kirsh, B. (2000b). Organizational culture, climate, and person-environment fit: Relationships with employment outcomes for mental health consumers. *Work: A Journal of Prevention, Assessment, and Rehabilitation, 14,* 1–14.

Kramer, P. J., & Gagne, C. (1997). Barriers to recovery and empowerment for people with psychiatric disabilities. In L. Spaniol, C. Gagne, & M. Koehler (Eds.), *Psychological and social aspects of psychiatric disability* (pp. 467–476). Boston: Center for Psychiatric Rehabilitation at Boston University.

Lazare, A., Eisenthal, S., & Wasserman, L. (1975). The customer approach to patienthood: Attending to patient requests in a walk-in clinic. *Archives of General Psychiatry, 32,* 553–558.

Lecomte, T., Wallace, C. J., Caron, J., Perreault, M., & Lecomte, J. (2004). Further validation of the Client Assessment of Strengths, Interests, and Goals. *Schizophrenia Research, 66,* 59–70.

Leviton, G. (1973). Professional and client viewpoints on rehabilitation issues. *Rehabilitation Psychology, 20,* 1–80.

Locke, E. A., Shaw, K. N., Saari, L. M., & Latham, G. P. (1981). Goal setting and task performance: 1969–1980. *Psychological Bulletin, 90,* 125–152.

Lysaker, P., Bell, M. D., Bryson, G., & Zito, W. (1993). *Rater's guide for the Work Behavior Inventory: Rehabilitation, research and development service.* West Haven, CT: Department of Veteran Affairs.

Mosher, L., & Burti, L. (1992). Relationships in rehabilitation: When technology fails. *Psychosocial Rehabilitation Journal, 15*(4), 11–17.

Mowbray, C. T., Collins, M., & Bybee, D. (1999). Supported education for individuals with psychiatric disabilities: Long-term outcomes from an experimental study. *Social Work Research, 23*(2), 89–100.

New Freedom Commission on Mental Health. (2003). *Achieving the promise: Transforming mental health care in America.* DHHS Pub. No. SMA-03-3832. Rockville, MD.

Noble, L. M., Douglas, B. C., & Newman, S. P. (2001). What do patients expect of psychiatric services? A systematic and critical review of empirical studies. *Social Science and Medicine, 52,* 985–998.

Orlinsky, D. E., Grawe, K., & Parks, B. K. (1994). Process and outcome in psychotherapy—Noch einmal. In A.E. Bergin & S.L. Garfield (Eds.), *Handbook of psychotherapy and behavior change* (4th ed., pp. 270–376). New York: John Wiley & Sons.

Patterson, T. L., Goldman, S., McKibbin, C. L., Hughs, T., & Jeste, D. V. (2001). UCSD Performance-Based Skills Assessment: Development of a new measure of everyday functioning for severely mentally ill adults. *Schizophrenia Bulletin, 27*(2), 235–245.

Phelan, M., Slade, M., Thornicroft, G., Dunn, G., Holloway, F., Wykes, T., et al. (1995). The Camberwell Assessment of Need: The validity and reliability of an instrument to assess the needs of people with severe mental illness. *British Journal of Psychiatry, 167,* 589–595.

Phelan, M., Wykes, T., & Goldman, H. (1994). Global function scales. *Social Psychiatry and Psychiatric Epidemiology, 29*(5), 205–211.

Pratt, C. W., Gill, K. J., Barrett, N. M., & Roberts, M. M. (2006). *Psychiatric rehabilitation* (2nd ed.). San Diego, CA: Academic Press.

Proctor, B. E., Prevatt, F., Adams, K., Hurst, A., & Petscher, Y. (2006). Study skills profiles of normal-achieving and academically-struggling college students. *Journal of College Student Development, 47*(1), 37–51.

Rapp, C. A., & Goscha, R. J. (2005). What are the common features of evidence-based practice? In R. E. Drake, M. R. Merrens, & D. W. Lynde (Eds.), *Evidence-based mental health practice* (pp. 189–216). New York: W.W. Norton.

Rogers, E. S., Anthony, W. A., Cohen, M., & Davies, R. R. (1997). Prediction of vocational outcome based on clinical and demographic indicators among vocationally ready clients. *Community Mental Health Journal, 33*(2), 99–112.

Rogers, E. S., Anthony, W. A., & Lyass, A. (2004). The nature and dimensions of social support among individuals with severe mental illnesses. *Community Mental Health Journal, 40*(5), 437–450.

Rogers, E. S., Hursh, N., Kielhofner, G. R., & Spaniol, L. (1990). *Situational assessment: Scales to assess work adjustment and interpersonal skills.* Boston: Center for Psychiatric Rehabilitation, Boston University.

Rogers, E. S., Sciarappa, K., & Anthony, W. A. (1991). Development and evaluation of situational assessment instruments and procedures for persons with psychiatric disability. *Vocational Evaluation & Work Adjustment Bulletin, 24*(2), 61–67.

Rosen, A., Hadzi-Pavlovic, D., & Parker, G. (1989). The Life Skills Profile: A measure assessing function and disability in schizophrenia. *Schizophrenia Bulletin, 15*(2), 325–337.

Ryan, W. (1976). *Blaming the victim.* New York: Vintage Books.

Salvi, G., Leese, M., & Slade, M. (2005). Routine use of mental health outcome assessments: Choosing the measure. *British Journal of Psychiatry, 186,* 146–152.

Sayers, M. D., Bellack, A. S., Wade, J. H., Bennett, M. E., & Fong, P. (1995). An empirical method for assessing social problem solving in schizophrenia. *Behavior Modification, 19,* 267–289.

Schmieding, N. J. (1968). Institutionalization: A conceptual approach. *Perspectives in Psychiatric Care, 6*(5), 205–211.

Scott, J. E., & Lehman, A. F. (1998). Social functioning in the community. In K. J. Mueser & N. Tarrier (Eds.), *Handbook of social functioning in schizophrenia* (pp. 1–19). Needham Heights, MA: Allyn & Bacon.

Sederer, L. I., & Dickey, B. (Eds.). (1996). *Outcomes assessment in clinical practice.* Baltimore: Williams & Wilkins.

Sederer, L. I., Dickey, B., & Hermann, R. C. (1996). The imperative of outcomes assessment in psychiatry. In L. I. Lederer & B. Dickey (Eds.), *Outcomes assessment in clinical practice* (pp. 1–7). Baltimore: Williams & Wilkins.

Shumway, M., Sentell, T., Chouljian, T., Tellier, J., Rozewicz, F., & Okun, M. (2003). Assessing preferences for schizophrenia outcomes: Comprehension and decision strategies in three assessment methods. *Mental Health Services Research, 5*(3), 121–135.

Slade, M., Phelan, M., & Thornicroft, G. (1998). A comparison of needs assessed by staff and by an epidemiologically representative sample of patients with psychosis. *Psychological Medicine, 28,* 543–550.

State of Alabama Department of Mental Health Services. (1984). *Utilization and needs assessment.* Unpublished manuscript, Birmingham, AL.

Stein, C. H. (2005). Aspirations, ability, and support: Consumers' perception of attending college. *Community Mental Health Journal, 41*(4), 451–468.

Stein, C. H., Rappaport, J., & Seidman, E. (1995). Assessing the social networks of people with psychiatric disability from multiple perspectives. *Community Mental Health Journal, 31*(4), 351–367.

Stiles, P. G., Poythress, N. G., Hall, A., Falkenbach, D., & Williams, R. (2001). Improving understanding of research consent disclosures among persons with mental illness. *Psychiatric Services, 52*(2), 780–785.

Substance Abuse and Mental Health Services Administration (SAMHSA). (2006). *National Consensus Statement on Mental Health Recovery.* Retrieved August 14, 2006, from http://www.mentalhealth.samhsa.gov/publications/allpubs/sma05-4129.

Sue, S., Zane, N., & Young, K. (1994). Research on psychotherapy with culturally diverse populations. In A. E. Bergin & S. L. Garfield (Eds.), *Handbook of psychotherapy and behavior change* (4th ed., pp. 783–817). New York: John Wiley & Sons.

Sullivan, G., Dumenci, L., Burnam, A., & Koegel, P. (2001). Validation of the Brief Instrumental Functioning Scale in a homeless population. *Psychiatric Services, 52*(8), 1097–1099.

Takahashi, M., Tanaka, K., & Miyaoka, H. (2006). Reliability and validity of communication skills questionnaire (CSQ). *Psychiatry and Clinical Neurosciences, 60*(2), 211–218.

Tryon, G. S., & Winograd, G. (2002). Goal consensus and collaboration. In J. C. Norcross (Ed.), *Psychotherapy relationships that work: Therapist contributions and responsiveness to patients* (pp. 109–125). New York: Oxford University Press.

Tsang, H., Lam, P., Ng, B., & Leung, O. (2000). Predictors of employment outcomes for people with psychiatric disabilities: A review of literature since the mid '80s. *Journal of Rehabilitation, 66,* 19–31.

Tsang, H., & Pearson, V. (2000). Reliability and validity of a simple measure for assessing the social skills of people with schizophrenia necessary for seeking and securing a job. *Canadian Journal of Occupational Therapy, 67*(4), 250–259.

Tsang, W. H. H., & Pearson, V. (1996). A conceptual framework for work-related social skills in psychiatric rehabilitation. *Journal of Rehabilitation, 62,* 61–66.

Unger, K., Anthony, W., Sciarappa, K., & Rogers, E. S. (1991). A supported education program for young adults with long-term mental illness. *Hospital and Community Psychiatry, 42,* 179.

Vaccaro, J. V., Pitts, D. B., & Wallace, C. J. (1992). Functional assessment. In R. P. Liberman (Ed.), *Handbook of psychiatric rehabilitation* (pp. 78–94). Boston: Allyn & Bacon.

Vermeire, E., Hearnshaw, H., Van Royen, P., & Denekens, J. (2001). Patient adherence to treatment: Three decades of research. A comprehensive review. *Journal of Clinical Pharmacy and Therapeutics, 26,* 331–342.

Vess, J. (2001). Development and implementation of a functional skills measure for forensic psychiatric patients. *Journal of Forensic Psychiatry, 12*(3), 592–609.

Waghorn, G., Chant, D., & King, R. (2005). Work-related self-efficacy among community residents with psychiatric disabilities. *Psychiatric Rehabilitation Journal, 29*(2), 105–113.

Walitzer, K. S., Dermen, K. H., & Connors, G. J. (1999). Strategies for preparing clients for treatment—A review. *Behavior Modification, 23*(1) 129–151.

Wallace, C. J. (1986). Functional assessment in rehabilitation. *Schizophrenia Bulletin, 12*(4), 604–630.

Wallace, C. J., Connie, J. N., Liberman, R. P., Aitchison, R. A., Lukoff, D., Eider, J. P., et al. (1980). A review and critique of social skills training with schizophrenic patients. *Schizophrenia Bulletin, 6*(1), 42–63.

Wallace, C. J., Lecomte, T., Wilde, J., & Liberman, R. P. (2001). CASIG: A consumer-centered assessment for planning individualized treatment and evaluating program outcomes. *Schizophrenia Research, 50,* 105–119.

Wallace, C. J., Liberman, R. P., Tauber, R., & Wallace, J. (2000). The Independent Living Skills Survey: A comprehensive measure of the community functioning of severely and persistently mentally ill individuals. *Schizophrenia Bulletin, 26*(3), 631–658.

Ware, J. E., Snow, K. K., Kosinski, M., & Gandek, B. (1993). *SF-36 health survey manual and interpretation guide.* Boston: New England Medical Center, The Health Institute.

Webster's Illustrated Encyclopedia Dictionary. (1990). Montreal, Canada: Tormont Publications.

Weiner, H. R. (1993). Multi-Function Needs Assessment: The development of a functional assessment instrument. *Psychosocial Rehabilitation Journal, 16*(4), 51–61.

Weinstein, C. E., & Palmer, D. R. (2002). *Learning and Study Strategies Inventory (LASSI): Users manual* (2nd ed.). Clearwater, FL: H & H.

Wewiorski, N. J., & Fabian, E. S. (2004). Association between demographic and diagnostic factors and employment outcomes for people with psychiatric disabilities: A synthesis of recent research. *Mental Health Services Research, 6*(1), 9–21.

Willer, B., & Miller, G. (1978). On the relationship of client satisfaction to client characteristics and outcome of treatment. *Journal of Clinical Psychology, 34,* 157–160.

World Health Organization. (2001). *International Classification of Functioning, Disability and Health.* Geneva: Author.

Wykes, T. (1998). Social functioning in residential and institutional settings. In K. T. Mueser & N. Tarrier (Eds.), *Handbook of social functioning in schizophrenia* (pp. 20–38). Needham Heights, MA: Allyn & Bacon.

Zimet, G. D., Dahlem, N. W., Simet, S. G., & Farley, G. K. (1988). The Multidimensional Scale of Perceived Social Support. *Journal of Personality Assessment, 52*(1), 30–41.

Chapter 20

Multicultural Issues in Assessment

Richard H. Dana

During the early 1960s and extending through the 1980s, there were initiatives by the U. S. government to remove barriers to access and equal opportunities for rehabilitation services. Rehabilitation reform (Middleton, Rollins, & Harley, 1999) included the Civil Rights Act of 1964, the Americans With Disabilities Act, and the 1973 Rehabilitation Act describing poverty as an anchor for priorities as well as a "critical marker for disability-related risks" (Middleton, Harley, Rollins, & Solomon, 1998, p. 14). The Rehabilitation Act recommended consumer control, equal access, independence, self-determination, and self-help, while the 1992 amendments of this Act embraced all Americans by establishing a cultural diversity initiative.

This legislative history provided the foundations for addressing the civil rights of people with disabilities (Jenkins, Ayers, & Hunt, 1996). However, early guidelines for culturally competent services and service delivery were not implemented due to "a culturally encapsulated ethnocentric focus" (Middleton et al., 2000, p. 220). A "call to action" by these authors proposed multicultural competences and standards because "the rehabilitation counseling profession lacks a clear, normative statement elucidating appropriate, culturally competent professional conduct" (p. 223). These proposed competencies and standards were consistent with the mainstream counseling psychology triad of operationalized multicultural competences (i.e., beliefs/attitudes, knowledge, skills). These competency areas contributed to understanding consumer world views, cultural values, and non–Western health and illness beliefs (Belgrave & Jarama, 2000). Relevant assessment issues included knowledge of community resources, interpreters/bilingual counselors, instrument translations, and interpretation of assessment findings, including the interaction of host and other ethnic minority cultures and the impact of oppression (Middleton et al., 2000). Culturally appropriate interventions were recently advocated as essential components of vocational rehabilitation services (Harley, 2005; Mpofu, Beck, & Weinrach, 2004).

To date, however, despite these efforts, "there has been no urgency to integrate cultural sensitivity into service delivery or rehabilitation education" (Mpofu, Beck, & Weinrach, 2004). The *Code of Professional Ethics for Rehabilitation Counselors* (2001) provides only a general context for respecting culture and diversity (including using caution in evaluating and interpreting test scores, developing and adapting interventions and services, and recruiting ethnic minority faculty and students) and conducting culturally sensitive research (Marshall, Leung, Johnson, & Busby, 2003).

Members of non–European American cultural/racial groups (African Americans, American Indians, Latinos) continue to have disproportionately higher disability and poverty rates (Leung, 2003). These individuals underutilize rehabilitation services as a result of perceived untrustworthiness and credibility deficits of service providers who are white (Belgrave & Jarama, 2000). For many persons, disability *per se* was secondary to an unremitting struggle for life necessities and maintaining security in the absence of adequate education, occupation, and health care benefits (Devlieger & Albrecht, 2000). Many African Americans who have lower socioeconomic status or lack formal education also prefer and rely on informal community counseling services in settings and with personnel who understand them racially and culturally. Other non-white populations experience similar continuing disparities in accessing and utilizing equitable and unbiased mental health services (Snowden & Yamada, 2005).

Chapter Revision Essentials

The corresponding chapter in the third edition of the *Handbook* (Dana, 2001) described awareness and historic advocacy of cultural issues in health, mental health, and social services within a rehabilitation reform climate providing limited implementation of the democratic ideals inherent in civil rights. During the interim between *Handbook* editions, national professional sensibilities and political consciousness coalesced concerning the necessity for culturally sensitive health/mental health care as the *sine qua non* for practice (e.g., Costantino, Dana, & Malgady, 2007; Dana, 2007; Huang et al., 2005). Culture now contributes an essential context for rehabilitation counselors in assessment, intervention, and research (Marshall, Sanderson, Johnson, Du Bois, & Kvedar, 2006).

A number of dimensions affect the contents and status of the multicultural assessment issues described in this chapter: (a) cultural competency: assessment and training; (b) comprehensive assessment renaissance; (c) standard and new multicultural assessment instruments; and (d) general and culture-specific research methodologies: interdisciplinary consensus. Prior to examining these dimensions, a brief description of two overarching issues—demographics of the cultural/racial national population and health/mental health professionals and an emergent professional confrontation of racism—is necessary.

Population Demographics/ Confronting Racism

A shift in population demographics evidenced by a 31% ethnic minority population (U. S. Census Bureau, 2004) may be partially responsible for a recent focus on implementation of cultural issues in training, practice, and research. Americans of European origins will be in a minority nationally at some point in this century as they are now in several states, including California, Texas, and New Mexico.

Prior to other areas of psychology, counseling psychology developed a "critical mass" of approximately 30% ethnic minority students/faculty. Exemplary programs include 38%/25% (Rogers, 2006), and all graduate psychology programs now contain 27%/12% (Norcross, Kohout, & Wichierski, 2005). The presence of greater numbers of prominent professionals of color who have experienced oppression provides evidence for their subsequent professional confrontation of racism (for autobiographical examples, see Ponterotto, Casas, Suzuki, & Alexander, 2001; Robinson & Ginter, 1999).

Counseling psychology remains preeminent in expanding awareness and knowledge concerning the pervasive and continuing impact of oppression and scientific racism on the nature and functioning of human services as well as advocating equity and social justice in health/mental health services for all persons predicated on ethical research with ethnocultural populations and communities (e.g., Carter, 2005; D. W. Sue, 2003; Holiday & Holmes, 2003; Ponterotto, Casas, Suzuki, & Alexander, 2001; Toporek, Gerstein, Fouad, Roysircar, & Israel, 2005; Trimble & Fisher, 2005).

Cultural Competence

Counseling Psychology championed cultural competency training (Pope-Davis, Liu, Toporek, & Brittan-Powell, 2003), expanded professional vistas by embracing resources in Cultural Psychology and Cross-Cultural Psychology (e.g., Bernal, Trimble, Burlew, & Leong, 2003), and penetrated Clinical Psychology by a shared emphasis on an empirical basis for practice with multicultural populations. An integration of culture and competence, defined by specific skills and training objectives, provided a complex transforming process in training counseling psychologists to understand clients as individuals who embody their cultural perspectives in all aspects of their lives (Ridley, Mendoza, & Kanitz, 1994). However, these explicit training goals and procedures for multicultural competency developed in counseling psychology are available primarily for counseling and psychotherapy rather than psychological assessment. In rehabilitation counseling, cultural competence recognizes "patterns of human behavior that include beliefs, values, and behaviors of a . . . group [linked to] . . . the capacity to function within the context of culturally-integrated patterns of human behavior" (Schaller, Parker, & Garcia, 1998, p. 40).

Early surveys of cultural competence, conducted in a predominantly European American system with professional psychologists who did not feel adequately trained to provide services to multicultural populations, were reported in the 3rd edition chapter version. When these surveys were replicated with vocational rehabilitation counselors, the counselors of European American origin lacked sufficient multicultural competency training, although counselors of color perceived themselves as providing responsible and ethical services to ethnic minority populations. This early survey literature, however, suffered from modest return rates of 30% to 60% using scales fostering socially desirable responding and reporting high scores that may not necessarily lead to more successful client outcomes of multicultural counseling (Ponterotto et al., 2000).

Recent vocational rehabilitation surveys examined multicultural competency correlates of counselors (Bellini, 2003), competency effects of white racial attitudes (Cumming-McCann & Accordino, 2005), and service outcomes (Bellini, 2003; Matrone & Leahy, 2005). These studies employed the

Multicultural Counseling Inventory (MCI; Sodowsky, Taffe, Gutkin, & Wise, 1994). Demographic variables, especially race and white racial attitudes, were associated with training effects for counselor–client relationship quality. However, age, agency experience, level of education, multicultural caseload, and research experience variables were not relevant, although positive effects were obtained by inclusion of a specific multicultural course and workshops. The MCI was criticized as a self-report instrument influenced by idealized and cultural social desirability responding in these studies. Rehabilitation client outcomes, defined as successful client closures, were not affected by MCI multicultural competency. However, a hierarchical linear modeling yielded significant effects for counselor race plus other factors (Matrone & Leahy, 2005), although an earlier study (Bellini, 2003) found very small magnitude group-specific outcomes as a function of race and MCI multicultural competency.

These vocational rehabilitation studies did not employ a new multicultural competency instrument constructed from the items contained in several earlier measures yielding the three original factors and an additional Sociocultural Diversity factor of particular relevance for disability clients, the *California Brief Multicultural Competence Scale* (CBMCS; Gamst et al., 2004). The CBMCS controls for social desirability, provides separate scores for service providers of differing cultural/racial origins (Der-Karabetian et al., 2002), and constitutes the training component of the *Multicultural Assessment-Intervention Process* (MAIP) model described later in this chapter.

Assessment Services in Rehabilitation

Individual assessment of clients for rehabilitation services includes using interviews; job tryouts; observations; medical examinations; standardized psychological tests; and ratings of physical, intellectual, and emotional skills by professionals, clients, and their significant others (Berven, 2004). In addition, beyond describing individuals, rehabilitation assessment has a broad scope for conceptualizing and identifying professional and individual career and life goals, barriers, intervention needs, specific strategies, and related programming for problem-solving requiring comprehensive service or treatment. Assessment and monitoring of health outcomes are mandatory for improving health care and rehabilitation (Heinemann, 2000; McAweeney & Crewe, 2000).

A new rehabilitation assessment paradigm honors these objectives by classifying 22 assessment instruments relevant for outcomes of services (Bolton, 2001, 2004). These instruments identified economic, employment, independent living, personality, and psychosocial variables as vocational rehabilitation objectives. A helpful table classified these instruments according to measurement issues (i.e., Variable class: economic, vocational, psychosocial; Perspective: agency/client/employer; Dimensions: Total scores: primary scales, second-order factors; Period use: pretest, case closure, and follow-up). Information on competencies as well as deficits is crucial for designing rehabilitation interventions and evaluating outcomes of rehabilitation services. In addition to psychiatric diagnoses and nondiagnostic information, functional assessment provides systematic approaches related to the skills and interests required for employment and independent living (Brown, Gordon, & Diller, 1983). Functional assessment measures designate areas of functioning and rely on face validity—an appearance of relevance to rehabilitation goals—as well as empirical validity or significant relationships to rehabilitation outcomes.

The importance of ethnicity, race, and culture in all human service areas, including rehabilitation, is now part of a renaissance of comprehensive assessment. However, assessment training for application of these varied instruments with a multicultural rehabilitation population has not been implemented by a multicultural competency training agenda. Such an agenda is required to facilitate bias reduction among assessors, in service delivery, and in standard instruments.

Bias

Fairness as well as responsible and ethical test usage can be facilitated by systematic approaches to reduce bias (Dana, 1994). Bias in standard tests and assessor attitudes toward clients is apparent by failure to exercise credible social etiquette during the entire rehabilitation counseling process including assessment, intervention services, and outcome evaluation (Dana, 2000, 2002a, 2002b). Assessor bias typically occurs as a consequence of stereotyping and ethnocentrism or minimizing differences among members of different racial/ethnic groups and European origin Americans, but it also can exist because of prejudice and racism. White counselors may minimize or deny client claims of discrimination and stereotypy and prefer nonracist explanations of client experience (Mpofu, 2005), although there are few evidence-based studies on perceptions of counselors by these clients (Redmond & Slaney, 2002; Thomas & Weinrich, 2002). Assessor evaluation bias on the MMPI, for example, also results in perception of unwarranted psychopathology (Whatley, Allen, & Dana, 2003) as well as underestimation of African American client potential in rehabilitation students and counselors (Rahimi, Rosenthal, & Chan, 2003; Rosenthal, 2004; Rosenthal & Berven, 1999). It is ethically mandatory for rehabilitation programs to provide training to reduce assessment bias in courses, practica, and internship experiences (Dana, 1994).

Service Delivery

In service delivery, bias is often exposed by an impersonal, task-oriented, formal European American style. The willingness of a client to comply with assessment tasks is related to absence of this form of bias. Client compliance is encouraged by use of culturally appropriate social etiquette, and descriptions of group-specific professional social etiquette are available (Dana, 1993, 1998a, 2005). Understanding and practicing respectful social etiquette facilitates rapport, fosters assessment compliance, and ensures continuous task involvement as a required component of culturally competent assessment and treatment services.

Standard Assessment Instruments

Historically, bias has also occurred in applications of standard personality and psychopathology instruments with populations from different cultures. Such bias may be present in the assessment instruments employed by vocational rehabilitation counselors whenever the norms are not relevant for a particular client as a consequence of race, ethnicity, and/or social class. Bias in standard tests used with clients in minority racial and ethnic groups potentially occurs in the absence of demonstrated cross-cultural equivalence (Van de Vijver, 2000). Whenever client response sets, test-taking expectations, and attitudes differ from normative populations, caution should be exercised in test interpretation (Dana, 2005). Bias may also be present in the form of stereotypy and caricature, particularly in instruments lacking objective scoring and relevant normative data.

Bolton's selected instruments exemplify low inference interpretation and face validity. Potential bias occurs in these assessment measures because of the unknown relevancy of available normative data for clients of racial or ethnic minority. Local norms and acculturation/racial identity status norms are needed to reduce assessor interpretation bias. Bias remediation among rehabilitation counselors requires explicit training initiated and evaluated by multicultural competency assessment (Ponterotto & Alexander, 1996).

Correction for Bias

Corrections for bias begin with good ethnic science to provide empirically derived knowledge as the basis for vocational rehabilitation practice with clients. Such mandatory knowledge includes research to provide a basis for understanding cultural competence training, assessment instruments, multicultural interventions, and a service delivery context illustrated by the MAIP model.

Research Issues with Multicultural Populations

Assessment services for clients for rehabilitation from different cultural origins and acculturation status are predicated on a number of assessment research issues germane to multicultural assessment applications (Dana, 2003, August). These issues include (a) selecting measures; (b) reformulation of assumptions; (c) definition of variables; (d) group comparisons; (e) normative data; and (f) research designs and strategies.

Selecting Measures

Cross-cultural psychologists have employed the terms *etic* and *emic* to specify the locus of investigation and origin of measuring instruments. These terms describe different but overlapping and symbiotic nondichotomous perspectives of equivalent value and importance (Berry, 1999). Etic implies a broad structure for description and comparison of cultures using instrumentation that is developed externally from a given culture. Emic pertains to discovery and understanding emerging within a particular language and culture pertinent to understanding individuals in their life contexts. Whenever a standard test, or emic constructed in the United States, is translated for non-English speakers, the test is employed as if it has the same meaning for individuals with other than European American cultural origins. Such a test may be erroneously assumed to be universally applicable, but in the absence of demonstrated cultural equivalence it should be described as an imposed etic.

Reformulation of Assumptions

Assessment-derived assumptions include myths that drive uninformed counseling practice with multicultural populations. Assessment examples include universal applications of standard tests constructed in the United States (Dana, 1993); objective tests as valid information resources than relatively higher inference projective methods (Meyers et al., 2001); and greater merit of quantitative than qualitative research designs (Camic, Rhodes, & Yardley 2003). Similarly, assessment research has been adversely affected by an overarching myth: the conventional null hypothesis (Malgady, 2000). Malgady's recommendation to reverse the null hypothesis of no cultural bias to specify bias and alter the practical implications of Type 1 and 2 errors dramatically affects the likelihood that multicultural assessment practice would include moderator variables as sources of cultural information, client language proficiency evaluation, and culture-specific interpretation strategies (Dana, 2005; Sue, 1998).

Definition of Variables

Multicultural research has been plagued by a failure to distinguish between distal and proximal variables. Distal variables such as "culture," "race," and "ethnicity" are complex, are burdened with surplus meaning, and lack consensual definition (APA, 2003a). Proximal variables provide linkages within the research process to transform these vague referents into concrete operations clarifying research-based conclusions. Whenever race or ethnicity is operationalized as a demographic variable, culture is rendered distally; in most ethnic minority research the demographic variable functions as a proxy variable for the underlying culturally based personality processes that mediate cultural difference as expressed in standard psychological tests (Okazaki & Sue, 1995; Sue & Sue, 2003). Whenever groups are described by overinclusive, misleading, and stereotypic "ethnic glosses," there is insufficient detail to understand the level of cultural identification (Trimble, Helms, & Root, 2003). Direct measures of the psychological processes affecting test performances and more adequate description of sample characteristics are mandatory.

Group Comparisons

Inaccurate and incomplete group identifications encourage invalid conclusions concerning the meaning of observed differences between groups on assessment measures (Azibo, 1988); these differences may be genuine cultural differences or simply illustrate bias. Comparative studies frequently employ groups that are too small, unrepresentative, or inadequately and incompletely matched. It remains unknown what magnitude of statistical difference is required for clinical interpretation of scores. Allen and Walsh (2000) noted that nonequivalence in instrument metric qualities or underlying construct definitions, in addition to genuine differences between groups, also serves to confound the meaning of obtained group differences. An Index of Correction for culture derived from comparing acculturation status scores with normative data has been suggested (Cuellar, 2000).

Normative Data

Normative data serving as comparative criteria for racial/ethnic minority and European origin populations often describe a sophisticated, privileged, primarily middle-class group (Lonner & Ibrahim, 2002). These quickly outdated normative studies have become the comparative standard despite existing methodologies for exploring the relation of group-specific test scores on test variables to a cross-culturally equivalent criterion variable as well as to the underlying nomological net through tests of convergent and divergent validity. These methodologies are less prone to the types of basic methodological flaws that can result in bias (Allen & Dana, 2004).

Norms for separate ethnic minority populations have been considered infeasible due to the magnitude of within-group and between-group differences in the absence of scale equivalence across groups. In this regard, Lezak (2002) notes that "some test norms developed for the dominant culture so skew their application to persons from other cultures that we cannot use them to evaluate ability levels in intact participants, much less make the finegrained intratest comparisons on which we base many of our test interpretations . . . (and) common sense dictates against developing a full set of age × sex × education norms for all the most commonly used tests for every local ethnic group or subgroup" (p. 343). Lezak also identifies activities of daily living providing useful norms and norms-in-our-heads or behavioral expectations with legitimate cross-cultural applications.

Nonetheless, local norms for some isolated, relatively unacculturated groups within larger societies have limited utility as practical markers of potential worldview and behavior differences. However, these norms distinguish between universal and local standards within a global society mediated by English language usage (Dana, 2003) and may provide information necessary to modify existing instruments (Lee & Sue, 2001).

Furthermore, corrections for acculturation, or racial/cultural identity status applied to scores from standard instruments, provide an alternative normative data resource. Acculturation refers to changes in traditional cultural patterns as a result of continuous, first-hand contact. Acculturation status describes outcomes to changes in individuals during this process as a result of cultural orientations identified by Berry (1999) and employed in the MAIP model (Dana, 1993, 1998a). Acculturation status remains a specific variable of interest underlying ethnic group membership by documentation as a major source of heterogeneity and identified as a performance correlate and a source of confounding with psychopathology on psychological instruments (Dana, 2000a). Acculturation status norms describe individuals who are either traditional or in the process of developing racial identities for whom existing test norms may be inappropriate.

Research Designs and Strategies

Opportunities for introducing alternative methods are limited by overreliance on comparative methodology coupled with employment of distal rather than proximal variables and selective utilization of scientific principles overemphasizing the importance of internal validity. This methodological focus defines elegance by the clarity of causal effects of one variable upon another and relative neglect of external validity, or the generality of findings to specific settings and populations (Sue, 1999). Cultural equivalence must be established for constructs, items, and methods (Allen & Walsh, 2000; Van de Vijver, 2000). Linguistic equivalence has been used as the sole cross-cultural equivalence exemplar. Unwarranted generalizations from competent translations in the absence of research-based construct and scalar equivalence are common (Dana, 2005). Construct validation is difficult and time consuming to design and implement, but this is not a legitimate excuse for failure to employ these methods. There has been underutilization of advances in factorial invariance through confirmatory factor analysis, tests of differential item functioning using item response theory, and regression analyses of cultural identity measures on test scores in published assessment research (Allen & Dana, 2004).

Rehabilitation research is now incorporating advanced methodologies such as multiple regression and other correlation methods, archival data for program evaluation, meta-analysis, structural equation modeling, measures of clinically significant change, item response theory, and qualitative research (Chan & Rosenthal, 2006). Rehabilitation researchers should also be familiar with recent guidelines for research on racial/ethnic populations (Council of National Psychological Associations for the Advancement of Ethnic Minority Research, 2000).

Multicultural Assessment Instruments

I have cherished the belief that cultural bias would be reduced by construction of new instruments for culture-specific populations with normative data for European Americans and ethnic minorities. However, with the exception of the *Tell-Me-a-Story Test* (TEMAS; Costantino, Malgady, & Rogler, 1988; Costantino et al., 2007), there are few multicultural assessment instruments despite the well-known limitations of standard instruments with non–European American populations (Dana, 1993, 2000a, 2005; Van de Vijver, 2000). As a remedy for the limited availability of multicultural instruments, a published symposium (Dana, 2002c) featured four successful multicultural assessment courses in Alaska, California, and Colorado describing different approaches to multicultural assessment training. Despite these exemplars, there is little support for such dedicated training in the United States, Latin America, and Europe (Dana, 2003).

Furthermore, the presence of guidelines (e.g., Dana, 2005; Ridley, Hill, Thompson, & Omerod, 2001; Roysircar-Sodowsky & Kuo, 2001) has not resulted in consensual multicultural assessment training analogous to the proliferation of training models, courses, and examples for multicultural competency training in counseling and psychotherapy. To further exacerbate the difficulty of offering specialized multicultural assessment courses, the quality of comprehensive assessment training *per se* is now insufficient to meet internship expectations for competent interpretation of standard tests (Clemence & Handler, 2001; Stedman, Hatch, & Schoenfeld, 2001).

Multicultural Interventions

Culture-specific intervention approaches predicated on adaptations and culturally based variables for ethnic minority populations are emerging from a matrix of cultural knowledge and experience within a research context designed to provide empirical documentation for cultural competence training (e.g., Bernal & Scharron-Del-Rio, 2001; Miranda et al., 2006; Vera, Vila, & Alegria, 2003; Weisman, 2005; Wong Kim, Zane, Kim, & Huang, 2003). In the absence of consensus on the kinds and extent of required adaptations, new intervention approaches for cognitive therapy and time-limited dynamic therapy provide distinctive findings by diagnostic categories and specific cultural/racial groups. Adaptations and culturally based variables are consistent with evidence-based practice, broadly defined as "the integration of the best available research with clinical expertise in the context of patient characteristics, culture, and preferences" (APA Presidential Task Force, 2006, p. 273).

An earlier description of culture-specific healing practices for some African American, African, and Afro-Caribbean populations (Dana, 1998a) has been supplemented by recent distinctive approaches to culture-specific interventions by rehabilitation authors (Harley, 2005; Mpofu, 2005). Harley (2005) provides guidelines for indigenous healing practices including herbs, rituals, and metaphysical processes conducted in an atmosphere of trust with evidence of effectiveness. "Finding the point of compromise between clinical protocol and indigenous philosophy regarding individual choice with respect to treatment protocol (traditional vs. scientific)" (Harley, 2005, p. 300) is a judgmental issue requiring counselor–client collaboration. Harley also suggests cultural assessment is necessary prior to integration of these practices with Western clinical healing systems and cites the ADDRESSING components to systematically organize cultural issues: Age and generational influences, Developmental and acquired Disabilities, Religion and spiritual orientation, Ethnicity, Socioeconomic status, Sexual orientation, Indigenous heritage, National origin, and Gender (Hays, 2001). These practices foster assumptions contained in an integrative multidimensional counseling model conducive to the uniqueness of human development (D'Andrea & Daniels, 2001). Mpofu (2005) cites prevention science strategies for population-level interventions that are *universal* (e.g., rehabilitation legislation for general population), *selective* (specified treatment impact for a subpopulation), and *indicated* (remedial for individuals who are at risk).

MAIP Model

The MAIP model, a clinical application of Malgady's reversal of the null hypothesis (2000), has origins in cultural identity assessment tools (Ponterotto, Gretchen, & Chauhan, 2001), cultural competence conceptual and empirical literature (e.g., Dana, 1997, 1998b, 2002a; Dana, Aragon, & Kramer, 2002), and research-driven MAIP applications in California public mental health settings (e.g., Gamst, Dana, Der-Karabetian, Meyers, & Guarino, 2007; Gamst, Rogers, Der-Karabetian, & Dana, 2006).

The MAIP model supports monitoring of clients and service providers with culturally tailored assessments, cultural competency training, empirically documented treatments/culturally based variables, and outcome evaluations. This framework incorporates cultural and racial issues into human services to increase the reliability and usefulness of assessment information designed and individualized to reduce client dropout rates and facilitate applications of relevant and effective interventions. Adapted for African Americans (Morris, 2000), the MAIP is applicable to other cultural/racial groups (Gamst, Dana,

Der-Karabetian, & Kramer, 2000, 2001; Gamst, Dana, Der-Karabetian, Aragon, Arellano, & Kramer, 2002).

Cultural orientation, assessment instruments, formulations/conceptualizations, and *interventions* designate potential cultural issues during the service delivery process. In Figure 20.1, these issues are identified by seven questions (Q1–Q7). These questions can increase the reliability of the entire rehabilitation process and provide more valid applications of cost-effective interventions amenable to empirical evaluation of service outcomes.

Q1: Etic instrument? Although the MAIP model was developed from the premise that universal, or genuine etic, tests/instruments may be developed in the future, at present there are none that can be unequivocally accepted and used by practitioners. The available imposed etic endeavors—described in this chapter in the *Handbook's* third edition (Dana, 2001)—remain fragmentary, equivocal, and controversial for both personality and psychopathology constructs.

Q2: Cultural Orientation? Cultural orientation refers to acculturation status and describes a client's relationship to a culture or origin and to mainstream American society. *Assimilated* people exhibit behaviors, values, and perceptions indistinguishable from those of mainstream Americans. *Marginal* indicates retention of some components from an original culture as well as selective incorporation of components from European American culture. A *bicultural* orientation implies equal knowledge of both an original culture and mainstream culture and the ability to function comfortably in either context. A *transitional* orientation for American Indians/Alaska Natives includes traditional individuals who question their traditional values and religion. *Traditional* people include migrants, sojourners, refugees, and persons living in the United States who have remained sufficiently apart from mainstream American culture to retain their languages and cultures in a relatively intact form. For African Americans, racial identity developmental status or cultural identity status determination may be necessary in order to develop rehabilitation interventions employing cultural components and necessitating matching counselors and clients for racial or cultural origins.

Acculturation or racial identity information is needed for decisions on the adequacy of standard tests for a client with or without modifications for culture or on whether dedicated emic measures, if available, are preferable. Acculturation status or racial identity information is mandatory for preparing cultural formulations relevant for psychopathology diagnoses as well as for culture-specific and identity-specific conceptualizations leading to interventions for various rehabilitation objectives. Cultural formulations and conceptualizations are difficult for European American origin counselors to prepare because familiarity with a client's first language, worldview, cultural self-concept, health/illness beliefs, and culture-bound syndromes may be required (e.g., Dana, 2000c, 2002b). In vocational rehabilitation counseling, conceptualizations provide information on cultural boundaries and components of the cultural self. This information may help to evaluate culturally derived and readily available motivational and coping resources (Dana, 1998c). Acculturation instruments are available for many ethnic and racial populations in the United States as are measures for

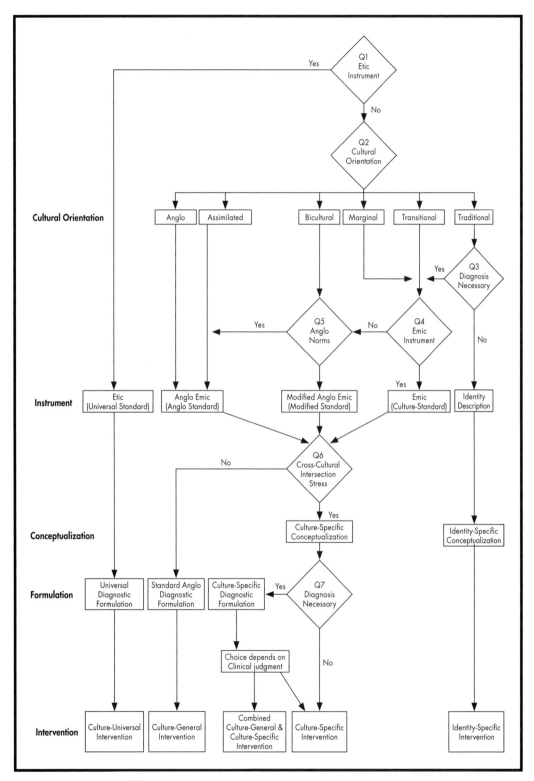

FIGURE 20.1. Multicultural assessment–intervention process model. *Note.* Adapted from *Multicultural Assessment, Applications, and Examples* (p. 70), by R. H. Dana, 2005, Mahwah, NJ: Erlbaum.

describing worldviews, values, and individualism/collectivism (Dana, 2005), including brief instruments (Van de Vijver & Phalet, 2004), although few professional psychologists include these measures in assessment.

Q3: Clinical Diagnosis? Vocational rehabilitation services in nonpsychiatric settings may only require a structured diagnostic interview to determine presence or history of a major psychiatric disorder.

Q4: Emic instruments? Relatively few emic instruments are available for multicultural populations except for African Americans (Jones, 1996) probably because African American psychologists have ignored the negative attitudes of the white assessment establishment toward emic measures. Jones includes potentially relevant measures for vocational rehabilitation cognition, language assessment and attitudes, personality characteristics and psychological well-being, coping skills, reactions to stress and racism, social supports, support in the work environment, and a chapter on methodological analysis of fair employment testing. Acculturative stress has been measured for African Americans (Anderson, 1991) and for Hispanics (Cervantes, Padilla, & Salgado de Snyder, 1991). The incorporation of information from emic instruments into individual appraisals facilitates recognition of how a European worldview can restrict awareness of problems shared on a daily basis by non-European Americans.

Q5: European American/Anglo norms? This question is posed in the absence of ethnic minority emic instruments or consensually accepted modifications for standard tests (i.e., Anglo emics/imposed etics). Norms for these standard tests may or may not be useful for traditional ethnic minority rehabilitation clients, although they can be used with assimilated or Anglo clients. Applications of these norms with clients who are bicultural or marginal should be done with extreme caution. For example, on the MMPI-2, if a non-Puerto Rican Spanish translation is used, more than 70 items will be misunderstood/misconstrued due to language differences, resulting in significant elevations on several clinical scales, and no similar scale elevations occur using the Puerto Rican translation for the same assessees.

Q6: Cross-cultural interaction stress? This source of stress is a daily experience for many ethnic minorities and can have pervasive biopsychosocial effects and adverse health outcomes. Culture-specific conceptualizations for individual appraisal lead to more effective utilization of available resources and can increase the probability that clients from multicultural populations will be retained for sufficient time periods to positively affect rehabilitation outcomes. Counselor cultural competence is now known to improve clinical outcomes as a consequence of cultural responsiveness rather than matching clients and providers *per se.*

Q7: Clinical Diagnosis? This question serves to provide an opportunity to reexamine the need for a clinical diagnosis as a consequence of preparing culture-specific formalizations and conceptualizations.

The MAIP model classifies interventions as culture-general, combined, and culture-specific. These interventions are applicable with client preference or knowledge of the status of client cultural orientation and/or racial identity development. Assessment for these interventions requires preparation of culture-specific formulations and identity-specific conceptualizations to provide relevant information for selecting interventions for problems-in-living and those resulting from stress, oppression, and discrimination.

Rehabilitation Cultural Competence: Multicultural Assessment Training

As a proposal to remedy training deficits, a set of multicultural assessment competencies contained in a cultural competency model for multicultural psychological assessment training (Allen, 2007) could be applied in a dedicated one-semester course for rehabilitation counselors. In Figure 20.2, this model incorporates basic knowledge in test construction, psychometric theory, classical measurement theory, and construct validity with a collaborative approach already present in rehabilitation assessment practice. Culturally congruent assessment includes acculturation/racial identity status evaluation, culturally grounded test interpretation, local norms to qualify test interpretation, and report-writing skills for communicating acculturation/racial identity status information affecting test data interpretations and requiring awareness of multicultural ethics.

The assessment subsections of the APA Ethical Code (2002) discuss limitations on instrument usage whenever established reliability and validity for multicultural populations do not exist. The code recognizes linguistic and cultural differences as well as instrument adaptations "in light of research on or evidence" (p. 1070) derived from cultural knowledge and clinical judgment in administration and interpretation (Rollins, 2005). These ethical code suggestions are consistent with the Middleton et al. (2000) delineation of rehabilitation counselor multicultural assessment competencies.

This course would introduce assessment supervision in use of the rehabilitation assessment instrument repertoire recommended by Bolton (2001, 2004) as exemplars for employment with multicultural client populations during practica, internship, and postdoctoral training experiences. This course would encourage bias reduction by development of cultural knowledge resources (e.g., Dana, 1998c; Hershenson, 2000; Lomay, & Hinkebein, 2006), augment self-knowledge of attitudes (Utsey, Gernat, & Bolden, 2003), and contribute to understanding good ethnic science requirements (Allen & Dana, 2004; Chan & Rosenthal, 2006; Sue & Sue, 2003).

Conclusion

Rehabilitation counseling has come of age in reconciling the nature of counselors' comprehensive and collaborative assessment services with their multi-problem, multicultural client populations. As described in this chapter, a

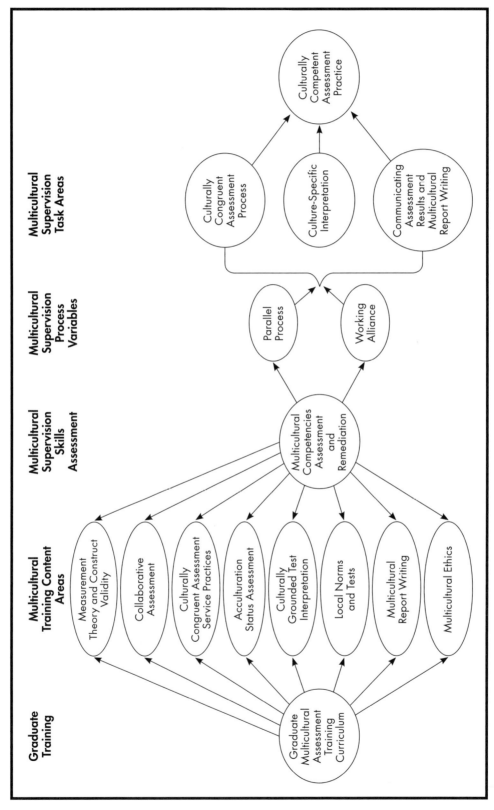

FIGURE 20.2. A cultural competency model for multicultural psychological assessment. *Note.* From *Multicultural Assessment Supervision: Process, Interpretation, and Report Writing.* Paper submitted for publication.

rehabilitation counseling perspective currently contains multicultural assessment and cultural competency knowledge and skills implementing an earlier idealism. Rehabilitation counseling is coalescing with a positive psychology and is "implemented by focusing on recovery criteria deemed critical by consumers, emphasizing the credibility of subjective outcomes, and examining the role of helper–consumer relationships as well as underlying humanistic values" (Costantino et al., 2007, p. 18). A majority of rehabilitation clients require quality care to nourish hope, encourage motivation, and provide continuing support for coping with functional limitations, pervasive poverty, and histories of discrimination encompassing all phases of living.

Quality care in rehabilitation services is predicated on using comprehensive assessment, employing culturally sensitive instruments, and training counselors for cultural competence. Comprehensive assessment, described by Bolton's 22 instruments, embraces economic, employment, independent living, personality, and psychosocial rehabilitation objectives. Hope theory promises a framework for understanding rehabilitation objectives and facilitating new interventions (Snyder, Lehman, Kluck, & Monsson, 2006). Marshalling assessment instruments for desired service outcomes demonstrates a necessary strategy otherwise available only in refugee assessment (Dana, 2007) but can be emulated in mental health (Dana, in press). One additional instrument measuring *Salutogenesis* and identified in the rehabilitation literature (Lustig, Rosenthal, Strauser, & Haynes, 2000) has an encouraging history with multicultural populations (e.g., Ying, Akutsu, Zhang, & Huang, 1997; Ying, Lee, Tsai, 2000). Bringing services directly to clients in their homes or places of residence by telerehabilitation can further simplify access for some ethnic minorities receiving substantial home care (Marshall, Sanderson, Johnson, Du Bois, & Kvedar, 2006).

The rationale, equivalence research, and training necessary for applying Bolton's lexicon of instruments with ethnic minority populations has not been established or made available to rehabilitation counseling students and practitioners. For example, access to quality health/mental health services for multicultural populations cannot occur in the absence of routine assessment of racial identity and acculturation status. This information affects problem identification, training culturally competent providers, and development of culturally sensitive interventions. Although quality care is dependent upon broadly defined evidence-based practices from quantitative and qualitative research implemented by cooperative, interdisciplinary endeavors, substantive research still needs to be accomplished using appropriate methodologies with culturally based variables related to service outcomes (e.g., Callahan & Barisa, 2005).

These issues suggest that a service delivery model such as the MAIP is necessary to provide an overall structure for rehabilitation services. A flexible structure permits equitable access for cultural minorities. Respectful attention to cultural issues is essential to maintenance of uninterrupted, collaborative, quality services leading to routine outcome evaluations of rehabilitation objectives. In this endeavor, training counselors to incorporate the current rehabilitation assessment knowledge necessary to serve multicultural client populations is now imperative. The ingredients specified by Allen (2006) can be used for multicultural assessment courses in vocational rehabilitation.

References

Allen, J. (in press). Multicultural assessment supervision: Process, interpretation and report writing. *Professional Psychology: Research and Practice.*

Allen, J., & Dana, R. H. (2004). Methodological issues in cross-cultural and multicultural Rorschach research. *Journal of Personality Assessment, 82*(2), 189–205.

Allen, J., & Walsh, J. A. (2000). A construct-based approach to equivalence: Methodologies for cross-cultural/multicultural personality assessment research. In R. H. Dana (Ed.), *Handbook of cross-cultural and multicultural personality assessment* (pp. 63–85). Mahwah, NJ: Erlbaum.

American Psychological Association. (2002). Ethical Principles of Psychologists and Code of Conduct. *American Psychologist, 57,* 1060–1073.

American Psychological Association. (2003). Guidelines on multicultural education, training, research, practice, and organizational change for psychologists. *American Psychologist, 58,* 377–402.

Americans With Disabilities Act of 1990, 42 U.S.C. § 12101 *et seq.* (1990).

Anderson, L. P. (1991). Acculturative stress: A theory of relevance to black Americans. *Clinical Psychology Review, 11,* 685–702.

APA Presidential Task Force. (2006). Evidence-based practice in psychology. *American Psychologist, 61,* 271–285.

Azibo, D. A. (1988). Understanding the proper and improper usage of the comparative framework. *Journal of Black Psychology, 15,* 81–91.

Belgrave, F. Z., & Jarama, S. L. (2000). Culture and the disability and rehabilitation experience: An African American example. In R. G. Frank & T. R. Elliott (Eds.), *Handbook of rehabilitation psychology* (pp. 558–600). Washington, DC: American Psychological Association.

Bellini, J. (2002). Correlates of multicultural counseling competencies of vocational rehabilitation counselors. *Rehabilitation Counseling Bulletin, 45,* 65–76.

Bellini, J. (2003). Counselors' multicultural competencies and vocational rehabilitation outcomes in the context of counselor-client racial similarity and difference. *Rehabilitation Counseling Bulletin, 46,* 164–173.

Bernal, G., & Scharron-Del-Rio, M. R. (2001). Are empirically supported treatments valid for ethnic minorities? Toward an alternative approach for treatment research. *Cultural Diversity and Ethnic Minority Psychology, 7,* 328–342.

Bernal, G., Trimble, J.E., Burlew, A. K., & Leong, F. T. L. (Eds.) (2003). *Handbook of racial & ethnic minority psychology.* Thousand Oaks, CA: Sage.

Berry, J. W. (1999). Psychology of acculturation. *Nebraska Symposium on Motivation, 39,* 201–234.

Berven, N. L. (2004). Assessment. In T. F. Riggar & D. R. Maki (Eds.), *Handbook of rehabilitation counseling.* New York: Springer.

Bolton, B. (2001). Measuring rehabilitation outcomes. *Rehabilitation Counseling Bulletin, 44*(2), 67–75.

Bolton, B. (2004). Counseling and rehabilitation outcomes. In F. Chan, N. L. Berven, & K. R. Thomas (Eds.), *Counseling theories and techniques for rehabilitation health professionals* (pp. 444–465). New York: Springer.

Brown, M., Gordon, W. A., & Diller, L. (1983). Functional assessment and outcome measurement: An integrative review. In E. L. Pan, T. E. Backer, & C. L. Vash (Eds.), *Annual Review of Rehabilitation* (Vol. 3, pp. 93–120). New York: Springer.

Callahan, C. D., & Barisa, M. T. (2005). Introduction to the Special Issue of Rehabilitation Psychology: Issues in outcomes measurement. *Rehabilitation Psychology, 50,* 5.

Camic, P. M., Rhodes, J. E., & Yardley, L. (Eds.), *Qualitative research in psychology: Expanding perspectives in methodology and design.* Washington, DC: American Psychological Association.

Carter, R. T (Ed.). (2005). *Handbook of racial-cultural psychology and counseling* (Vols. 1, 2). New York: Wiley.

Cervantes, R. C., Padilla, A. M., & Salgado de Snyder, N. (1991). The Hispanic Stress Inventory: A culturally relevant approach to psychosocial assessment. *Psychological Assessment, 3,* 438–447.

Chan, F., & Rosenthal, D. A. (2006). Introduction to the Special Series: Advanced research methodology in rehabilitation. *Rehabilitation Counseling Bulletin, 49,* 219–222.

Civil Rights Act of 1964 42 U.S.C §§ 2000d 2000d-7 (P. L. 88-352) (1964).

Clemence, A. J., & Handler, L. (2001). Psychological assessment on internship: A survey of training directors and their expectations for students. *Journal of Personality Assessment, 76,* 18–47.

Code of Professional Ethics for Rehabilitation Counselors (1995). *Journal of Applied Rehabilitation Counseling, 18*(4), 26–31.

Costantino, G., Dana, R. H., & Malgady, R. (2007). *Tell-Me-A-Story assessment of children in multicultural societies.* Mahwah, NJ: Lawrence Erlbaum Associates.

Council of National Psychological Associations for the Advancement of Ethnic Minority Interests. (2000). *Guidelines for research in ethnic minority communities.* Washington, DC: American Psychological Association..

Cuellar, I. (2000). Acculturation as a moderator of personality and psychological assessment. In R. H. Dana (Ed.), *Handbook of cross-cultural and multicultural personality assessment* (pp. 113–129). Mahwah, NJ: Lawrence Erlbaum Associates.

Cumming-McCann, A., & Accordino, M. P. (2005). An investigation of rehabilitation counselor characteristics, White racial attitudes, and self-reported multicultural counseling competencies. *Rehabilitation Counseling Bulletin, 48,* 167–176.

Dana, R. H. (1993). *Multicultural professional perspectives for professional psychology.* Boston: Allyn & Bacon.

Dana, R. H. (1994). Testing and assessment ethics for all persons: Beginning and agenda. *Professional Psychology: Research and Practice, 25,* 349–354.

Dana, R. H. (1998a). *Understanding cultural identity in intervention and assessment.* Thousand Oaks, CA: Sage.

Dana, R. H. (1998b). Multicultural assessment in the United States, 1997: Still art, not yet science, and controversial. *European Journal of Personality Assessment, 14,* 62–70.

Dana, R. H. (1998c). Personality assessment and the cultural self: Emic and etic contexts as learning resources. In L. Handler & M. Hilsenroth (Eds.), *Teaching and learning personality assessment* (pp. 325–345). Hillsdale, NJ: Lawrence Erlbaum Associates.

Dana, R. H. (2000a). Culture and methodology in personality assessment. In I. Cuellar & F. Paniagua (Eds.), *Handbook of multicultural mental health: Assessment and treatment of diverse groups* (pp. 97–120). San Diego, CA: Academic Press.

Dana, R. H. (2000b). Multicultural assessment of adolescent and child personality and psychopathology. In A. L. Comunian & U. P. Gielen (Eds.), *Human development in international perspective* (pp. 233–258). Lengerich, Germany: Pabst Science Publishers.

Dana, R. H. (2000c). The cultural self as locus for assessment and intervention with American Indians/Alaska Natives. *Journal of Multicultural Counseling & Development, 28,* 66–82.

Dana, R. H. (2001). Multicultural issues in assessment. In B. Bolton (Ed.), *Handbook of measurement and evaluation in rehabilitation* (3rd ed., pp. 449–469). Gaithersburg, MD: Aspen.

Dana, R. H. (2002a). Mental health for African Americans: A cultural/racial perspective. *Cultural Diversity and Ethnic Minority Psychology, 8,* 3–18.

Dana, R. H. (2002b). Examining the usefulness of DSM-IV. In K. Kurasaki, S. Okazaki, & S. Sue (Eds.), *Asian American mental health: Assessment methods and theories* (pp. 29–46). New York: Kluwer Academic/Plenum Publishers.

Dana, R. H. (2002c). Introduction to Symposium-Multicultural assessment: Teaching methods and competence evaluation. *Journal of Personality Assessment, 79,* 195–199.

Dana, R. H. (2003). Assessment training, practice, and research in the new millennium: Challenges and opportunities for professional psychology. *Ethical Human Sciences and Services, 5,* 127–140.

Dana, R. H. (2003, August). *Bridging the gap between standard and multicultural assessment practice: An agenda for research and training.* Invited address presented at the meeting of the American Psychological Association, Toronto, Canada.

Dana, R. H. (2005). *Multicultural assessment principles, applications, and examples.* Mahwah, NJ: Lawrence Erlbaum Associates.

Dana, R. H. (2007). Refugee assessment practices and cultural competency training. In J. P. Wilson & C. Tang (Eds.), *The cross-cultural assessment of psychosocial trauma and posttraumatic stress disorder* (pp. 91–112). New York: Springer.

Dana, R. H. (in press). Clinical diagnosis of multicultural populations. In L. A. Suzuki, J. G. Ponterotto, & P. J. Meller (Eds.), *Handbook of multicultural assessment* (3rd ed.). San Francisco: Jossey-Bass.

Dana, R. H., Aragon, M., & Kramer, T. (2002). Public sector mental health services for multicultural populations: Bridging the gap from research to clinical practice. In M. N. Smyth (Ed.), *Health care in transition* (Vol. 1, pp. 1–13). Hauppauge, NY: Nova Science Publishers.

D'Andrea, M., & Daniels, J. (2001). Respectful counseling: An integrated multidimensional model for counselors. In D. B. Pope-Davis, & H. L. C. Coleman (Eds.), *The intersection of race, class, and gender in multicultural counseling* (pp. 417–466). Thousand Oaks, CA: Sage.

Der-Karabetian, A., Gamst, G., Dana, R. H., Aragon, M., Arellano, L., Morrow, G., et al. (2002). *California Brief Multicultural Competence Scale (CBMCS) User Guide.* La Verne, CA: University of La Verne.

Devlieger, P.J., & Albrecht, G. L. (2000). Your experience is not my experience. *Journal of Disability Policy Studies,* 11(1), 51–60.

Gamst, G., Dana, R. H., Der-Karabetian, A., & Kramer, T. (2000). Ethnic match and client ethnicity effects on global assessment and visitation. *Journal of Community Psychology, 28,* 547–564.

Gamst, G., Dana, R. H., Der-Karabetian, A., & Kramer, T. (2001). Asian American mental health clients: Cultural responsiveness and global assessment. *Journal of Mental Health Counseling, 23,* 57–71.

Gamst, G., Rogers, R., Der-Karabetian, A., & Dana, R. H. (2006). Addressing mental health disparities: A preliminary test of the Multicultural Assessment Intervention Process (MAIP) model. In E. V. Metrosa (Ed.), *Racial and ethnic disparities in health and healthcare* (pp. 1–18). Hauppauge, NY: Nova Science Publishers.

Gamst, G., Dana, R. H., Der-Karabetian, A., Meyers, L. S., & Guarino, A. J. (2007). *A structural analysis of the Multicultural Assessment Intervention Process model.* Submitted for publication.

Gamst, G., Dana, R. H., Der-Karabetian, A., Aragon, M., Arellano, L., & Kramer, T. (2002). Effects of Latino acculturation and ethnic identity status on mental health outcomes. *Hispanic Journal of Behavioral Sciences, 24,* 479–504.

Gamst, G., Dana, R. H., Der-Karabetian, A., Aragon, M., Arellano, L., Morrow, G., et al. (2004). Cultural competency revised: The California Brief Multicultural Competence Scale. *Measurement and Evaluation in Counseling and Development, 37,* 163–183.

Harley, D. A. (2005). African Americans and indigenous counseling. In D. A. Harley & J. M. Dillard (Eds.), *Contemporary mental health issues among African Americans* (pp. 293–306). Alexandria, VA: American Counseling Association.

Hays, P. A. (2001). *Addressing cultural complexities in practice: A framework for clinicians and counselors.* Washington, DC: American Psychological Association.

Heinemann, A. W. (2000). Functional status and quality-of-life measures. In R. G. Frank & T. R. Elliott (Eds.), *Handbook of rehabilitation psychology* (pp. 261–286). Washington, DC: American Psychological Association.

Hershenson, D. R. (2000). Toward a cultural anthropology of disability and rehabilitation. *Rehabilitation Counseling Bulletin, 43,* 150–157.

Holiday, B. G., & Holmes, A. L. (2003). A tale of challenge and change: A history and chronology of ethnic minorities in the United States. In G. Bernal, J. E. Trimble, A. K. Burlew, & F. T. L. Leong (Eds.), *Handbook of racial & ethnic minority psychology* (pp. 15–64). Thousand Oaks, CA: Sage.

Huang, L., Stroul, B., Friedman, R., Mrazek, R., Friesen, B., Pires, S., et al. (2005). Transforming mental health care for children and their families. *American Psychologist, 60,* 615–627.

Jenkins, A. E., Ayers, G. E., & Hunt, B. (1996). Cultural diversity and rehabilitation: The road traveled. *Rehabilitation Education, 10,* 83–103.

Jones, R. (1996). *Handbook of tests and measurements for black populations* (Vols. 1 & 2). Hampton, VA: Cobb & Henry.

Lee, J., & Sue, S. (2001). Clinical psychology and culture. In D. Matsumoto (Ed.), *The handbook of culture and psychology* (pp. 287–305). New York: Oxford University Press.

Leung, P. (2003). Multicultural competencies and Rehabilitation Counseling/Psychology. In D. B. Pope-Davis, H. L. K. Coleman, W. M. Liu, & R. L. Toporek (Eds.), *Handbook of multicultural competencies in counseling and psychology* (pp. 439–455). Thousand Oaks, CA: Sage.

Lezak, M.D. (2002). Responsive assessment and the freedom to think for ourselves. *Rehabilitation Psychology, 47,* 339–353.

Lomay, V. T., & Hinkebein, J. H. (2006). Cultural considerations when providing rehabilitation services to American Indians. *Rehabilitation Psychology, 51,* 36–42.

Lonner, W. J., & Ibrahim, F. A. (2002). Appraisal and assessment in cross-cultural counseling. In P. B. Pedersen, J. G. Draguns, W. J. Lonner, & J. E. Trimble (Eds.), *Counseling across cultures* (5th ed., pp. 355–378). Thousand Oaks, CA: Sage.

Lustig, D. C., Rosenthal, D. A., Strauser, D. R., & Haynes, K. (2000). The relationship between sense of coherence and adjustment in persons with disabilities. *Rehabilitation Counseling Bulletin, 43,* 134–141.

Malgady, R. G. (2000). Myths about the null hypothesis and the path to reform. In R. H. Dana (Ed.), *Handbook of cross-cultural and multicultural personality assessment* (pp. 49–62). Mahwah, NJ: Lawrence Erlbaum Associates.

Marshall, C. A., Leung, P., Johnson, S. R., & Busby, H. (2003). Ethical practice and cultural factors in rehabilitation. *Rehabilitation Education, 17,* 55–65.

Marshall, C. A., Sanderson, P. R., Johnson, S. R., Du Bois, B., & Kvedar, J. C. (2006). Considering class, culture, and access in rehabilitation intervention and research. In K. J. Hagglund & A. W. Heinemann (Eds.), *Handbook of applied disability and rehabilitation research* (pp. 25–44). New York: Springer.

Matrone, K. F., & Leahy, M. J. (2005). The relationship between vocational rehabilitation client outcomes and rehabilitation counselor multicultural counseling competencies. *Rehabilitation Counseling Bulletin, 48,* 233–244.

McAweeney, M., & Crewe, N. (2000). Evaluating outcomes research: Statistical concerns and clinical relevance. In R. G. Frank & T. R. Elliott (Eds.), *Handbook of rehabilitation psychology* (pp. 311–326). Washington, DC: American Psychological Association.

Meyer, G. J., Finn, S. E., Eyde, L. D., Kay, G. G., Moreland, K. I., Dies, R. R., et al. (2001). Psychological testing and psychological assessment: A review of evidence and issues. *American Psychologist, 56,* 128–165.

Middleton, R. A., Harley, D. A., Rollins, C. W., & Solomon, T. (1998). Affirmative action, cultural diversity, and the disability policy reform: Foundations to the civil rights of persons with disabilities. *Journal of Applied Rehabilitation Counseling, 29*(3), 9–18.

Middleton, R. A., Rollins, C. W., & Harley, D. (1999). The historical and political context of the civil rights of persons with disabilities: A multicultural perspective for counselors. *Journal of Multicultural Counseling and Development, 27*(2), 105–120.

Middleton, R. A., Rollins, C. W., Sanderson, P. L., Leung, P., Harley, D. A., Ebener, D., et al. (2000). Endorsement of professional multicultural rehabilitation competencies and standards: A call to action. *Rehabilitation Counseling Bulletin, 43,* 219–240.

Miranda, J., Bernal, G., Lau, A., Kohn, L., Hwang, W-C., & LaFromboise, T. (2005). State of the science on psychosocial interventions for ethnic minorities. *Annual Review of Clinical Psychology, 1,* 113–142.

Morris, E. F. (2000). Assessment practice with African Americans: Combining standard assessment measures within an Africentric orientation. In R. H. Dana (Ed.), *Handbook of cross-cultural and multicultural personality assessment* (pp. 573–603). Mahwah, NJ: Lawrence Erlbaum Associates.

Mpofu, E. (2005). Selective interventions in counseling African Americans with disabilities. In D. A. Darley & J. M. Dillard (Eds.), *Contemporary mental health issues among African Americans.* Alexandria, VA: American Counseling Association.

Mpofu, E., Beck, R., & Weinrach, S. G. (2004). In F. Chan, N. L. Berven, & K. R. Thomas (Eds.), *Counseling theories and techniques for rehabilitation health professionals* (pp. 386–402). New York: Springer.

Norcross, J. C., Kohout, J. L., & Wicherski, M. (2005). Graduate study in psychology 1971 to 2004. *American Psychologist, 60,* 959–975.

Okazaki, S., & Sue, S. (1995). Methodological issues in assessment research with ethnic minorities. *Psychological Assessment, 7,* 367–375.

Ponterotto, J. G., & Alexander, C. M. (1996). Assessing the multicultural competence of counselors and clinicians. In L. A. Suzuki, P. J. Meller, & J. G. Ponterotto (Eds.), *Handbook of multicultural assessment: Clinical, psychological, and educational applications* (pp. 651–672). San Francisco: Jossey-Bass.

Ponterotto, J. G., Fuertes, J. N., & Chen, E. C. (2000). Models of multicultural counseling. In S. A. Blour & R. W. Lent (Eds.), *Handbook of counseling psychology* (3rd ed., pp. 639–669). San Francisco: Jossey-Bass.

Ponterotto, J. G., Gretchen, D., & Chauhan, R. V. (2001). Cultural identity and multicultural assessment: Quantitative and qualitative tools for the clinician. In L. A. Suzuki, J. G. Ponterotto, & P. J. Meller (Eds.), *Handbook of multicultural assessment: Clinical, psychological, and educational applications* (2nd ed., pp. 67–99). San Francisco: Jossey-Bass.

Ponterotto, J. G., Casas, J. M., Suzuki, L. A., & Alexander, C. M. (Eds.). (2001). *Handbook of multicultural counseling* (2nd ed.). Thousand Oaks, CA: Sage.

Pope-Davis, D. B., Liu, W. M., Toporek, R. L., & Brittan-Powell, C. S. (2003). *Handbook of cultural competencies in counseling and psychotherapy.* Thousand Oaks, CA: Sage.

Rahimi, M., Rosenthal, D. A., & Chan, F. (2003). Effects of client race on clinical judgment of African American undergraduate students in rehabilitation. *Rehabilitation Counseling Bulletin, 46,* 157–163.

Rehabilitation Act of 1973, 29 U.S.C. § 701 *et seq.* (1973).

Ridley, C. R., Hill, C. L., Thompson, C. E., & Omerod, A. J. (2001). Clinical practice of assessment: Toward an idiographic perspective. In D. B. Pope-Davis, & H. L. K. Coleman (Eds.), *The intersection of race, class, and gender in multicultural counseling* (pp. 191–211). Thousand Oaks, CA: Sage.

Ridley, C. R., Mendoza, D. W., & Kanitz, B. E. (1994). Multicultural training: Reexamination, operationalization, and integration. *Counseling Psychologist, 22*(2), 227–289.

Robinson, T. L., & Ginter, E. J. (1999). Introduction to the Journal of Counseling & Development's special issue on racism. *Journal of Counseling & Development, 44,* 3.

Rogers, M. R. (2006). Exemplary multicultural training in school psychology programs. *Cultural Diversity and Ethnic Minority Psychology, 12,* 115–133.

Rollins, W. W. (2005). Ethical implications in mental health counseling with African Americans. In D. A. Harley & J. M. Dillard (Eds.), *Contemporary mental health issues among African Americans* (pp. 307–316). Alexandria, VA: American Counseling Association.

Rosenthal, D. A. (2004). Effect of client race on clinical judgment of practicing European American vocational rehabilitation counselors. *Rehabilitation Counseling Bulletin, 47*(3), 131–141.

Rosenthal, D. A., & Berven, N. L. (1999). Effects of client race on clinical judgment. *Rehabilitation Counseling Bulletin, 42,* 243–264.

Roysircar-Sodowsky, G., & Kuo, P. Y. (2001). Determining cultural validity of personality assessment: Some guidelines. In D. B. Pope-Davis, & H. L. K. Coleman (Eds.), *The intersection of race, class, and gender in multicultural counseling* (pp. 213–239). Thousand Oaks, CA: Sage.

Schaller, J., Parker, R., & Garcia, S. M. (1998). Moving toward culturally competent rehabilitation counseling services: Issues and practices. *Journal of Applied Rehabilitation Counseling, 29*(2), 40–48.

Snowden, L. R., & Yamada, A-M. (2005). Cultural differences in access to care. *Annual Review of Clinical Psychology, 1,* 143–166.

Snyder, C.R., Lehman, K. A., Kluck, B., & Monsson, Y. (2006). Hope for rehabilitation and vice versa. *Rehabilitation Psychology, 51,* 89–112.

Stedman, J. M., Hatch, J. P., & Schoenfeld, L. S. (2001). The current status of psychological assessment training in graduate and professional schools. *Journal of Personality Assessment, 77,* 398–407.

Sue, D. W. (2003). *Overcoming our racism: The journey to liberation.* San Francisco: Jossey-Bass.

Sue, S. (1998). In search of cultural competence in psychotherapy and counseling. *American Psychologist, 53,* 440–448.

Sue, S. (1999). Science, ethnicity, and bias: Where have we gone wrong? *America Psychologist, 54,* 1070–1077.

Sue, S., & Sue, L. (2003). Ethnic science is good science. In G. Bernal, J. E. Trimble, A. K. Burlew, & F. T. Leong (Eds.), *Handbook of racial and ethnic minority psychology* (pp. 198–207). Thousand Oaks, CA: Sage.

Toporek, R. L., Gerstein, L., Fouad, N., Roysircar, G., & Israel, T. (2005). *Handbook for social justice in counseling psychology.* Thousand Oaks, CA: Sage.

Trimble, J. E., & Fisher, C. B. (Eds.). (2005). *The handbook of ethical research with ethnocultural populations and communities.* Thousand Oaks, CA: Sage.

Trimble, J. E., Helms, J. E., & Root, M. P. P. (2003). Social and psychological perspectives on ethnic and racial identity. In G. Bernal, J. E. Trimble, A. K. Burlew, & F. T. L. Leong (Eds.), *Handbook of racial and ethnic minority psychology* (pp. 219–275). Thousand Oaks, CA: Sage.

U. S. Census Bureau. (2004). *U. S. interim projections by age, sex, race, and Hispanic Origin.* Retrieved December 8, 2005, from hppt://www.census.gov/ipcwww/usintrerimroj/.

Utsey, S. O., Gernat, C. A., & Bolden, M. A. (2003). Teaching racial identity development and racism awareness: Training in professional psychology programs. In G. Bernal, J. E. Trimble, A. K. Burlew, & F. T. L. Leong (Eds.), *Handbook of racial and ethnic minority psychology* (pp. 147–166). Thousand Oaks, CA: Sage.

Van de Vijver, F. (2000). The nature of bias. In R. H. Dana (Ed.), *Handbook of cross-cultural and multicultural personality assessment* (pp. 87–106). Mahwah, NJ: Lawrence Erlbaum Associates.

Van de Vijver, F. J. R., & Phalet, K. (2004). Assessment of multicultural groups: The role of acculturation. *Applied Psychology: An International Review, 53*(2), 215–236.

Vera, M., Vila, D., & Alegria, M. (2003). Cognitive-behavior therapy: Concepts, issues, and strategies for practice with racial/ethnic minorities. In G. Bernal, J. E. Trimble, A. K. Burlew, & F. T. L. Leong (Eds.), *Handbook of racial and ethnic minority psychology* (pp. 521–538). Thousand Oaks, CA: Sage.

Weisman, A. (2005). Integrating culturally based approaches with existing interventions for Hispanic/Latino families coping with schizophrenia. *Psychotherapy: Theory, Research, Practice, Training, 42,* 178–197.

Whatley, R., Allen, J., & Dana, R. H. (2003). Racial identity and the MMPI in African American male college students. *Cultural Diversity and Ethnic Minority Psychology, 8,* 344–352.

Wong, E. C., Kim, B. S., Zane, N. W. S., & Huang, J. S. (2003). Examining culturally based variables associated with ethnicity: Influences on credibility perceptions of empirically supported interventions. *Cultural Diversity and Ethnic Minority Psychology, 9,* 88–96.

Ying, Y-W, Akutsu, P. D., Zhang, X., & Huang, L. N. (1997). Psychological dysfunction in Southeast Asian refugees as mediated by sense of coherence. *American Journal of Community Psychology, 25,* 839–859.

Ying, Y-W., Lee, P. A., & Tsai, J. L. (2000). Cultural orientation and racial discrimination: Predictors of coherence in Chinese American young adults. *Journal of Community Psychology, 25,* 427–442.

Index

About The Editors

Brian F. Bolton, PhD (University of Wisconsin–Madison), was a University Professor of Rehabilitation and Adjunct Professor of Psychology at the University of Arkansas–Fayetteville. He is a Fellow of the Division of Evaluation, Measurement, and Statistics and of the Division of Rehabilitation Psychology of the American Psychological Association, Fellow of the Society for Personality Assessment, and Fellow of the American Psychological Society. He received the Burlington Northern Faculty Achievement Award for scholarly research from the University of Arkansas, the Roger Barker Distinguished Research Award from the Division of Rehabilitation Psychology of the American Psychological Association, the Distinguished Career in Rehabilitation Counseling Research Award from the American Rehabilitation Counseling Association, an Alumni Achievement Award from the University of Wisconsin, and the Buros Institute Distinguished Reviewer Award. He has received 12 research project awards from the American Rehabilitation Counseling Association. His 10 edited and authored books include *Psychology of Deafness for Rehabilitation Counselors, Psychosocial Adjustment to Disability, Rehabilitation Counseling Research, Rehabilitation Client Assessment,* and *Special Education and Rehabilitation Testing: Current Practices and Test Reviews.* He has contributed 20 chapters to books, including *Functional Psychological Testing, Encyclopedia of Clinical Assessment, Annual Review of Rehabilitation, Handbook of Multivariate Experimental Psychology, Rehabilitation Counseling: Basics and Beyond, Rehabilitation Outcomes: Analysis and Measurement, Psychology for Health Science Students, Improving Assessment in Rehabilitation and Health,* and *Counseling Theories for Rehabilitation Health Professionals.* He has written 36 test reviews for the *Mental Measurements Yearbook* and *Test Critiques,* and he has authored more than 100 articles in psychology and rehabilitation journals. His assessment instruments include the *Work Personality Profile, Employability Maturity Interview, Vocational Personality Report, Work Temperament Inventory,* and *Functional Capacities Computer Report.* He was previously editor of the *Rehabilitation Counseling Bulletin* and co-editor of *Rehabilitation Education.* He is a past president of the Society for Applied Multivariate Research. He is a licensed psychologist, Humanist minister, and Distinguished Toastmaster.

Randall M. Parker, PhD (University of Missouri at Columbia), is the Melissa Elizabeth Stuart Centennial Professor of Education, a Professor of Special Education, and the Director of Rehabilitation Counselor Education at the University of Texas at Austin. He is a Fellow of the American Psychological Association, Division 22, Rehabilitation Psychology, and Division 17,

Counseling Psychology. In addition, he received the School of Education Alumni Achievement Award from the University of Wisconsin–Madison; the College of Education Outstanding Faculty Award from the College of Education at the University of Texas at Austin; and the Distinguished Career in Rehabilitation Counseling Research Award from the American Rehabilitation Counseling Association. He has published more than 100 refereed articles, book chapters, book reviews, and journal editorials. His assessment instruments include the *Occupational Aptitude Survey and Interest Schedule*. He is a past editor and co-editor of the *Rehabilitation Counseling Bulletin* and is a past president of the American Rehabilitation Counseling Association and the Texas Psychological Association. He is a licensed psychologist in Texas and is also a Certified Rehabilitation Counselor.